Progress in

Obstetrics and Gynaecology

Progress in Obstetrics and Gynaecology
Edited by John Studd

Contents of Volume 14

ISBN 0 443 064075
ISSN 0261 0140

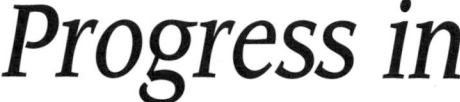

Progress in

Obstetrics and Gynaecology

VOLUME 15

Edited by

John Studd DSc MD FRCOG

Professor of Gynaecology and Consultant Gynaecologist
Academic Department of Obstetrics and Gynaecology,
Chelsea and Westminster Hospital, London, UK

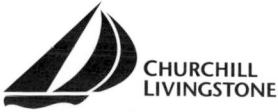

CHURCHILL
LIVINGSTONE

EDINBURGH LONDON NEW YORK OXFORD PHILADELPHIA ST LOUIS SYDNEY TORONTO 2003

CHURCHILL LIVINGSTONE
An imprint of Elsevier Science Limited

First published 2003
  Reprinted 2003

ISBN 0 443 072221
ISSN 0261 0140

British Library Cataloguing in Publication Data
A catalogue record for this book is available from the British Library

Library of Congress Cataloging in Publication Data
A catalog record for this book is available from the Library of Congress

Note
Medical knowledge is constantly changing. As new information becomes available, changes in treatment, procedures, equipment and the use of drugs become necessary. The editor, contributors and the publishers have taken care to ensure that the information given in this text is accurate and up to date. However, readers are strongly advised to confirm that the information, especially with regard to drug usage, complies with the latest legislation and standards of practice.

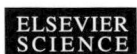

ELSEVIER
SCIENCE
your source for books,
journals and multimedia
in the health sciences

www.elsevierhealth.com

Commissioning Editor – Ellen Green
Project Manager – Frances Affleck
Designer – Sarah Russel
Editorial services and Typeset – BA & GM Haddock
Printed in Spain

The publisher's policy is to use paper manufactured from sustainable forests

Contents

Contributors

Paul E. Adinkra MB BS DFFP
Department of Obstetrics and Gynaecology, Norwick Park Hospital, Harrow, Middlesex, UK

Tom Bourne PhD MRCOG
Consultant, The Early Pregnancy, Gynaecological Ultrasound and Minimal Access Surgery Unit, St George's Hospital Medical School, London, UK

Deborah C.M. Boyle MD MRCOG DFFP
Specialist Registrar in Obstetrics and Gynaecology, Hillingdon Hospital, Uxbridge, Middlesex, UK

Charlotte Chaliha MB BChir MA MD MRCOG
Specialist Registrar, East Surrey Hospital, Redhill, Surrey, UK

Shiao Chan BA(Camb) MB BChir MRCOG
MRC Clinical Training Fellow, Department of Maternal and Fetal Medicine, Birmingham Women's Hospital, Birmingham, UK

George Condous MRCOG
Clinical Research Fellow, The Early Pregnancy, Gynaecological Ultrasound and Minimal Access Surgery Unit, St George's Hospital Medical School, London, UK

Gerard Conway MD FRCP
Consultant Endocrinologist, Department of Endocrinology, Middlesex Hospital, London, UK

Sarah Creighton MD MRCOG
Consultant Gynaecologist, Department of Obstetrics and Gynaecology, University College London Hospitals, London, UK

Wilhelm H. Cronje MB ChB
Research Fellow, Academic Department of Obstetrics and Gynaecology, Chelsea and Westminster Hospital, London, UK

Steven Dobbs MD MRCOG
Consultant Gynaecologist and Gynaecological Oncologist, Belfast City
Hospital, Belfast, UK

Claudine L. Domoney MA MRCOG
Research Fellow, Academic Department of Obstetrics and Gynaecology,
Chelsea and Westminster Hospital, UK

Peter L. Dwyer MB BS FRCOG FRACOG CU
Head of Department of Urogynaecology, The Royal Women's Hospital and
Mercy Hospital for Women, Melbourne, Victoria, Australia

Joanne Ellison MB ChB
Specialist Registrar, Glasgow University Department of Obstetrics and
Gynaecology, Glasgow Royal Infirmary, Glasgow, UK

Robert Fox MD MRCOG
Consultant Gynaecologist, Maternity Unit, Directorate of Obstetrics,
Gynaecology & Paediatrics, Taunton & Somerset Hospital, Taunton, UK

Colin G. Fink BSc MB ChB PhD FRCPath
Micropathology Ltd, University of Warwick Science Park, Barclays Venture
Centre, Coventry, UK

Jayne Franklyn MD PhD FRCP FMedSci
Professor of Medicine and Honorary Consultant Endocrinologist, Division of
Medical Sciences, University of Birmingham, Birmingham, UK

Ian A. Greer MD FRCP(Glas) FRCP(Edinb) FRCP(Lond) FRCOG MFFP
Regius Professor and Head of Division of Developmental Medicine,
University of Glasgow, Glasgow Royal Infirmary, Glasgow, UK

Joyce Harper BSc PhD
Senior Lecturer in Human Genetics and Embryology, Department of
Obstetrics and Gynaecology, University College London, London, UK

Annie P. Hawkins MRCOG DFFP Diploma of the Institute of Psychosexual Medicine
Research Fellow, Academic Department of Obstetrics and Gynaecology,
Chelsea and Westminster Hospital, London, UK

Pauline A. Hurley BMedSci BM BS MRCOG
Consultant in Obstetrics and Fetal Medicine, The Women's Centre, The John
Radcliffe Hospital, Oxford, UK

Sharif I.M.F. Ismail MSc MBA MA MMedSci(Ed) LLM MRCOG
Specialist Registrar in Obstetrics and Gynaecology, Royal Glamorgan
Hospital, Ynysmaerdy, Llantrisant, Nr Pontyclun, Mid-Glamorgan, Wales

Mark Kilby MD MRCOG
Consultant and Clinical Reader in Fetal Medicine, Department of Maternal
and Fetal Medicine, Division of Reproductive and Child Health, University
of Birmingham, Birmingham, UK

Charles R. Kingsland MD FRCOG
Consultant Gynaecologist, Head of Reproductive Medicine Unit, Liverpool
Women's Hospital, Merseyside, UK

Ronnie F. Lamont BSc MD FRCOG
Consultant in Obstetrics and Gynaecology, Norwick Park Hospital, Harrow,
Middlesex, UK and Honorary Lecturer, Institute of Obstetrics and
Gynaecology, Imperial College Medical School, Hammersmith Hospital,
London, UK

Iwan Lewis Jones MD
Consultant Andrologist and Senior Lecturer, Department of Obstetrics and
Gynaecology, Liverpool Women's Hospital, Merseyside, UK

Adrian M. Lower FRCOG
Consultant Gynaecologist, St Bartholomew's Hospital, London, UK

Raj Mathur MRCOG
Subspecialty Trainee in Reproductive Medicine, University Department of
Obstetrics and Gynaecology, The Rosie Hospital, Cambridge, UK

Catherine L. Minto MB ChB
Specialist Registrar and Clinical Research Fellow, Academic Department of
Obstetrics and Gynaecology, University College London, London, UK

David Nunns MD MRCOG
Consultant Gynaecological Oncologist, Nottingham City Hospital,
Nottingham, UK

Emeka Okaro MRCOG
Clinical Research Fellow, The Early Pregnancy, Gynaecological Ultrasound
and Minimal Access Surgery Unit, St George's Hospital Medical School,
London, UK

Miguel Oliveira da Silva MD PhD
Departments of Obstetrics-Gynaecology & Preventive Medicine, Consultant
at Hospital de Santa Maria, Professor of Lisbon Faculty of Medicine,
University of Lisbon, Lisbon, Portugal

Barry O'Reilly MD MRCOG
Fellow in Urogynaecology and Pelvic Floor Reconstructive Surgery, The
Royal Women's Hospital and Mercy Hospital for Women, Melbourne,
Victoria, Australia

Chris W.G. Redman MA FRCP
Professor of Obstetric Medicine, The John Radcliffe Hospital, Oxford, UK

Charles H. Rodeck DSc FRCOG FRCPath FMedSci
Professor and Head, Department of Obstetrics and Gynaecology, University
College London, London, UK

Gavin P. Sacks MA DPhil MRCOG
Specialist Registrar, Department of Obstetrics and Gynaecology, Chelsea and Westminster Hospital, London, UK

Hassan N. Sallam MD FRCOG PhD(Lond)
Professor in Obstetrics and Gynaecology, Department of Obstetrics and Gynaecology, The University of Alexandria, Egypt

Ian L. Sargent BSc PhD
University Reader, Nuffield Department of Obstetrics and Gynaecology, The John Radcliffe Hospital, Oxford, UK

Jai B. Sharma MD DNB MRCOG MFFP MAMS
Associate Professor, Department of Obstetrics and Gynaecology, Maulana Azad Medical College, and Associated Lok Nayak Hospital, New Delhi, India

Stuart L. Stanton FRCS FRCOG
Professor and Director, Urogynaecology Unit, Department of Obstetrics and Gynaecology, Lanesborough Wing, St George's Hospital Medical School, London, UK

John W.W. Studd DSc MD FRCOG
Professor of Gynaecology and Consultant Gynaecologist, Academic Department of Obstetrics and Gynaecology, Chelsea and Westminster Hospital, London, UK

Paul Symonds TD MD FRCP FRCR
Reader in Oncology and Consultant in Clinical Oncology, University of Leicester, Leicester Royal Infirmary, Leicester, UK

Alexander Taylor MBBS MRCOG
Clinical Research Fellow, Minimally Invasive Therapy Unit and Endoscopy Training Centre, University Department of Obstetrics and Gynaecology, Royal Free Hospital, London, UK

Kevin Thomas MRCOG
Specialist Registrar, Liverpool Women's Hospital, Merseyside, UK

Simon Wood MRCOG
Subspecialty Trainee in Reproductive Medicine, Liverpool Women's Hospital, Merseyside, UK

Sharif I.M.F. Ismail

The learning problems of overseas Part 2 MRCOG candidates

Overseas doctors taking the Part 2 Membership examination tend to have a lower pass rate than their British colleagues, despite having good level of knowledge and experience from their own countries.[1] As a result, they take longer to pass their examination, which causes them distress and delays their progress in training. This article looks at the learning problems they might encounter and explores how these can be improved.

THE ORGANISATION OF OVERSEAS TRAINING

Overseas candidates can take the examination from their home countries, after training in hospitals recognised for this purpose, with at least two College fellows/members to guide candidates preparing for the examination. Some have training in the UK as well, which requires registration with the General Medical Council in London. This registration is granted either by passing the Professional and Linguistic Assessment Board (PLAB) Test or getting exemption, usually through sponsorship by the College, as part of the Overseas Doctors Training Scheme (ODTS). Sponsored doctors take the International English Language Testing System (IELTS), which is used to assess the ability of overseas students to undertake university studies.[2]

THE SPECIAL NEEDS OF OVERSEAS DOCTORS

Although overseas training has been running for decades, little has been written about it and most of literature about international education relates to overseas university students.[3] The special needs of such candidates relate to differences in perceptions and expectations.[4] Just as a 10-year-old child is considered abnormal if he/she can not count, because a child at this age is

Dr Sharif I.M.F. Ismail MSc MBA MA MMedSci(Ed) LLM MRCOG, Specialist Registrar in Obstetrics and Gynaecology, Royal Glamorgan Hospital, Ynysmaerdy, Llantrisant, Nr Pontyclun, Mid-Glamorgan, Wales CF72 8XR, UK, Tel: 0144 344 3526; Fax: 0144 344 3178

expected to count, overseas doctors are assessed according to the perceived norms of the examination. These doctors are good achievers who did well to join medical schools and even better to go to another country for more training. They are not, therefore, disabled in that they can not learn, but rather in that their performance may not match that expected in the examination.

THE RANGE OF PROBLEMS FACING OVERSEAS DOCTORS

The problems facing overseas university students include living in a foreign culture, language difficulties, separation reactions, racial discrimination, accommodation problems, dietary restrictions, financial stress, loneliness, problems of late adolescents and early adulthood as well as academic problems.[5] Whilst overseas doctors may encounter some of these problems, they tend to be more mature and their difficulties centre around those related to learning, language as well as living problems, such as sorting out accommodation and education for their children.[6]

Language problems

Overseas students will inevitably have features that distinguish them from native English speakers, such as accent, intonation, grammar and vocabulary. Yet there are subtle ones that affect communication and these might be culturally-related, including readiness to ask questions, expressing disagreement, and asking for clarification, which could indicate patterns of behaviour in a particular society where students are not expected to disagree with their tutors. Taking this example into the oral section of the Membership examination, where the examiner expects the candidate to justify his/her management, an overseas candidate might find it difficult to disagree with the examiner, as he/she is used to agreeing with teachers, as a source of authority.[7]

The same applies to written English, as indicated by the expectations of Chinese students in British universities.[8] For example, starting an essay with an introduction is a common requirement by British tutors. Yet, Chinese students are used to establishing common ground before tackling specified issues, and their writings might, therefore, seem unclear and full of waffle. Although an inductive answer, giving an introduction that outlines direction, might be as good as a deductive one, that states the idea just before the conclusion, it is the expectation of the examiner, who can not find the information where it is usually found, that makes the difference and leaves the overseas candidate with a poor mark.[7] Applying this observation to the Membership examination, which includes 10 short essays to be answered on a maximum of two sides of A4 paper each, an overseas candidate could waste half the available space going round the question, instead of targeting it straight away.

Impact of language problems

Language, as a vehicle of communication, can affect the learning of overseas doctors. For example, the perception of language as a barrier can affect overseas students' ability to express themselves and cause them anxiety about making friends.[9] Foreign medical graduates in the US feared rejection by patients, experienced difficulties in communicating emotional support to them and, on occasion, felt depressed as a result.[10] Similarly, poor command of English can lead to difficulties in adapting to the British culture,[11] which can affect learning and preparing for the Membership examination.

Relative role of language problems

Although the majority of overseas doctors, who come to the UK for clinical training, are from countries where English is not the first language, most of them will have read English medical textbooks, and some will have studied medicine in English as well. With the insistence that doctors score 7 in each component of the International English Language Testing System (IELTS),[1] all sponsored doctors should have a reasonable command of English language. The same applies to those taking the Professional and Linguistic Assessment Board (PLAB) Test. Bearing in mind that English language is the most commonly used language in international settings (e.g. in conferences and the medical literature) as well as in the media (e.g. films and songs), it is unlikely that overseas doctors would have serious deficiency in this area.

Cultural problems

A concept of culture

The word 'culture' refers to the customs of a particular group.[12] Whilst the term generally refers to the traditions of a society, such as shopping and visiting friends,[13] it relates to patterns of learning and professional work when considered in relation to training and examinations. Consequently, learning cultures are systems of beliefs, practices and expectations that constitute the norm for a specified group of learners, according to which individuals will be judged and evaluated. Despite being so obvious to the insider, such systems might be so strange to an outsider, who might come from another group with a totally different set of norms.[7]

Culture shock

Culture shock refers to the impact of facing a new environment upon moving from one place to another. It is common to all types of such change, including travel and training. The term 'shock' indicates that such a change can be serious enough to cause inability to function properly and even require urgent and serious help. Whilst a clinically shocked person would show unmistakable signs, such as rapid pulse and low blood pressure, and similarly, first aid measures needed to save him/her are physical ones, including intravenous fluids and medications, the manifestations of culture shock are more subjective and subtle, such as feeling confused and making inadequate progress, and the same applies to the help required in these circumstances, which could involve guidance and explanation.[14]

Learning culture shock

Whilst modern life in Britain, as part of the Western style of living, might not be a new encounter to most people, given the volume of films, news and books available, it is the culture of learning as well as preparing for and taking examinations that overseas candidates might not be very familiar with.

Consequently, they might get confused as a result of being unable to recognise the way in which examinations are devised and answers are marked. This confusion could lead to mental as well as emotional strain, and even the perception that the examination is designed specifically to fail overseas candidates, which might imply racism,[15] and giving up trying for the examination altogether.[16]

Features of culture shock

Culture shock is characterised by mental and emotional strain, whilst trying to understand and adapt to the new environment. This strain might be associated with a sense of deprivation, having lost usual company and friends, which in turn could lead to detachment from the new environment to the extent of rejecting it, or feeling rejected by it. There is often some ambiguity regarding roles, duties and values, which are different to those of the old environment, leading to surprise on facing new features, anxiety about how to react to them, and feeling unable to deal with new situations.[17]

Overseas candidates mastered techniques appropriate for the examinations in their home countries and got used to certain patterns of patient care that are relevant to the case mix as well as the organisation of care. As they face the examination and/or have training in the UK, they loose these familiar signs and have to work from scratch to identify new signs that they can read and understand. It is the confusion, worry and anxiety that surround this searching phase that represent the learning culture shock. This can lead to uncertainty as to how to handle situations, such as which material to read, which courses to attend, how to prepare for the examination, and so on.

Even differences in social life can affect learning. For example, alcohol, which is a prominent social activity for British people, is not allowed in certain cultures. As result, overseas doctors belonging to these cultures may feel pressurised to follow patterns they do not approve of, or feel isolated and possibly misunderstood, if they adhere to their values. Likewise, having relationships, partners, parties, discos and dances may not be acceptable for some backgrounds.[18] The implications of this on making friends and getting help is something worth consideration, as it may affect how overseas doctors cope with their new environment. Handling these rather sensitive issues requires skill in explaining oneself, whilst understanding the views of others.

Risk factors

Attempts have been made to identify those likely to face more difficulties upon changing places, so as to identify those who need most help. The incidence of home-sickness amongst first-year English psychology students was found to be related to independence prior to coming to university, and also the ability to relate to others and seek help.[19] For example, those who always relied on their parents were more likely to feel helpless upon moving to university. Likewise, girls were more open about their home-sickness, and thus get help from colleagues and mentors, than boys, who tended to keep their problems to themselves, and thus have higher incidence of anxiety and depression. Whilst it is unlikely that doctors in active practice are still dependent on their parents, it is possible that some are still dependent on their colleagues and friends.

Similarly, practising doctors could differ in their readiness to discuss their perceived problems with others, in order to get help and advice.

Having high expectations was associated with worse reactions, upon failing to fulfil these expectations, amongst West Indian immigrants to the UK.[20] Accordingly, overseas candidates who come aspiring to make quick progress might feel frustrated as they find themselves unable to progress at the speed they were hoping to. Whilst high expectations have disadvantages, having low expectations can lead to less overall achievement.[21] A candidate who thinks it would take him/her 2 years to get to know how to prepare for the Membership examination, may take even longer to take it and, if he/she is anticipating several goes before passing, it might well be that he/she will go home without it. It is important, therefore, that candidates have realistic expectations, so as to put in reasonable effort, but without getting very frustrated on facing difficulties.

Friends

Friendship represents a source of care to the individual as well as a forum for communication.[22] For overseas students, this can be of value during the transitional period, when an overseas doctor is adapting to the new environment. Friends from the same country or region, especially those who passed the examination, may help explaining new situations and provide an idea about examination and how to prepare for it.[23] It is to be noted here that being limited to friends from the same country could reflect poor adaptation to the new environment. For example, a group of American pupils visiting France ended up staying together because they could not get on with the French or understand their habits.[13] Likewise, friends from the same country can propagate the wrong advice, as a result of bad experience that may not necessarily apply to the newcomer. There is why some recommended that groups are led, even informally, by an experienced participant.[24] Friends from the host country might be of help as well. For example, British students in Australia were found to have faced less problems when they have at least a close Australian friend.[25] It is, therefore, the help, rather than the nationality, that counts and overseas doctors would benefit from their colleagues regardless of their country of origin.

Positive aspects of culture shock

Whilst changing the place of learning can have bad aspects, it can have good ones, such as looking into differences, making comparisons and drawing conclusions on which action is more suitable for which circumstances.[26] As overseas candidates get to know their new environment, they should reflect on areas of difference, identify positive aspects of their learning mechanisms and reading back home, that are still relevant to their new environment, which they will have to keep, and also mark ones where change or modification would be necessary. There is no point, therefore, in eroding the sense of shock altogether, as it helps understanding differences in learning practice and developing methods to adapt to these differences. What is important is to help these candidates pass through this phase smoothly so as to identify their way through the British postgraduate clinical training.

Adaptation

The adaptation of overseas students to the British academic environment could be seen as a four-stage process, that is equally applicable to overseas doctors.[11]

Orientation

During this stage, students explore the physical environment around them, such as clothes and housing, and may face stressful situations, arising from non-familiarity with new ways, such as commercial transactions. Likewise, overseas doctors would get used to the parts of the examination, and layout of their hospital wards.

Transitions of self worth

During this stage, students come to realise value differences between their original background and the new one. For example, having to write an assignment in a new way can be a difficult task, as the student will have to change the way of expressing him/herself. Similarly, overseas doctors would realise differences in answering questions and dealing with cases.

Consolidation of identity and roles

During this stage, the student would have developed some kind of arrangement to cope with the new situation. This could be showing every assignment to a colleague or tutor, without necessarily understanding the value of a particular way of writing. The same applies to overseas doctors, who might discuss their answers in the examination with College members and check the management of cases with their colleagues.

Maturity

During this stage, the student not only knows how to negotiate the new tasks, but understands the underlying value as well. For example, the student will now realise the significance of relating literature to practical applications relevant to the scenarios posed in the assignment. Similarly, overseas doctors would know how to tackle questions and deal with cases, on the basis of realising the skills tested for in the examination and the clinical case mix encountered in British hospitals.

Overseas students, and doctors, vary in how they pass through these phases. Whilst most candidates gain insight promptly, and progress satisfactorily in their studies and training, there are those who may never pass beyond the role-crisis phase of adaptation. Helping overseas doctors would, therefore, benefit from locating where they are in the process of adaptation.

ASPECTS OF LEARNING CULTURE

Learning styles

In order to understand how overseas doctors could adapt to their new environment of learning and assessment, it is important to look at key features of the type of learning expected in the UK.

Deep learning

Deep learning indicates that the learner tries not only to store facts and concepts, but relate them to his/her prior experience and daily practice as well. It is a mature phase that requires judgement and ability to link different areas together and relates to assessment methods that specifically test ability to evaluate concepts in terms of their practical value and require reflection on one's experience. In contrast, superficial learning is prevalent where assessment requires recall of facts and figures, such as lists of indications and contra-indications. The questions encountered in the Membership examination target opinion and application, rather than mere recall of figures. Consequently, overseas doctors preparing for this examination may have to change from surface learning, which might be more suitable for the examinations in their home countries, to deep learning.[15] It is to be noted that deep learning should not preclude mastering basic facts and figures, which define clinical conditions, but rather lead to a better understanding of the value of these figures in real life. Whilst rote learning is to discouraged, failure to give a straightforward definition of a common condition is certainly unacceptable.[27]

Experiential learning

Strongly related to deep learning is the fact that learning is gained from experience, as distinct from simply reading books and articles. As deep learning relies on relating facts to practice and developing one's own opinion, it requires reflection on performance so as to relate observations to concepts in order to develop one's own judgement, rather than mere memorising of information.[28] For example, candidates might be asked about their opinion of the methods used in investigating abnormal uterine bleeding and this will require considering the merits of these methods, as experienced by the candidate, rather than stated in books. It is interesting that one of the common causes of failure in the examination is that candidates abandon their day-to-day practice in an effort to impress the examiner.[29] Focusing on one's experience is a process that will require time, thinking as well as discussion with colleagues and can not be done if candidates are busy trying to read every paper and remember each figure.

Constructive learning

For learning to be experiential, new information and skills will have to be assessed in the light of existing ones. This marks the understanding of the value of these new skills and their application in day-to-day practice, as compared to superficial learning, which centres on simple recall of concepts without realising their significance.[30] Learning can, therefore, be seen as a process of assimilation during which the learner fits different pieces together, as he/she gains experience in day-to-day practice, a concept commonly referred to as constructivism.[31] The Membership examination tests the ability to construct answers from multiple sources, and overseas doctors will have to learn how to integrate new knowledge gained in the UK, with their existing knowledge and experience, gained whilst in their home countries. Candidates should not discredit their existing knowledge and start from scratch, as this destructivism could lea d to retardation, rather than progression. The idea is like 'do not through the baby with the bath water'.

Differences in clinical care

Alongside the change in learning style, overseas doctors face a change in the clinical environment. This will represent the background in which they will learn and demonstrate their experience in the examination, which is geared to clinical practice in the UK. Adapting to this practice has been emphasised by The Royal College of Obstetricians and Gynaecologists, as central to being prepared for the examination.[1] Examples of differences include:

1 Case mix could be different to that encountered overseas. For example, high parity, with its associated problems, is common in non-industrialised countries, whereas old age, with its clinical presentations, is more common in industrialised world. As a result, menopausal problems are more common in the UK whereas obstetric complications are more common in non-industrialised countries. Consequently, candidates may deal with obstetric problems in a different way to that adopted in the UK. The same applies to areas of special interest, such as urodynamics and colposcopy, which are available in many British hospitals, though they might be limited to specialised centres overseas.

2 The organisation of maternal health care in some non-industrialised countries may be different to that in the UK. For example, antenatal care might be patchy such that complications could present late, leading to higher rate of problems such as rupture uterus. This will have influenced the way in which overseas doctors deal with presentations like antepartum haemorrhage, where rupture uterus might be high on the differential diagnosis list, though it is rarely seen in the UK. Re-ordering such lists will take time and effort. Similarly, some countries do not have midwives and for doctors coming from such countries, the provision of most care in the UK by midwives, with doctors only needed upon the occurrence of complications, might be a strange situation, that requires adaptation in itself.

3 The prominence of areas like management, litigation, research, audit as well as communication. For example, litigation is less prevalent in most non-industrialised countries, such that medico-legal areas are totally new to most overseas doctors. Similarly, communication skills, like those involved in counselling and using information leaflets, are quite important for patient care in the UK, given the high level of patient awareness of heath matters. For doctors coming from countries with lower rates of literacy, and thus patient awareness of health issues, communication with patients takes a different form, such that acquiring new communication skills might be a bit of a challenge.

4 Family codes and patterns of sexual conduct might be different in some of the non-industrialised countries, such that sexually transmitted diseases, teenage contraception, single mothers, abortion, gametes donation and surrogacy are rarely encountered. These areas will require special adaptation, as they relate to moral and cultural values.

One particular source of confusion is that overseas doctors might have preconceived ideas about practice in British hospitals from College members back home or reading books. When the reality proves to be different from such ideas, they might lose confidence in their friends and what they have read and, as a result, have a worse degree of culture shock. For example, British books published in the 1980s indicated that the use of forceps is preferred to the ventouse as a method of instrumental delivery.[32] This changed in the 1990s, with the introduction of the soft sialistic cup, such that the vacuum extractor became more popular.[33] For those who come to the UK unaware of this change, this discrepancy might lead to discrediting the reading made overseas and having to read again from scratch, which, aside from aggravating the shock and confusion, is a waste of time and effort.

Candidate–supervisor interaction

The relation between overseas students and their tutors reflects learning patterns. For example, the expectations of Chinese students in British universities contrasted with those of their tutors.[8] The students relied on their tutors as sources of knowledge and expected not only to get well prepared handouts, but also clear guidance as to how problems could be solved. On the other hand, the tutors expected the students to develop their independence, look for material themselves and ask for help if needed. This matches the styles of learning, where superficial learners aim at memorising facts and expect these to be dictated by tutors. Deep, experiential and constructive learning requires a degree of independence so as to seek the appropriate information, appraise its value in relation to practice and relate it to existing knowledge.[30] Similarly, an overseas doctor might expect his/her consultant to identify the material to read for the examination and give training for the oral and clinical sections. The consultant, on the other hand, would expect the candidate to look for material him/herself, select the ones that he/she prefers, think independently about what he/she reads and seek help, if and when needed.

Having these opposite roles in mind can only lead to frustration. Following their learning style, of memorisation and reproduction of material, overseas students expect their tutors to provide them with the one correct answer. Seeing these tutors as the ultimate source of knowledge, the students do not challenge their ideas, even when the tutors adopt an inappropriate line, to stimulate thinking, which is central to deep learning.[34] Taking this scenario to clinical training, overseas doctors would presume that their consultants will provide them with everything they need, and do not disagree with them no matter what they say. If this pattern is followed in the oral examination, where examiners might adopt a line of management different to that suggested by the candidate, to assess his/her reasons as well as confidence, the outcome could be dire if the candidate follows the examiner and changes his/her mind. This might be compounded by the perception of cultural values, such as Islamic values, which are prevalent in Malaysia and endorse respect for the parents and teachers.[11]

An even more interesting distinction between overseas and British cultures of student–tutor interaction lies in the way in which students ask for help.[7] Overseas students may hint at their problems in an indirect way, expecting their tutors to know the problem and its solution, whereas the tutor might presume that the student does not have any problem, as he/she is not asking for help. Taking this to the Membership examination, a candidate might ask about the oral section in general terms, when in reality he/she is looking for help in relation to this part. The consultant, unaware of this hidden agenda, may tell stories about his/her own experience as a candidate, which may not be what the candidate was looking for.

The same applies to feedback, where tutors might be used to group discussion to elicit comments whilst the students might feel uncomfortable with making negative comments in public. As a result, they commonly feel that the whole exercise is a waste of time and a rather perverted way to getting the students to say that everything is fine. Taking this to clinical training, overseas doctors may not appreciate the value of audit and perinatal mortality meetings as methods of providing feedback on performance, and expect to be told what they did wrong and how to improve on one-to-one basis. Bearing in mind that their expression of dissatisfaction may not be a direct one, it is no surprise that consultants may never get the message.

Similarly, there is a difference in preferred teaching methods. Overseas students, used to superficial learning, prefer lectures to tutorials and discussions. Their tutors, on the other hand, keen on developing the ability of these students to think independently, rely on seminars and group work and yet may receive little co-operation from the students, ending in clashing approaches and failure of the educational interaction.[34] Taking this to clinical training, overseas doctors might expect local teaching to provide them with answers to examination questions, rather than building their ability to think about their practice and explore relevant literature accordingly, with minimal participation in discussions. Clearly, this will frustrate both sides, as consultants supervising teaching sessions and overseas doctors attending them have diverse expectations.

A more important difference is that overseas candidates tend to have considerable anxiety about their training. As highly motivated candidates, they are keen on making the most of their training and return home with the inner satisfaction and outward measure of success.[35] They are usually concerned about the possibility of failure, which is one of the main worries for them, and consider it as 'losing face', which indicates the link to social status and self-esteem. Failure can, therefore, be a very stressful experience, especially when overseas trainees come to the UK after making significant progress in their own countries and are not thus used to failure. Whilst this anxiety motivates them to learn, the stress it can cause might cause ill health and depression, and lead to inappropriate preparation for the examination and even failure, as a result of information overload and inadequate relaxation.[23] Moreover, it will make it difficult for candidates to get help, as communication will be rather muted.

As overseas candidates take failure badly, it is quite important to support them upon failure. Misery breeds under-performance and moral support is vital to enabling candidates to look into the reasons behind failure so as to do better next time. Failure in the examination should not be regarded as a failure in life and career, as some successful doctors recovered from failure through focused work. In fact, the ability to take failure and know how to deal with it is an important feature of mature and adult learners, who are able to deal with life's ups and downs smoothly. It is important to outline that failure is likely to be due to inability to demonstrate basic attitudes, skills and knowledge, usually because of failure to acquire them through experience, as a result of worry as well as factual overload. If overseas candidates, who are suffering from exhaustion and information overload, try harder, they are likely to fail even worse, with negative effects on their health, clinical performance as well as their friends and families.[23]

IMPROVING OVERSEAS LEARNING

Intercultural skills

Intercultural skills mark the ability to handle and understand cultural differences. These skills will enable both candidates as well as supervising consultants to understand and deal with the differences between clinical care and assessment styles in the UK and those encountered overseas, and thus ease culture shock and allow adaptation to the new clinical and learning environment.[21] For example, relying on the library and regular meetings in British hospitals reflects the need to read from multiple sources, without necessarily buying them, and discussing what is read with colleagues, to maintain the link to practice. On the other hand, reading from a limited number of sources, usually owned by the candidate, might be a familiar pattern in some non-industrialised countries, where assessment tests merely recall of facts and figures. This understanding of variation should assist guiding overseas doctors in their home countries as well as in British hospitals. What follows here relates primarily to training in the UK, though it also applies to overseas doctors preparing for the examination in their home countries.

Induction

The induction of overseas doctors represents an opportunity to highlight potential problems and how to avoid them. Induction days are held for new doctors and, since 1995, the College has required an acclimatisation period of 2 weeks prior to the start of their training in the UK.[1] It is important that this induction addresses differences in clinical care as well as assessment methods, alongside other areas such as lay out and rota arrangements. Given their contrasting learning expectations, consultants might leave overseas doctors to explore their new environment whereas these doctors expect their tutors to know their needs and provide them without request.[36] It is not uncommon for doctors to do nothing during these 2 weeks, making them a complete waste of time. The recently introduced induction days for overseas doctors could be improved by including sessions about learning and assessment styles as well as patterns of clinical care, alongside financial aspects, audit, communication and legal areas.[37]

Learning style modification

Awareness of the learning styles of overseas doctors should guide the acquisition of the skills conducive to the deep, constructive and experiential learning necessary to pass the examination.[6]. Examples of selective skill building are included below.

Improving small group teaching

Overseas doctors might regard local teaching and audit meetings as boring commitments rather than opportunities for reflective thinking and experiential learning. It is useful for supervising consultants to engage these doctors in the discussion by asking them for their views and inviting them to comment on the ideas expressed by others, so as to ensure that they develop critical skills, appreciate relevance, and relate theory to practice.

Improving private study

By stimulating overseas doctors to pursue focused project-like learning activity, such as doing an audit, consultants can guide overseas doctors to acquire skills like developing a focused task, so as not to copy work that have been done before, but try to relate audit standards to local practice and identify relevance as well as limitations. These skills are central to experiential learning expected in the Membership examination.

Improving reading and critical thinking

The way in which overseas doctors take notes whilst in lectures can be improved from writing every thing, to summarising the main points, through active engagement in discussions. The same applies to reading skills, so that overseas doctors do not simply learn what they read by heart, but weigh it in the light of their practice. This will be of value in those sections of the examination that rely on the ability to evaluate ideas and options, rather than simply recall of investigation and treatment methods. This level of thinking would include identifying the evidence behind various options, evaluating these options in the light of day-to-day practice as well as considering the requirements for, and the implications of, each option, so as to demonstrate the thought behind answers.

Improving problem solving

Problem solving has become prominent in the new Objective Structured Clinical Examination, which replaced the old clinical and oral sections in 1998. Training in problem solving would include working from answers, working from assumptions, thinking of practical implications, and identifying alternatives.

Courses

Preparatory courses are commonly attended by overseas candidates. These could help in outlining the differences in clinical care as well as learning and assessment styles, by looking at a range of answers and how they are marked and evaluated, rather than trying to cover many topics and include several mock examinations. Showing candidates the criteria of a good answer, in terms of focusing on day-to-day practice in British hospitals, rather than simple recall of literature no matter how detailed or updated it can be, will avoid false impressions commonly gained from comparing performance to other candidates.[38] The emphasis should, therefore, be on the depth of understanding as well as realisation of aspects of difference, so as to guide the candidate in his/her preparation for the examination.

Feedback

As overseas students and doctors might not understand their new environment, providing a mechanism for discussion helps clarifying vague areas, dealing with problems and ensuring that adequate progress is being made. To illustrate, a weekly meeting was arranged between the Saudi nurses and their tutors at George Mason University in the US to enable early management of problems.[39] A number of warning indicators has been identified for research students, such as making excuses for unfinished work and focusing on the next stage, rather than the current one.[6] Similar indicators for overseas doctors would include poor adaptation to the practice in the UK, obsession with figures, pre-occupation with journals and books, low profile in local meetings, and simple reproduction of previous audits. Feedback is even more important upon failure and this should highlight areas of weakness, showing which answers were considered the best and which ones were considered the worst. The availability of past questions and answers on the College website is a significant step in guiding training to the level and scope of answers expected.

General help

Helping overseas students also extends to areas related to living in a foreign country, without necessarily focusing on learning. Most British universities nowadays have special officers to deal with overseas affairs and do provide facilities for worship for different religions. The same approach was adopted at George Mason University in the US in training the Saudi nurses, where students were allowed a break for Friday prayers and arrangements were made for them to contact their families regularly.[39] This eases the sense of isolation amongst overseas candidates and helps them to concentrate better on their learning. Along the same lines, it would be helpful to pay attention to praying and dialling facilities, married accommodation, child care as well as spouse education and professional development for overseas doctors.

Requirements

Supervising overseas doctors will require time, effort and skill.[6] Changes can not be made overnight and overseas doctors will need time to adapt to their new environment and change their learning style. It is promising that education is now part of the curriculum of specialist registrars, so that future consultants will be prepared for their educational role. Yet, they will need time to gain experience in dealing with overseas candidates and develop intuition.[40] It is equally encouraging that postgraduate deaneries are appointing special advisers for overseas doctors and producing handbooks, so that information can be available though differences in learning need to be specifically outlined. Written material, computer packages and electronic sources of knowledge are especially useful as they do not require a tutor and are available overseas.

Improving overseas training will also require commitment and follow-up. Universities have given special attention to overseas students and their special needs as part of trying to provide education for all types of students, including mature and disabled students. Similarly, the College should underline the importance of catering for all trainees, including those from overseas, to maintain its global role. Likewise, monitoring of the quality of training provided to overseas doctors should help ensure that improvements are being made[41] and the hospital recognition scheme could be of value in this respect.[42] Just as external examiners and student representatives assist educational boards in monitoring the educational process in universities,[43] the representation of overseas doctors in the College should enable paying attention to the needs of overseas doctors world-wide.

Variation

Not withstanding the observations made here, it is important to remember that many overseas candidates do exceptionally well and manage to gain experience and also contribute to their clinical and learning environments. Variations are commonly seen and some tutors have reported their encounter with Asian students with very high analytical skills and British students with poor structuring abilities.[34] It is worth mentioning here similar differences in learning and assessment methods exist even amongst European countries. For example, there is more emphasis on acquisition of facts, regular attendance and reliance on teachers in France.[41] Overseas doctors should, therefore, be assessed as individuals, without being limited to a stereotyped image that might apply to some, rather than all, of them.

CONCLUSIONS

The learning problems of overseas doctors taking the Part 2 Membership examination relate to their familiarity with clinical care in British hospitals as well as their awareness of the style of the examination. As the examination is geared to clinical practice in the UK, candidates will have to adapt to the case mix and pattern of care encountered in British hospitals. They also need to change their learning style from mere focus on facts to deep understanding of their value in the light of the experience they accumulate through their day-to-day practice, so as to demonstrate the right level of competence required to pass the examination. They pass through a form of culture shock as they face this new clinical and learning environment and easing this requires skills in understanding and explaining differences in clinical and learning cultures.

Ideally, orientation should begin back home, through College members and fellows as well as printed guides and electronic sources of information should address differences in clinical care and assessment methods. Training in British hospitals should target them as well as in induction, local teaching as well as preparatory courses. Supervising consultants should guide candidates to link theory to practice, base their knowledge on their daily experience and reflect on patterns of care. Experience gained in the UK should supplement that gained back home and warning signs, such as obsession with facts and low participation in meeting, should be taken seriously. Overseas doctors should be encouraged to become more independent in their thought and pro-active in seeking guidance. Their anxiety regarding the examination should be taken into account, especially upon failure, when feedback should outline the differences in clinical care and assessment style.

Awareness of cultural differences in socialising as well as helping in areas like accommodation and professional development for spouses would help candidates get on with their colleagues and settle down so as to concentrate on their learning. Training overseas doctors will require teaching experience, which in return will be enriched by supervising a variety of candidates. Likewise, it requires commitment and monitoring so as to enhance the global role of the College. Enhanced representation of overseas doctors will enable addressing their needs and co-operation with international organisations will strengthen the College profile. Training of overseas doctors should be regarded as an example for other forms of international exchange, where trainees are regarded as individuals so as to meet their special needs, without being limited by patterns or stereotypes.

References

1 Royal College of Obstetricians and Gynaecologists. Report of the RCOG Working Party on Overseas Affairs. London: RCOG, 1995
2 Gupta R, Lingham S. The overseas doctors training scheme. BMJ Classified, 9 January 1999; 2–3
3 McNamara D, Harris R. Overseas Students in Higher Education: Issues in Teaching and Learning. London: Routledge, 1997
4 Luxford M. Children with Special Needs. Edinburgh: Floris Books, 1994
5 Furnham A, Tresize L. The mental health of foreign students. Soc Sci Med 1983; 17: 365–370
6 Brown G, Atkins M. Effective Teaching in Higher Education. London: Routledge, 1988
7 Cortazzi M, Jin L. Communication for learning across cultures. In: McNamara D, Harris R. (eds) Overseas Students in Higher Education: Issues in Teaching and Learning. London: Routledge, 1997; 76–90
8 Jin L. Academic cultural expectations and second language use; Chinese postgraduate students in the UK, A cultural synergy model, PhD Thesis, University of Leicester.
9 Beaver B, Tuck B. The adjustment of overseas students at a tertiary institution in New Zealand. N Z J Ed Stud 1988; 33: 167–179
10 Fiscella K, Roman-Diaz M, Lue B et al. Being a foreigner, I may be punished if I make a small mistake: assessing transcultural experiences in caring for patients. Fam Pract 1997; 14: 112–116
11 Mohamed O. Counselling for excellence: adjustment development of South-East Asian students. In: McNamara D, Harris R. (eds) Overseas Students in Higher Education: Issues in Teaching and Learning. London: Routledge, 1997; 156-172.
12 Cowie AP. Oxford Advanced Learners' Dictionary of Current English, 4th edn. Oxford: Oxford University Press, 1989
13 Wilkinson S. Study abroad from participants' perspective: a challenge to common beliefs. Foreign Lang Ann 1998; 31: 23–29
14 Mumford DB. The measurement of culture shock. Soc Psychiatry Psychiatr Epidemiol 1988; 33: 149–154
15 Harris R. Overseas students in the United Kingdom university system: a perspective from social work. In: McNamara D, Harris R. (eds) Overseas Students in Higher Education: Issues in Teaching and Learning. London: Routledge, 1997; 30–45
16 Gloria AM, Kurpius SER, Hamilton KD et al. African American students' persistence at a predominantly white university: influences of social support, university comfort and self beliefs. J Coll Stud Dev 1999; 40: 257–268
17 Oberg J. Cultural shock; adjustment to new cultural environments. Pract Anthropol 1960; 7: 177–182
18 Wright C. Gender matters: access, welfare, teaching and learning. In: McNamara D, Harris R. (eds) Overseas Students in Higher Education: Issues in Teaching and Learning. London: Routledge, 1997; 91–107

19 Brewin C, Furham A, Howe M. Demographic and psychological determinants of homesickness and confiding among students. Br J Psychol 1989; 80: 467–477

20 Cochrane R. The Social Creation of Mental Illness. London: Longman, 1983

21 Furnham A. The experience of being an overseas student. In: McNamara D, Harris R. (eds) Overseas Students in Higher Education: Issues in Teaching and Learning. London: Routledge, 1997; 13–29

22 Cobb A. Social support as a moderator of life stress. Psychomat Med 1976; 38: 300–314

23 Gray C. Challenging the 'F' word: redefining failure in medical careers. BMJ Classified on 12 June 12 1999; 2–3

24 Yates P, Cunningham J, Moyle W, Wollin J. Peer mentorship in clinical education; outcomes of a pilot programme for first year students. Nurse Educ Today 1997; 17: 508–514

25 Sellitz C, Cook S. Factors influencing attitudes of foreign students towards the host country. J Soc Iss 1962; 18: 7–23

26 Adler P. The transition experience: an alternative view of culture shock. J Hum Psychol 1975; 15: 13–23

27 Hanretty KP. A Handbook for Clinical Examinations in Obstetrics and Gynaecology. West Sussex: Eurocommunica, 1994

28 Rogers A. Teaching Adults, 2nd edn. Buckingham: Open University, 1996

29 Wagstaff TI. Case Presentations in Obstetrics and Gynaecology. Oxford: Butterworth-Heinemann, 1991

30 Whitman N. A review of constructivism: understanding and using a relatively new theory. Fam Med 1993; 25: 517–521

31 Duffy TM, Jonassen DH. Constructivism: new implications for instructional technology. Educ Technol 1991; 31: 7–12

32 Hibbard BM. Principles of Obstetrics. London: Butterworths, 1988

33 Johanson R. Choice of instrument for vaginal delivery. Curr Opin Obstet Gynecol 1997; 9: 361–365

34 Todd ES. Supervising overseas students: problem or opportunity?. In: McNamara D, Harris R. (eds) Overseas Students in Higher Education: Issues in Teaching and Learning. London: Routledge, 1997; 173–186

35 Elsey B. Teaching and learning. In: Kinnell M. (ed) The Learning Experience of Overseas Students. Buckingham: Society for Research into Higher Education and Open University, 1990

36 Hofstede G. Cultures and Organisations, London: Harper Collins, 1994

37 Holcombe C, Watters DK. Training of overseas qualified doctors in Britain: new report recommends improvements. BMJ 1995; 311: 642–643

38 Salter R, Smith S. How to pass the MRCP (UK) examination: ask a successful candidate!. Postgrad Med J 1998; 74: 33–34

39 Carty RM, Hale JE, Carty GM et al. Teaching international nursing students: challenges and strategies. J Prof Nurs 1998; 14: 34–42

40 Tomlinson P. Understanding Mentoring: Reflective Strategies for School-based Teacher Preparation, Buckingham: Open University, 1995

41 Brennan J. Studying in Europe. In: McNamara D, Harris R. (eds) Overseas Students in Higher Education: Issues in Teaching and Learning. London: Routledge, 1997; 62–75

42 Harvey L. The new collegialism: improvement with accountability. Tertiary Educ Manag 1995; 1: 153–160

43 Ackers J. Evaluating UK courses: the perspective of the overseas student. In: McNamara D, Harris R. (eds) Overseas Students in Higher Education: Issues in Teaching and Learning. London: Routledge, 1997; 187–200

Gavin P. Sacks   Chris W.G. Redman   Ian L. Sargent

The immunology of human pregnancy

Recent advances in reproductive immunology have caused a fundamental shift in our appreciation of the very nature of human pregnancy. For nearly 50 years, the subject has been dominated by Medawar's 'fetal allograft' hypothesis, in which an analogy is assumed between the fetus and a tissue transplant (an allograft). In this framework, all maternal immune mechanisms are considered potentially harmful for the fetus and, therefore, must be overcome, bypassed or suppressed. Much progress has been made in elucidating the ways in which the fetus evades specific immunological attack. However, it has also become clear that fetal–maternal interaction is a much more complex affair. In particular, a hitherto relatively neglected area of interest is the non-specific, or innate, arm of the maternal immune system. An understanding of these wide-spread changes is relevant to all pregnancy-related phenomena.

FUNDAMENTAL OBJECTIVES IN PREGNANCY

Reproduction is obviously essential for the propagation of life, and yet for the individual pregnancy can be extremely dangerous, if not fatal. The commonest causes of maternal deaths – infection, haemorrhage, pre-eclampsia and thrombosis – are direct results of physiological changes wrought on the mother by the fetus. Indeed, it is argued that 'fetal' genes are selected to promote anything that is necessary to serve the development of the fetus (e.g. maternal

Dr Gavin P. Sacks MA DPhil MRCOG, Specialist Registrar, Department of Obstetrics and Gynaecology, Chelsea and Westminster Hospital, 369 Fulham Road, London SW10 9NH, UK (for correspondence)

Prof. Chris W.G. Redman MA FRCP, Professor of Obstetric Medicine, The John Radcliffe Hospital, Oxford OX3 9DU, UK

Dr Ian L. Sargent BSc PhD, University Reader, Nuffield Department of Obstetrics and Gynaecology, The John Radcliffe Hospital, Oxford OX3 9DU, UK

> **Box 1** Possible aims of the maternal immune adaptation to pregnancy
>
> - To avoid fetal rejection whilst maintaining immune competence
> - To aid fetal–maternal communication and maternal recognition of pregnancy
> - To provide local growth factors

immune suppression, raised blood pressure and blood glucose) and result in the tendency to maternal disease (e.g. severe infection, pre-eclampsia and diabetes).[1] 'Maternal' genes will be selected to guard the interests of the mother, and may conflict with some fetal objectives. Arising out of this conflict will be a delicate balance or compromise – the maternal adaptation to pregnancy.

The balance for the maternal immune system is some element of suppression to minimise the risk of rejection of fetal (paternal) tissues whilst maintaining enough immune competence to fight infection. In addition, though, there are other potential functions of immune cells and their products (cytokines; Box 1). Immune cells are the body's main means of recognising foreign antigens, but the reaction to them can be tailored depending on the background of other signals received. 'Immune rejection' is not the only possible response. For example, some cytokines at the maternal–fetal interface act as local growth factors and encourage fetal growth. More wide-spread activation of inflammatory pathways can affect other maternal targets, including the clotting system and the vascular endothelium. Thereby, the adaptation of the maternal immune system to pregnancy may be not just a means to avoid fetal rejection, but also a mechanism for the maternal recognition of pregnancy so that appropriate physiological changes can be made.

THE MEDAWAR–SHWARTZMAN PARADOX

The origin of the 'fetal allograft' hypothesis was Medawar's observation that rejection of skin grafts could be prevented by administration of cortisone.[2] He was aware that steroid levels are raised in pregnancy, and so made the analogy

> **Box 2** Medawar's postulates for survival of a 'fetal allograft'
>
> - Anatomical separation of the fetus from its mother
> - Antigenic immaturity of the fetus
> - Immunological inertness of the mother

between pregnancy and a tissue graft. In his influential paper, he proposed possible mechanisms by which the antigenically foreign body of the fetus avoids maternal immunological attack (Box 2).

This useful approach has been extensively reviewed in a previous chapter in this series[3] and elsewhere,[4] and provides the framework for much of the forthcoming discussion. However, a more dynamic maternal-fetal relationship is suggested by an alternative and paradoxical model of pregnancy which was discovered at a similar time as Medawar's pioneering work, but has, until recently, received rather less attention.

The localized Shwartzman reaction of haemorrhagic necrosis is induced in some animals by a priming injection of endotoxin in the footpad followed 24 h later by a sublethal intravenous endotoxin injection.[5] An intravenous priming injection causes a similar but more generalised and fatal reaction, characterised by bilateral renal cortical necrosis.[6] In pregnant animals, identical pathological lesions are observed after just a single intravenous injection of endotoxin; the priming injection is not required.[6,7] Thus, pregnant women may be similarly prone to exaggerated responses to endotoxin during pregnancy.

It is not known how pregnancy 'primes' animals for the Shwartzman reaction. But in non-pregnant animals, an alternative 'priming agent' is cortisone, and other 'provocative factors' include starch and glycogen.[8,9] Recent workers have identified non-specific mechanisms mediating the reaction,[10] and monocytes and natural killer cells in particular.[11,12]

Thus there is a paradox that in Medawar's model of pregnancy, cortisone causes the maternal immune system to be less responsive to foreign antigens,[2] while in the experimental Shwartzman reaction cortisone, like pregnancy itself, increases sensitivity to a range of non-specific stimuli including endotoxin.[8] The maternal immune system is suppressed in one model, but primed to respond in another.

The explanation for this paradox lies in the potential for differential modulation of the two main arms of the immune system: adaptive (immune) and non-specific (inflammatory).

IMMUNE SYSTEM OVERVIEW

There are two arms of the immune system: the innate (non-specific) and adaptive (specific), both of which have cellular and humoral components (Table 1).

The adaptive system, often synonymous with 'immunity', has been studied most because of its specificity, effectiveness at eliminating infection, and

Table 1 Cellular and humoral components of innate and adaptive immunity

Component	Innate	Adaptive
Cellular	Monocytes/macrophages, granulocytes, NK cells, mast cells, γδ T-cells	T- and B-cells
Humoral	Complement, acute phase proteins, mannose binding lectin, clotting cascade	Antibodies

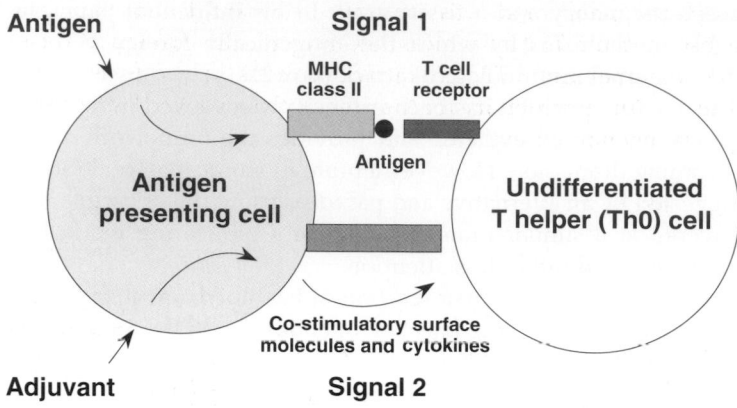

Fig. 1 Stimulation of an immune response. Antigen presenting cells such as macrophages not only process and present antigen to T-cells (in association with MHC class II proteins), but also have receptors for adjuvant (e.g. endotoxin). Adjuvant 'activates' these cells to produce cytokines (e.g. IL-12) and surface molecules (e.g. CD86) which determine the type and extent of the T cell response.

presence in higher multicellular organisms only. Essentially, antigen displayed on the cell surface in association with major histocompatibility complex (MHC) proteins triggers the activation of helper T-cells which produce co-stimulatory molecules (e.g. cytokines) which in turn co-ordinate the effector response. As part of 'routine' immune surveillance, most cells (with few exceptions, such as red blood cells) express MHC class I protein (HLA-A, HLA-B or HLA-C), and professional 'antigen presenting cells' such as macrophages express MHC class II protein (HLA-D). Foreign class II MHC can itself stimulate a host immune response, and is the main mechanism of the immune rejection of tissue allografts. The innate system is a first line of defence, but also, crucially, instigates the immune response by processing and presenting antigen in association with MHC class II molecules, the so called 'signal 1' (Fig. 1).[13]

But it is now recognised that signal 1 alone is not enough to generate a full immune response which also requires 'adjuvants' (such as endotoxin). Adjuvants interact with the innate immune system to produce 'signal 2', in the form of co-stimulatory surface molecules or cytokines (Fig. 1).[13–16] Thus it is believed that signal 2 determines the biological significance of antigens, and communicates this information to the adaptive system. In the absence of signal 2, T-cells would be unable to appreciate the dangerous nature of new antigens they encounter. For example, endotoxin, a by-product of all Gram-negative bacterial infections, is readily recognized by the innate system, and the subsequent production of signal 2 (e.g. the cytokine IL-12) encourages the differentiation of antigen-specific lymphocytes. Signal 2 'interprets' the environment in which antigens are encountered and then 'instructs' the adaptive system to respond appropriately.[15] There are basically two kinds of subsequent adaptive response: cell-mediated and antibody-mediated.

The adaptive response is co-ordinated by activated helper T lymphocytes (Th cells) which can differentiate into either Th1 or Th2 cells defined by their patterns of cytokine production (Table 2).[17] Th1 cells produce cytokines which stimulate macrophage phagocytic activity and cytotoxic T-cells (i.e. cell-mediated responses); while Th2 cells stimulate B-cells and eosinophils (i.e. antibody-mediated responses).[18] The characteristic cytokine products of Th1 and Th2 cells are mutually inhibitory for the differentiation and effector functions of the reciprocal phenotype (Fig. 2).

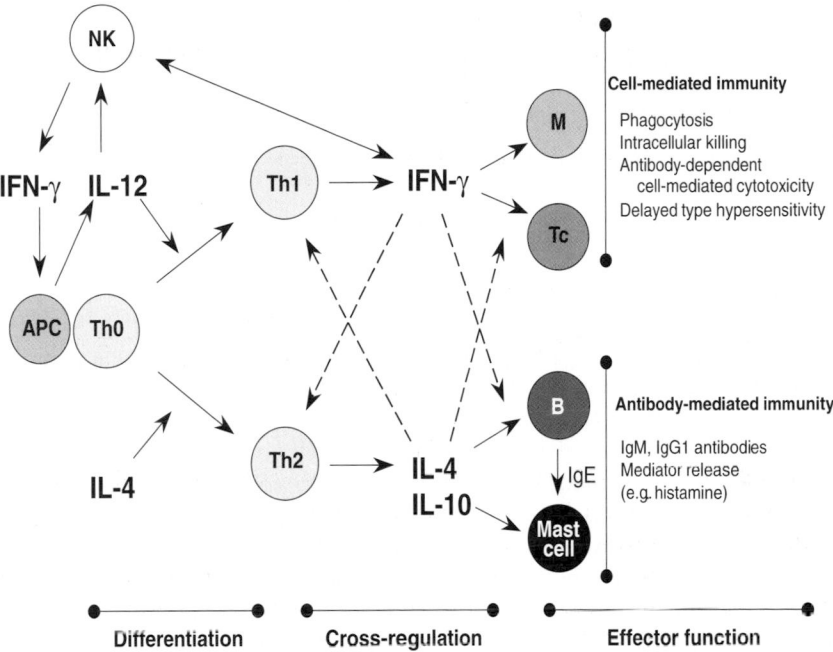

Fig. 2 A schematic representation of critical cytokines in Th1 and Th2 immune responses. Antigen is presented to undifferentiated T-cells (Th0) by antigen presenting cells (APCs) which may be monocytes, macrophages or dendritic cells. APCs which are activated by endotoxin or other products release IL-12 which induces Th0 cells to differentiate to Th1 cells. IL-12 also stimulates natural killer (NK) cells, resulting in the early release of IFN-γ, and subsequent positive feedback on APCs and an additional stimulus for Th1 cell differentiation. In other circumstances (e.g. parasitic infection), the early presence of IL-4 initiates Th2 differentiation. Th1 cells produce IFN-γ (and other cytokines such as TNF-β and IL-2) which stimulate NK cells, macrophages (M), and cytotoxic CD8⁺ T-cells. These are the main effector cells of a Th1 response. Th2 cells produce IL-4 and IL-10 which induce B-cells to produce antibodies. Th2 cytokines and IgE also stimulate mast cells and eosinophils (not shown) which release mediators of allergic-type responses (e.g. histamine). Inhibitory cross-regulatory pathways are shown by dashed arrows. IFN-γ inhibits the proliferation of Th2 cells, while IL-10 and IL-4 inhibit APCs, the development of Th1 cells, and monocyte and cytotoxic T cell responses.

Table 2 Cytokines produced by Th1 and Th2 cells

Th1 cytokines	Th2 cytokines
IFN-γ	IL-4
TNF-β	IL-5
*IL-2	*IL-6
*TNF-α	*IL-10
	*IL-13

*Preferential Th1 or Th2 production in mice, but less restricted in humans.

Box 3 Placental products that may modulate innate immunity in vivo

- Syncytiotrophoblast microvillous membranes
- Progesterone
- Corticotrophin releasing hormone
- Human chorionic gonadotrophin
- Human placental lactogen
- Vascular endothelial growth factor
- Interleukin-4

The discovery of this interplay between innate and adaptive immunity has changed the perception of what the immune system is actually doing. Classically, as in the 'fetal allograft' model of pregnancy, it has been assumed that the immune system distinguishes between self and non-self,[19] and it must, therefore, either be turned on or off. But this view has never been entirely satisfactory – the fetus is patently not a tissue allograft or infective organism, and shares many maternal antigens. But in signal 2, the innate system appears to be able to distinguish between dangerous and non-dangerous,[14] an insight that is a significant shift away from the all-or-none constraints of specific immunity. It has also led us to speculate that the innate arm of the immune system may even be able to distinguish the pregnant from the non-pregnant state,[20] and is discussed further below.

THE ANATOMY OF FETAL–MATERNAL INTERACTION

One of the survival mechanisms of the fetus against maternal immune attack is the anatomical separation imposed by the placenta which restricts access of the maternal immune system to fetal cells.[21] However, this important barrier is not perfect. Fetal nucleated erythrocytes can enter the maternal blood in early pregnancy,[22] and fetal leukocytes, though less frequent, have also been detected.[23] Their presence is presumed to result from fetal–maternal haemorrhage which may take place as part of the normal development of the placenta or as a sporadic event. The maternal immune system is likely to be stimulated by these trafficking fetal cells.

While the placenta is not a perfect barrier, it still forms the primary interface between fetal and maternal tissues. There are two main areas of consideration. First, in the uterine decidua (pregnant endometrium), there is direct contact between extravillous cytotrophoblast cells and maternal immune cells. These are primarily components of innate immunity: macrophages and large granular lymphocytes (closely related to natural killer [NK] cells); there are relatively few T-cells.[24,25]

Second, maternal blood is in direct contact with trophoblast tissues, either in the intervillous space where it bathes the syncytiotrophoblast lining the villi, or in the systemic circulation where fragments of syncytiotrophoblast, cytotrophoblast cells[26] and syncytiotrophoblast microvillous membrane particles[27] are detectable. The latter may occur as a consequence of apoptosis or programmed cell death, which is known to occur in the normal syncytium.[28,29] The subsequent formation of 'syncytial sprouts' may result in 'breaks' in the syncytiotrophoblast and shedding of both membrane particles and exposed whole villous cytotrophoblast cells directly into maternal blood.[30] Most of the embolised cells lodge in the pulmonary capillaries, but some have been detected in the peripheral circulation.[26] The deportation of syncytiotrophoblast micro-villous membrane particles into the peripheral circulation is more common[27] and, whether by default or design, may be an important signalling mechanism between the placenta and maternal immune system. The extrapolation of the maternal–fetal interface to include the entire maternal circulation is key to understanding the overall immunological response to human pregnancy.

TROPHOBLAST EXPRESSION OF MHC

Whether in the decidua or maternal circulation, trophoblast is the fetal tissue most commonly exposed to the maternal immune system. All forms of trophoblast are negative for MHC class II antigens[31] and, therefore, unable to stimulate maternal lymphocytes directly, as occurs in classical tissue transplant rejection reactions. The syncytiotrophoblast and underlying villous cytotrophoblast are also negative for class I MHC antigens[32] and are, therefore, unable to be attacked by maternal cytotoxic T-cells.

Class I MHC expression on extravillous cytotrophoblast in the placental bed and chorionic membrane is more complicated. In brief, both non-classical HLA-G[33,34] and HLA-E,[35] and classical HLA-C[36] are expressed. Decidual NK cells express receptors for these class I molecules, and this is therefore a potential mechanism for recognition of trophoblast cells. Whether NK function is thereby suppressed, or NK cells play a part in limiting trophoblast invasion is uncertain.[35] Furthermore, as those class I antigens are less polymorphic than other class I antigens (HLA-A, HLA-B), they may also prevent attack by maternal cytotoxic T-cells.[4]

CYTOKINES AT THE PLACENTAL–DECIDUAL INTERFACE

In the event of exposure of fetal cells, and possibly even of non-classical MHC antigens, Medawar's 'fetal allograft' model proposed that there must be some element of maternal immune suppression to prevent a rejection reaction.[4,17,37] As most pregnant women are clearly not immunocompromised, it is hypothesised that there is a subtle immunological shift to Th2-type cytokine responses in pregnancy that would minimise potentially more harmful cell-mediated (Th1 type) responses.[38]

Animal studies have shown that Th2-type cytokines are indeed released spontaneously from placental tissue in culture,[39] and that pregnancy loss can be caused by Th1 cytokines,[40] but prevented by Th2 cytokines.[41] In addition, other powerful Th2 promoting factors such as progesterone[42] and prostaglandin E$_2$[43] are present in high concentrations at the maternal–fetal interface.

Less is known about cytokines at the maternal–fetal interface in human pregnancy, but a wide variety (including both Th1- and Th2-types) have been detected.[44] It has, therefore, been argued that an altered cytokine balance may be achieved by the absence of particular cytokines, the most striking being the Th1-type cytokine IL-2.[45] We have used cell-specific methods that have shown preferential production by trophoblast cells of IL-4 rather than IFN-γ, IL-12 or TNF-α.[46]

However, it is still not yet known whether Th2 cytokines predominate in vivo, or whether the presence of Th1 cytokines is necessarily harmful. For example, it is hypothesised that cytokines have other essential non-immune functions – in particular, they can stimulate placental growth.[47,48] Cytokines such TNF-α, IL-6, IFN-γ and IL-4 bind to specific receptors on trophoblast cells and can stimulate trophoblast production of human chorionic gonadotrophin.

SYSTEMIC CYTOKINE RESPONSES IN PREGNANCY

Wegmann et al.[38] also hypothesised that there is a similar bias to Th2 responses in the maternal immune system away from the maternal-fetal interface – that pregnancy is a 'Th2 phenomenon'. This would account for the remission during pregnancy of cell-mediated autoimmune diseases such as rheumatoid arthritis,[49] the flare-up of systemic lupus erythematosus (SLE) which is principally mediated by autoantibodies,[50] and the increased incidence of some intracellular infections during pregnancy, including malaria, tuberculosis, leprosy and coccidioidomycosis.[38]

There is some support for this hypothesis. First, in an animal model, pregnancy impairs resistance to *Leishmania major* infection in mice (normally eliminated by cell-mediated immunity), and is associated with predominantly Th2 cytokine production by stimulated peripheral lymphocytes.[51] Second, in humans, peripheral blood mononuclear cells from pregnant women produce more Th2 cytokines than Th1 cytokines after stimulation in vitro.[52] It is still uncertain whether this is due to a relative suppression of Th1 responses, or whether Th2 responses are actually enhanced (Sacks et al., in preparation).

A pregnancy Th2 bias is consistent with older data showing suppression of maternal cell-mediated immunity.[53,54] Also, in contrast to the evidence for only sporadic T-cell sensitisation to fetal antigens, antifetal (paternal) HLA allo-antibodies are more commonly detected in about 15% of women in their first pregnancies, and in 60% of multiparous women.[4] This indicates that when the maternal immune system is confronted with fetal antigens (a consequence of fetal-maternal haemorrhage, or possibly trophoblast shedding), it responds with a Th2-type antibody-mediated bias.

A Th2-type response is less likely to cause immune rejection and, moreover, potentially harmful antibodies to fetal MHC antigens appear to be effectively filtered out by binding to antigens in the placental villous stroma – the concept of the 'placental sponge'.[4]

INNATE ACTIVATION IN PREGNANCY

Although hitherto given relatively scant attention, there is extensive evidence that maternal innate (cellular and humoral) systems are activated in normal pregnancy.[20] The maternal decidua is infiltrated by macrophages[24,55] and large granular lymphocytes,[25] and in peripheral maternal blood there are increased numbers of monocytes[56] and granulocytes[57] from the first trimester onwards.

In normal pregnancy, circulating monocytes have activated phenotypes, including increased expression of the endotoxin receptor CD14.[58] When stimulated with endotoxin in vitro, monocyte production of IL-12 is increased in pregnancy (unpublished). This appears of direct relevance to the particular sensitivity of pregnant animals to endotoxin and the Shwartzman reaction,[7] and supports other evidence of monocyte activation in pregnancy.[20]

Circulating granulocytes are also activated in some ways, including increased cell migration[59] and phagocytosis,[60,61] increased surface antigen expression,[58] and raised blood levels of the granulocyte activation products elastase,[62] lactoferrin[63] and alkaline phosphatase.[64]

In normal pregnancy there are increased levels of acute phase proteins and activation of clotting factors typical (albeit to a lesser degree) of an inflammatory reaction.[65–67] There are also reports of increased levels of some complement components[68] which are consistent with activation of the classical complement pathway.[69]

Not all components of the innate system are activated in the maternal circulation. Most notably, the number of circulating NK cells is reduced and their function is suppressed.[70] There may be specific inhibitory factors released by trophoblast such as soluble HLA-G.[71]

THE INFLAMMATORY MODEL OF PREGNANCY

We have hypothesised that the activation of innate immunity occurs in part to compensate for the Th2-type bias of adaptive immunity, and is presumably driven by factors released by the placenta.[20] There are several candidate factors (soluble and particulate) which are released from the placenta directly into the maternal circulation, and many have already been shown to have contrasting effects on lymphocytes (suppressed) and monocytes (activated) in vitro (Box 3). The overall release of placental soluble and particulate factors into the maternal circulation is the 'adjuvant' that stimulates the inflammatory reaction of pregnancy (Fig. 3).

We are particularly interested in the role of particle shedding from the syncytiotrophoblast into maternal blood.[30] Fetal DNA in maternal blood[72] could be derived from such degraded trophoblast. Such placentally-derived particles would almost certainly be eliminated by phagocytes and may lead to their activation; or, even in the absence of phagocytosis, membrane lipids may stimulate innate systems via lipid receptors such as CD14, CD11b, L-selectin and the mannose receptor.[15,73] We have shown that syncytiotrophoblast microvillous membrane particles isolated from a perfused placental lobule stimulate monocytes to produce TNF-α and IL-12 in vitro (unpublished). Certain sequences of bacterial DNA are able to stimulate TNF-α and IL-12 production from monocytes,[74] and this may also occur with fetal DNA. Therefore, in vivo, inflammatory responses may be produced directly in the maternal circulation by products of the fetus and placenta, analogous to the experimental stimulation of cytokine production following an intravenous injection of endotoxin[75,76] or, indeed, the Shwartzman reaction.

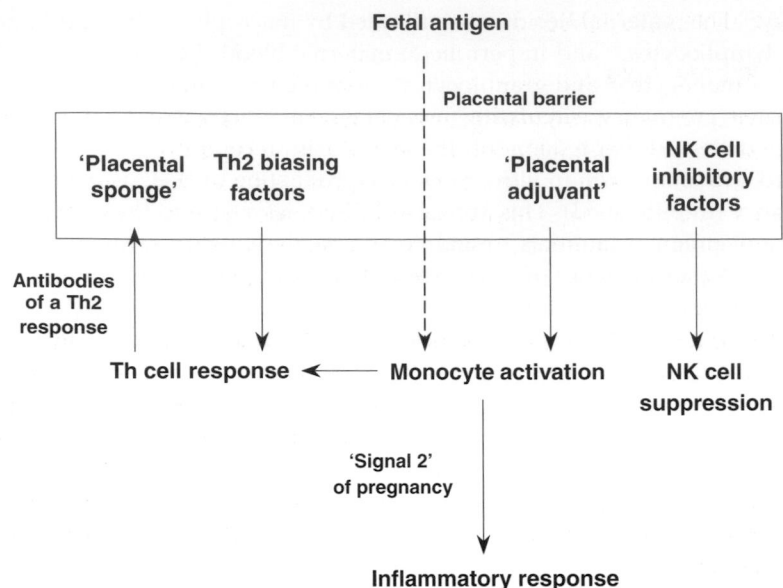

Fig. 3 The placenta and the maternal immune response. The placenta effectively regulates all aspects of the maternal immunological adaptation to pregnancy. Fetal-specific antigens are largely denied access to maternal immune cells, and if presentation does occur (e.g. in the decidua or blood), placental factors bias the response to a less damaging antibody (Th2) type. Anti-fetal antibodies are 'absorbed' by antigens in the placenta. NK cells are specifically inhibited, but factors comprising 'placental adjuvant' stimulate monocytes. This is the 'signal for pregnancy' and results in an inflammatory response. See text for details.

THE 'SIGNAL FOR PREGNANCY' HYPOTHESIS

It is hypothesised that placental 'adjuvant' stimulates signal 2 (Fig. 1), but, in contrast with a classical immune response, signal 1 (i.e. antigen presentation) is largely avoided in pregnancy (Fig. 3). Moreover we hypothesise that signal 2 in pregnancy is unique.[20] Whereas endotoxin, for example, is an adjuvant that signals infection and danger, lipid components on fetal-trophoblast membranes, perhaps in conjunction with other soluble circulating factors (Box 3), may generate specific pregnancy signals through interaction with the innate system.

The signal for pregnancy, or 'signal P' refers to the instruction given by a stimulated innate system to lymphocytes.[20] This instruction may be via the expression of surface antigens or cytokine release, or even by a more indirect effect. There is much interest in the recent finding that monocytes from pregnant women inhibit lymphocyte proliferation in vitro,[77] and that this 'suppressor' effect is due to the over-consumption of tryptophan (an essential amino acid in culture media) by monocytes.[78] In vivo, it has now been shown that there is high activity of the enzyme indoleamine 2,3 dioxygenase (IDO) which catabolises tryptophan in the placenta, and that inhibition of IDO leads to increased pregnancy loss in mice.[79] This has been proposed as a mechanism for lymphocyte suppression in pregnancy.

CLINICAL IMPLICATIONS

Infection in pregnancy

Physiological changes of pregnancy such as increased tissue fluid and urinary stasis increase the risk of infection, and the developing fetus itself has a poorly developed immune system. One would expect overall maternal immunity to be enhanced rather than suppressed to cope with these changes. Nevertheless, some elements of the maternal immune system are certainly suppressed, and an alteration in the incidence and severity of infections in pregnancy would be expected.

The shift towards Th2-type responses results in a slight increase in viral infections which are normally eliminated by Th1-type cell-mediated immune responses.[80,81] But this effect is smaller than would be expected because of the activation of innate immunity. It is now accepted that most infections are eliminated by the combined efforts of the innate and adaptive systems,[82,83] and we hypothesise that enhanced innate immunity eliminates many early infections *more* rather than less efficiently during pregnancy, and these might not even present clinically.

However, in some virulent infections which are not rapidly cleared, the innate immune system may become over-stimulated. Thus, some infections during pregnancy have been reported to have more severe clinical presentations, including pyelonephritis, group B *Streptococcus*, *Listeria monocytogenes*, infectious hepatitis, varicella zoster, influenza, coccidioidomycosis, and malaria. In these cases, the immunological balance required for a response which avoids damaging immune attack on the placenta may result in an over-reliance on innate rather than adaptive cell-mediated immunity, with non-specific tissue damage compounding the effects of persistent infection

Pre-eclampsia

The concept[38] that normal pregnancy is a 'Th2 phenomenon' has spurred some investigators to hypothesise that abnormal pregnancy is caused by an 'immune shift' to Th1-type responses. In pre-eclampsia, it has been reported that maternal blood levels of the Th1-type cytokine IL-12 are raised,[84] although we were unable to confirm those results, and there are other reports that Th2-type cytokines are also raised.[85] Such measurements of circulating cytokines are inevitably difficult to interpret as the source of cytokine production is not known. Since cytokines act at a cellular level (and are not, by definition, hormones) detection in the circulation can do no more than confirm that some form of immunological or inflammatory reaction is occurring somewhere or other. However, using cell-specific flow cytometric techniques it has recently been reported that the ratio of Th1:Th2 cells in circulating blood is increased in pre-eclampsia compared to normal pregnancy.[86] We hypothesise that this represents an increased and thereby decompensated systemic inflammatory response to pregnancy.[87]

It is established that there is increased activation of circulating leukocytes in pre-eclampsia.[58] But since normal pregnancy is itself an inflammatory state, we have hypothesised that pre-eclampsia is what happens when, towards the end of pregnancy, the systemic inflammatory response of normal pregnancy becomes decompensated.[87] Endothelial cell dysfunction[88] may be one part of a more extensive intravascular inflammatory response that, in total, is characteristic of pre-eclampsia.

Excessive inflammatory stimuli released from the placenta will be related to placental size, and hence the increased incidence of pre-eclampsia with advancing gestational age, multiple pregnancy and diabetic pregnancy. In some cases, the inflammatory stimulus is excessive even from a small placenta. This would most typically be in relation to early onset pre-eclampsia, and might be induced by placental hypoxia secondary to uteroplacental arterial insufficiency, which amplifies release of inflammatory stimuli into the maternal circulation.[30,87] In other cases, the maternal inflammatory response is excessive. Such women will include those with genetic predispositions,[89] or where there are concurrent alternate stimuli to the inflammatory response such as malaria[90] and disseminated lupus erythematosus.[91]

The hypothesis accounts for some other frustrating features of pre-eclampsia, such as the lack of a single cause or screening test, or a single treatment that will be more effective than delivery and termination of the pregnancy.[87]

Miscarriage and recurrent miscarriage

There is less evidence for the inflammatory model in early pregnancy, although there are increased numbers of circulating monocytes[56] and granulocytes,[57] and innate cell infiltration of the decidua from as early as 6 weeks' gestation. Inflammatory responses may be initiated by human chorionic gonadotrophin,[92] which is one of the earliest hormones detectable in pregnancy. It has been hypothesised that early inflammatory responses against the trophoblast may be necessary, in evolutionary terms, to eliminate those fetuses which are 'less fit'.[93] We have described how an inflammatory response may be an important signalling mechanism for pregnancy, and failure to produce an appropriate response may be one cause of miscarriage and recurrent miscarriage. Thus, more Th1-type cytokines are produced by stimulated leukocytes from women who have an early miscarriage compared with those from normal pregnant women,[52] and similarly for stimulated leukocytes from women with recurrent miscarriages compared with normal parous women.[94]

'Immunotherapy' for recurrent miscarriage is currently out of vogue[95] and not yet proven to be effective.[96] But future immunological therapies might involve the stimulation of innate immunity (in which the timing and intensity of such stimulation may be critical), and more specific immune modulation to bias maternal immune responses to a Th2-type pattern.

CONCLUSIONS

Medawar's original concepts of the 'fetal allograft' and maternal 'immunosuppression' have presented a rather benign view of pregnancy which appears at odds with other substantial changes in maternal physiology. The Shwartzman reaction is one particularly striking paradox. Thus, this new inflammatory model emphasises a dynamic immunological relationship between mother and fetus, accounting for the considerable mixing of maternal and fetally-derived cells, and the activation rather than suppression of some elements of the maternal immune system. This is relevant to most conditions of pregnancy, whether infective, autoimmune, or specific to pregnancy.

References

1 Haig D. Genetic conflicts in human pregnancy. Q Rev Biol 1993; 68: 495–532
2 Medawar PB. Some immunological and endocrinological problems raised by the evolution of viviparity in vertebrates. Symp Soc Exp Biol 1953; 7: 320–338
3 Nicholas NS. Human fetal allograft survival. In: Studd J. (ed) Progress in Obstetrics and Gynaecology, vol. 7. Edinburgh: Churchill Livingstone, 1989; 1–25
4 Sargent IL. Maternal and fetal immune responses during pregnancy. Exp Clin Immunogenet 1993; 10: 85–102
5 Shwartzman G. A new phenomenon of local skin reactivity to B. typhosus culture filtrate. Proc Soc Exp Biol Med 1928; 25: 560–561
6 Apitz K. A study of the generalized Shwartzman phenomenon. J Immunol 1935; 29: 255–266
7 Beller FK, Schmidt EH, Holzgreve W, Hauss J. Septicemia during pregnancy: a study in different species of experimental animals. Am J Obstet Gynecol 1985; 151: 967–975
8 Thomas L, Good RA. Studies on the generalized Shwartzman reaction. I General observations concerning the phenomenon. J Exp Med 1952; 96: 605–624
9 Stetson CA. Studies on the mechanism of the Shwartzman phenomenon. Certain factors involved in the production of the local hemorrhagic necrosis. J Exp Med 1953; 93: 489–504
10 Mori W. The Shwartzman reaction: a review including clinical manifestations and proposal for a univisceral or single organ third type. Histopathology 1981; 5: 113–126
11 Ozmen L, Pericin M, Hakimi J et al. Interleukin 12, interferon gamma, and tumor necrosis factor alpha are the key cytokines of the generalized Shwartzman reaction. J Exp Med 1994; 180: 907–915
12 Heremans H, Dillen C, van Damme J, Billiau A. Essential role for natural killer cells in the lethal lipopolysaccharide-induced Shwartzman-like reaction in mice. Eur J Immunol 1994; 24: 1155–1160
13 Fearon DT. Seeking wisdom in innate immunity. Nature 1997; 388: 323–324
14 Matzinger P. Tolerance, danger, and the extended family. Annu Rev Immunol 1994; 12: 991–1045
15 Fearon DT, Locksley RM. The instructive role of innate immunity in the acquired immune response. Science 1996; 272: 50–53
16 Medzhitov R, Janeway Jr CA. Innate immunity: impact on the adaptive immune response. Curr Opin Immunol 1997; 9: 4–9
17 Mosmann TR, Sad S. The expanding universe of T-cell subsets: Th1, Th2 and more. Immunol Today 1996; 17: 138–146
18 Roitt IM. Essential Immunology, 9th edn. Oxford: Blackwell, 1997
19 Janeway Jr CA, Goodnow CC, Medzhitov R. Danger – pathogen on the premises! Immunological tolerance. Curr Biol 1996; 6: 519–522
20 Sacks GP, Sargent IL, Redman CWG. An innate view of human pregnancy. Immunol Today 1999; 20: 114–118
21 Redman CWG. The fetal allograft. Fetal Med Rev 1990; 2: 21–43
22 Bianchi DW, Zickwolf GK, Yih MC et al. Erythroid-specific antibodies enhance detection of fetal nucleated erythrocytes in maternal blood. Prenat Diagn 1993; 13: 293–300
23 Yeoh SC, Sargent IL, Redman CWG, Wordsworth BP, Thein SL. Detection of fetal cells in maternal blood. Prenat Diagn 1991; 11: 117–123
24 Hunt JS, Robertson SA. Uterine macrophages and environmental programming for pregnancy success. J Reprod Immunol 1996; 32: 1–25
25 King A, Loke YW, Chaouat G. NK cells and reproduction. Immunol Today 1997; 18: 64–66
26 Johansen M, Redman CWG, Wilkins T, Sargent IL. Trophoblast deportation in human pregnancy – its relevance for pre-eclampsia. Placenta 1999; 20: 531–539

27 Knight M, Redman CWG, Linton EA, Sargent IL. Syncytiotrophoblast microvilli are shed into the maternal circulation in increased amounts in pre-eclamptic pregnancy. Br J Obstet Gynaecol 1998; 105: 632–640

28 Nelson DM. Apoptotic changes occur in syncytiotrophoblast of human placental villi where fibrin type fibrinoid is deposited at discontinuities in the villous trophoblast. Placenta 1996; 17: 387–391

29 Huppertz B, Frank HG, Kingdom JC, Reister F, Kaufmann P. Villous cytotrophoblast regulation of the syncytial apoptotic cascade in the human placenta. Histochem Cell Biol 1998; 110: 495–508

30 Redman CWG, Sargent IL. Placental debris, oxidative stress and pre-eclampsia. Placenta 2000; 21: 597–602

31 Giacomini P, Tosi S, Murgia C et al. First-trimester human trophoblast is class II major histocompatibility complex mRNA⁺/antigen. Hum Immunol 1994; 39: 281–289

32 Sunderland CA, Naiem M, Mason DY, Redman CWG, Stirrat GM. The expression of major histocompatibility antigens by human chorionic villi. J Reprod Immunol 1981; 3: 323–331

33 Ellis SA, Sargent IL, Redman CWG, McMichael AJ. Evidence for a novel HLA antigen found on human extravillous trophoblast and a choriocarcinoma cell line. Immunology 1986; 59: 595–601

34 Kovats S, Main EK, Librach C, Stubblebine M, Fisher SJ, DeMars R. A class I antigen, HLA-G, expressed in human trophoblasts. Science 1990; 248: 220–223

35 King A, Hiby SE, Gardner L et al. Recognition of trophoblast HLA class I molecules by decidual NK cell receptors – a review. Placenta 2000; 21: S81–S85

36 King A, Boocock C, Sharkey AM et al. Evidence for the expression of HLA-C class I mRNA and protein by human first trimester trophoblast. J Immunol 1996; 156: 2068–2076

37 Romagnani S. The Th1/Th2 paradigm. Immunol Today 1997; 18: 263–266

38 Wegmann TG, Lin H, Guilbert L, Mosmann TR. Bidirectional cytokine interactions in the maternal–fetal relationship: is successful pregnancy a Th2 phenomenon? Immunol Today 1993; 14: 353–356

39 Lin H, Mosmann TR, Guilbert L, Tuntipopipat S, Wegmann TG. Synthesis of T helper 2-type cytokines at the maternal–fetal interface. J Immunol 1993; 151: 4562–4573

40 Chaouat G, Menu E, Clark DA, Dy M, Minkowski M, Wegmann TG. Control of fetal survival in CBA x DBA/2 mice by lymphokine therapy. J Reprod Fertil 1990; 89: 447–458

41 Chaouat G, Assal Meliani A, Martal J et al. IL-10 prevents naturally occurring fetal loss in the CBA x DBA/2 mating combination, and local defect in IL-10 production in this abortion-prone combination is corrected by in vivo injection of IFN-tau. J Immunol 1995; 154: 4261–4268

42 Piccinni MP, Giudizi MG, Biagiotti R et al. Progesterone favors the development of human T helper cells producing Th2-type cytokines and promotes both IL-4 production and membrane CD30 expression in established Th1 cell clones. J Immunol 1995; 155: 128–133

43 Kelly RW, Critchley HO. A T-helper-2 bias in decidua: the prostaglandin contribution of the macrophage and trophoblast. J Reprod Immunol 1997; 33: 181–187

44 Robertson SA, Seamark RF, Guilbert LJ, Wegmann TG. The role of cytokines in gestation. Crit Rev Immunol 1994; 14: 239–292

45 Vince GS, Johnson PM. Is there a Th2 bias in human pregnancy? J Reprod Immunol 1996; 32: 101–104

46 Sacks GP, Clover L, Bainbridge D, Redman CWG, Sargent IL. Flow cytometric measurement of intracellular Th1 and Th2 cytokine production by human villous and extravillous cytotrophoblast. Placenta 2001; 22: 550–559

47 Wegmann TG, Athanassakis I, Guilbert L et al. The role of M-CSF and GM-CSF in fostering placental growth, fetal growth, and fetal survival. Transplant Proc 1989; 21: 566–568

48 Guilbert L, Robertson SA, Wegmann TG. The trophoblast as an integral component of a macrophage-cytokine network. Immunol Cell Biol 1993; 71: 49–57

49 Da Silva JA, Spector TD. The role of pregnancy in the course and aetiology of rheumatoid arthritis. Clin Rheumatol 1992; 11: 189–194

50 Varner MW. Autoimmune disorders and pregnancy. Semin Perinatol 1991; 15: 238–250

51 Krishnan L, Guilbert LJ, Russell AS, Wegmann TG, Mosmann TR, Belosevic M. Pregnancy impairs resistance of C57BL/6 mice to *Leishmania major* infection and causes decreased antigen-specific IFN-gamma response and increased production of T helper 2 cytokines. J Immunol 1996; 156: 644–652

52 Marzi M, Vigano A, Trabattoni D et al. Characterization of type 1 and type 2 cytokine production profile in physiologic and pathologic human pregnancy. Clin Exp Immunol 1996; 106: 127–133

53 Gehrz RC, Christianson WR, Linner KM, Conroy MM, McCue SA, Balfour Jr HH. A longitudinal analysis of lymphocyte proliferative responses to mitogens and antigens during human pregnancy. Am J Obstet Gynecol 1981; 140: 665–670

54 Strelkauskas AJ, Davies IJ, Dray S. Longitudinal studies showing alterations in the levels and functional response of T and B lymphocytes in human pregnancy. Clin Exp Immunol 1978; 32: 531–539

55 Starkey PM, Sargent IL, Redman CWG. Cell populations in human early pregnancy decidua: characterization and isolation of large granular lymphocytes by flow cytometry. Immunology 1988; 65: 129–134

56 Smarason AK, Gunnarsson A, Alfredsson JH, Valdimarsson H. Monocytosis and monocytic infiltration of decidua in early pregnancy. J Clin Lab Immunol 1986; 21: 1–5

57 Barden A, Graham D, Beilin LJ et al. Neutrophil CD11b expression and neutrophil activation in pre-eclampsia. Clin Sci Colch 1997; 92: 37–44

58 Sacks GP, Studena K, Sargent IL, Redman CWG. Normal pregnancy and pre-eclampsia both produce inflammatory changes in peripheral blood leukocytes akin to those of sepsis. Am J Obstet Gynecol 1998; 179: 80–86

59 Berge LN, Ostensen M, Revhaug A. Phagocytic cell activity in pre-eclampsia. Acta Obstet Gynecol Scand 1988; 67: 499–504

60 Shibuya T, Izuchi K, Kuroiwa A, Okabe N, Shirakawa K. Study on non-specific immunity in pregnant women: increased chemiluminescence response of peripheral blood phagocytes. Am J Reprod Immunol Microbiol 1987; 15: 19–23

61 Barriga C, Rodriguez AB, Ortega E. Increased phagocytic activity of polymorphonuclear leukocytes during pregnancy. Eur J Obstet Gynecol Reprod Biol 1994; 57: 43–46

62 Greer IA, Haddad NG, Dawes J, Johnstone FD, Calder AA. Neutrophil activation in pregnancy-induced hypertension. Br J Obstet Gynaecol 1989; 96: 978–982

63 Rebelo I, Carvalho Guerra F, Pereira Leite L, Quintanilha A. Lactoferrin as a sensitive blood marker of neutrophil activation in normal pregnancies. Eur J Obstet Gynecol Reprod Biol 1995; 62: 189–194

64 Polishuk WZ, Diamant YZ, Zuckerman H, Sadovsky E. Leukocyte alkaline phosphatase in pregnancy and the puerperium. Am J Obstet Gynecol 1970; 107: 604–609

65 Fagan EA. Disorders of the liver, biliary system and pancreas. In: De Swiet M (ed) Medical Disorders in Obstetric Practice. Oxford: Blackwell, 1989; 426–520

66 Letsky EA. Coagulation defects. In: De Swiet M (ed) Medical Disorders in Obstetric Practice. Oxford: Blackwell, 1989; 104–165

67 Wisdom SJ, Wilson R, McKillop JH, Walker JJ. Antioxidant systems in normal pregnancy and in pregnancy-induced hypertension. Am J Obstet Gynecol 1991; 165: 1701–1704

68 Adelsberg BR. The complement system in pregnancy. Am J Reprod Immunol 1983; 4: 38–44

69 Hopkinson ND, Powell RJ. Classical complement activation induced by pregnancy: implications for management of connective tissue diseases. J Clin Pathol 1992; 45: 66–67

70 Gregory CD, Lee H, Rees GB, Scott IV, Shah LP, Golding PR. Natural killer cells in normal pregnancy: analysis using monoclonal antibodies and single-cell cytotoxicity assays. Clin Exp Immunol 1985; 62: 121–127

71 Munz C, Holmes N, King A et al. Human histocompatibility leukocyte antigen (HLA)-G molecules inhibit NKAT3 expressing natural killer cells. J Exp Med 1997; 185: 385–391

72 Lo YM, Corbetta N, Chamberlain PF et al. Presence of fetal DNA in maternal plasma and serum. Lancet 1997; 350: 485–487

73 Malhotra R, Bird MI. L-Selectin – a signalling receptor for lipopolysaccharide. Chem Biol 1997; 4: 543–547

74 Lipford GB, Sparwasser T, Bauer M et al. Immunostimulatory DNA: sequence-dependent production of potentially harmful or useful cytokines. Eur J Immunol 1997; 27: 3420–3426

75 LeMay DR, LeMay LG, Kluger MJ, D'Alecy LG. Plasma profiles of IL-6 and TNF with fever-inducing doses of lipopolysaccharide in dogs. Am J Physiol 1990; 259: R126–R132

76 Jansen PM, van der Pouw Kraan TC, de Jong IW et al. Release of interleukin-12 in experimental *Escherichia coli* septic shock in baboons: relation to plasma levels of interleukin-10 and interferon-gamma. Blood 1996; 87: 5144–5151

77 Bjercke S, Bertheussen K, Maltau JM. Increased relative frequency of suppressor monocytes in peripheral blood in early pregnancy. APMIS 1989; 97: 125–130

78 Munn DH, Zhou M, Attwood JT et al. Prevention of allogeneic fetal rejection by tryptophan catabolism. Science 1998; 281: 1191–1193

79 Mellor AL, Munn DH. Tryptophan catabolism and T-cell tolerance: immunosuppression by starvation? Immunol Today 1999; 20: 469–473

80 Brabin BJ. Epidemiology of infection in pregnancy. Rev Infect Dis 1985; 7: 579–603

81 Chapman ST. Prescribing in pregnancy. Bacterial infections in pregnancy. Clin Obstet Gynaecol 1986; 13: 397–416

82 Unanue ER. Studies in listeriosis show the strong symbiosis between the innate cellular system and the T-cell response. Immunol Rev 1997; 158: 11–25

83 Xiong H, Ohya S, Tanabe Y, Mitsuyama M. Persistent production of interferon-gamma (IFN-gamma) and IL-12 is essential for the generation of protective immunity against *Listeria monocytogenes*. Clin Exp Immunol 1997; 108: 456–462

84 Dudley DJ, Hunter C, Mitchell MD, Varner MW, Gately M. Elevations of serum interleukin-12 concentrations in women with severe pre-eclampsia and HELLP syndrome. J Reprod Immunol 1996; 31: 97–107

85 Sacks GP, Scott D, Tivnann H, Mire-Sluis T, Sargent IL, Redman CWG. Interleukin-12 and pre-eclampsia. J Reprod Immunol 1997; 34: 155–158

86 Saito S, Sakai M, Sasaki Y, Tanebe K, Tsuda H, Michimata T. Quantitative analysis of peripheral blood Th0, Th1, Th2 cells and the Th1:Th2 cell ratio during normal human pregnancy and pre-eclampsia. Clin Exp Immunol 1999; 117: 550–555

87 Redman CWG, Sacks GP, Sargent IL. Pre-eclampsia: an excessive maternal inflammatory response to pregnancy. Am J Obstet Gynecol 1999; 180: 499–506

88 Roberts JM, Taylor RN, Musci TJ, Rodgers GM, Hubel CA, McLaughlin MK. Pre-eclampsia: an endothelial cell disorder. Am J Obstet Gynecol 1989; 161: 1200–1204

89 Chen G, Wilson R, Wang SH, Zheng HZ, Walker JJ, McKillop JH. Tumour necrosis factor-alpha (TNF-alpha) gene polymorphism and expression in pre-eclampsia. Clin Exp Immunol 1996; 104: 154–159

90 Sartelet H, Rogier C, Milko Sartelet I, Angel G, Michel G. Malaria associated pre-eclampsia in Senegal. Lancet 1996; 347: 1121

91 Jones WR. Autoimmune disease and pregnancy. Aust N Z J Obstet Gynaecol 1994; 34: 251–258

92 Shibuya T, Izuchi K, Kuroiwa A, Harada H, Kumamoto A, Shirakawa K. Study on non-specific immunity in pregnant women: effect of hormones on chemiluminescence response of peripheral blood phagocytes. Am J Reprod Immunol 1991; 15: 19–23

93 Schuiling GA, Koiter TR, Faas MM. Why pre-eclampsia? Hum Reprod 1997; 12: 2087–2091

94 Hill JA, Polgar K, Anderson DJ. T-helper 1-type immunity to trophoblast in women with recurrent spontaneous abortion. JAMA 1995; 273: 1933–1936

95 Christiansen OB. A fresh look at the causes and treatments of recurrent miscarriage, especially its immunological aspects. Hum Reprod 1996; 2: 271–293

96 Scott JR. Immunotherapy for recurrent miscarriage. Cochrane database of systematic reviews 2000; 2: CD000112

Joyce Harper Charles Rodeck

Pre-implantation genetic diagnosis

Pre-implantation genetic diagnosis (PGD) was developed more than a decade ago as an alternative to prenatal diagnosis for couples at risk of transmitting an inherited disease to their offspring (reviewed in Harper & Delhanty[1]). Patients are required to go through in vitro fertilisation (IVF) procedures so that embryos can be generated in vitro. In the majority of cycles, 1–2 embryonic cells (blastomeres) are biopsied from the 6–10 cell stage embryo (day 3 after insemination). The biopsied blastomeres can then be used for the diagnosis. The polymerase chain reaction (PCR) is used for the diagnosis of single gene defects or triplet repeat disorders, and fluorescent in situ hybridisation (FISH) is used to analyse chromosomes. Embryos unaffected by the disease examined are replaced in the patient's uterus and, hopefully, the pregnancy is started knowing that the fetus is free from disease. However, single cell diagnosis is technically challenging and added problems, such as PCR contamination, allele dropout and chromosomal mosaicism have made PGD more difficult than was originally envisaged. Added to this are the ethical concerns of how such a procedure could develop in the future. In recent years, through the European Society of Human Reproduction and Embryology (ESHRE), an international PGD consortium has been established to report annually on the referrals for PGD, PGD cycles performed, pregnancies and deliveries, as well as to discuss the methods used in PGD and ethical concerns. The most recent data from the consortium will be discussed throughout this chapter.[2,3]

Dr Joyce Harper BSc PhD, Senior Lecturer in Human Genetics and Embryology, Department of Obstetrics and Gynaecology, Gower Street Campus, University College London, 86–96 Chenies Mews, London WC1E 6HX, UK (for correspondence)

Prof. Charles H. Rodeck DSc FRCOG FRCPath FMedSci, Head, Department of Obstetrics and Gynaecology, Gower Street Campus, University College London, 86–96 Chenies Mews, London WC1E 6HX, UK

REFERRALS

The patients referred for PGD are mostly those for whom prenatal diagnosis is also offered. Couples may discover they are carrying a genetic disease due an affected family member, after the delivery of an affected child or, in the case of chromosomal abnormalities, after a karyotype is performed due to recurrent miscarriage. In some cases, as part of their genetic counselling, PGD will be discussed. Some couples that opt for PGD have already had prenatal diagnosis and repeated terminations of pregnancy, but do not wish to undergo a further prenatal diagnosis. However, there are also patients who have moral or religious objections to termination of pregnancy and wish to opt for PGD as their first reproductive choice. Patients who have had repeated miscarriages due to chromosome imbalances often feel that PGD is their only hope of achieving a normal child. However, for fertile patients, PGD is not an easy option, and the cost of PGD has to be taken into consideration, as not all health authorities will fund this treatment. Therefore, natural conception is always an alternative. The infertile patient, who is also carrying a genetic or chromosomal abnormality, is in a very different position and so adding PGD to their fertility treatment is a sensible option.

PGD is not available in all cases where prenatal diagnosis would be available. It is technically challenging to develop a single cell diagnosis for a particular mutation or chromosome abnormality, which often takes many months and has a high cost. The ESHRE PGD consortium data show that only a few genetic defects and chromosomal abnormalities have been diagnosed by PGD.[2]

Patients opting for PGD require the same preliminary investigations as IVF couples, such as semen assessment, examination of the uterus, etc. For a PGD cycle, the IVF stimulation and treatment is the same as a standard IVF cycle, except that it is important to try and obtain at least 9 oocytes to ensure that after the diagnosis, there will be some good quality, unaffected embryos to transfer.[4]

BIOPSY

Embryo biopsy is not a difficult procedure when performed by an experienced embryologist. Since many embryologists already perform micromanipulation procedures, such as intracytoplasmic sperm injection (ICSI) for the treatment of male infertility, embryo biopsy is a relatively easy addition to their skills.

Theoretically, there are three stages that cells can be removed from the pre-implantation embryo: (i) polar bodies from the oocyte and zygote; (ii) blastomeres from cleavage stage embryos; and (iii) trophectoderm cells from the blastocyst. In practice, the majority of PGD centres use cleavage stage biopsy. From the ESHRE PGD Consortium data,[3] 755 cycles used cleavage stage biopsy, 3 used polar body only and 1 used both. There have been no reports on the use of blastocyst biopsy for clinical PGD cases.

Cleavage stage biopsy

This was the original method used for PGD and the technique has remained almost unchanged.[5,6] Cleavage stage biopsy involves two steps – zona drilling and blastomere aspiration (Fig. 1). The majority of centres use acid Tyrodes' solution for zona drilling. Acid Tyrodes' solution (pH 2.2) dissolves the zona

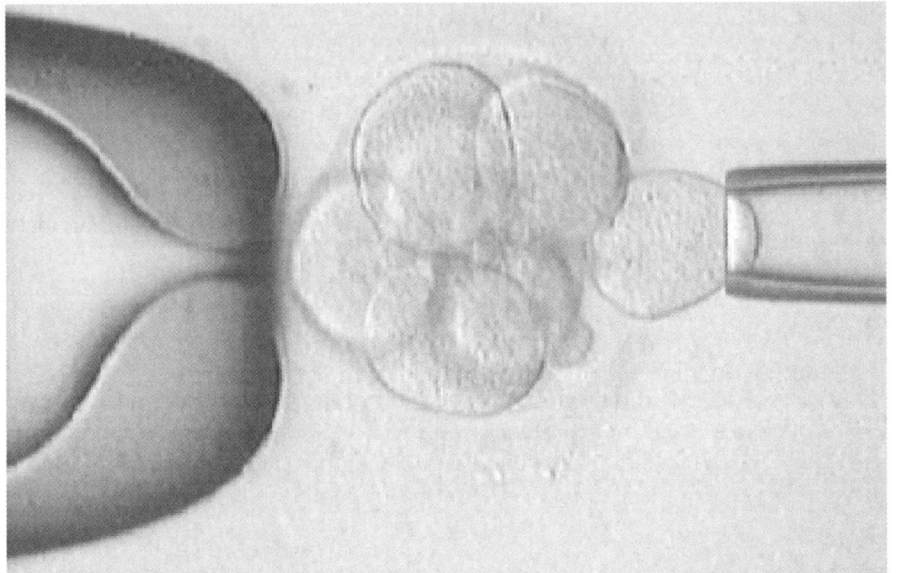

Fig. 1 Cleavage stage embryo biopsy. Removal of one cell from an 8-cell embryo. [Courtesy of Alpesh Doshi, University College London, UK – first published on <www.fertilityconfidential.com> and reproduced with permission.]

pellucida. However, the technique does not allow accurate control over the size of the hole drilled. The use of a non-contact laser for zona drilling in embryo biopsy has been suggested.[7] The laser has been used by many IVF centres as a technique aimed to increase the chances of implantation, termed assisted hatching. However, the use of the laser for PGD cycles has been slow,[6,7] as it is currently not approved by the Food and Drug Administration in the US and is very expensive to purchase. However, the control over the size of the hole is very accurate using a laser, and often smaller holes are possible, which may be an advantage for implantation. A third method of zona breaching, partial zona dissection, has also been reported.[8] The advantage of this method is that a flap is made in the zona to enable the blastomeres to be aspirated, but no hole as such is formed in the zona. Very few groups have reported using this method.[8]

Once the zona is breached, 1–2 blastomeres can be aspirated from the embryo. At the 8-cell stage, human embryos start to undergo compaction, whereby they increase their cell:cell contacts and a number of intercellular junctions are formed. Therefore, trying to biopsy blastomeres at this stage has sometimes proved difficult and blastomere lysis can occur. Recently, the use of Ca^{2+}/Mg^{2+}-free culture medium has reduced blastomere lysis during biopsy.[9] The junctions set up between blastomeres are Ca^{2+}-dependent and so removal of the Ca^{2+} reduces junction formation. This reaction is reversible and during biopsy allows for easy removal of blastomeres.

Polar body biopsy

When this method was originally developed it was thought that removal of just the first polar body from the oocyte (preconception diagnosis) would be possible, but it was soon realised that removal of both the first and second polar body are required for an accurate diagnosis. However, the second polar body is only extruded from the oocyte after fertilisation, at the zygote stage, and so the term preconception diagnosis cannot be used. The first polar body degenerates quite rapidly in the human and so this should be removed as soon as possible after collection. However, this would require two manipulator procedures and so both simultaneous[10] and sequential[11] biopsy have been reported. Besides being quite labour intensive, the main drawback of polar body biopsy is that only maternal chromosomes are examined, and so diseases carried by the male partner cannot be diagnosed. However, it has been used by two groups for the diagnosis of the common aneuploidies in patients undergoing IVF procedures.[10,12]

Acid Tyrodes' solution is not used for drilling the zona in polar body biopsy as acid Tyrodes' solution has been found to affect adversely the oocyte meiotic spindle.[13] Therefore, either a bevelled pipette can be used or a laser,[14] and three dimensional mechanical zona dissection has recently been reported.[8]

Blastocyst biopsy

This procedure has not been applied clinically as yet as up to 60% of human embryos arrest in culture and do not reach the blastocyst stage. Therefore, a high number of embryos would be lost before the PGD procedure and this would reduce the chances of good quality, normal embryos for transfer. However, there have been several reports on the method of blastocyst biopsy.[15,16] A hole is made in the zona pellucida using acid Tyrodes' solution or a laser and the blastocyst is returned to culture for several hours during which time it will start to hatch. Some of the trophectoderm cells can be removed from the hatching blastocyst and used for diagnosis. Once the blastocyst has hatched it would need to be transferred to the uterus quite rapidly as this is the stage that it would start to implant. Blastocyst biopsy would, therefore, give more cells for diagnosis, but less time. Also, the trophectoderm cells are involved in implantation and so reduction in their number may reduce pregnancy rates.

SINGLE CELL DIAGNOSIS

Whether polar body, cleavage stage or blastocyst biopsy has been performed, the diagnosis for PGD is essentially a single cell diagnosis. This is the most technically challenging part of PGD and a high number of embryos are required to ensure that, after the diagnosis, there are some good quality, unaffected embryos for transfer.[4] PCR and FISH are both excellent techniques in which to study single cells but both require a substantial amount of work to ensure an accurate diagnosis.

Polymerase chain reaction (PCR)

PCR is used throughout science and medicine for research and diagnostic work. PCR amplifies fragments of DNA many thousands of times and a number of techniques can be used to differentiate the fragments of DNA. One

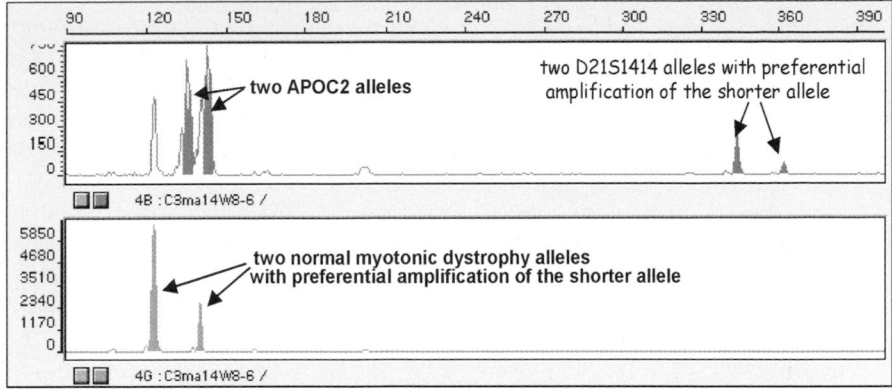

Fig. 2 Informative markers by fluorescent PCR. Result from GeneScan™ analysis on ABI Prism 310™ for myotonic dystrophy, APOC2 and D21S1414 primers triplex amplified from a single buccal cell of a heterozygote subject for the 3 loci. Lane 4B shows 2 APOC2 alleles and 2 D21S1414 alleles, lane 4G shows two normal myotonic dystrophy alleles. [From Piyamongkol et al.,[19] with permission.]

of the early methods used for PGD was heteroduplex analysis, but more recent techniques include single strand conformational polymorphism, restriction endonuclease digestion and fluorescent PCR (reviewed by Wells & Sherlock[17]). Since PCR for PGD was developed to amplify DNA from a single blastomere, two problems have arisen – contamination and allele dropout.[17] Contamination is generally a problem for PCR as DNA from the air, the personnel performing the procedure, or cells from other samples can contaminate any PCR reaction. In PGD, contamination can result from sperm or cumulus cells. During fertilisation, sperm will become embedded in the zona pellucida and during zona drilling these can become dislodged and inadvertently contaminate PCR reactions. To ensure that this does not happen, ICSI is used for all PCR PGDs. Since ICSI injects a single sperm into the oocyte, the zona is free from sperm. Maternal contamination can occur due to cumulus cells as these surround the oocyte and embryo. Therefore, these must be removed before all PGD cases as they can contaminate PCR and FISH diagnosis. The second difficulty with PCR diagnosis is a phenomenon termed allele dropout (ADO) or preferential amplification. This occurs when one allele amplifies preferentially. For example, in carriers there should always be a normal and mutated PCR fragment, but, if ADO occurs, only one of the fragments may be detected. Therefore, PCR conditions must be optimal to ensure that ADO is eliminated or reduced to a minimum. ADO is mainly a problem for dominant disorders, as if the mutated allele drops out, the embryo would be diagnosed as normal.

Since contamination and allele dropout have probably been responsible for all the PCR misdiagnosis in PGD (reviewed by Harper & Delhanty[1] and Lissens & Sermon[18]), methods to eliminate these problems are currently being developed. One method is to use informative markers, to ensure that the DNA examined is embryonic.[19] Figure 2 shows PGD for myotonic dystrophy using polymorphic markers which were informative for this couple. Since the parents have different alleles for these markers, the embryo should inherit one

Table 1 Reported PCR diagnosis for single gene disorders up to 2000

Recessive disorders
        Cystic fibrosis (various mutations)
        Tay Sachs disease
        β-Thalassaemia
        Sickle cell anaemia
        Rhesus blood typing
        Spinal muscular atrophy
        Adrenogenital syndrome
        Congenital adrenal hyperplasia
        Plakophilin-1 (PKP1)
        Medium chain acyl CoA dehydrogenase deficiency
Dominant disorders
        Marfans syndrome
        Familial adenomatous polyposis coli
        Charcot-Marie-Tooth disease (type 1A)
        Osteogenesis imperfecta
        Crouzon's syndrome
Triplet repeat disorders
        Myotonic dystrophy
        Huntington's chorea
        Fragile X
Specific diagnosis of X-linked disease
        Lesch Nyhan syndrome
        Duchenne muscular dystrophy
        Charcot-Marie-Tooth disease
        Retinitis pigmentosum
        Ornithine transcarbamylase deficiency

allele from each parent. Therefore, maternal or paternal contamination, or that from another source, can be detected.

As single cell PCR diagnosis is so technically challenging, the diseases that have been diagnosed by this method are still very limited. Table 1 shows all the reported PCR diagnosis. In the future, PCR diagnosis may become more technically challenging rather than easier (see below).[20]

Fluorescent in situ hybridisation (FISH)

For the diagnosis of chromosome abnormalities, the ideal method to use would be karyotyping, but obtaining a karyotype from pre-implantation embryos is very problematic. Therefore, the method of choice is interphase fluorescent in situ hybridisation (FISH). FISH uses fluorescently tagged DNA probes that bind to specific chromosomes. Analysis under a fluorescent microscope is performed and the FISH signals appear as coloured dots. FISH using probes for the sex chromosomes and an autosome (usually chromosome 18) is the preferred method of embryo sexing for patients at risk of X-linked disease as the exact number of sex chromosomes can be determined.[21–23] This is important in the case of XO embryos as these are at risk of X-linked disease.[21]

A high proportion of referrals for PGD are for patients carrying chromosomal abnormalities, usually Robertsonian or reciprocal translocations. These patients usually have balanced chromosome arrangements, but during gametogenesis, chromosomally unbalanced sperm or oocytes are produced which will give rise to chromosomally unbalanced embryos. Most of these

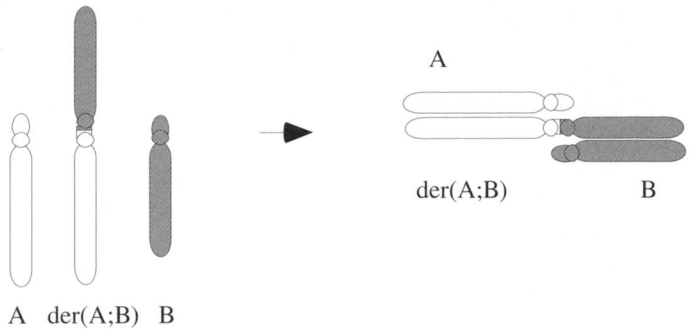

Fig. 3 Robertsonian translocation – fusion of two acrocentric chromosomes with varying loss of centromeric and short-arm material. (B) Pairing arrangement (trivalent) adopted by Robertsonian translocations during early meiosis allowing pairing of most homologous regions. [From Harper JC, Delhanty JDA, Handyside AH. *Preimplantation Genetic Diagnosis*. London: Wiley, with permission.]

chromosome abnormalities will be incompatible with life and so these couples often experience repeated miscarriages. Robertsonian translocations involve the acrocentric chromosomes (13, 14, 15, 21, 22) which contain a satellite and long arm (Fig. 3). In a Robertsonian translocation, the satellites are lost and the long arms join together. PGD for Robertsonian translocations is relatively straightforward, as FISH probes are available for all the acrocentric chromosomes.[24] Reciprocal translocations can involve any two chromosomes. DNA breakage occurs in two chromosomes and the chromosomes re-join incorrectly (Fig. 4). Reciprocal translocations are more technically difficult to examine by PGD.[25] A probe combination needs to be designed for each particular translocation being examined, which is usually specific for each couple. This is made technically more challenging, as commercial probes are not available to cover all possible reciprocal translocations. PGD can also be offered for inversions,[26] gonadal mosaicism,[27] Klinefelter's syndrome[28] insertions, and ring chromosomes.

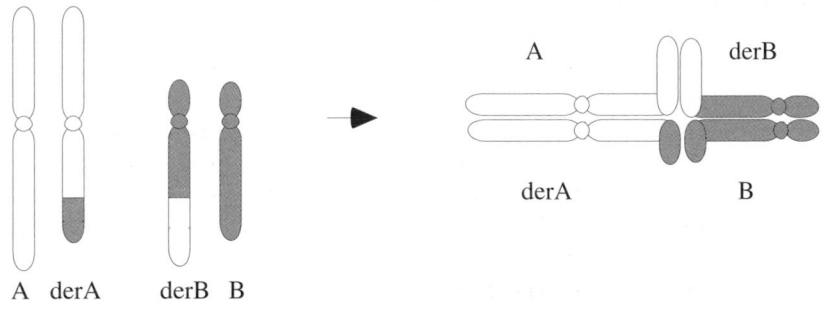

Fig. 4 Reciprocal translocation – reciprocal exchange of material between two non-homologous chromosomes. (B) Cross-shaped arrangement (quadrivalent) adopted by reciprocal translocations during early meiosis allows pairing of homologous chromosomes. [From Harper JC, Delhanty JDA, Handyside AH. *Preimplantation Genetic Diagnosis*. London: Wiley, with permission.]

In recent years, the possible use of PGD and FISH to screen embryos for the chromosomes commonly involved in aneuploidy (13, 18, 21, X and Y) in IVF patients has been reported.[10,12] Data currently suggest that the miscarriage rate may be decreased after pre-implantation screening in infertile women over 35 years of age going through IVF.[12] Only one blastomere is taken for the diagnosis as it is felt that taking 2 may decrease the pregnancy rates. However, only 9 chromosomes have so far been examined and to have a significant effect, probably all of the chromosomes have to be analysed.[29] This procedure may also be helpful for patients experiencing recurrent miscarriage, whose chromosomes are normal.[30]

One important phenomenon seen in PGD is that of chromosomal mosaicism. Examination of whole embryos for research purposes has shown that human pre-implantation embryos are highly mosaic.[31–33] The most common abnormalities seen at the cleavage stages are haploid or tetraploid nuclei, with up to 50% of human embryos showing mosaicism. At the blastocyst stage, the most common abnormality seen is tetraploid mosaicism, with almost all blastocysts analysed in one study showing some tetraploid nuclei.[34] Chromosomal mosaicism has important consequences for PGD as the concept of PGD was that 1–2 cells removed from the embryo would be representative of the rest of the embryo. This is clearly not the case. However, mosaicism is not a problem for sexing (there would have to be female nuclei in a male embryo), or autosomal recessive disorders. It is mainly a problem for PGD of chromosomal abnormalities and was probably the cause of a misdiagnosis of trisomy 21 when screening for aneuploidy. However, most centres offering PGD biopsy 2 blastomeres to increase the likelihood of detecting mosaicism, but this cannot be ruled out.[6] Therefore, patients have to be aware that there is a slight chance that abnormal embryos will be replaced.

THE FUTURE AND ETHICAL CONSIDERATIONS

There are three reasons why PGD is not currently widely available. The first is the technical challenge of establishing a single cell diagnosis for different patients and diseases. This is time consuming and expensive and, at the current time, a number of misdiagnoses have been reported (reviewed by Harper & Delhanty[1] and Lissens & Sermon[18]). The second is the low pregnancy rate. The ESHRE PGD consortium reports a pregnancy rate of 17%[2] and 19%[3] per cycle. Therefore, patients may need to undergo several cycles before establishing a pregnancy. Finally there is the cost. Already mentioned is the time to work-up the specific diagnosis for each patient, but the IVF, biopsy, and diagnosis itself are all expensive procedures, and the personnel and extra equipment involved also have to be taken into consideration. In the UK, some health authorities may pay for 1–2 cycles of PGD, but the majority will not fund this treatment.

The majority of research into PGD is to develop more sophisticated diagnostic procedures.[20] For PCR, these have mainly involved being able to undertake more than one PCR reaction for each single cell. This is essential if informative markers (to reduce the risk of contamination) are going to be used. Therefore, a multiplex PCR, where more than one set of PCR primers is used in one reaction, has recently been developed.[20] The use of whole genome amplification has also been used for some PCR PGD cycles.[17,20] In this procedure, the whole genome is randomly amplified, and aliquots removed and used for specific PCR reactions. However, the whole genome may not amplify uniformly. An increase in the use of fluorescent PCR has been reported[19] as this is a highly sensitive technique that can be successfully used for multiplex PCR reactions. In the future, the use of DNA chips or arrays may enable multiple genes to be analysed from a single cell.[20]

For FISH, the original methods of using 2 probes have now improved to those using up to 9 probes. However, with the addition of more probes, the FISH efficiency decreases.[35] Therefore, the use of alternative methods to interphase FISH have been suggested to analyse all the chromosomes. One of these is to convert the interphase nucleus to metaphase chromosomes[36] so that all of the chromosomes can be analysed. The best way to analyse such chromosomes would be spectral karyotyping. However, recently two groups have reported using comparative genomic hybridisation (CGH)[37,38] on blastomeres with the view to offer PGD for chromosome abnormalities. In this technique, the DNA of the blastomere is labelled with a fluorochrome (e.g. red) after whole genome amplification and control DNA is labelled in another fluorochrome (e.g. green) and the two are co-hybridised on to a control metaphase spread. The intensity of the two fluorochromes on the metaphase spread is digitally analysed and up to six metaphases compared. If the blastomere has a chromosome missing, the metaphase will show more green and if it has an extra chromosome, it will show more red. Even fragments of chromosome imbalance can be analysed in this way. However, the procedure takes at least 72 h to perform and so cannot currently be used for PGD.

It is important to consider the ethical aspects of PGD.[39] In the UK, all PGD treatment cycles have to first be approved by the Human Fertilisation and Embryology Authority. PGD has been performed for some late onset disorders, such as inherited cancer predisposition, Huntington's chorea, etc. Prenatal diagnosis is often offered to couples at risk of transmitting late onset disorders, but ethical debates concerning using PGD for late onset disorders have arise. Internationally, there is concern that PGD will develop into the diagnosis of characteristics and non-disease genes. PGD for sexing for social reasons is already offered in Jordan and Australia but this procedure is not possible in the UK due to ethical constraints set by the Human Fertilisation and Embryology Authority. The main arguments against sex selection is that it is sexist and would undermine the female as in most situations a male pregnancy would be requested (the majority of cases in Jordan are for male sex selection).[40] Also the concern is that PGD could be used for selecting for certain characteristics. In some cases, a number of genes may be involved with the predisposition of a characteristic, but with procedures such as DNA chips and arrays, a diagnosis may be technically possible.

CONCLUSIONS

PGD is technically a very challenging procedure and couples have to undergo IVF procedures, even though they may be fertile. However, the procedure is a useful option for some couples at risk of transmitting an inherited disease to their offspring, as an alternative to prenatal diagnosis.

References

1 Harper JC, Delhanty JDA. Preimplantation genetic diagnosis. Curr Opin Obstet Gynaecol 2000; 12: 67–72

2 ESHRE Preimplantation Genetic Diagnosis (PGD) Consortium. Preliminary assessment of data from January 1997 to September 1998. ESHRE PGD Consortium Steering Committee. Hum Reprod 1999; 14: 3138–3148

3 ESHRE PGD Consortium. 2000 Human Reproduction Handyside AH, Pattinson JK, Penketh RJ, Delhanty JD, Winston RM, Tuddenham EG. Biopsy of human preimplantation embryos and sexing by DNA amplification. Lancet 1989; 1: 347–349

4 Vandervorst M, Liebaers I, Sermon K et al. Successful preimplantation genetic diagnosis is related to the number of available cumulus-oocyte complexes. Hum Reprod 1998; 13: 3169–3176

5 Handyside AH, Kontogianni EH, Hardy K, Winston RM. Pregnancies from biopsied human preimplantation embryos sexed by Y-specific DNA amplification. Nature 1990; 344: 768–770

6 Van de Velde H, De Vos A, Sermon K, Saesseb C, De Rycke M, Van Assche E, Lissens W et al. Embryo implantation after biopsy of one or two cells from cleavage-stage embryos with a view to preimplantation genetic diagnosis. Prenat Diagn 2000; 1030–1037

7 Boada M, Carrera M, De La Iglesia C, Sandalinas M, Barri PN, Veiga AJ. Successful use of a laser for human embryo biopsy in preimplantation genetic diagnosis: report of two cases. Assist Reprod Genet 1998; 15: 302–307

8 Cieslak J, Ivakhnenko V, Wolf G, Sheleg S, Verlinsky Y. Three-dimensional partial zona dissection for preimplantation genetic diagnosis and assisted hatching. Fertil Steril 1999; 71: 308–313

9 Dumoulin JC, Bras M, Coonen E, Dreesen J, Geraedts JP, Evers JL. Effect of Ca^{2+}/Mg^{2+}-free medium on the biopsy procedure for preimplantation genetic diagnosis and further development of human embryos. Hum Reprod 1998; 13: 2880–2883

10. Verlinsky Y, Cieslak J, Ivakhnenko V et al. Preimplantation diagnosis of common aneuploidies by the first- and second-polar body FISH analysis. J Assist Reprod Genet 1998; 15: 285–289

11 Strom C, Rechitsky S, Cieslak J et al. Preimplantation diagnosis of single gene disorders by two-step oocyte genetic analysis. J Assist Reprod Genet 1997; 14: 469–475

12 Munné S, Magli C, Cohen J et al. Positive outcome after preimplantation diagnosis of aneuploidy in human embryos. Hum Reprod 1999; 14: 2191–2199

13 Malter HE, Cohen J. Partial zona dissection of the human oocyte: a non-traumatic method using micromanipulation to assist zona pellucida penetration. Fertil Steril 1989; 51: 139–148

14 Montag M, van der Ven K, Delacretaz G, Rink K, van der Ven H. Laser-assisted microdissection of the zona pellucida facilitates polar body biopsy. Fertil Steril 1998; 69: 539–542

15 Muggleton-Harris AL, Glazier AM, Pickering SJ. Biopsy of the human blastocyst and polymerase chain reaction (PCR) amplification of the B-globin gene and a dinucleotide repeat motif from 2–6 trophectoderm cells. Hum Reprod 1993; 8: 2197–2205

16 Veiga A, Sandalinas M, Benkhalifa M et al. Laser blastocyst biopsy for preimplantation genetic diagnosis in the human. Zygote 1997; 5: 351–354

17 Wells D, Sherlock JK. Strategies for preimplantation genetic diagnosis of single gene disorders by DNA amplification. Prenat Diagn 1998; 18: 1389–1401

18 Lissens W, Sermon K. Preimplantation genetic diagnosis: current status and new developments. Hum Reprod 1997; 12: 1756–1761

19 Piyamongkol W, Harper JC, Sherlock JK et al. A successful strategy for preimplantation genetic diagnosis of myotonic dystrophy using multiplex fluorescent PCR. Prenat Diagn 2001; 21: 223–232

20 Harper JC, Wells D. Recent advances and future developments in PGD. Prenat Diagn 1999; 19: 1193–1199

21 Delhanty J, Griffin D, Handyside AH et al. Detection of aneuploidy and chromosomal mosaicism in human embryos during preimplantation sex determination by fluorescent in situ hybridisation (FISH). Hum Mol Genet 1993; 2: 1183–1185

22 Griffin DK, Handyside AH, Harper JC et al. Clinical experience with preimplantation diagnosis of sex by dual fluorescent in situ hybridisation. J Assist Reprod Genet 1994; 11: 132–143

23 Staessen C, Van Assche E, Joris H et al. Clinical experience of sex determination by fluorescent in-situ hybridization for preimplantation genetic diagnosis. Mol Hum Reprod 1999; 5: 382–389

24 Conn CM, Harper JC, Winston RM, Delhanty JD. Infertile couples with Robertsonian translocations: preimplantation genetic analysis of embryos reveals chaotic cleavage divisions. Hum Genet 1998; 102: 117–123

25 Van Assche E, Staessen C, Vegetti W et al. Preimplantation genetic diagnosis and sperm analysis by fluorescence in-situ hybridization for the most common reciprocal translocation t(11;22). Mol Hum Reprod 1999; 5: 682–690

26 Iwarsson E, Ahrlund-Richter L, Inzunza J et al. Preimplantation genetic diagnosis of a large pericentric inversion of chromosome 5. Mol Hum Reprod 1998; 4: 719–723

27 Conn CM, Cozzi J, Harper JC, Winston RM, Delhanty JD. Preimplantation genetic diagnosis for couples at high risk of Down syndrome pregnancy owing to parental translocation or mosaicism. J Med Genet 1999; 36: 45–50

28 Reubinoff BE, Abeliovich D, Werner M, Schenker JG, Safran A, Lewin A. A birth in non-mosaic Klinefelter's syndrome after testicular fine needle aspiration, intracytoplasmic sperm injection and preimplantation genetic diagnosis. Hum Reprod 1998; 13: 1887–1892

29 Bahce M, Cohen J, Munne S. Preimplantation genetic diagnosis of aneuploidy: were we looking at the wrong chromosomes? J Assist Reprod Genet 1999; 16: 176–181

30 Pellicer A, Rubio C, Vidal F et al. In vitro fertilization plus preimplantation genetic diagnosis in patients with recurrent miscarriage: an analysis of chromosome abnormalities in human preimplantation embryos. Fertil Steril 1998; 71: 1033–1039

31 Harper JC, Coonen E, Handyside AH, Winston RML, Hopman AHN, Delhanty JDA. Mosaicism of autosomes and sex chromosomes in morphologically normal monospermic preimplantation human embryos. Prenat Diagn 1995; 15: 41–49

32 Delhanty JDA, Harper JC, Ao A, Handyside AH, Winston RML. Multicolour FISH detects frequent chromosomal mosaicism and chaotic division in normal preimplantation embryos from fertile patients. Hum Genet 1997; 99: 755–760

33 Munné S, Grifo J, Cohen J, Weier HUG. Chromosome abnormalities in human arrested preimplantation embryos, a multiple-probe FISH study. Am J Hum Genet 1994; 55: 150–159

34 Ruangvutilert P, Delhanty JDA, Serhal P, Rodeck CH, Harper JC. FISH analysis on day 5 post insemination of human arrested and blastocyst stage embryos. Prenat Diagn 2000; 20: 552–560

35 Ruangvutilert P, Delhanty JDA Rodeck CH, Harper JC. Relative efficiency of FISH on metaphase and interphase nuclei from non-mosaic trisomic or triploid fibroblast cultures. Prenat Diagn 2000; 20: 159–162

36 Willadsen S, Levron J, Munne S et al. Rapid visualization of metaphase chromosomes in single human blastomeres after fusion with in-vitro matured bovine eggs. Hum Reprod 1999; 14: 470–475

37 Wells D, Delhanty JDA. Comprehensive chromosome analysis of human preimplantation embryos using WGA & single cell CGH. Mol Hum Reprod 2000; 6: 1055–1062

38 Vouliare L, Slater H, Williamson R, Wilton L. Chromosome analysis of blastomeres from human embryos by using CGH. Hum Genet 2000; 105: 210–217

39 Viville S, Pergament D. Results of a survey of the legal status and attitudes towards preimplantation genetic diagnosis conducted in 13 different countries. Prenat Diagn 1998; 18: 1374–1380

40 Berkowitz JM. Sexism and racism in preconceptive trait selection. Fertil Steril 1999; 71: 415–417

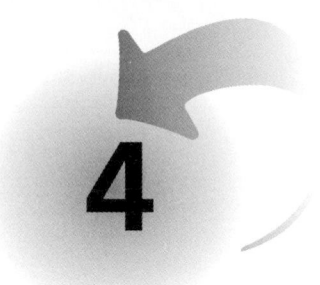

Pauline A. Hurley

International travel and the pregnant woman

The world seems to be becoming a smaller place. More women and their families are taking holidays abroad rather then in the UK, with long-haul destinations becoming more popular. International travel now forms an important part of the lives of professional women and, therefore, obstetricians and general practitioners are more frequently asked for advice regarding travelling in pregnancy. This chapter gives an overview of what needs to be considered and provides guidance for immunisation, malaria prophylaxis and answers some of the more commonly asked questions.

PREPARATION

Medical insurance and airline regulation

Each airline will have its own restrictions regarding the gestation time at which they are prepared to carry the pregnant traveller. For some it may be as early as 28 weeks and for others as late as 36 weeks. These limits apply to the return flight and many will require a doctor's letter to confirm fitness to travel. Each traveller must check with the airline for its particular regulations.

Travel insurance does not usually cover 'pre-existing medical conditions' and this will include pregnancy. Any policy taken out needs to be checked carefully; additional policies which cover delivery abroad and special care facilities for the child may prove to be prohibitively expensive. Within the European Union, reciprocal arrangements are available and women should be advised to take with them a E111 form in order to make use of free, or reduced-cost medical treatment.

Those with pre-existing medical conditions which may be exacerbated by pregnancy should be advised against long distance travel. If they require

Ms Pauline A. Hurley BMedSci BM BS MRCOG, Consultant in Obstetrics and Fetal Medicine, The Women's Centre, The John Radcliffe Hospital, Headley Way, Oxford OX3 9DU, UK

Table 1 Commonly recommended vaccinations

Area of the world	Recommended for all areas	Recommended for some areas
Indian subcontinent	Hepatitis A Polio Tetanus Typhoid Tuberculosis	Yellow fever Meningococcal meningitis
Far East	Cholera Hepatitis A Tetanus Polio Tuberculosis	Japanese encephalitis
Middle East	Hepatitis A Tetanus Polio Tuberculosis	Meningococcal meningitis
Africa	Cholera Hepatitis A Typhoid Tetanus Tuberculosis	Yellow fever Meningococcal meningitis Polio
Central and South America	Hepatitis A Tuberculosis Typhoid Tetanus Polio	Cholera Yellow fever
Eastern Europe	Hepatitis A Polio Tetanus	
Areas out of immediate medical attention or rural stays > 30 days	Rabies Hepatitis B	

medically prescribed drugs, they should be taken in their original containers and a check made that there are no restrictions on taking them out of this country or into another.

For those travelling in early pregnancy, an ultrasound scan to confirm an intra-uterine, on-going pregnancy may be prudent and is recommended by the American College of Obstetricians and Gynecologists.[1]

Vaccinations

The more commonly recommended vaccinations for foreign travel are: cholera, hepatitis A, typhoid, tetanus, tuberculosis and polio. Diphtheria, meningococcal meningitis, rabies and yellow fever may be recommended for some destinations (Table 1).

It should be remembered that no vaccine toxoid or immunoglobulin can be regarded as entirely safe, particularly in the first trimester. There must be a clear indication for vaccination after the risks and benefits have been considered and whether travel to an endemic area is really necessary. Acute illness, either as a result of giving a vaccine[2] or as a result of contracting an infection, brings with it the risk of premature labour or in utero infection, with its consequent morbidity and mortality.

Cholera

Cholera vaccination is no longer recommended by the World Health Organization (WHO) for international travellers and it should no longer be an entry requirement into any foreign country.[3] There is a significant risk of both fetal and maternal morbidity with cholera infection, but the heat-killed bacterial vaccine only gives limited personal protection against this acute diarrhoeal disease and does not contain the spread of disease which relies on scrupulous personal hygiene and avoidance of contaminated water. It has no place in the treatment of outbreaks and the risks of giving the vaccine in pregnancy are unknown. Taking into account the above, cholera vaccination should not be given in pregnancy.

Hepatitis A

Hepatitis A is most commonly associated with travel to rural areas in non-industrialised countries, but it has been reported in destinations closer to home. There is some evidence that infection occurring in the third trimester is more severe and, whilst maternal infection is said not to be associated with transmission to the fetus, there are reports of placental abruption and preterm delivery[4] plus the theoretical risk to the neonate if the mother is acutely ill at the time of delivery.

Protection against hepatitis A is usually conveyed by giving human normal immunoglobulin (HNIG) which gives protection for up to 4 months and carries no apparent risk in pregnancy. HAV, a formaldehyde-inactivated hepatitis A vaccine is available, but only recommended for the frequent traveller. There are no data regarding its use in pregnancy. The risk is probably small, but there are concerns about its use because of the febrile response to vaccination which is common.

Typhoid

Typhoid, caused by the Gram-negative bacillus *Salmonella typhi*, has high mortality and morbidity rates and results from poor sanitation and contaminated food or water sources. No vaccine is 100% effective or a substitute for careful hygiene and food preparation. Whilst there are vaccines available (a monovalent whole cell vaccine, which is heat-killed and phenol-preserved, a typhoid Vi polysaccharide antigen and an oral, live, attenuated vaccine), none has an established safety in pregnancy and the fetal risks are unknown.

Tetanus

Tetanus toxoid has not been associated with any adverse effects when given in pregnancy and the American College of Obstetricians and Gynecologists endorses its use in pregnancy, particularly for those women likely to give birth in less than satisfactory hygienic circumstances.[1] The morbidity rates associated with tetanus are high and neonatal mortality is in the region of 60%.

Since the 1950s, tetanus vaccination has been given routinely and is now combined with diphtheria and pertussis for a more effective response. Toxoid should, however, be given to any traveller who has not recently been vaccinated.

Tuberculosis

Tuberculosis (TB) vaccination should only be given to those who have no characteristic scar from previous immunisation and are tuberculin-test negative on two occasions. It is recommended for travellers to Asia, Africa and Central and Southern America but only for those who are intending a protracted stay. The Bacillus Calmette-Guerin vaccine (BCG) is a live, attenuated vaccine. No harmful effects have been observed during pregnancy, but the advice is to not give in early pregnancy and preferably to defer immunisation until after delivery. Transplacental transmission of TB with congenital infection is rare.[5]

Poliomyelitis

Poliomyelitis may be more severe in pregnancy with fetal/neonatal infections and anoxic fetal damage. Sabine vaccine (live, oral vaccine) is the preferred method of immunisation and there is no evidence that its administration affects pregnancy outcome.[6] Its use, however, should be limited to those travelling to endemic areas.

Diphtheria

The vast majority of women in the UK will have received vaccination against diphtheria and it has been virtually eliminated from this country. Administration of diphtheria toxoid is now the most commonly used form of protection for travellers to endemic areas if neither vaccination or booster has been given in the last 10 years. The advice is not altered by pregnancy.

Rabies

Rabies vaccine and immunoglobulin have both been given to pregnant women with no reported cases of congenital abnormality or infection.[7] Post-exposure vaccination is the normal recommendation and, therefore, it should not be given in pregnancy at any other time.

Yellow fever

Yellow fever vaccination is contra-indicated in pregnancy being a live, attenuated vaccine. Fatality for unimmunised adults in epidemics, however, is 50% and, in certain circumstances, the benefit of vaccination may outweigh the risk of infection.

Meningitis

Vaccines are only available for serogroups A and C of *Neiseria meningitides*, with none developed against the more common serogroup B. The available vaccine should only be given in pregnancy if there is a significant risk of infection, which includes travel to Sub-Saharan Africa, Delhi, Nepal, Pakistan and for Haj pilgrims travelling to Saudi Arabia.

Malaria prophylaxis

No drug regimen ensures complete protection against malaria and the best protection is to avoid the mosquito bite. There is no vaccine available against malaria. In pregnancy, all the complications of malaria are more severe. These include haemolytic anaemia, jaundice, hepatorenal syndrome and cerebral malaria. In addition, there is an increased risk of mid-trimester abortion, preterm delivery and low birth weight as direct complications in pregnancy. Transplacental transmission is also a possibility which may have devastating consequences for the neonate, splenic rupture, seizures and profound thrombocytopenia have all been reported. There is evidence that placental malaria increases the risk of vertical transmission of HIV to the fetus.[8]

Chloroquine, given in a dosage of 300 mg weekly, is regarded as safe to prescribe in pregnancy, but many malarial areas are now not only chloroquine resistant but multidrug resistant. These areas include East Africa, Thailand, Papua New Guinea and the Thai-Cambodian and Myanmar borders. Women who are pregnant should strongly be advised not to travel to these areas.

It should also be remembered that malaria prophylaxis must start one week before travel to an infected area and continue for a further 4 weeks on return.

Other drugs used either singly or in combination for malaria prophylaxis include: Proguanil, Mefloquine, Fansidar (pryimethamine sulfadoxine), Maloprim (pyrimethamine and Dapsone), Doxycycline and the chinca alkaloids.

Proguanil, marketed as Paludrine, given in a dose of 200 mg daily, is usually combined with chloroquine and together they convey 70% protection in areas where the transmission rate is said to be highest, i.e. Sub-Saharan Africa. The combination is said to be safe in pregnancy, but folate supplementation is recommended.

Mefloquine (Larium) is said to convey 90% protection for visits to high-risk areas. It is given in a dosage of 250 mg weekly and would appear to be safe in pregnancy, but monitoring continues.[9] It is, however, best to avoid its use during the first trimester and around the time of conception as there have been reports of teratogenicity in animal studies. Some trials have suggested an increase in the number of stillbirths associated with mefloquine usage.[10,11] More recently, concern has been expressed with regard to serious central nervous system events, including seizures and psychosis, occurring in up to 1 in 10,000 users. Mood swings, headaches, dizziness, and insomnia are reported to occur more frequently in females than males (7.6% compared to 1.8%) As a result, the use of mefloquine is contra-indicated in patients at risk of seizure, who have epilepsy or any other recognised psychiatric illness.[12] Its use in pregnancy must, therefore, be considered very carefully.

Fansidar (pyrimethamine sulfadoxine) is no longer recommended for malaria prophylaxis because of its associations with agranulocytosis and skin reactions including Stevens-Johnson syndrome and toxic epidermal necrolysis.[13]

Maloprim is also not recommended in pregnancy because of its possible teratogenic effects and the risk of neonatal haemolysis. Doxycycline is said to convey some protection against malaria, but is not licensed for use as prophylaxis. The problems of incorporation of the tetracyclines into fetal teeth and bones is also well recognised and, therefore, its use certainly in the last trimester cannot be recommended.

The chinca alkaloids, quinine and quinidine, have both been linked to stillbirth and congenital abnormality.[14] They have no place in prophylaxis, but continue to have a place in the treatment of severe infection when risk must be weighed against benefit to mother and her fetus.

It should be remembered that the mosquito is not always nocturnal and, in high-risk areas, physical protection in the form of trousers and long-sleeved shirts is to be recommended together with the use of a good insect repellent. Burning coils, candles and using mosquito nets are also recommended where they are provided. The most effective insect repellents, unfortunately, contain DEET (14C-N,N,diethyl-*m*-tolumide) which not only may cause skin reactions but is readily absorbed through the skin and, in animal studies, crosses the placental barrier.[15] The safety of DEET has not been established in pregnancy. There is some evidence that it accumulates in fatty tissues and the brain and there is a report of a child with mental retardation, impaired sensorimotor co-ordination and craniofacial dysmorphology being born to a woman who had applied DEET on a daily basis throughout her pregnancy.[16] Insect repellents bought locally in the country of destination may be the most effective.

TRAVELLING

Advice for the pregnant traveller should not be confined to airline travel. Long journeys in cars or buses must also be taken into account, and the pregnant woman reminded that she is not exempt from seat belt regulations. Most accidents which befall travellers are of the vehicular type, and a seat belt worn 'between the breast and under the bump' must be used when travelling even for short distances as recommended for the general population. The advice regarding seating position and duration of travel apply as much to car journeys as they do to airline travel.

When travelling by air, there is no danger for the pregnant woman from the X-ray security devices either for international or internal flights.

Commercial airlines, cruising at high altitude, maintain a pressure equivalent to that of between 5000–8000 feet above sea level. Travel in unpressurised aircraft is contra-indicated in pregnancy. At this altitude, there is a relative oxygen deprivation which, because of the oxygen dissociation curve of fetal haemoglobin, does not endanger the fetus. However, women with a sickling trait (SS, SC, sickle/β-thalassaemia) or severe anaemia (less than 8.5 g/dl) may require supplemental oxygen for which some airlines impose an additional charge that may be as high as the price of an addition seat (personal communication).

Humidity on most commercial airlines is low and maintained at approximately 8%. This promotes dehydration and a liberal intake of non-alcoholic fluids is recommended.

An association between deep vein thrombosis (DVT) and long distance air travel is well recognised.[17,18] As pregnancy is a hypercoagulable state (with an increase in clotting factors VII, IX and X, an increase in fibrinogen and decrease in endogenous anticoagulants anti-thrombin III and protein S[19]), there is an increased risk of thrombosis. Those who have a factor V Leiden gene mutation or are known to have protein S and protein C deficiencies are at further increased risk. Women with SLE or the antiphospholipid syndrome should also be advised that they are at increased risk of DVT.

Immobility, a cramped seating position, compression of the popliteal vein by the edge of the seat together with dehydration all increase the risk of venous thrombosis. Most DVTs occur after flights of greater than 12 h duration, but the risk probably starts to increase with journeys of greater than 5 h.[20]

It is important for pregnant women to maintain adequate hydration. Alcoholic drinks should be avoided because they promote diuresis by suppression of antidiuretic hormone. It is also important to maintain lower limb mobility. Flexion and extension of the ankles will improve lower limb circulation and regular deep breathing will assist venous return to the heart. An aisle seat rather than a window seat gives more leg room and facilitates taking short walks around the aircraft.

For those with added risk factors, consideration should be given to wearing TED stockings, at least below the knee. Some would advocate the use of low-dose aspirin prior to a long haul flight. The part played by platelets in venous thrombosis is far from clear and, therefore, the usefulness of aspirin must be questioned. It is, however, unlikely to be harmful. For those with an underlying thrombophilia, a single dose of low molecular weight heparin before and after the flight should be considered.[21]

Travel sickness and antemetics

Travel may exacerbate the nausea and vomiting associated with early pregnancy. Many therapeutic agents have been tried and some are more effective than others. Vitamin B$_6$ (pyridoxine) is useful, but its effects may decline with time. Cyclizine, a piperazine derivative with both antemetic and antihistaminic properties, is effective and has not been shown to be associated with any adverse outcomes. Dimenhydrinate (another antihistamine used for motion sickness and marketed under several different names) may have some oxytocic activity and is best avoided in pregnancy.[22]

Prochlorperazine, chlorpromazine and promethazine have all been used extensively in pregnancy without adverse effect. However, they may be associated with extrapyramidal effects in both the mother and fetus and should be used sparingly.

Jet lag

Problems accommodating to changes in time should be anticipated travelling west to east. The use of melatonin has been recommended by some to help with the change, but this should be avoided in pregnancy as should fad diets. Tranquillisers of any sort, including sleeping pills, should only be taken on medical advice. A gradual change to local time is recommended, taking frequent small meals and avoiding caffeine.

HAVING REACHED THE DESTINATION

Food and water safety, traveller's diarrhoea, sun, sport and exercise are all things that should be considered and planned for in advance. Poor sanitation is, unfortunately, a common problem in many areas of the world and exposes the traveller to the risk of typhoid, hepatitis, cholera and polio. Even if the traveller has been vaccinated, this should not be an excuse to take risks with personal safety. No water should be regarded as entirely safe unless it is bottled and the seal is secure at the point of purchase. Boiling, filtering, chlorinating or iodine purification can be used short-term if necessary. In areas of high-risk, bottled water should also be used for tooth brushing.

Ice should not be placed in drinks and salads avoided as they will have been washed, if at all, in local water. Fruit juices may have been diluted with contaminated water and, therefore, it is safer to take drinks directly from a can or bottle opened at the table. Drinking straws cannot be considered as safe. The author has personally witnessed the gathering of straws from the floor at a 'café' which were washed and returned to a dispenser.

Steaming, smoking, stir-frying and microwaving as methods of cooking may not kill some parasites. Undercooking of meat is a potential danger as well as spicing of food which may disguise the taste of tainted/contaminated cuisine. Soft cheeses, paté and shellfish are best avoided in pregnancy. Short-term, a vegetarian diet is not harmful.

Diarrhoea and other infections

Traveller's diarrhoea may be more common in pregnancy and with it comes the risk of dehydration and premature labour. It needs to be treated early and aggressively. Loperamide (Imodium) should be used in preference to diphenylate with atropine (Lomotil) and should be used combined with fluid replacement which can usually be achieved by using Dioralyte sachets or a home-made version of this as substitute.[23] Intravenous fluids may be required if dehydration is severe.

Although traveller's diarrhoea is usually self-limiting, infections such as giardiasis and amoebiasis may need to be considered. Metronidazole is a useful antiparasitic, but is known to cross the placenta and in mice has been associated with teratogenicity. It is also reported to cause mutation in some bacteria,[24] and should, therefore, be used with caution. Similarly, ciprofloxacin has been used with good effect to treat diarrhoea, but its safety in pregnancy has not been established. Trimethoprim is a better alternative.

Piperazine is contra-indicated in pregnancy. Treatment of worm infestation susceptible to piperazine is best deferred until after delivery.

Urinary tract infections are common in pregnancy with increased risk in a hot climate. Although the penicillins and cephalosporins cross the placenta readily, neither have been reported as unsafe in pregnancy. Erythromycin does not cross the placenta readily and only low levels are found in the fetus providing another safe option in pregnancy.[25]

Antifungals such as nystatin and clotrimazole (Canesten) can be used topically in pregnancy and all pregnant women should be advised to take this as part of their first aid kit.[26] Advice should also be given regarding analgesia.

Many over-the-counter analgesics contain aspirin and should be avoided in pregnancy because of the risk of placental abruption.[1] Paracetamol is safe and should be used as a first line but, as with all drugs in pregnancy, in moderation.

The prostaglandin synthetase inhibitors are effective analgesics and also have some tocolytic properties. There is concern that indomethecin may cause premature closure of the fetal ductus arteriosus and it should, therefore, be avoided.[27] The same concerns have not been demonstrated with ibuprofen or sulindac, but they have been associated with decreased amniotic fluid volume and may also be best avoided as self-administered drugs.[28]

Codeine phosphate can safely be used for short periods as can meperidine (Demerol and hydromorphone).

Sun, sea, sand and sport

Acclimatisation to heat takes approximately 2 weeks. Hyperthermia with strenuous exercise is a risk. In general, women should be advised that their heart rate should not be raised above 140 beats/min and that strenuous exercise should not be undertaken for longer than 15 min. Loose clothing is recommended as heat tolerance is less in pregnancy.

Pregnancy is not a time for taking up new energetic sports. Swimming is good exercise, but fresh water should be avoided because of the risk of infection, e.g. schistosomiasis. Chlorinated pools or salt water are safer. Water skiing and water slides are potentially dangerous with the risk of forcing contaminated water into the vagina and through the cervix; such activities are, therefore, best advised against.

There is no consensus regarding safe depth/time profiles for scuba diving in pregnancy. Experienced divers may dive up to 60 feet, but certainly this is not the time to dive for the first time. It is, however, unlikely that responsible diving schools would take the risk of renting equipment to a pregnant diver.

In case of emergency

All pregnant travellers should be advised to take their hospital notes or co-operation card with them to provide their basic medical history and results of blood tests, including blood group, and details of how their medical practitioners in the UK can be contacted. Suggestions for a basic medical pack are given in Table 2.

A sterile medical pack, which can be bought over-the-counter, is recommended and should be used if there is any doubt about the standards of hygiene encountered.

Complications can arise in any pregnancy and it is advisable to make sure that contact numbers for local maternity units or the hotel doctor are sought on

Table 2 The pregnant travellers first aid kit

Indication	Suggestion
General	Sterile medical pack
Travel sickness	Vitamin B_6 or Cyclizine
Malaria prophylaxis	Proguanil and Chloroquine
Diarrhoea	Loperamide (and metronidazole)
Thrush	Canesten pessary and cream
Urinary tract or upper respiratory tract infection	Erythromycin
Analgesic	Paracetamol and codeine phosphate

arrival. Embassy or Consulate numbers may be needed if there is any question regarding transfer home.

KEY POINTS FOR CLINICAL PRACTICE

- International travel can never be made completely safe.

- Adherence to the guidelines provided in this chapter should, however, reduce the risks for the pregnant traveller and ensure a safe journey for both her and her fetus.

References

1 Rose SR. Pregnancy and travel. Emerg Med Clin North Am 1997; 15: 93–111
2 Samuel BU, Barry M. The pregnant traveller. Infect Dis Clin North Am 1998; 12: 325–354
3 Hurley PA. Vaccination in pregnancy. Curr Obstet Gynaecol 1998; 8: 169–175
4 Watson JC, Fleming DW, Bordella AJ et al. Vertical transmission of hepatitis A resulting in an outbreak in a neonatal intensive unit. J Infect Dis 1993; 167: 567–571
5 Nelson-Piercy C. Respiratory disease, Ch 4. In: Handbook of Obstetric Medicine. Isis Medical Media, 1997; 56–59
6 Harjulehto-Mervaala T, Hovi T, Aro T, Jaxen H, Hiilesmaa HK. Oral poliovirus vaccination and pregnancy complications. Acta Obstet Gynaecol Scand 1995; 74: 262–265
7 Chutivongse S, Wilde H. Post exposure rabies vaccination during pregnancy: experience with 21 patients. Vaccine 1989; 7: 546-548
8 Bloland PB, Wirima JT, Steketree RW et al. Maternal HIV infection and infant mortality in Malawi: evidence for increased mortality due to placental malaria. AIDS 1995; 9: 721–726
9 Consumer Association Report. Clarification: Fansidar – not for malaria prophylaxis. DTB 1998; 36: 24
10 Nosten F, ter Kuile F, Maelankiri L et al. Mefloquine prophylaxis prevents malaria during pregnancy: a double-blind, placebo controlled-study. J Infect Dis 1994; 169: 595–603
11 Phillips-Howard PA, Steffen R, Kerr L et al. Safety of mefloquine and other antimalarial agents in the first trimester of pregnancy. J Travel Med 1998; 5: 121–126
12 Winstanley P, Behrens R. Malaria prophylaxis with mefloquine: neurological and psychiatric adverse drug reactions. Prescribers J 1999; 39: 161–165
13 Consumer Association Report. Mefloquine and malaria prophylaxis. DTB 1998; 36: 20–22
14 McEvoy GK, Litvak K, Welsh OH et al. (eds) American Hospital Formulary Service Drug Information. Bethesda, MD; American Society of Health-System Pharmacists, 1997
15 Blomquist L, Thorsell W. Distribution and fate of insect repellent 14C-N,N diethyl-m-tolumide in the animal: II Distribution and excretion after cutaneous application. Acta Pharmacol Toxicol 1977; 41: 235–243
16 Sheafer C, Peters PW. Intrauterine diethyltoluamide exposure and fetal outcome. Reprod Toxicol 1992; 6: 175–176
17 Collins REC, Castleden WM. Thrombosis of leg arteries after prolonged travel. BMJ 1979; iv: 147–148
18 Cruickshank JM, Gorlin R, Jennett B. Air travel and thrombotic episodes: the economy class syndrome. Lancet 1988; ii: 497–498
19 Mercer A, Brown JD. Venous thrombosis associated with air travel: a report of 33 patients. Aviat Space Environ Med 1998; 69: 154–157
20 Giangrande PLF. Thrombosis and Air Travel (pamphlet). Aviation Air Institute, 1999

21 Antiplatelet Trialists' Collaboration. Collaborative overview of randomised trials of antiplatelet therapy III. Reduction in venous thrombosis and pulmonary embolism by antiplatelet prophylaxis against surgical and medical patients. BMJ 1994; 308: 235–246

22 Little BB, Gilstrap LC. Antihistamines, decongestants and expectorants during pregnancy. In: Little BB, Gilstrap LC. (eds) Drugs and Pregnancy. London: Chapman and Hall, 1998

23 Hurley PA. Travelling in pregnancy. Diplomate 1999; 5: 254

24 Hammill HA. Metronidazole, clindamycin and quinolones. Obstet Gynecol Clin North Am 1989; 16: 531–540

25 Rosa FW, Baum C, Shaw M. Pregnancy outcomes after first-trimester vaginitis drug therapy. Obstet Gynecol 1987; 69: 751–755

26 Sibai BM, Caritis SN, Thom E et al. Prevention of pre-eclampsia with low dose aspirin in healthy, nulliparous pregnant women. N Engl J Med 1993; 329: 1213–1218

27 Moise KJ, Huhta JC, Sharif DS et al. Indomethecin in the treatment of premature labour: effects on the fetal ductus arteriosus. N Engl J Med 1988; 319: 327–331

28 Hickok DE, Hollenbch KA, Reilley SD, Nyberg DA. The association between decreased amniotic fluid volume and treatment with non-steroidal anti-inflammatory agents for preterm labour. Am J Obstet Gynecol 1989; 160: 1525–1530

Joanne Ellison Ian A. Greer

Thrombo-embolism in pregnancy: problems, prevention and treatment

The most recent *Report on Confidential Enquiries into Maternal Deaths* cites venous thrombo-embolism (VTE) as the leading direct cause of maternal death in the UK.[1] These findings appear to support a study which highlighted a lack of appreciation of risk factors for VTE in pregnancy by a significant minority of obstetricians, which may lead to a failure to institute appropriate thromboprophylaxis.[2] There is a need to educate all healthcare professionals involved in the care of pregnant women, not just obstetricians, that the risk of thrombo-embolism is increased from early pregnancy until the late puerperium and to promote awareness of risk factors.[1] This is important since many thrombotic events occur following discharge from hospital. Venous thrombo-embolism is a multicausal disease and each woman's risk should be individually assessed by taking into account any family or personal history of venous thrombo-embolism, the presence of congenital or acquired thrombophilia(s) and acquired risk factors such as immobility, dehydration, obesity and any concomitant medical illness(es).[3] The role of acquired thrombophilia in the pathogenesis of venous thrombo-embolic disease has been well documented. In the last decade, our understanding of the aetiology and pathogenesis of venous thrombo-embolism has increased with the identification of several heritable genetic mutations affecting coagulation system factors and co-factors and which predispose affected individuals to thrombosis – the so called 'congenital thrombophilias'. The natural history of many of these thrombophilic defects in pregnancy is not yet known and, at present, women with congenital thrombophilia(s) should be referred to

Dr Joanne Ellison, Specialist Registrar, Glasgow University Department of Obstetrics and Gynaecology, Glasgow Royal Infirmary, 10 Alexandra Parade, Glasgow G31 2ER, UK (for correspondence)

Prof. Ian A. Greer MD FRCP(Glas) FRCP(Edinb) FRCP(Lond) FRCOG MFFP, Regius Professor and Head of Division of Developmental Medicine, University of Glasgow, Glasgow Royal Infirmary, 10 Alexandra Parade, Glasgow G31 2ER, UK

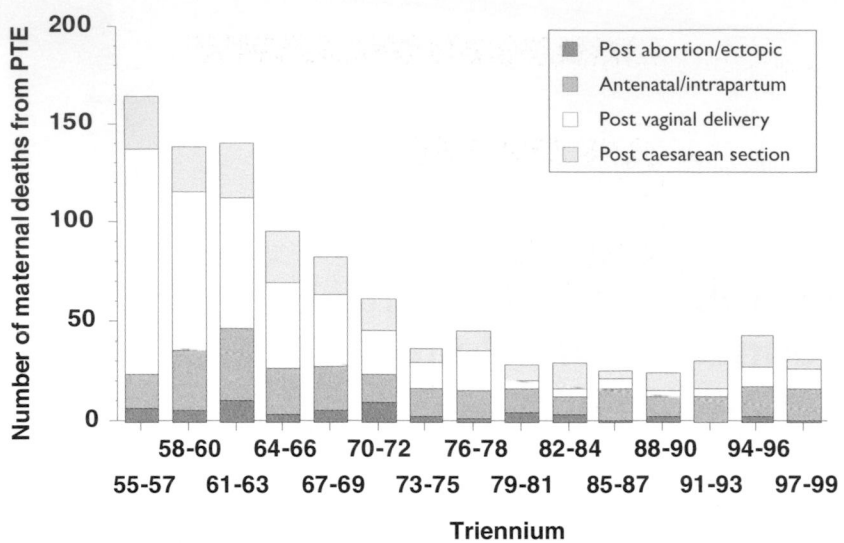

Fig. 1 Incidence of fatal PTE in pregnancy in England 1955–1984, UK 1985–1996 (figures taken from Confidential Enquiries into Maternal Deaths, 1955–1996).

specialist units for maternity care. The importance of objective diagnosis of deep venous thrombosis or pulmonary embolism cannot be over-emphasised – the diagnosis of either has profound implications, not only for management of a current pregnancy, but also for future contraceptive choices and pregnancy management.[4] Heparin remains the best, and the most commonly used, agent for treatment and prophylaxis of venous thrombo-embolism in pregnancy, despite its potential hazards: allergy, osteoporosis and heparin-induced thrombocytopenia.[4] The introduction of low molecular weight heparin use in obstetric practice has been a significant development as it minimises the risk of such complications without conceding clinical effectiveness.[5]

EPIDEMIOLOGY OF VENOUS THROMBO-EMBOLISM IN PREGNANCY AND ASSOCIATED RISK FACTORS

Since the 1950s, we have witnessed a dramatic reduction in the incidence of death from VTE (Fig. 1).[6] Nevertheless, it remains the commonest direct cause of maternal death in the UK today.[1] This reduction is mainly attributable to a reduction in the incidence of fatal pulmonary thrombo-embolism (PTE) following vaginal delivery. The numbers of antenatal, peripartum and PTE following caesarean section having changed little since the early 1950s. However, since the 1980s, there has been a reversal of this downward trend in fatality following vaginal delivery, highlighting the need for thrombo-prophylaxis even after vaginal delivery in women at risk of VTE. In the past, postpartum deaths were commoner than those occurring antenatally. The incidence is now approximately equal, although the rate is higher postpartum due to the shorter time period of the puerperium compared to the antenatal period. It is important to be aware, as demonstrated in the most recent *Confidential Enquiries Report*, that deaths occur in the first trimester in

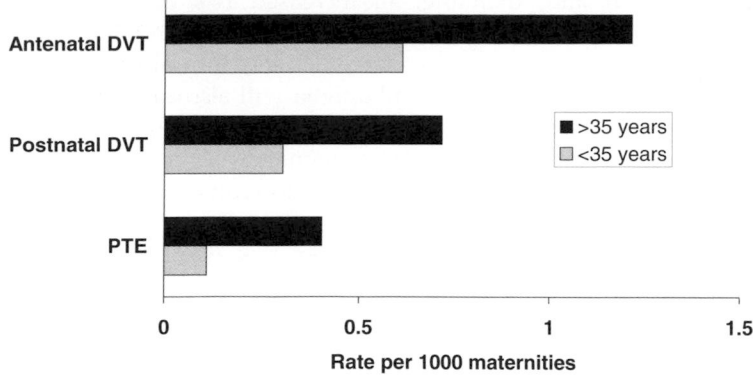

Fig. 2 The age specific incidence of VTE in pregnancy in Scotland 1983–1992.

association with complications such as hyperemesis or ectopic pregnancy. Caesarean delivery carries an increased risk of fatal PTE as compared to vaginal delivery. Data from the mid-1980s estimate this elevated risk at 26:1,[7] although emergency procedures carry a higher risk than elective ones. The most recent report demonstrates a substantial reduction in deaths following Caesarean section. This reduction may relate to the introduction of the RCOG guidelines for thromboprophylaxis in 1995. The majority of these deaths occurred in the first 2 weeks of the puerperium; however, a significant proportion occur at 2–6 weeks' postpartum often following discharge from hospital. It is, therefore, important that health workers in the community are aware of this risk.

It is more difficult to estimate the incidence of non-fatal VTE owing to the difficulty in screening. Clinical judgement is unreliable in the detection of deep venous thrombosis (DVT). A prospective study from the 1960s using radiolabelled fibrinogen following vaginal delivery suggested that clinical underdiagnosis was occurring.[8] Studies using venous plethysmography have estimated the risk of VTE antenatally and following caesarean section to be 0.07% and 1.8%, respectively.[9,10] A retrospective review of 72,000 deliveries found the overall incidence of objectively confirmed DVT to be 0.71 per 1000 deliveries, 0.50 per 1000 occurring antenatally and 0.21 per 1000 occurring in the postpartum period.[11]

Advanced maternal age and operative delivery increase a woman's risk VTE.[11] For women under 35 years old, the risk of antenatal DVT is 0.615 per 1000 compared to 1.216 per 1000 for older women.[12] Similarly, the risk of postpartum DVT is 0.304 per 1000 in women under the age of 35 years, and 0.72 for those above this threshold (Fig. 2).[12,13] However, it is important to remember that data for postpartum DVT may not be complete since 40% of postpartum DVTs occur following discharge from hospital and often these women present to general practitioners rather than obstetric units. Other significant risk factors include high parity (> 4), obesity, and reduced physical activity, surgical procedures during pregnancy or immobility, which may occur as a consequence of hospitalisation, and bed rest. Pre-eclampsia, excessive blood loss or anaemia, sickle cell anaemia and dehydration are also risk factors. Blood groups other than 'O' are associated with higher circulating levels of factor VIII and, therefore, an increased risk of VTE.[7] Medical conditions such as inflammatory bowel disease, cancer and the nephrotic syndrome all contribute to the risk of developing a thrombus. A family or personal history of thrombosis or thrombophilia will also carry an increased risk. It is essential to enquire about such details at the first visit. Finally, a significant number of thrombotic events in pregnancy occur in the absence of any obvious clinical risk factor.[11] It is important to remember that pregnancy itself constitutes a major risk factor for VTE.

Pregnancy-associated VTE carries a greater risk of a future thrombo-embolic event than VTE occurring outwith pregnancy, and it has been suggested that this risk may be as high as 12–15% for pregnancy and the puerperium and 33% for DVT outwith pregnancy over a mean follow-up time of 10 years.[14] McColl et al.[15] have recently performed a case control study of women with previous VTE. They found that after a median follow-up period of just over 4 years, over 70% had symptoms consistent with the post-thrombotic syndrome, although there was no difference in the prevalence of deep venous insufficiency between pregnancy-associated events and those occurring outwith pregnancy. Furthermore, the risk of developing deep venous insufficiency was several-fold higher with DVT than with PTE.

THE PATHOGENESIS OF VENOUS THROMBO-EMBOLISM

The three components of Virchow's triad – hypercoagulability, venous stasis and vascular damage – are all features of normal pregnancy. Pregnancy is associated with a dramatic increase in the plasma concentration of coagulation factors I, V, VII, VIII, IX, X, XII, and von Willebrand factor.[7,16] There are also significant changes in the natural anticoagulant system. Protein C and antithrombin concentrations remain unchanged, but there is a reduction in the concentration of protein S, a co-factor necessary for the anticoagulant action of activated protein C, and, in addition, around 40% of women develop an acquired resistance to activated protein C.[16] The activated protein C sensitivity ratio, a measure of activated protein C resistance, decreases with advancing gestation, and this may be related to increases in procoagulant factors V and VIII. Fibrinolysis is reduced in pregnancy by the secretion of plasminogen activator inhibitor II (PAI-II) by the placenta and also increased circulating concentrations of PAI-I, which is produced in the endothelium and the liver.[7,17] These changes appear to constitute a physiological adaptation of the body to the haemostatic challenge of delivery. Indeed, one study has shown pathological hypercoagulability in association with the factor V Leiden mutation to be associated with reduced blood loss at delivery and reduced incidence of postpartum anaemia.[18]

Relative stasis occurs in the deep venous system of the legs during normal pregnancy, a substantial reduction in blood flow becoming evident by the early part of the second trimester, reaching a nadir by 36 weeks' gestation.[19] Following delivery, it takes 6 weeks for blood flow to return to normal. This stasis is partly due to the mass of the enlarging uterus impeding blood flow in the pelvic venous system, but it is also related to the progressive dilatation of the deep leg veins. This increase in the diameter of the major leg veins occurs to a greater degree on the left side as compared to the right. In pregnancy, the majority of DVTs occur on the left side (85% as compared to 55% outwith pregnancy).[11,15] This may be as a consequence of the right iliac artery and the right ovarian artery crossing the left iliac vein. In pregnancy, the majority of DVTs occur in the iliofemoral segments rather than the deep calf veins. This is important since iliofemoral thromboses are more likely to embolise.

DVT in pregnancy may present with lower abdominal pain, owing to the development of a peri-ovarian collateral venous circulation or extension of the clot into the pelvic veins. When accompanied by the mild pyrexia and leukocytosis, which commonly accompanies venous thrombo-embolism, it is easy to see how DVT may be misdiagnosed as a urinary tract infection or acute appendicitis.

Passage of the fetal head through the birth canal inevitably causes trauma to the pelvic veins. This trauma is increased in operative delivery, whether abdominal or vaginal. Thus, all aspects of Virchow's triad, hypercoagulability, venous stasis and vascular damage come together in the course of normal pregnancy and delivery, so setting the scene for VTE.

THROMBOPHILIA

Thrombophilias are heritable or acquired abnormalities that predispose individuals to thrombosis. Thrombophilia may also confer an increased risk of pregnancy complications such as miscarriage, pre-eclampsia and intra-uterine growth restriction.

Acquired thrombophilia

While there are a number of acquired thrombotic risk factors such as medical conditions like ulcerative colitis, systemic lupus erythematosus, myeloproliferative disorders and the nephrotic syndrome, acquired thrombophilia is a term usually reserved for the antiphospholipid antibody syndrome. This is termed primary antiphospholipid syndrome when it occurs in isolation and secondary antiphospholipid syndrome when in association with systemic lupus erythematosus. Clinical features consistent with the antiphospholipid syndrome are: arterial or venous thrombosis, recurrent miscarriage, thrombocytopenia, haemolytic anaemia, mitral valve disruption, hypertension, pulmonary hypertension and livedo reticularis. Women who have had a clinical episode suggestive of the antiphospholipid syndrome should be screened for anti-phospholipid antibodies. Women who test positive should be screened again 3 months later to confirm the diagnosis and exclude false positives which may be caused by viral infection and exposure to certain drugs.

Congenital thrombophilia

A familial tendency to VTE has been observed for some time. Over the last 10 years or so, several genetic defects which predispose individuals to thrombosis have been identified. Heritable defects associated with thrombosis include antithrombin deficiency, protein C deficiency, protein S deficiency, the factor V Leiden mutation, the prothrombin gene variant and homozygosity for the so-called thermolabile variant of the enzyme methylene tetrahydrofolate

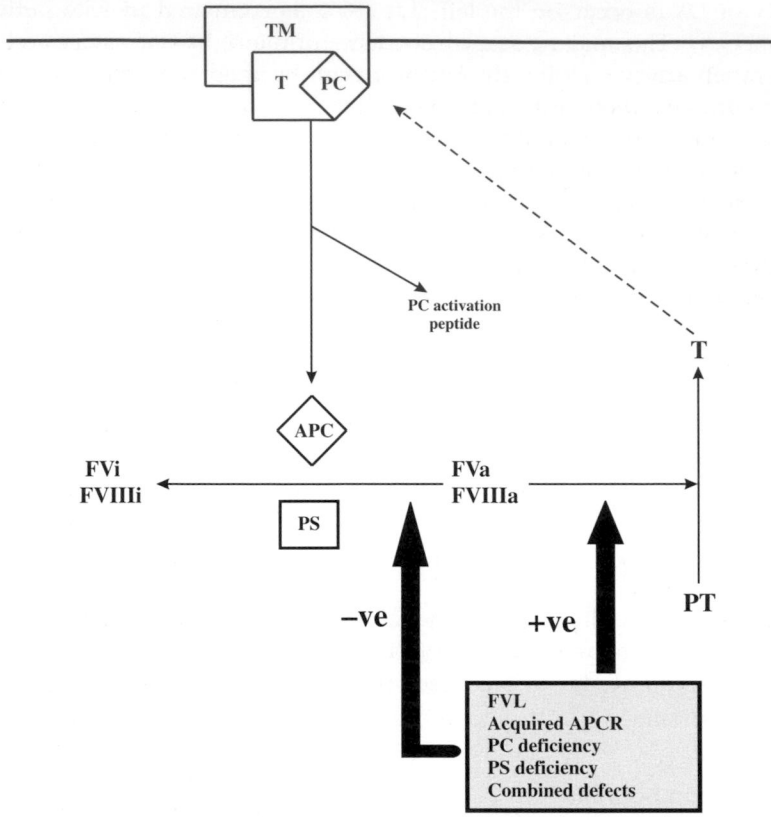

Fig. 3 Thrombin (T) generation from the coagulation cascade is dependent on activated coagulation factors V and VIII (FVa and FVIIIa). Factor V Leiden, acquired activated protein C resistance (APCR), protein C (PC) deficiency, protein S (PS) deficiency and combined defects have a positive effect on thrombin generation. When thrombin and protein C bind to thrombomodulin (TM) expressed on the endothelial surface, PC is activated (APC). APC converts activated FV and FVIII (Va and FVIIIa) to their inactive forms (FVi and FVIIIi).

reductase (MTHFR C677T) which regulates homocysteine, metabolism and leads to hyperhomocysteinaemia.

Physiological haemostasis is maintained by a delicate equilibrium between procoagulant, anticoagulant and fibrinolytic systems. The congenital thrombophilias largely affect the two major endogenous anticoagulant systems, the antithrombin system and the protein C/protein S system. Antithrombin is the most important physiological inhibitor of thrombin. It binds directly to thrombin to inhibit coagulation. Antithrombin deficiency is the least common of the thrombophilic traits, occurring in only 0.02% of the population; however, it confers the greatest risk of thrombosis, with about 50% of affected patients having had a thrombotic event before the age of 25 years.[20] Type I antithrombin deficiency is a quantitative deficiency of functionally normal antithrombin. Type II antithrombin deficiency is where there are normal levels of circulating antithrombin, but, owing to a mutation resulting in a single amino acid substitution, the antithrombin is qualitatively abnormal, so disturbing its function.

The natural anticoagulant protein C/protein S system is responsible for the inactivation of the activated coagulation factors Va and VIIIa. When thrombin is generated, it binds to thrombomodulin expressed on the surface of endothelial cells. The thrombin–thrombomodulin complex converts circulating (inactive) protein C to activated protein C (APC). Activated protein C together with its co-factor protein S cleave activated factor V and VIII so inactivating these factors. This results in a negative feedback loop leading to down-regulation of the coagulation system and a reduction in thrombin and fibrin generation. Adequate generation and function of APC depends upon intact functioning of the endothelium, adequate levels of the components of the protein C/protein S system and normal sensitivity to the effects of APC (Fig. 3). Resistance to the anticoagulant effect of APC is a common finding in familial thrombosis, being present in 20–70% of individuals who have had a venous thrombo-embolic event.[21] In most individuals, this is due to a G->A 1691 mutation in the gene coding for coagulation factor V.[22] This mutation destroys one of the APC cleavage sites in activated factor V by replacement of Arg506 by Gln (factor V R506Q). This is the most highly prevalent of the thrombophilic defects, being present in 2–7% of Caucasian populations. Other defects in factor V, such as factor V Cambridge, have also been identified. Congenital protein C deficiency has been estimated to occur in 1:300–500 of the population.[23,24] Approximately 50% of affected individuals in thrombophilic families will have had a venous thrombotic event by the age of 40 years.[25] The relative risk of thrombosis in population-based studies for unselected patients with protein C deficiency was 6.5.[20] Protein S is a vitamin K dependent single chain glycoprotein and is a co-factor for the anticoagulant action of APC. Heterozygous protein S deficiency causes a significant risk of thrombosis,[26] but the prevalence of protein S deficiency in the general population has not been established.

Recently, a mutation in the prothrombin gene has been described in association with venous thrombosis.[27] This mutation is found in 1–2% of the general population, but is found in 16.9% of women with pregnancy-associated venous thrombo-embolism.[27] This gives a relative risk for VTE in pregnant women with the prothrombin gene mutation of 15.2 (95% confidence intervals [CI] 4.2–52.6) compared to the normal pregnant population. This finding was confirmed by a study by McColl et al., where the odds ratio for VTE in pregnancy with the mutation was 4.4 (95% CI 1.2–16) compared to the pregnant non–carriers.[28]

Hyperhomocysteinaemia is an established risk factor for venous and arterial thrombosis. It is most commonly caused by the thermolabile variant of MTHFR.[31] However, in pregnancy, homozygotes for MTHFRC677T do not have an increased risk of venous thrombosis.[29,31,32] This may be because homocysteine levels normally fall in pregnancy and folic acid, which is widely taken in pregnancy, reduces levels of homocysteine.

A thrombophilic trait on its own may not lead to a clinical thrombotic event. Thrombosis is a multicausal disease. Many thrombophilias are common in the general population – such as factor V Leiden, the prothrombin gene mutation, high concentrations of factor VIII and hyperhomocysteinaemia – and can occur together in one individual. Acquired risk factors for VTE such as pregnancy, the puerperium, use of oral contraceptive pills, and immobilisation are also common. Clinical VTE tends to occur when risk factors are combined.[3] Combinations of risk factors may exhibit synergy, where the effect of two or more risk factors exceeds their separate effects.

ANTITHROMBOTIC TECHNIQUES USED IN PREGNANCY

Unfractionated and low molecular weight heparins do not cross the placenta and are not secreted in breast milk.[33,34] Therefore, they pose no direct risk to fetal well-being when used antenatally in addition to being suitable for use by lactating mothers. There are, however, hazards associated with the use of heparin – osteoporosis, heparin-induced thrombocytopenia and allergy. The long-term use of unfractionated heparin is associated with a significant risk of osteoporosis. This risk relates poorly to dose and duration of therapy. The incidence of osteoporotic fracture in women receiving unfractionated heparin as long-term antenatal prophylaxis has been estimated at 2.2%.[35] However, the use of low molecular weight heparin (dalteparin) for long-term thromboprophylaxis during pregnancy induces a smaller decrease in bone mineral density compared to the use of unfractionated heparin ($P < 0.02$) and the reduction. The reduction in bone mineral density for women receiving low molecular weight heparin is no greater than that in healthy pregnant women.[36] Allergy to heparin usually manifests as cutaneous plaque-like, erythematosus lesions which are usually itchy. It is important to distinguish this from bruising owing to faulty injection technique. Sometimes switching heparin preparations or switching to a low molecular weight heparin may solve this problem; however, a degree of cross-reactivity does exist. The most serious complication of heparin, although rare, is heparin-induced thrombocytopenia (HIT). There are two forms of this: type I is an immediate onset idiosyncratic reaction where platelets clump together but function remains intact. This is of little clinical significance. Type II has a delayed onset (5–15 days from commencement of therapy) and is associated with the development of antibodies to heparin-platelet factor 4 complexes.[34-39] This is associated with profound thrombocytopenia and the development of potentially life-threatening paradoxical thrombosis. Cessation of heparin administration is the only solution to type II HIT. With unfractionated heparin, the incidence of type II HIT is 1–3%. With low molecular weight heparin, it is considerably lower.[40] When HIT does arise, unfractionated heparin or low molecular weight heparin should be stopped and replaced with the heparinoid Orgaran or warfarin.

Warfarin crosses the placenta and is associated with a specific warfarin embryopathy with first trimester exposure, particularly between 6–9 weeks' gestation.[41] This occurs in up to 6% of fetuses and may be avoided by substituting heparin for warfarin in the first trimester. Warfarin therapy has also been associated with the development of neurological abnormalities. This may be due to an increased incidence of intracerebral haemorrhage in utero. The fetal liver is immature and less proficient at producing coagulation factors. Maternal warfarin therapy, even when within the therapeutic range, may lead to a relatively larger reduction in vitamin K dependent coagulation factors in the fetus predisposing it to haemorrhage. Warfarin should not be used beyond 36 weeks' gestation as this places both mother and fetus at risk of haemorrhagic complication during labour and delivery. Warfarin is not secreted in breast milk and may be useful for thromboprophylaxis postpartum to minimise long-term exposure to heparin and risk of osteoporosis.

Dextran has been used for peripartum thromboprophylaxis in the past. It is, however, associated with maternal anaphylactic and anaphylactoid reactions. Its use should be avoided prior to delivery since anaphylactoid reactions are associated with uterine hypertonus, and a high incidence of fetal distress, neurological abnormalities and death.[42]

Thrombo-embolic deterrent stockings are useful in pregnancy where they can be combined with other techniques. They prevent overdistension of the veins and the resultant exposure of subendothelial collagen.[43] Similarly, intermittent pneumatic compression and other mechanical techniques are of value in the intra-operative situation.

Aspirin has an antithrombotic effect[44] and is not harmful to the fetus when used in low doses (60–75 mg once daily). It is particularly useful when prophylaxis is required, but the risk is not deemed sufficiently high to warrant heparin therapy. Recombinant hirudin has been used in the non-pregnant situation for patients who develop heparin-induced thrombocytopenia but should not be used in pregnancy as it crosses the placenta.

THROMBOPROPHYLAXIS IN PREGNANCY AND THE PUERPERIUM

Antenatal thromboprophylaxis

It is important to identify patients at risk of VTE. Patients with either a family or personal history of thrombosis should be identified when they book for antenatal care. This should be part of the antenatal booking assessment. Women with a positive family or personal history of VTE should be offered screening for thrombophilia. In addition, women with acquired risk factors for VTE such as immobility, obesity, hyperemesis, dehydration, surgery, pre-eclampsia and medical conditions such as the nephrotic syndrome, inflammatory bowel disease and infection, should be considered for thromboprophylaxis.

Women with a single previous VTE
Whether or not a woman who has had only one previous VTE should be treated with heparin prophylaxis, given the associated hazards, is controversial. Women with a history of VTE (with or without thrombophilia) have generally been considered to have a higher risk of recurrence in subsequent pregnancies. Estimates of the rate of recurrent venous thrombosis during pregnancy in a woman with a history of VTE have varied between 0–13%.[45–47] The higher estimates of the frequency of recurrence come from retrospective studies of non-consecutive patients,[47,48] whereas the lower estimates come from prospective, albeit small (n = 20, n = 59), studies.[45,46] In a prospective study by Brill-Edwards et al., 125 pregnant women with a single previous episode of objectively diagnosed VTE were monitored through pregnancy.[49] Antepartum heparin was withheld. Anticoagulants (usually warfarin with a target INR of 2–3 with an initial short course of unfractionated or LMW heparin) were given in the post-partum period for 4–6 weeks. The recurrence rate of VTE was 2.4% (95% CI 0.2–6.9%). Ninety-five patients had

blood testing to identify a thrombophilia. There were no recurrences in the 44 patients who did not have an identifiable thrombophilia (0%, 95% CI 0.0–8.0%) and had a previous episode associated with a transient risk factor. Patients with abnormal test results and/or a previous episode of thrombosis that was idiopathic (unprovoked) had an antepartum recurrence rate of 5.9% (95% CI 1.2–16.2%). Based on these results, the absolute risk of antepartum recurrent VTE in women without thrombophilia and whose previous episode of thrombosis was associated with a temporary risk factor is low and antepartum heparin prophylaxis with heparin is not routinely justified provided there are no new or additional risk factors and the implications are discussed with patients. However, she should be treated with thromboprophylaxis for 6 weeks after delivery. In addition, some thromboprophylactic strategy should be put in place for such women and consideration given to thrombo-embolic deterrent stockings or low dose aspirin where the previous VTE has been idiopathic or there is an underlying thrombophilic defect.

Idiopathic previous VTE, when the woman is not on long-term anticoagulants, has a higher risk of recurrence and there is a stronger case for antenatal heparin prophylaxis in this situation, with postpartum thromboprophylaxis for 6 weeks.

For patients with the factor V Leiden mutation, prothrombin gene variant, protein C or protein S deficiency and a past history of one VTE not on long-term anticoagulants, LMWH should usually be employed However, women with a hereditary deficiency of antithrombin and a past history of thrombosis have a substantially increased risk of venous thrombo-embolism and, accordingly, should usually receive adjusted dose heparin or LMWH throughout pregnancy. At the time of delivery, when these women are at particular risk of thrombosis, antithrombin preparations can be added.

Recurrent VTE

Women with recurrent VTEs (> 2) are at high risk of antenatal thrombosis and require prophylaxis with unfractionated heparin or low molecular weight heparin with or without thrombo-embolic deterrent stockings. Those normally maintained on long-term anticoagulation outwith pregnancy are likely to require adjusted dose heparin or LMWH.

Thrombophilia but no episode of VTE

Women with an identified congenital thrombophilia may require antenatal thromboprophylaxis. Usually, they will have been identified because they have a family history and, therefore, come from a symptomatic kindred. This, itself, is likely to be an additional risk factor for thrombosis. Those who are asymptomatic but carry factor V Leiden, protein C, protein S or the prothrombin variant can be managed with careful observation or unfractionated or low molecular weight heparin, particularly if they come from a symptomatic kindred. Antithrombin deficiency has a higher risk of VTE and usually merits specific thrombo-prophylaxis with heparin or LMWH. The timing of commencement of thrombo-prophylaxis will depend on the underlying thrombophilic disorder. As our understanding of thrombophilia is rapidly changing, it is appropriate for women with congenital thrombophilias to be managed at specialist units, particularly, as the risk of VTE varies with the type of thrombophilia, and some women may have multiple thrombophilic defects.

For unfractionated heparin, a dose of 10,000 IU twice daily is appropriate for thromboprophylaxis in pregnancy and, where low molecular weight heparin is used, the dosage recommended for high risk situations is employed. For enoxaparin, this is 40 mg once daily and for dalteparin 5000 IU once daily. Women who weigh less than 50 kg, may be treated with lower doses (2500 IU dalteparin once daily; 20 mg enoxaparin once daily) and higher doses may be necessary for very obese women. It is generally considered unnecessary to adjust these dosages with advancing gestation,[5,50,51] although one study has suggested that the maximum plasma concentration achieved decreases with advancing gestation.[52]

Peripartum and postnatal thromboprophylaxis

Some form of thromboprophylaxis should be continued during labour and delivery. This will include LMWH, TED stockings and intermittent pneumatic compression. Careful attention should be paid to the timing of heparin/LMWH injections if regional anaesthesia is to be used. To avoid the rare complication of an epidural haematoma, catheter placement and removal should be avoided at the time of peak plasma concentrations of heparin.[53] This involves a delay of at least 4 h following the injection of unfractionated heparin. The delay following injection of low molecular weight heparin is arbitrary. In our unit, we currently recommend a delay of 12 h and have not experienced complications and this appears to be a common practice. The injection of unfractionated or low molecular weight heparins should be avoided until at least 2 h after catheter removal.

Data from the US have led to controversy over the use of low molecular weight heparin preparations in combination with regional anaesthesia, following a report by the Food and Drug Administration of an association with epidural haematoma. However, this report was concerned, for the most part, with elderly women undergoing orthopaedic surgery and a dosage of 30 mg of enoxaparin twice daily was used rather than 40 mg once daily. In addition to this, there were no guidelines regarding timing of injection relative to placement or removal of an epidural catheter. Many of the women were concomitantly using non-steroidal anti-inflammatory drugs and often these women had multiple puncture attempts at siting the epidural catheter. It is, therefore, impossible to extrapolate information from this very different population and clinical situation and apply it to pregnant women on prophylactic dosages of low molecular weight heparin. It is, however, prudent to be watchful for signs of cord compression in women on heparin or low molecular weight heparin with regional anaesthesia in labour or for caesarean section.

Women who undergo caesarean delivery have an increased risk of VTE, those who have an emergency caesarean in labour being at particular risk. The Royal College of Obstetricians and Gynaecologists' Working Party 1995, defined the risk of VTE for women post-caesarean section in combination with other variables and made recommendations for their management (Table 1). Patients undergoing elective caesarean delivery with no other risk factors are deemed to be low risk. Good hydration and early mobilisation are recommended. Those with an additional risk factor (e.g. obesity, age > 35 years) in

Table 1 Risk assessment profile for thrombo-embolism in Caesarean section

Low risk: early mobilisation and hydration

> Elective Caesarean section – uncomplicated pregnancy and
> no other risk factors

Moderate risk: consider one of a variety of prophylactic measures

> Age > 35 years
> Obesity (> 80 kg)
> Para 4 or more
> Labour 12 hours or more
> Gross varicose veins
> Current infection
> Pre-eclampsia
> Immobility prior to surgery (> 4 days)
> Major current illness, e.g. heart or lung disease, cancer, inflammatory
> bowel disease, nephrotic syndrome
> Emergency caesarean section in labour

High risk: heparin prophylaxis with or without leg stockings

> A patient with three or more moderate risk factors from above
> Extended major pelvic or abdominal surgery;
> e.g. Caesarean hysterectomy
> Patients with a family or personal history of deep vein thrombosis,
> pulmonary embolism or thrombophilia, paralysis of the
> lower limbs
> Patients with antiphospholipid antibodies (cardiolipin antibody
> or lupus anticoagulant)

addition to caesarean delivery, or where the caesarean was performed as an emergency procedure in labour, are considered to be at moderate risk of VTE and one of a variety of thromboprophylactic measures should be considered. These measures include thrombo-embolic deterrent stockings, low molecular weight heparin or prophylactic doses of unfractionated heparin. Women with 3 or more risk factors in addition to caesarean section, or with severe problems such as thrombophilia or paralysis of the lower limbs are considered to be at high risk and thromboprophylaxis with unfractionated or low molecular weight heparin should be commenced.

This is best combined with thrombo-embolic deterrent stockings. There is a need for management guidelines for women at risk of VTE following vaginal delivery. Consideration of specific prophylaxis should be given to women with multiple risk factors following vaginal delivery.

Women who are on heparin following caesarean section usually continue this for 5 days or until they are discharged home. Following delivery, women who require thromboprophylaxis antenatally usually continue on the same regimen until at least 6 weeks post-partum, by which time plasma levels of coagulation factors have returned to their prepregnancy values. Women who have an on-going risk factor (e.g. immobility) or who are at particular risk of VTE, such as those with antithrombin deficiency, should continue thromboprophylaxis until 3 months post-partum. Those at very high risk will continue warfarin indefinitely. Warfarin may be used postnatally to minimise the risk of osteoporosis from long-term unfractionated heparin; however, many women prefer to remain on low molecular weight heparin as this avoids the need for monitoring.

THROMBOPROPHYLAXIS FOR PREGNANT WOMEN WITH ARTIFICIAL HEART VALVES

Pregnancy in a woman with a mechanical heart valve is not benign. It carries a 1–4% risk of maternal mortality, mainly attributable to complications of valve thrombosis.[53] The management of pregnancy in women with mechanical heart valves is controversial as there are few controlled trials to guide optimal antithrombotic therapy. Continuing anticoagulation with warfarin offers, on the basis of the available evidence, the best protection against thrombo-embolic complications.[54] However, as discussed earlier, there are risks associated with the use of warfarin in pregnancy. Recently, it has been proposed that, when warfarin is used at doses of 5 mg or less, there is minimal risk of fetal abnormality.[55] This suggests that the fetal risk may not be attributable to the degree of anticoagulation per se. Furthermore, at least some of the problems associated with warfarin were reported when the anticoagulant control was poorly standardised and higher doses of warfarin employed.[55] Thus, some authorities advocate continuing warfarin throughout pregnancy on the basis that the risk of fetal problem has been overstated in the past; however, reports of embryopathy continue in contemporary practice.[57] Others, particularly in North America, consider that the risk of litigation is unacceptable and advocate adjusted dose heparin throughout.[58] In the most comprehensive analysis to date on the use of anticoagulation in pregnant women with mechanical heart valves, Chan et al.[54] have compared the three most commonly used regimens for thrombopropylaxis. Oral anticoagulants (warfarin) alone, the use of unfractionated heparin between 6–12 weeks' gestation, and unfractionated heparin for the duration of pregnancy. Their principal findings were that thromboprophylaxis was most effective with oral anticoagulation alone, but the risk of fetal embryopathy was 6% with this management. Substituting unfractionated heparin for oral anticoagulants between 6–12 weeks' gestation eliminated this risk, but was, in turn, associated with an increased risk of thrombo-embolic complications (9.2%). Their results on the use of heparin alone throughout the duration of pregnancy must be interpreted with caution. While they found the risk of thrombo-embolic complication on this regimen to be unacceptably high (33.3%), only 5 pregnancies are included in their analysis and, of these, 3 pregnancies involved the use of low dose unfractionated heparin (< 15,000 U/day), while the remaining 2, which employed adjusted dose heparin, did not report their respective target activated partial thromboplastin time (APTT) ratios. Thus, there is no accurate assessment of the risks associated with the use of appropriate adjusted dose unfractionated heparin in pregnancy in these cases. We have recently reported a case where enoxaparin was used in therapeutic dosage in a pregnant woman with a mechanical heart prosthesis.[59] This woman had no thrombotic or haemorrhagic complications and no episodes of thrombocytopenia using therapeutic doses of enoxaparin and low dose aspirin throughout pregnancy. To date, 3 cases have been reported describing the use of LMWH in pregnant women with prosthetic heart valves.[60,61] In 2 of these, nadroparin calcium was used at a dosage of 0.1 ml/10 kg twice daily, the manufacturer's recommended dosage for treatment of venous thrombo-embolic disease and no thrombotic or haemorrhagic complications were encountered in either case.[60] The third reported case describes the use of enoxaparin, in thromboprophylaxis dosage 40 mg once daily.[61] This pregnancy was complicated by the development of a valve thrombus at 35 weeks' gestation leading to severe haemodynamic decompensation which necessitated emergency caesarean section and simultaneous mitral valve replacement. This case underlines the need for LMWHs to be used at the recommended therapeutic dosage in pregnant women with heart valves. Further studies are required to confirm the role of LMWHs during pregnancy in women with mechanical prosthetic heart valves. In the management of such women, it is important to discuss the risks and benefits of each form of anticoagulation with her, ideally pre-pregnancy.

Thus, there is no ideal management plan based on sound evidence for the management of the woman with mechanical heart valves requiring anticoagulants in pregnancy. She may be maintained on warfarin until 36 weeks' gestation or have adjusted dose heparin or LMWH in the first trimester and throughout pregnancy.

DIAGNOSIS AND TREATMENT OF VENOUS THROMBO-EMBOLISM IN PREGNANCY

In women with suspected VTE, it is critical to obtain an objective diagnosis. Such a diagnosis not only has implications for the management of the current pregnancy, but will also affect other aspects of the woman's life, such as future contraceptive options. Duplex or real time ultrasonography are the first-line diagnostic tools in diagnosing DVT.[62] If initial investigations are negative, but there is continuing concern about the possibility of DVT, then the woman should be treated and a repeat ultrasound scan performed a week later. Alternatively, limited X-ray venography could be considered. Pulmonary thrombo-embolism is traditionally diagnosed using ventilation perfusion scanning. This issue of ventilation perfusion scanning in pregnancy inevitably raises concern over fetal well-being due to radiation exposure. However, the risk to the fetus from V/Q scan, limited venography and chest radiography with abdominal shielding is minimal and appears insignificant compared to the maternal and fetal risk from an untreated PTE. If ventilation perfusion scanning is inconclusive, the results of venous ultrasonography may be useful as a positive leg scan will lead to treatment in any event.

Pulmonary angiography is considered the gold standard for diagnosing PTE but is rarely necessary. It may be used if there is a high probability of PTE on clinical grounds, but an inconclusive ventilation perfusion test result. If there is persistent clinical suspicion of VTE in the face of negative test results, then the patient should be treated and the tests repeated after 7 days. If the tests are again negative, then it is appropriate to discontinue treatment at this stage. Newer imaging techniques such as MRI, helical CT and digital subtraction angiography may facilitate the diagnosis in the future.

D-dimer levels in plasma are being used as a screening test for VTE outwith pregnancy, a high level of D-dimer leading to objective testing for DVT or PTE. In pregnancy, D-dimer increases. It also increases in conditions such as pre-eclampsia, which is, itself, a risk factor for VTE. Thus, an increased D-dimer does not have the same implication for the diagnosis of VTE in pregnancy. However, a low D-dimer level is likely to suggest the absence of VTE in pregnancy.

With objectively confirmed VTE, a woman should receive therapeutic dosages of unfractionated or LMWH and these should be continued throughout pregnancy. Thrombo-embolic deterrent stockings should be worn. Unfractionated heparin should be administered intravenously or by subcutaneous injection twice daily and may be administered by patient self-injection. The increase in factor VIII and fibrinogen which accompanies pregnancy effects a relative resistance to the activated partial thromboplastin time (APTT). It is more accurate to measure the anticoagulant effects of heparin using an assay for anti-factor-Xa activity during pregnancy. LMWHs exhibit better absorption and bioavailability and have a longer half-life than unfractionated heparin. Therefore, they need only be administered once daily for treatment of VTE outwith pregnancy. As their half-life in the circulation is shorter in pregnancy, twice daily administration may be preferred until more information is available. Therapeutic dosages are based on the maternal weight and, while experience in this setting is limited, peak anti-factor-Xa levels should be monitored aiming for a target range of 0.4–1.0 µg/ml.[64] Our own regimen is to use enoxaparin 1 mg/kg body weight, twice daily. At the time of delivery, the dose of unfractionated or LMWHs should be reduced to prophylactic levels and the timings adjusted to allow spinal or epidural anaesthesia, as described above. Warfarin may be substituted for heparin postnatally to avoid the risk of osteoporosis, though some women may prefer to continue with LMWH. Treatment should continue for at least 6 weeks postnatally and sometimes for 3 months for severe problems with ongoing risk factors.

KEY POINTS FOR CLINICAL PRACTICE

- Pulmonary thrombo-embolism remains the commonest direct cause of maternal mortality and there is a need for constant vigilance in identifying those at risk.

- Venous thrombo-embolism is a multicausal disease – both hereditary predisposition to thrombosis and acquired risk factors must be considered.

- A personal or family history of VTE should be investigated by thrombophilia screening. Heritable thrombophilias relevant to VTE in pregnancy include factor V Leiden, protein C deficiency, protein S deficiency and the prothrombin gene mutation.

- Heparin is usually the most suitable agent for both prophylaxis and treatment of venous thrombo-embolism in pregnancy and LMWH offers several advantages over unfractionated heparin.

- However, we need more information on the natural history of the thrombophilias in pregnancy and evidence from randomised trials on which to base and consolidate clinical practice.

References

1 National Institute of Clinical Excellence for England and Wales, Scottish Programme for Clinical Effectiveness in Reproductive Health, Department of Health, Social Services and Public Safety for Northern Ireland. The Confidential Enquiries into Maternal Deaths in the United Kingdom 1997–99. London: RCOG Press, December 2001

2 Greer IA, de Swiet M. Thrombosis prophylaxis in obstetrics and gynaecology. Br J Obstet Gynaecol 1993; 100: 37–40

3 Rosendaal FR. Venous thrombosis : a multicausal disease. Lancet 1999; 353: 1167–1173

4 Greer IA. Thrombosis in pregnancy : maternal and fetal issues. Lancet 1999; 353: 1258–1265

5 Nelson-Piercy C. Hazards of heparin: allergy, heparin-induced thrombocytopenia and osteoporosis. In: Greer IA. (ed) Baillière's Clinical Obstetrics and Gynaecology. Thromboembolic Disease in Obstetrics and Gynaecology. London: Baillière Tindall, 1997; 489–509

6 Greer IA. Epidemiology, risk factors and prophylaxis of venous thrombo-embolism in obstetrics and gynaecology. In: Greer IA. (ed) Baillière's Clinical Obstetrics and Gynaecology. Thromboembolic Disease in Obstetrics and Gynaecology. London: Baillière Tindall, 1997; 403–430

7 Greer IA. Special case of venous thrombo-embolism in pregnancy. In: Tooke JE, Lowe GDO. (eds) A Textbook of Vascular Medicine. London: Arnold, 1996; 538–561

8 Friend JR, Kakkar VV. The diagnosis of deep venous thrombosis in the puerperium. J Obstet Gynaecol Br Common 1970; 77: 820–824

9 Bergqvist A, Bergqvist D, Hallbook T. Deep vein thrombosis during pregnancy – a prospective study. Acta Obstet Gynaecol Scand 1983; 62: 443–448

10 Bergqvist A, Bergqvist D, Hallbook T. Acute deep venous thrombosis (DVT) after caesarean. Acta Obstet Gynaecol Scand 1979; 58: 473–476

11 McColl MD, Ramsay JE, Tait RC et al. Risk factors for pregnancy associated venous thrombo-embolism. Thromb Haemostas 1997; 78: 1183–1188

12 Macklon NS, Greer IA. Venous thromboembolic disease in obstetrics and gynaecology: the Scottish experience. Scot Med J 1996; 41: 83–86

13 Rutherford S, Montoro M, McGhee W, Strong T. Thromboembolic disease associated with pregnancy: an 11 year review. Am J Obstet Gynecol 1991; 164: 286–286

14 Bergqvist D, Bergqvist A, Lindhagen A, Matzsch T. Long term outcome of patients with venous thrombo-embolism during pregnancy. In: Greer IA, Turpie AGG, Forbes CD. (eds) Haemostasis and Thrombosis in Obstetrics and Gynaecology. London: Chapman and Hall, 1992; 349–359

15 McColl MD, Ellison J, Greer IA, Tait RC, Walker ID. Prevalence of the post thrombotic syndrome in young women with previous venous thrombo-embolism. Br J Haematol 2000; 108: 272–274

16 Clark P, Brennand J, Conkie JA, McCall F, Greer IA, Walker ID. Activated protein C sensitivity, protein C, protein S and coagulation in normal pregnancy. Thromb Haemostas 1998; 79: 1166–1170

17 Forbes CD, Greer IA. Physiology of haemostasis and the effect of pregnancy. In: Greer IA, Turpie AGG, Forbes CD. (eds) Haemostasis and Thrombosis in Obstetrics and Gynaecology. London: Chapman and Hall, 1992; 1–25

18 Lindqvist PG, Svensson PJ, Dahlback B, Masal K. Factor V Q^{506} mutation (activated protein C resistance) associated with reduced intrapartum blood loss – a possible evolutionary selection mechanism. Thromb Haemostas 1998; 79: 69–73

19 Macklon NS, Greer IA, Bowman AW. An ultrasound study of gestational and postural changes in the deep venous system of the leg in pregnancy. Br J Obstet Gynaecol 1997; 104: 191–197

20 Walker ID. Inherited coagulation and thrombophilia and pregnancy. In: Bonnar J. Recent Advances in Obstetrics and Gynaecology, vol. 20. Edinburgh: Churchill Livingstone, 1998; 35–64

21 Dahlback B, Carlsson M, Svensson PJ. Familial thrombophilia due to a previously unrecognised mechanism characterised by poor anticoagulant response to activated protein C: prediction of a co-factor activated protein C. Proc Natl Acad Sci USA 1993; 90: 1004–1008

22 Bertina RM, Koeleman BPC, Koster T et al. Mutation in blood-coagulation factor V associated with resistance to activated protein-C. Nature 1994; 369: 64–67

23 Miletich JP, Sherman I, Broze G. Absence of thrombosis in subjects with heterozygous protein C deficiency. N Engl J Med 1987; 317: 991–996

24 Tait RC, Walker ID, Reitsma PH. Prevalence of protein C deficiency in the healthy population. Thromb Haemostas 1995; 73: 87–93

25 Allaart CF, Poort SR, Rosendaal F. Increased risk of venous thrombosis in carriers of hereditary protein C deficiency defect. Lancet 1993; 341: 134–138

26 Cooper DN, Tudenham EGD. The molecular genetics of familial venous thrombosis. In: Meade TW. (ed) Clinical Haematology: Thrombophilia. London: Baillière Tindall, 1994; 637–674

27 Poort SR, Rosendaal FR, Reitsma PH, Bertina RM. A common genetic variation in the three untranslated region of the prothrombin gene is associated with elevated plasma prothrombin levels and an increase in venous thrombosis. Blood 1996; 88: 36–38

28 McColl MD, Walker ID, Greer IA. The role of inherited thrombophilia in venous thrombo-embolism associated with pregnancy. Br J Obstet Gynaecol 1999; 106: 756–766

29 McColl MD, Ellison J, Reid R, Tait RC, Walker ID, Greer IA. Prothrombin 20210G->A, MTHFR C677T mutations in women with venous thrombo-embolism associated with pregnancy. Br J Obstet Gynaecol 2000; 107: 565–569

30 Den Heijer M, Koster T, Blom HJ et al. Hyperhomocysteinemia as a risk factor for deep vein thrombosis. N Engl J Med 1998; 334: 759–762

31 Gerhardt A, Scharf RE, Beckmann MW et al. Prothrombin and factor V mutations in women with a history of thrombosis during pregnancy and the puerperium. N Engl J Med 2000; 342: 374–380

32 Greer IA. The challenge of thrombophilia in maternal-fetal medicine. N Engl J Med 2000; 342: 424–425

33 Matzsch T, Bergqvist D, Bergqvist A et al. No transplacental passage of standard heparin or an enzymatically depolymerized low molecular weight heparin. Blood Coag Fibrinol 1991; 2: 273–278

34 Melissari E, Parker CJ, Wilson NV et al. Use of low molecular weight heparin in pregnancy. Thromb Haemostas 1992; 68: 652–656

35 Dahlman TC. Osteoporotic fractures and the recurrence of thrombo-embolism during pregnancy and the puerperium in 184 women undergoing thromboprophylaxis with heparin. Am J Obstet Gynecol 1993; 168: 1265–1270

36 Pettila V, Leinonen P, Markkola A, Hillesmaa V, Kaaja R. Postpartum bone mineral density in women treated for thromboprophylaxis with unfractionated heparin or LMW heparin. Thromb Haemost 2002; 87: 182–186

37 Amiral J, Bridey F, Wolf M et al. Antibodies to macromolecular platelet factor 4-heparin complexes in heparin induced thrombocytopenia: a study of 44 cases. Thromb Haemostas 1995; 73: 21–28

38 Aster RH. Heparin-induced thrombocytopenia and thrombosis. N Engl J Med 1995; 332: 1374–1376

39 Chong H. Heparin-induced thrombocytopenia. Br J Haematol 1995; 89: 431–439

40 Warkentin TE, Levine MN, Hisch J et al. Heparin-induced thrombocytopenia in patients treated with low molecular weight heparin or unfractionated heparin. N Engl J Med 1995; 332: 1330–1335

41 Ginsberg JS. Fetal abnormalities and anticoagulants. In: Greer IA, Turpie AGG, Forbes CD. (eds) Haemostasis and Thrombosis in Obstetrics and Gynaecology. London: Chapman and Hall, 1992; 361–370

42 Barbier P, Jongville AP, Autre TE, Coureau C. Fetal risks with dextran during delivery. Drug Safety 1992; 7: 71–73

43 Macklon NS, Greer IA. Technical note: compression stockings and posture – a comparative study of their effects on the proximal deep veins in the leg at rest. Br J Radiol 1995; 68: 515–518

44 Thromboembolic Risk Factors (THRIFT) Consensus Group. Risk of and prophylaxis for venous thrombo-embolism in hospital patients. BMJ 1992; 305: 567–574

45 de Swiet M, Floyd E, Letsky E. Low risk of recurrent thrombo-embolism in pregnancy. Br J Hosp Med 1987; 38: 264

46 Howell R, Fidler J, Letsky E et al. The risk of antenatal subcutaneous heparin prophylaxis: a controlled trial. Br J Obstet Gynaecol 1983; 90: 1124–1128

47 Badaracco MA, Vessey M. Recurrent venous thromboembolic disease and the use of oral contraceptives. BMJ 1974; 1: 215–217

48 Tengborn L. Recurrent thrombo-embolism in pregnancy and puerperium: is there a need for thromboprophylaxis? Am J Obstet Gynecol 1989; 160: 90–94

49 Brill-Edwards P, Ginsberg JS, Gent M et al. Safety of withholding antepartum heparin in women with a previous episode of venous thrombo-embolism. N Engl J Med 2000; 343: 439–444

50 Brennand JE, Walker ID, Greer IA. Anti-activated factor X profiles in pregnant women receiving antenatal thromboprophylaxis with enoxaparin. Acta Haematol 1999; 101: 53–55

51 Ellison J, Walker ID, Greer IA. Antenatal use of enoxaparin for prevention and treatment of thrombo-embolism in pregnancy. Br J Obstet Gynaecol 2000; 107: 1116–112

52 Casele HL, Laifer SA, Woelkers DA, Venkataramanan R. Changes in the pharmacokinetics of the low-molecular-weight heparin enoxaparin sodium during pregnancy. Am J Obstet Gynecol 1999; 181: 1113–1117

53 Letsky EA. Peripartum prophylaxis of thrombo-embolism. In: Greer IA. (ed) Baillière's Clinical Obstetrics and Gynaecology. Thromboembolic Disease in Obstetrics and Gynaecology. London: Baillière Tindall, 1997; 523–543

54 Chan WS, Anand S, Ginsberg JS. Anticoagulation of pregnant women with mechanical heart valves. Arch Intern Med 2000; 160: 191–196

55 Vitale N, De Feo M, De Santo LS, Pollice A, Tedesco N, Contrufo M. Dose-dependent fetal complications of warfarin in pregnant women with mechanical heart valves. J Am Coll Cardiol 1999; 33: 1642–1645

56 Sbarouni E, Oakley CM. Outcome of pregnancy in women with valve prostheses. Br Heart J 1994; 71: 196–201

57 Wellesley D, Moore I, Heard M, Keeton B. Two cases of warfarin embryopathy – a re-emergence of this condition ? Br J Obstet Gynaecol 1998; 105: 805–807

58 Ginsberg JS, Greer IA, Hirsh J. Sixth American College of Chest Physicians (ACCP) Consensus Conference on Antithrombotic Therapy: Use of Antithrombotic Agents During Pregnancy. Chest 2001; 119 (Suppl. 1): 1225–1315

59 Ellison J, Thomson AJ, Walker ID, Greer IA. Use of enoxaparin in a pregnant woman with a mechanical heart valve prosthesis. Br J Obstet Gynaecol 2001; 108: 757–759

60 Lee LH, Liauw PC, Ng AS. Low molecular weight heparin for thromboprophylaxis during pregnancy in 2 patients with mechanical mitral valve replacement. Thromb Haemostas 1996; 76: 628–630

61 Lev-Ran O, Kramer A, Gurevitch J, Shapira I, Mohr R. Low-molecular weight heparin for prosthetic heart valves: treatment failure. Ann Thorac Surg 2000; 69: 264–266

62 Macklon NS. Diagnosis of deep venous thrombosis and pulmonary embolism. In: Greer IA. (ed) Baillière's Clinical Obstetrics and Gynaecology. Thromboembolic Disease in Obstetrics and Gynaecology. London: Baillière Tindall, 1997; 463–477

63 RCOG Green Top Guideline, No. 28 – Thromboembolic disease in pregnancy and the puerperium: acute managemenr. http://www.rcog.org.uk/guidelines

64 Thomson AJ, Walker ID, Greer IA. Low molecular weight heparin for immediate management of thromboembolic disease in pregnancy. Lancet 1998; 352: 1904

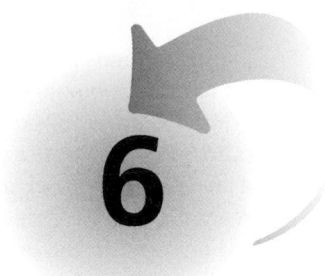

S. Chan J.A. Franklyn M.D. Kilby

6

Thyroid hormones in pregnancy and the fetus

Thyroid disorders are amongst the commonest endocrine disorders in women of childbearing age and are, therefore, encountered commonly in pregnancy. Disorders of thyroid hormone production and their treatment can affect fertility, maternal well-being, fetal growth and development. Furthermore, pregnancy-induced physiological changes may themselves exacerbate or improve thyroid disorders.

THYROID HORMONE REGULATION AND METABOLISM

The thyroid gland synthesises and releases thyroxine (T_4) and tri-iodothyronine (T_3), in a ratio of about 4:1.[1] The production of thyroid hormones is controlled by serum thyrotrophin (TSH) synthesised by the anterior pituitary gland and released in response to thyrotrophin-releasing hormone (TRH) secreted from neurons of the paraventricular nucleus into the hypophyseal portal circulation. TRH and TSH synthesis and release are regulated by negative feedback of circulating thyroid hormones (free T_4 and free T_3; Fig. 1).

Most circulating thyroid hormone is in the form of T_4, with 99.7% being protein bound. The main protein involved is thyroxine-binding globulin (TBG).[1] Unbound hormones are termed free T_4 (FT_4) and free T_3 (FT_3) and are available for tissue uptake (*vide infra*).

Dr Shiao Chan BA(Camb) MB BChir MRCOG, MRC Clinical Training Fellow, Department of Maternal and Fetal Medicine, Birmingham Women's Hospital, Edgbaston, Birmingham B15 2TG, UK

Professor Jayne Franklyn MD PhD FRCP FMedSci, Professor of Medicine and Honorary Consultant Endocrinologist, Division of Medical Sciences, University of Birmingham, Edgbaston, Birmingham B15 2TT, UK

Dr Mark Kilby MD MRCOG, Consultant and Clinical Reader in Fetal Medicine, Department of Maternal and Fetal Medicine, Division of Reproductive and Child Health, University of Birmingham, Edgbaston, Birmingham B15 2TG, UK (for correspondence)

Intracellular T_3 is, however, generated and modulated by a group of three selenoprotein enzymes. T_4 requires mono-de-iodination of the outer ring of the iodothyronine molecule to produce T_3, the active metabolite. Type I and II de-iodinase (DI) enzymes are able to do this. Type I DI is responsible for production of most of the peripheral circulating T_3 and is expressed predominantly in the liver and kidney. Type II DI activity is important for the local tissue supply of T_3 and is found in the brain, brown adipose tissue and pituitary. Conversely, type III DI is responsible for inner ring de-iodination, which converts T_4 to reverse T_3 (rT_3) and T_3 to di-iodothyronine (T_2), both of which are inactive metabolites.

Type III DI activity is stimulated by T_3,[1,2] so T_3 concentrations can be regulated locally. There is an abundance of this enzyme in trophoblast, which accounts for the high circulating levels of rT_3 in the fetus. The specific role for rT_3 in humans is unclear. In rodents, rT_3 has been shown to stimulate adipocyte metabolism, amino acid uptake, hepatic amino-transferase and growth hormone secretion.[3]

T_4 and T_3 can also be reversibly conjugated with glucuronide and sulphate, with excretion via bile or urine which allows the retention of iodine. Conjugated T_3 has no affinity for thyroid receptors and very low levels are found in the adult.[4]

THYROID HORMONES AND THE MOTHER

In the UK, many thyroid disorders will have been diagnosed and treated prepregnancy and a good obstetric outcome may be anticipated. Overt hypothyroidism and severe thyrotoxicosis are frequently encountered in the UK and are associated with anovulation, subfertility and pregnancy loss.[5–7] Milder forms of both hypothyroidism and hyperthyroidism do not render a woman infertile, but they may still be associated with an increased risk of miscarriage.[7,8] Pregnant women with thyroid disorders should be managed jointly by obstetricians and physicians with an interest in thyroid disease.

The physiology of maternal thyroid hormone metabolism

Iodine is a major component of thyroid hormones with dietary requirements increasing in pregnancy due to the enhanced transplacental uptake of iodide[9]

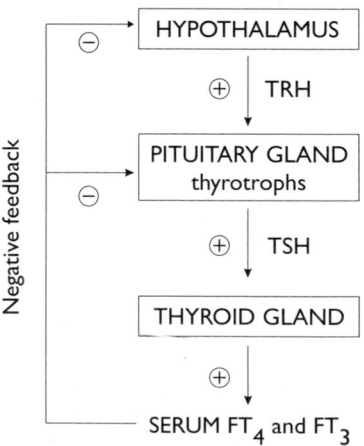

Fig. 1 Thyroid hormone regulation by the hypothalamic-pituitary-thyroid axis.

and increased maternal renal clearance.[6,10] Hence pregnancy is a state of relative iodine-deficiency. Furthermore, the placenta is rich in type III DI, which inactivates thyroid hormones.[1] As a result, homeostatic mechanisms compensate for this by increasing thyroid iodine uptake and synthesis of thyroid hormones, with associated glandular enlargement.[11] In areas where women experience dietary iodine insufficiency, noticeable diffuse enlargement of the thyroid gland in pregnancy may occur. Even in iodine-sufficient parts of the world, there is normally a physiological increase in the size of the thyroid gland by an average of 10–20%.[12]

A rise in serum TBG concentration (induced by oestrogen[13]) occurs in the first trimester and is sustained at this high level throughout pregnancy. As a consequence, the serum total T_4 and T_3 concentrations increase, but circulating FT_4 and FT_3 concentrations are largely unchanged.

In addition, production of human chorionic gonadotrophin (hCG) by the placenta reaches a peak towards the end of the first trimester. hCG is a bipeptide that has an identical α-subunit to TSH and a β-subunit with limited sequence homology to TSH, and has weak thyrotrophic activity.[14,15] This alone may not wholly account for the observed slight decrease in serum TSH and a marginal increase in FT_4 level in the first trimester.[15,16] Even so, in most cases, TSH and FT_4 are maintained within the limits of non-pregnancy values.

It has been postulated that there is a transient resetting of the hypothalamic-pituitary-thyroid axis negative feedback system in early gestation aimed at increasing T_4 supply to the fetus. Maternal supply of T_4 could be critical to fetal development before the fetal thyroid gland secretes hormone.[1] It has also been documented that T_3 can stimulate the production of 17β-oestradiol and epidermal growth factor in human placenta, and an increased supply of thyroid hormone may have a particular role at this crucial stage of trophoblast invasion, placental tissue differentiation and development.[17,18]

In gestational trophoblastic disease, there may be an abnormally high level of hCG resulting in clinical hyperthyroidism in 2% of cases.[19] In hyperemesis gravidarum, which occurs in 0.1–0.2% of pregnant women with singleton pregnancies,[20] there is no associated rise in hCG levels, but 40–70% of them still display biochemical hyperthyroidism.[21,22] A few studies have disputed this finding as the authors found no significant difference in thyroid function tests when pregnancies with hyperemesis were compared with normal first trimester pregnancies.[23] Molecular variants of hCG with greater thyrotrophic activity have been documented in hyperemesis and gestational trophoblastic disease which could explain the hyperthyroidism.[24] Some have also postulated that the hyperthyroidism may be due to an over-exaggerated resetting of the hypothalamic-pituitary-thyroid axis.[1] The majority of these cases will resolve spontaneously by the second trimester without treatment of hyperthyroidism, requiring only supportive measures.

Maternal serum TSH and FT_4 return to normal in the second trimester and it is now generally accepted that there is a slight decrease in FT_4 and also a slight rise in TSH levels in the third trimester. Reference ranges for FT_4, FT_3 and TSH significantly overlap those of the non-pregnant ones.[12,25] This tendency for biochemical hypothyroidism towards the end of pregnancy is normally well-tolerated with no clinical features of hypothyroidism. Clinical euthyroidism is maintained by an increased sensitivity of tissues to thyroid hormones at this time.[26] This is supported by the finding that the maximal nuclear binding capacity for thyroid hormones in maternal tissues progressively rises with gestation.[27] The apparent mild biochemical hypothyroidism may be a dilutional effect as there is a 50% increase in maternal blood volume.[25] This alone cannot be the only explanation as most of the increase in blood volume occurs in the first trimester of pregnancy. Mild hypothyroidism could be a physiological adaptation to try to conserve energy in preparation for parturition.[28] It could also be a reflection of an inability to compensate for the increased fetal demand for iodide with more active fetal thyroid hormone synthesis, increased breakdown of maternal thyroid hormones by a larger placenta, and transfer of maternal T_4 to the fetus. The corresponding rise in TSH reflects a normally functioning negative feedback system with the pituitary sensitivity to thyroid hormones remaining unchanged compared with other tissues.[25]

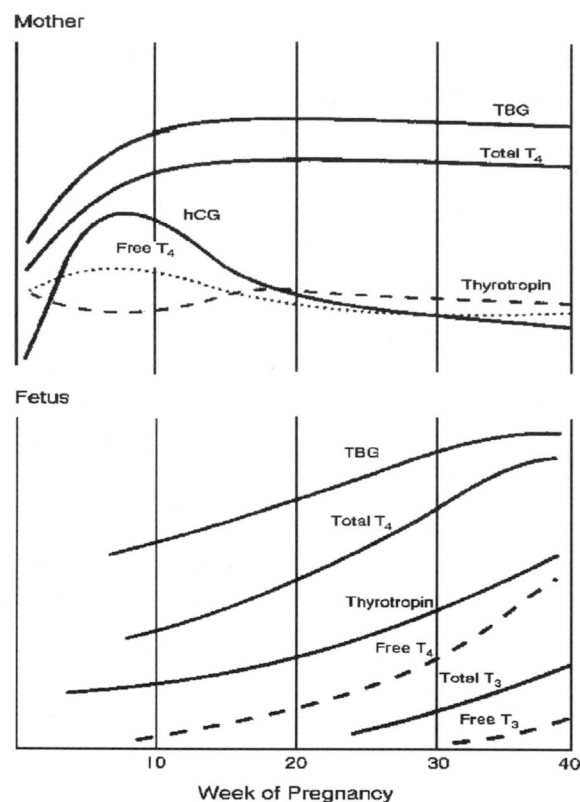

Fig. 2 Relative changes in maternal and fetal thyroid function during pregnancy. The effects of pregnancy on the mother include a marked and early increase in hepatic production of thyroxine-binding globulin (TBG) and placental production of human chorionic gonadotrophin (hCG). The increase in serum TBG, in turn, increases serum T_4 concentrations; hCG has thyrotrophin-like activity and stimulates maternal T_4 secretion. The transient hCG-induced increase in serum free T_4 inhibits maternal secretion of thyrotrophin.[2] (Reproduced with permission from the *New England Journal of Medicine*.)

Thyroid hormone assays

There are many different assays used to measure FT_4, FT_3 and TSH world-wide. FT_4 and FT_3 can be quantified with direct or indirect assays. Direct assays are theoretically better, but they pose technical challenges[29] so indirect assays are used in many laboratories. Albumin can interfere with indirect free thyroid hormone assays to a variable extent and newer assays have been developed to overcome this.[25] Older laboratory methods used to quantify TSH may be less able to distinguish TSH from hCG, which is present in significant concentrations in the first half of pregnancy. This assay interference may explain a slight rise in serum TSH in the first trimester of normal pregnancies described in some studies. Newer, more specific immunometric assays of thyrotrophin concentrations are now commonly used so interference by hCG is negligible.[29] In view of the biochemical variations of pregnancy (Fig. 2), TSH should not be considered in isolation, but always be measured in conjunction with FT_4 and FT_3 levels.[10] Appropriate reference ranges according to the assay techniques used and for gestation must be followed to avoid misdiagnosis and over-treatment.

MATERNAL HYPOTHYROIDISM

In the UK, the incidence of hypothyroidism diagnosed before pregnancy is about 1%. It is 3 times more common in white women than black women. Overt hypothyroidism during pregnancy is rare, occurring in about 0.05% of women.[7] It is most commonly a result of primary thyroidal failure due to chronic autoimmune thyroiditis associated with anti-thyroid peroxidase antibodies. Other rarer causes of hypothyroidism are listed in Table 1.

In primary thyroidal failure, investigations will reveal an elevated TSH and low FT_4 and FT_3 concentrations. Normocytic anaemia is an association in 30–40% of cases. Secondary consequences – such as hyperlipidaemia and mild, reversible abnormalities in liver function tests – may also be noted.[7] In two studies,[30,31] subclinical hypothyroidism (defined as raised TSH with normal serum FT_4 and FT_3) was found in over 2% of pregnancies, with apparently two-thirds of these resolving spontaneously within 10 weeks of diagnosis.[32]

The diagnosis of hypothyroidism in pregnancy may be difficult due to the non-specific symptoms. Up to 20% of biochemically hypothyroid women are

Table 1 Causes of hypothyroidism	
Autoimmune	Hashimoto's thyroiditis (chronic) de Quervain's thyroiditis (subacute, transient)
Iatrogenic	Thyroidectomy Previous radio-iodine or iodide treatment Drug therapy (e.g. lithium, amiodarone)
Congenital hypothyroidism	Thyroid dysgenesis Thyroid dyshormongenesis Genetic mutations of thyroid receptors
Iodine deficiency (probably commonest cause world-wide)	
Infiltrative disorders (e.g. sarcoidosis)	

asymptomatic.[33] Furthermore the presence of thyroid autoantibodies is non-specific, being present in up to 20% of biochemically euthyroid pregnant women.[34] A high index of suspicion is required in women treated previously for hyperthyroidism, those with previous head or neck irradiation, previous postpartum thyroiditis, and those with a goitre, or those on drug therapies with side-effects on the thyroid gland.

Treatment of hypothyroidism

Treatment is with thyroxine replacement. Some have found that thyroxine requirements in the first trimester of pregnancy increase by 50–100%.[35,36] This increased thyroxine requirement is usually sustained throughout pregnancy. Some hypothesise that this increased requirement, even in the third trimester, may be due to increased transfer of T_4 to the fetus, increased maternal clearance, placental catabolism and maternal weight gain.[2] Others claim that many women could go through pregnancy on the same prepregnancy thyroxine dose and any increase in pregnancy is a reflection of inadequate treatment prepregnancy.[37] Roti et al.[5] and Mandel et al.[36] have recommended that thyroid function tests are performed in each trimester as mild hypothyroidism may be asymptomatic and could have potentially deleterious consequences. Using these results with appropriate reference ranges, together with maternal signs and symptoms as a guide, the dose of thyroxine can be adjusted accordingly. Following a dose adjustment, the thyroid function should be checked again in a month's time.[6,10] Drugs commonly used in pregnancy, like iron supplements and aluminium hydroxide antacids, interfere with thyroxine absorption and should be taken at different times of the day.[38,39]

With maternal thyroxine therapy, the fetus is not at risk of thyrotoxicosis (as the placenta metabolises most of the thyroxine presented to it) and breast-feeding is safe. Pregnant women on adequate replacement from the start of pregnancy should expect a good obstetric outcome. However, they are still at increased risk of postpartum thyroiditis regardless of control during pregnancy.[7]

Obstetric outcome in hypothyroidism

Inadequate thyroxine replacement, on the other hand, can lead to maternal and fetal complications. Interestingly, women who are hypothyroid at the start of pregnancy are more at risk of pre-eclampsia, and possibly fetal distress in labour, despite subsequent euthyroidism with treatment during pregnancy.[40,41] Hypothyroidism at term is also associated with an increased risk of pregnancy-induced hypertension with the subsequent need for premature delivery, placental abruption, postpartum haemorrhage and cardiac dysfunction.[33] Increased risks of fetal distress in labour, low birth weight, stillbirths and reduced intellect in the offspring have all been reported in maternal hypothyroidism.[42] There does not appear to be an increased risk of major congenital anomalies associated with hypothyroidism.[33,41,43] The majority of infants are healthy and are without any evidence of thyroid dysfunction. In general, the poorer the control of hypothyroidism the more at risk the pregnancy.

It is possible that decreased maternal thyroid hormone levels mediate obstetric complications in the mother and fetus through a combination of factors including a reduced feto–maternal transfer of thyroid hormones and iodide, maternal metabolic impairment, anaemia, maternal cardiovascular changes, and through detrimental effects on placental function.

In hypothyroidism with an autoimmune aetiology, maternal anti-thyroid antibodies could theoretically be transferred across the placenta to affect the fetus. Glinoer et al. found that 40% of new-borns from euthyroid mothers with thyroid autoimmunity had an elevated thyroid peroxidase antibody titre at birth, with levels significantly correlated with those of maternal peroxidase antibody titres. The thyroid function in these new-borns was not, however, significantly different from controls who had mothers without thyroid pathology.[8] One study reported an increased incidence of transient congenital hypothyroidism in offspring of mothers with subclinical autoimmune hypo-thyroidism.[44] It is still widely believed, however, that the incidence of clinically relevant neonatal hypothyroidism due to anti-thyroid autoantibodies is low.

It is important to remember that, in women with previously treated Graves' disease who are currently on thyroxine replacement, transplacental passage of thyroid-stimulating antibodies could potentially cause neonatal thyrotoxicosis. Maternal euthyroidism secondary to good medical treatment gives no indication of autoantibody levels. Furthermore, 10% of women with Graves' disease may also have thyroid-blocking antibodies[45] which may give rise to transient neonatal hypothyroidism.

MATERNAL HYPERTHYROIDISM

The incidence of thyrotoxicosis in pregnancy is 0.05–0.2%, with over 90% due to Graves' disease.[5,11,46] This autoimmune condition is caused by antibodies that can stimulate the TSH receptor (TSAbs) resulting in thyroid hyperactivity and glandular enlargement. Other rarer causes of thyrotoxicosis are listed in Table 2.

Pregnant women can tolerate mild thyrotoxicosis quite well. Weight loss despite increased food intake, tremor, anxiety, and lid lag are all characteristic of thyrotoxicosis whilst pretibial myxoedema and exophthalmos are extrathyroidal manifestations of Graves' disease. A goitre associated with hyperthyroidism can further expand in pregnancy and may cause retrosternal obstruction resulting in enhanced anaesthetic risks.[10]

Investigations will reveal a significantly raised serum FT_4 and FT_3, with a suppressed TSH. The diagnosis may be confused in hyperemesis gravidarum and trophoblastic disease. The presence of TSAbs can be helpful in distinguishing

Table 2 Causes of thyrotoxicosis	
Autoimmune	Graves' disease
	Subacute thyroiditis
Thyroid tumours	Toxic nodular goitre
	Toxic adenoma
Iatrogenic	Drug therapy (e.g. iodine, amiodarone, lithium)
Pituitary thyrotrophic adenomas	
Gestational trophoblastic disease	

these from the diagnosis of new cases of Graves' disease. All women with past and present hyperthyroidism, whether on treatment or not, should have their thyroid function monitored in each trimester.

Graves' disease often improves in the second and third trimesters due to the general relative immune suppression in pregnancy, although hyperthyroidism can be transiently exacerbated in the first trimester possibly due to hCG stimulation.[47,48] Over half the women will have a recurrence of disease postpartum due to a rebound in the levels of antibodies.[47] In fact, new cases of Graves' disease are frequently diagnosed within the first 12 months following parturition.[49]

Treatment of hyperthyroidism and thyrotoxicosis

Medical treatment is very effective in the majority of pregnant women. Carbimazole and propylthiouracil (PTU) inhibit thyroid hormone synthesis and are equally effective in pregnancy.[50] The aim of treatment is to maintain the maternal serum FT_4 at the upper end of the normal range using as low a dose of the drug as possible in order to minimise the side-effects on the fetus.[51]

Both carbimazole and PTU can cross the placenta. As clearance of these drugs is very slow in the fetus, they tend to accumulate with the risk of fetal hypothyroidism and goitrogenesis. The reported incidence of goitre in neonates is 10% following in utero exposure to either drug.[52,53] Therefore, block and replace regimens (combined carbimazole or PTU and thyroxine) have no place in pregnancy because inadequate amounts of thyroxine are transferred to the fetus to compensate for the effect of the antithyroid drug. Neither carbimazole nor PTU is teratogenic.[54,55] Up to 1997, there had been fewer than 20 case reports of aplasia cutis, a benign scalp condition, in the fetus associated with maternal carbimazole ingestion.[6,56] Some of the cases of aplasia cutis may have a familial link.[6] Therefore, its use should not be precluded in pregnancy. In the US, PTU, which is more protein bound, is preferred to carbimazole in pregnancy, as it is believed that there is less transplacental transfer and less is secreted in breast milk.[54] More recent evidence has, however, shown no significant difference between the fetal hypothyroidism-inducing potential between the two drugs.[57]

Overall, 2% of patients taking carbimazole or PTU suffer side-effects, the most serious of which is agranulocytosis, a rapidly developing idiosyncratic phenomenon which occurs in 0.3% of patients on PTU.[58] It can also occur with high doses of carbimazole.[51] Hepatitis and vasculitis are also recognised side-effects of PTU.[59] A drug rash or urticaria occurs in 1–5% of patients on either drug. Carbimazole, which is more widely used in the UK during pregnancy, has a longer half-life so patient compliance is improved with less frequent dosing. There are fewer major toxic side-effects with carbimazole and it is cheaper.[53,60] Women who are already stable on one drug need not switch over to the other during pregnancy.

Transient biochemical hypothyroidism, which was claimed as being of little clinical consequence, has been reported in 1–5% of neonates whose mothers are on PTU.[6] In one study, cord blood T_4 levels at birth were found to be generally lower if mothers were still being treated compared with those mothers who were treated previously during pregnancy. The serum T_4

concentrations did not, however, correlate with either the dose or duration of treatment. None of the neonates was clinically hypothyroid at birth. Notably, there was a good correlation between maternal and fetal thyroid hormone levels.[61] Long-term follow-up after in utero exposure to either drug has not revealed any growth or intellectual impairment in the off-spring in several studies.[62-64] It is possible, however, that more subtle developmental problems may have been missed in these studies. Breast-feeding is safe with low maintenance doses of each drug.[65] Doses may be split or taken post-feeding to try to reduce secretion in breast milk.[66]

Newly diagnosed thyrotoxicosis in pregnancy is usually successfully controlled medically and serious complications are rare. Initially, aggressive treatment with high doses of carbimazole or PTU may be appropriate for a few weeks before the dose is gradually reduced.[10] If the disease is severe and control is poor, the mother is at risk of significant morbidity like congestive cardiac failure and a thyroid storm.[11]

Thyroid storm

Thyroid storm is very rare and complicates less than 1–2% of thyrotoxic pregnancies. It is a serious condition with maternal mortality rates of up to 25%.[67] Adequate fluid replacement, thermoregulation and aggressive treatment of concurrent illnesses, like hypertension, infection and anaemia, are key in the management of severely thyrotoxic patients.[6,11] PTU may be preferred as it also blocks peripheral conversion of T_4 to T_3. A short course of β-blockers, like propranolol, may be safely used for more rapid symptomatic control.[68,69] Dexamethasone or hydrocortisone may also be used to block the peripheral conversion of T_4 to T_3 and to prevent acute adrenal insufficiency.[66] Fetal monitoring should be performed continuously after 24 weeks' gestation during the acute crisis.[66]

Obstetric outcome in thyrotoxicosis

If thyrotoxicosis is well controlled, a good obstetric outcome can be expected. There are reports of increased obstetric complications in uncontrolled thyrotoxicosis, especially in the second half of pregnancy, like preterm labour, intra-uterine death, intra-uterine growth restriction, low birth-weight, pre-eclampsia, placental abruption, and maternal infection.[66,67,70] Overall, there is increased perinatal and neonatal mortality associated with maternal thyrotoxicosis.[67]

Radioactive iodine and non-radioactive iodides

These should not be used in the routine management of thyrotoxicosis or in diagnostic scans as they are transferred and taken up avidly by the fetal thyroid gland and may cause permanent thyroid damage and congenital hypothyroidism.[71,72] The risk is greatest from the tenth week of gestation when the fetal thyroid gland begins to accumulate iodide.

Inadvertent radio-iodine therapy in the first trimester has not been associated with congenital anomalies,[5] but there may be an associated increased risk of pregnancy loss and mental retardation in the off-spring.[72] In a separate case report, inadvertent radio-iodine therapy at 19 weeks' gestation resulted in a neonate who was clinically euthyroid at birth, but required thyroxine replacement to normalise TSH levels. The child was neuro-developmentally normal at 36 months.[73] Even though in many case reports infants appear to be clinically unaffected, their long-term prognosis, including the risk of developing hypothyroidism and thyroid malignancies later in life, is not known. It is recommended that pregnancy should be avoided for at least 4 months following treatment of thyrotoxicosis with radioactive iodine.[10]

Thyroidectomy

Thyroidectomy is rarely indicated in pregnancy. The anaesthetic and surgical risks to the mother are deemed to be higher than the risk of negative effects of antithyroid therapy on the fetus.[74] Surgery would be indicated if there is failure or intolerance of antithyroid drugs, suspected carcinoma or a large goitre causing tracheal or oesophageal compression. A short course of iodides can be safely used pre-operatively in pregnancy to control hyperthyroidism.[66] It is traditionally believed and a widely held view that, if needed, surgery is best performed in the second trimester as the risk of miscarriage is lowest. One study has, however, suggested that there is no increased risk of spontaneous abortions following surgery in the first trimester.[74] In the third trimester, postoperative hypocalcaemia can precipitate preterm labour.[75,76] Regular follow-up with thyroid function tests is needed postoperatively as a significant proportion will require thyroxine replacement eventually.[10]

THYROID NODULES

These are present in 1% of women of reproductive age. A cytological diagnosis should be made from cyst aspirate or fine-needle aspiration (FNA) of solid lesions, especially if there are other suspicious features like rapid enlargement, fixation to underlying tissues, and lymphadenopathy.[77,78] Ultrasonography can be used to measure and distinguish cystic from solid lesions, but is not indicated routinely. Most nodules are benign, 5% are malignant, and 20% have an indeterminate cytology result.[78]

Malignant lesions should be surgically removed, preferably in the second trimester. Surgery on indeterminate lesions diagnosed late in pregnancy may be deferred till after parturition as 80% are benign.[79,80] Following thyroidectomy for malignant lesions, high dose thyroxine is given to suppress endogenous TSH secretion as residual tumours may be TSH-dependent. Radioactive iodine treatment should be delayed until postpartum. Serum thyroglobulin, a marker of functioning thyroid tissue, is modestly elevated in normal pregnancy. Following total thyroidectomy for malignant disease and with adequate suppression of TSH, thyroglobulin should remain low in pregnancy and is, therefore, a useful tumour marker for evaluating the completeness of therapy and for monitoring residual or recurrent disease during gestation.[81] Pregnancy is believed not to have any effect on the natural history of thyroid cancers, but some pregnant women do develop tumours that are more aggressive than usual.[82,83]

POSTPARTUM THYROIDITIS

Biochemical evidence of postpartum thyroid dysfunction has a world-wide prevalence of about 5%,[84] usually developing 1–8 months postpartum.[85] There is wide geographical variation in prevalence rates. Amongst the highest reported is 16.7% in Mid-Glamorgan (UK), but most of these women were asymptomatic with only biochemical evidence of the condition.[86] About 70% of women who are positive for thyroid anti-microsomal antibodies in early pregnancy[87] and about 25% of women with type I diabetes mellitus[88] develop postpartum thyroiditis. Women with a family history of autoimmune hypothyroidism are also at increased risk of this condition.[89]

The condition is characterised by a transient subacute destructive lymphocytic thyroiditis resulting initially in biochemical evidence of thyrotoxicosis, due to an excessive release of preformed thyroid hormone, followed by hypothyroidism. This biphasic biochemical pattern is seen in 90% of patients.[90] Other patterns observed include hypothyroidism followed by hyperthyroidism, or hypo- or hyperthyroidism alone. About 50% of patients develop a small, painless goitre. The underlying aetiology is thought to be due to the postpartum rebound in the maternal immune system, resulting in a transient increase in anti-thyroid antibodies, which in most cases were already present before parturition.

Symptoms, if present, are often vague and non-specific, and are frequently attributed to the normal postpartum state. Fatigue is most typical, and can occur in both phases. About 20% of patients develop symptoms in both phases. A further 40% of patients experience symptoms in only the thyrotoxic phase and the remaining 40% in only the hypothyroidism phase. The thyrotoxic phase usually lasts for less than 2 months,[79] and can be distinguished from hyperthyroidism due to Graves' disease by a low thyroidal radioactive iodine uptake and the absence of TSAbs. The majority of women do not require treatment in this phase and the condition resolves spontaneously. If symptoms are marked, they can be treated with β-blockade.[6] The hypothyroidism phase is more likely to require treatment.[46] Thyroxine replacement may be required for 6–12 months and should be withdrawn gradually to re-assess thyroid status. At the end of the first year post-parturition, most women would have returned to euthyroidism spontaneously but 3–4% will remain permanently hypothyroid from this stage.[89,91]

Postpartum depression may be more common in women with postpartum thyroiditis.[89] Almost 70% of women will develop a recurrence of postpartum thyroiditis in subsequent pregnancies.[92] Long-term follow-up of these women with yearly thyroid function testing is recommended as 25% of them will develop permanent hypothyroidism within the next 5 years.[93] Current consensus opinion is that screening all women for postpartum thyroiditis is not justified as only a minority develop symptoms that require treatment and for most the disease is self-limiting. Some have recommended that those at increased risk should be screened at 3 and 6 months' postpartum.[94]

THYROID HORMONES AND THE FETUS

The fetal thyroid gland begins as an epithelial proliferation of the floor of the buccopharynx at 6 weeks' gestation. This thyroid primordium forms a bilobed diverticulum as it descends in front of the pharyngeal gut, reaching its final location anterior to the hyoid bone and laryngeal cartilages in the neck by 9 weeks' gestation. The thyroglossal duct that connects the gland to the pharyngeal gut then disappears.[95] It begins accumulating iodide at 10–12 weeks' gestation and thyroid hormone synthesis can be demonstrated at this time.[96,97] TRH can be detected in the fetal hypothalamus by 10 weeks' gestation.[95] TSH can be found in the anterior pituitary at 10–12 weeks' gestation, with serum levels rising towards term to values exceeding those of the adult.[96,98] The portal system that connects the hypothalamus to the pituitary is developed by 16 weeks' gestation and continues to mature with gestation. Thyroid hormones are released in appreciable amounts from around 16–18 weeks onwards.[9,99] From 20 weeks' gestation, the thyroid gland comes under pituitary TSH control.[9,100]

The placenta itself, and the fetal pancreas, also produce TRH. This, together with slow fetal degradation of TRH, results in high circulating fetal TRH concentrations, in contrast to low maternal levels. Increased TRH stimulation of the pituitary to produce more TSH is required, as thyroid follicular sensitivity to TSH develops only gradually with gestation and is not completely mature until term. Furthermore, the TSH response to TRH in the fetus and premature infant is prolonged, reflecting a relative hypothalamic hypothyroid state. The fetal thyroid is poor at autoregulation of iodide uptake and is very sensitive to iodide depletion and iodine inhibition.[101] In contrast to the adult with a working negative feedback loop, TSH and thyroid hormones rise concurrently over the course of gestation in the fetus. Even though the function of the fetal hypothalamic-pituitary-thyroid axis is largely auto-nomous, the negative feedback system only reaches full maturity a few weeks into its postnatal life and it is not completely independent of the maternal thyroid status in utero.[9,100]

The placenta is thought to be freely permeable to TRH (although several studies have disputed this) and iodide, but impermeable to TSH. Maternally-derived TRH may have a role in controlling fetal thyroid function[102] before the maturation of the hypothalamic-pituitary-thyroid axis. It has been demonstrated in humans that maternal thyroid hormones cross the placenta into the fetal circulation.[103] This is despite the placenta's inherent relative impermeability to thyroid hormones and its high type III DI levels which rapidly break down most T_4 and T_3 presented to it. The fetus is dependent on placentally transferred thyroid hormones before the onset of fetal thyroid function. Physiologically critical amounts of maternal T_4 are transferred to the fetus.[9] Thyroid hormones can be detected in the fetal circulation and brain in the first trimester, and these hormones have been shown to be of maternal origin.[99] In the second and third trimesters, circulating thyroid hormones in the human fetus are of both maternal and fetal origin, their presence being dependent on a functioning placenta for T_4 transport and supply of iodide substrate.

Fetal thyroid hormone levels are always significantly less than maternal levels, and the difference between them decreases with gestation as circulating concentrations of both thyroid hormones and TBG rise in the fetus.[100] There is a gradual increase in FT_4 levels with gestation approaching adult levels by 36 weeks' gestation.[3] Significant increases in serum FT_3 in the fetal circulation is

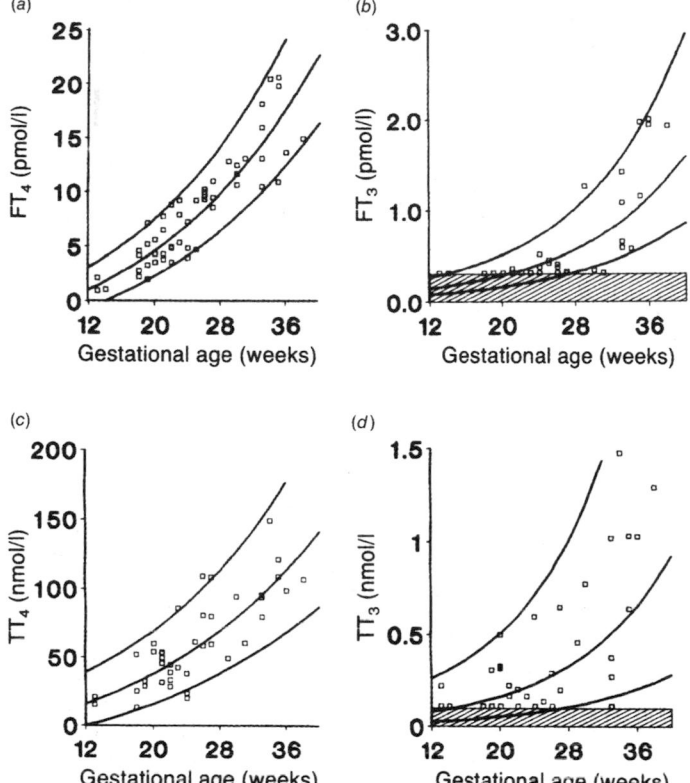

Fig. 3 The ontogeny of fetal concentrations of circulating FT_4, FT_3, total T_4 and total T_3 during gestation. Data from fetal blood samples obtained by cordocentesis.[98] (Reproduced with permission from Prof. K. Nicolaides.)

most evident in the third trimester as type I DI activity rises, hence peripheral conversion from T_4 increases.[2,3,18] At parturition, there is an acute rise in TSH secretion with a corresponding 2–6-fold rise in thyroid hormone levels, peaking 24–36 h after birth. Even so, at full-term birth, approximately 30% of thyroid hormones measured in cord blood are still derived from the mother;[9] fetal serum FT_3 concentrations are 2–3-fold less than those in the mother[104] and only become comparable to those of the adult several weeks later (Fig. 3).

Thyroid hormone metabolism in the fetus

It appears that there is a critical level of circulating thyroid hormone that must be maintained to facilitate optimal fetal development at each stage of fetal development. The placenta, which is rich in DIs, is ideally suited to play an important role in maintaining fetal thyroid hormone levels within a critical limit[9] and ensuring a continuing supply of iodide substrate to the fetus.

Type II DI activity is evident in early gestation in the rodent fetal brain and is thought to be important in normal brain development.[105] When there is hypothyroxaemia in the fetus, the activity of type I DI in peripheral tissues decreases to try to maintain circulating T_4 levels used to supply the more important organs such as the brain. Conversely, type II DI activity in the fetal brain, placenta and brown adipose tissue increases to try to maintain an adequate local supply of T_3.[106] A similar system may be operating in human fetuses and we have demonstrated type II DI activity in the human fetal brain in the first trimester.[106a]

Apart from converting T_4 to T_3, type I DI is also capable of the inactivating process of inner ring de-iodination of T_4 and T_3, a process which is 200- or 40-fold faster, respectively, if the thyroid hormones are sulphated.[107] Unlike the adult, type I DI activity is low in mammalian fetal tissues resulting in a high circulating level of sulphated T_4 and T_3, which may represent a reservoir of thyroid hormones in the fetus. It has been hypothesised that this system serves to protect organs that do not require high levels of thyroid hormone for their development, whilst maintaining adequate thyroid hormone supply to T_3-dependent tissues which also contain sulphatases to reactivate thyroid hormones, for example the brain.[4]

Therefore, local T_3 availability is not only determined by circulating levels of thyroid hormone, but also by differential tissue expressions of the various enzymes involved in thyroid hormone metabolism,[4] so that the limited transfer of thyroid hormones from the mother can have significant and diverse physiological effects at target organs.

Thyroid hormone action

T_3 activity is mediated primarily through thyroid hormone receptors (TRs). Four important TR isoforms have been characterised in humans. The *erbAα* locus on chromosome 17 encodes TRα1 and TRα2 proteins, whilst the *erbAβ* locus on chromosome 3 expresses TRβ1 and TRβ2, by alternate and spliced variants of mRNA.[99,108] TRα1, TRβ1 and TRβ2 bind T_3. The T_3–TR complex binds to specific DNA sequences or thyroid hormone response elements (TRE) found in the regulatory regions of target genes.[109] T_3 can, therefore, promote or inhibit the transcription of these genes. The α2 protein does not bind T_3 and has a postulated modulatory role mediated by competitive binding of protein to TRE.[110,111] The transcriptional action of TRs is also controlled by other DNA-binding nuclear proteins and related hormone receptors that can dimerise with TR independently of DNA-binding. These proteins can act as co-activators or co-repressors of TR function,[112–114] thus dictating an orderly schedule for thyroid hormone augmentation of specific genes to occur at appropriate times during gestation.

There are also temporal and anatomical variations in the expression of these TR isoforms throughout fetal life which determine thyroid responsiveness of each individual organ during development. The existence of specific TR isoforms implies the presence of specific roles for each of them.[115,116] For example, patients with homozygous deletion of the *TRβ* gene suffer with deaf-mutism, but demonstrate normal cognitive function,[117] implying a specific role for the TRβ protein in the development of the auditory apparatus and cortex. Post-transcriptional, translational and post-translational control of TR expression will also influence the ultimate phenotypic expression of T_3 activity.

The TRs are also known to function and bind to DNA and protein independently of T_3 binding,[118,119] and may have a non-thyroid hormone dependent role. The possibility of extranuclear thyroid hormone action has also been raised, even though definitive evidence is lacking to date.[120]

Interestingly, deletion of all known TRs in mice (knockout mice) has resulted in a milder overall phenotype than the debilitating ones of severe hypothyroidism.[121] Such mice only have a very hyperactive pituitary-thyroid axis, poor female fertility, and retarded growth and bone maturation. This raises the possibility that the effects of thyroid hormones in the development of the mouse central nervous system may also be mediated by other proteins apart from TRs. The case may be entirely different in humans.

Fetal hypothyroidism

Defective embryogenesis or dysfunction of one or more of the organs of the hypothalamic-pituitary-thyroid axis is responsible for 80% of cases of fetal hypothyroidism in iodine-sufficient areas.[122] The most common is thyroid dysgenesis occurring in 1:4000 pregnancies and the majority of these cases are sporadic. Some cases of thyroid dyshormonogenesis and TR or TSH receptor mutations display autosomal recessive or dominant traits. The other causes of fetal hypothyroidism include maternal ingestion of anti-thyroid drugs, transplacental passage of maternal antibodies and iodine deficiency.[9,122] The latter remains the commonest cause of neonatal hypothyroidism world-wide.[9]

The limited transplacental passage of thyroid hormones can mask the phenotypic effects of congenital hypothyroidism at birth and diagnosis can be delayed. These neonates still have higher TSH and lower thyroid hormone concentrations compared with normal neonates indicating that maternal compensation is inadequate.[123] All neonates in the UK are screened for congenital hypothyroidism, which has an incidence of 1:4000–7000. The diagnosis must not be missed as treatment is easy, cheap, and will prevent long-term developmental problems. Fetal hypothyroidism may result in the development of a fetal goitre, impaired bone maturation, and, more significantly, suboptimal brain development.[124,125] Delayed ossification of the distal femoral or proximal tibial epiphyses can be seen on X-ray films. There are reported cases of successful intra-uterine therapy with injections of thyroid hormones into amniotic fluid or through cordocentesis in overt hypothyroidism in utero.[126,127]

Thyroid hormones and fetal brain development

It is well established that the thyroid status of neonates and children has a significant long-term impact on their behaviour, locomotor ability, speech, hearing, and cognition.[124] Delay in restoring normal thyroid status in the neonate can lead to irreversible damage. Prompt thyroid supplementation following the diagnosis of neonatal hypothyroidism can restore neuro-development to within the normal range.[128] Even so, there are still subtle demonstrable language delay, visual–spatial impairments and lower mean IQ scores later in childhood compared with euthyroid controls, implying that brain development may be thyroid hormone sensitive not only in the neonatal period, but also prior to birth.[129,130]

Maternal T_4 transferred to the fetus confers some, but probably incomplete, protection of fetal brain development. Both maternal and fetal thyroid status in utero may be important in brain development. We know that some degree of compensation occurs if one or other is lacking, but differences in the neuropsychological development are still demonstrable in either case compared with euthyroid controls.

Long-standing neurodevelopmental defects are more prevalent in iodine-deficient parts of the world.[131,132] Observational studies performed in these areas have shown that iodine supplementation before pregnancy and in the first and second trimesters reduces the incidence of cretinism, but supplementation beginning later in pregnancy does not improve the neurodevelopmental status of the off-spring.[132,133] Even children of marginally iodine-deficient mothers show psychomotor and cognitive impairment.[134] Such data indicate the sensitivity of the developing central nervous system in the first half of pregnancy to maternal thyroid metabolism in utero.

Maternal hypothyroidism, not necessarily due to iodine deficiency, has also been associated with poorer neuropsychological outcome in off-spring. In The Netherlands, 220 mothers with a low serum FT_4 concentration at 12 weeks' gestation gave birth to babies who at 19 months of age had scores at or below the tenth percentile on the Psychomotor Developmental Index of Bayley Scales of Infant Development.[135] In the US, mothers who had a low serum butanol-extractable iodine (a measure of circulating thyroid hormones employed in the 1960s) before 24 weeks' gestation and who were not adequately treated, had infants with lower Bayley scores. These children were later shown to have lower IQ scores at 4 and 7 years of age.[136] Recently, another study performed in the US on the off-spring of 62 women with TSH concentrations above the 98th percentile during pregnancy, compared them with 124 matched controls. None of the neonates had hypothyroidism at birth. The children were assessed at 7–9 years of age. Those with hypothyroid mothers performed less well on all 15 of the neuropsychological tests and had, on average, a 4 point lower IQ score on the Wechsler Intelligence Scale for Children than the controls. Of the 62 biochemically hypothyroid women, 48 were not treated during the pregnancy as they were clinically euthyroid, and the children of this subgroup of women performed less well, with an average of 7 point lower IQ scores than controls; of these, 19% scored 85 or less. Interestingly, the serum total T_4 and FT_4 concentrations in the treated and the non-treated clinically euthyroid women were similar during pregnancy. This study demonstrates that subclinical hypothyroidism in women can result in neuropsychological deficits in their off-spring, and thyroxine supplementation can improve the outcome even when supplementation is inadequate.[137] In another study in Toronto, children at the extreme end of the spectrum including those with absent thyroid glands or who show evidence of hypothyroidism in utero performed less well in neurodevelopmental tests compared with others with congenital hypothyroidism. Different areas of ability were associated with the timing and duration of thyroid hormone deficiency, suggesting that there are critical periods over which various parts of the brain are sensitive to thyroid hormone supply.[125]

Clinical observations of neurodevelopmental delay can be explained by accompanying histological and biochemical changes within the brain. In the rat, thyroid hormones have been shown to be involved in the regulation of the processes of terminal brain differentiation such as dendritic and axonal growth, synaptogenesis, neuronal migration and myelination.[138–140] We know that in humans, T_3, T_4 and thyroid hormone receptors can be detected in the first trimester brain before the fetal thyroid gland becomes active, and T_3 is not detectable in other fetal tissues apart from the brain at this stage.[98,141,142] This is consistent with the theory that there is a specific role for maternally derived thyroid hormones in very early brain development. Initial studies suggest increasing TR expression (defined at mRNA and protein levels) in the human fetal brain with gestation,[142,143] perhaps reflecting the increasing role of thyroid hormones in the development of the central nervous system. In the human fetal brain, immunostaining of TR protein has been found principally within cortical pyramidal cells and cerebellar Purkinje cells.[142] The mere presence of TRs at any time does not, however, necessarily indicate that thyroid hormone-dependent action is occurring at the same time as other proteins may exert post-translational control on TR action. The precise timing for thyroid hormone-dependent central nervous system development in the human fetus is still unclear, and may be phasic and different for specific areas of the brain.

Potentially functional TREs have been found in the promoters of the rodent myelin basic protein (MBP) gene and human neurogranin gene, suggesting direct regulation by the T_3–TR complex.[144–146] The mRNA of MBP expressed in oligodendrocytes is reduced by at least 50% in hypothyroid fetal rats.[108] The lack of these proteins may be implicated in the delayed myelination observed histologically. The capacity of cultured cells to enhance MBP expression in response to T_3 has been reported to coincide with the appearance of TRβ1 mRNA.[147] The differentiation of cerebellar Purkinje cells is also thyroid hormone dependent. These cells express genes including calbindin, myo-inositol-triphosphate (IP_3) receptor and Purkinje-cell protein-2 (PCP-2), all of which show significantly delayed mRNA expression in neonatal hypothyroid rats. Interestingly, despite ultimate normalisation of these mRNA levels, the pups demonstrated a marked deficit in Purkinje cell maturation, confirming the importance of timing in thyroid hormone dependent neurodevelopment.[148]

Intra-uterine growth restriction and prematurity

Fetal development and growth depend on several endocrine, paracrine and autocrine events within the fetoplacental unit.[149] Malfunction of this unit can result in intra-uterine growth restricted (IUGR) fetuses, with brain-weight usually maintained relative to body-weight while other organs, like the liver, are significantly smaller. IUGR babies are significant contributors of perinatal and neonatal mortality and morbidity; 10% of low birth-weight babies suffer some degree of physical handicap[150] and 5% show neurodevelopmental delay at aged 9 years.[151]

In utero fetal blood sampling has shown that fetuses with severe IUGR have significantly lower levels of circulating FT_4, FT_3 and a slight elevation in TSH.[18,152] The thyroid status is also significantly correlated to the degree of fetal hypoxaemia and acidosis that are found in IUGR associated with uteroplacental insufficiency. Low levels of thyroid hormones may contribute to reduced oxygen consumption by peripheral tissues to maintain viability at the expense of disrupting neurodevelopment.[3] This is accompanied by a reduction in the expression of all thyroid receptor (TR) isoforms in the cerebellum and cerebral cortices of IUGR fetuses.[142] Very low birth-weight (VLBW) infants also have lower serum total T_4 and T_3 concentrations.[153] Histological abnormalities, which are similar to those described in thyroid deficiency, have also been noted in the cerebral and cerebellar cortices of growth restricted animal models.[154] Therefore, fetal thyroid status in utero has been postulated to play a role in the pathogenesis of neurodevelopmental impairment in IUGR and VLBW infants.

Premature infants of less than 30 weeks' gestational age (not necessarily with IUGR) also experience a transient period of hypothyroxinaemia with a fall in serum FT_4 concentrations without TSH elevation. FT_4 concentrations appear to reach a nadir during the second week of life and recover to expected values by the third or fourth week.[155,156] This period of 'transient hypothyroxinaemia' corresponds to a time of negative iodine balance in the neonate.[157] All this suggests that premature neonates have a problem with autoregulation of thyroidal iodine uptake and hence low thyroxine production. This is associated with lack of maturity of the hypothalamic-pituitary-thyroid axis resulting in an absence of a TSH surge in response to the hypothyroxinaemia.[158] Such neonates are unable to compensate for the loss of maternal T_4 and iodide supply in the short-term. Comparison of FT_4 concentrations of premature infants with intra-uterine fetuses of similar gestational age has revealed a 50% difference initially, a phenomenon not observed in term babies.[157] This difference is regarded by many to represent a physiological response, as thyroid hormone supplementation in premature infants has not demonstrated clear benefit to the long-term neurodevelopment of these infants.[159]

Therapeutic uncertainties

A few studies of thyroxine supplementation in premature infants aimed at restoring concentrations of thyroid hormone to those of their in utero counterparts have been performed. In one such study, the analysis of a subgroup of neonates delivered at 25–26 weeks' gestational age showed a higher mean IQ score in childhood in the thyroxine treated group compared with placebo treated controls. Conversely, over-supplementation in neonates older than 27 weeks' gestational age has been associated with hyperactive behaviour and a reduction in mean IQ relative to controls.[156] These few studies of thyroxine supplementation in premature infants, however, recruited only small numbers of patients, and these initial results need further verification. Furthermore, the optimal thyroid hormone levels for premature neonatal development at different gestational ages are not well defined, even though normal ranges for in utero fetuses across gestation have been published.[98] There is also uncertainty about the form in which thyroid hormones should be administered. Perhaps sulphated thyroxine is preferable to thyroxine or tri-iodothyronine.

Administrating iodine supplementation to pregnant women is also not straightforward. In Denmark, where there is a prevalence of mild-to-moderate iodine deficiency, maternal iodine supplementation of about 150 mg daily, as normally found in regular vitamin and mineral tablets, reduced maternal TSH but increased fetal TSH concentrations, whilst reducing thyroglobulin levels in cord blood at term. The observed mild biochemical hypothyroidism in neonates is unlikely to be of marked clinical significance, but biochemical findings do imply an inhibitory effect of iodine on the highly sensitive fetal thyroid function.[160] So, whilst iodine supplementation is of great benefit in reducing endemic cretinism in areas of severe iodine deficiency, this approach may be potentially harmful in areas of mildly deficient or normal dietary iodine intake.

Fetal and neonatal hyperthyroidism

This is usually observed in association with maternal Graves' disease. Transplacental passage of TSAbs is most likely to occur if the mother has active disease in the third trimester as this is when the most active placental transfer of maternal antibodies occur. Neonatal Graves' disease occurs in about 1–10% of infants born to mothers with Graves' disease.[3,161] The risk of developing this is increased if there are very high levels of TSAbs in the maternal circulation and where there is a history of an affected sibling.[162] The different affinities of the stimulating, and sometimes also blocking antibodies and their rates of clearance in the neonate, and levels of anti-thyroid drugs are probably factors determining the clinical manifestation of thyrotoxicosis in the off-spring.[163]

Clinically evident fetal thyrotoxicosis can also develop in utero, but is extremely rare as the high levels of type III DI in placenta, high thyroid hormone conjugation and low type I DI in the fetus favour a state of low T_3, the active metabolite, in fetal tissues.[122] Fetal thyrotoxicosis can result in fetal tachycardia, hydrops, intra-uterine growth restriction, goitrogenesis, and advanced bone maturation with resultant craniosynostosis.[164,165] Serial ultrasound scans of the fetus can be performed to detect these features. The definitive diagnosis is obtained by in utero fetal blood sampling.[166] Severe thyrotoxicosis in utero may result in fetal demise. Premature delivery occurs in up to 90% of cases and perinatal mortality may reach 50% if untreated.[167] Maternally administered anti-thyroid drugs can successfully treat fetal thyrotoxicosis.[168] Uncontrolled thyrotoxicosis in the first trimester has also been associated with an increased risk of minor congenital abnormalities in a few studies,[54] but this finding is disputed by others.[50,169]

At birth, thyroid function tests may be performed on the cord blood of babies with suspected thyrotoxicosis or with a particularly high risk of developing the condition. Levels of TSAbs in cord blood may also help to predict neonates at risk of developing thyrotoxicosis. These two tests are not recommended routinely for all Graves' disease cases. All these neonates, however, should be watched for signs of thyrotoxicosis like jitteriness, poor feeding, tachycardia, weight loss, a goitre, and, in severe cases, congestive cardiac failure. The half-life of TSAbs, which are IgG antibodies, are longer than anti-thyroid drugs. As the clearance of transplacental anti-thyroid drugs may take a few days, these drugs may still have an effect and result in a delay in the manifestation of hyperthyroidism by up to a week. Affected neonates may require anti-thyroid treatment for weeks or months until maternal TSAbs are metabolised.[6] Prognosis is poor if neonatal thyrotoxicosis is not recognised and treated promptly. Mortality rates are about 15% if untreated.[3] Generally, infants born to women who remain thyrotoxic despite therapy and infants who receive inadequate neonatal care sustain the greatest morbidity and mortality rates.

Fetal goitre

This may be a result of hypothyroidism or hyperthyroidism and can be detected by ultrasonography. It may also be associated with a raised maternal serum α-fetoprotein. A large goitre may cause tracheal or oesophageal obstruction resulting in polyhydramnios and neonatal asphyxia. It may also cause hyperextension of the neck making vaginal delivery difficult.[170] The aetiology of the goitre may be determined through analysis of samples from amniocentesis or cordocentesis. The latter is more reliable, but has a higher morbidity and mortality rate for the fetus.[166] Therapies are aimed at treating the underlying thyroid abnormality to resolve the goitre.[122,170,171]

KEY POINTS FOR CLINICAL PRACTICE

- The majority of pregnancies with a history of maternal thyroid disease are uncomplicated and result in good fetal outcomes.

- Most thyroid diseases are diagnosed and controlled preconceptually.

- Subclinical hypothyroidism is often missed and there are epidemiological data suggesting an association with lower IQ scores and subtle neurodevelopmental defects in the off-spring.

- There is, however, still insufficient evidence at this time to indicate screening of all women for thyroid disorders preconceptually or during pregnancy.

- No cost-effectiveness studies have been done, and the long-term impact of obstetric complications and fetal maldevelopment related to thyroid disorders in the population as a whole has not been well studied.

- Women with symptoms, or at increased risk of thyroid disorders because of previous or family history, should be tested for thyroid dysfunction.

- Newly diagnosed thyroid disorders must be treated promptly to reduce the risk of maternal and fetal complications.

- Overt fetal hypothyroidism and hyperthyroidism requiring in utero therapy are extremely rare.

- Despite good maternal management of thyroid disorders, neonatal hypothyroidism and hyperthyroidism still occur.

- Screening for neonatal hypothyroidism and increased surveillance of neonates at risk of hyperthyroidism is strongly recommended in order that prompt treatment can be instituted to prevent serious consequences.

- There is evidence at histological, biochemical and molecular levels pointing towards a crucial role for thyroid hormones in fetal brain development.

- There is a suggestion that reduction in circulating thyroid hormone concentrations is one of the factors mediating impaired neurological development in IUGR, VLBW and premature babies.

- More research is required into the precise role of thyroid hormones during the course of human fetal brain development. This will guide us in developing appropriate therapeutic interventions for mothers and neonates with thyroid disorders. Then, we can ultimately show if altering the thyroid status of pregnant women and their fetuses can reduce the prevalence of neurodevelopmental delay in non-endemic areas.

References

1 Brent GA. Maternal thyroid function: interpretation of thyroid function tests in pregnancy. Clin Obstet Gynecol 1997; 40: 3–15

2 Burrow GN, Fisher DA, Larsen PR. Maternal and fetal thyroid function. N Engl J Med 1994; 331: 1072–1078

3 Thorpe-Beeston JG, Nicolaides KH. Maternal and fetal thyroid function in pregnancy. In: Nicolaides K. (ed) Frontiers in Fetal Medicine Series. London: Parthenon, 1996; 10–11, 36–37

4 Visser TJ. Role of sulfate in thyroid hormone sulfation. Eur J Endocrinol 1996; 134: 12–14

5 Roti E, Minelli R, Salvi M. Management of hyperthyroidism and hypothyroidism in pregnant woman. J Clin Endocrinol Metab 1996; 81: 1679–1682

6 Ecker JL, Musci TJ. Treatment of thyroid disease in pregnancy. Prescribing in Pregnancy 1997; 24: 575–589

7 Montoro MN. Management of hypothyroidism during pregnancy. Clin Obstet Gynecol 1997; 40: 65–80

8 Glinoer D, Soto MF, Bourdoux PTTG et al. Pregnancy in patients with mild thyroid abnormalities: maternal and neonatal repercussions. J Clin Endocrinol Metab 1991; 73: 421–427

9 Fisher DA. Fetal thyroid function: diagnosis and management of fetal thyroid disorders. Clin Obstet Gynecol 1997; 40: 16–31

10 Nelson-Piercy C. Thyroid and parathyroid disease. In: Handbook of Obstetric Medicine. Oxford: ISIS Medical Media, 1997; 80–94

11 ACOG Technical Bulletin Number 181 – June 1993. Thyroid disease in pregnancy. Int J Gynecol Obstet 1993; 43: 82–88

12 Glinore D, de Nayer PT, Bourdeoux TG. Regulation of maternal thyroid during pregnancy. J Clin Endocrinol Metab 1990; 71: 276–287

13 Ain KB, Mori Y, Refetoff S. Reduced clearance rate of thyroxine-binding globulin (TBG) with increased sialylation: a mechanism for estrogen-induced elevation of serum TBG concentration. J Clin Endocrinol Metab 1987; 65: 689–696

14 Harada A, Hershman JM, Reed AW et al. Comparison of thyroid stimulators and thyroid hormone concentrations in the sera of pregnant women. J Clin Endocrinol Metab 1979; 48: 793–797

15 Ballabio M, Poshyachinda M, Ekins RP. Pregnancy-induced changes in thyroid function: role of hCG as putative regulator of maternal thyroid. J Clin Endocrinol Metab 1991; 73: 824–831

16 Glinoer D. The thyroid function during pregnancy: maternal and neonatal aspects. In: Beckers C, Reinwein D. (eds) The Thyroid and Pregnancy. Stuttgart: Schattauer, 1991, 35–43

17 Maruo T, Matsuo H, Mochizuki M. Thyroid hormone as a biological amplifier of differentiated function in early pregnancy. Acta Endocrinol (Copenh) 1991; 125: 58–66

18 Kilby MD, Verhaeg J, Gittoes N et al. Circulating thyroid hormone concentrations and placental thyroid hormone receptor expression in normal human pregnancy and pregnancy complicated by intrauterine growth restriction. J Clin Endocrinol Metab 1998; 83: 2964–2971

19 Amir SM, Osathanondh R, Berkowitz RS. hCG and thyroid function in patients with hydatidiform mole. Am J Obstet Gynecol 1984; 150: 723–728

20 Lazarus JH. Pregnancy, hCG, thyrotoxicosis and hyperemesis gravidarum. Clin Endocrinol 1993; 38: 343

21 Kaplan MM. Assessment of thyroid function during pregnancy. Thyroid 1992; 2: 57–61

22 Goodwin TM, Montoro M, Mestman JH. Transient hyperthyroidism and hyperemesis gravidarum. Clinical aspects. Am J Obstet Gynecol 1992; 167: 648–652

23 Wilson R, McKillop JH, McLean M et al. Thyroid function tests are rarely abnormal in patients with severe hyperemesis gravidarum. Clin Endocrinol 1992; 37: 331–334

24 Kimura M, Amino N, Tanaki H et al. Gestational thyrotoxicosis and hyperemesis gravidarum: possible role of hCG with higher stimulating activity. Clin Endocrinol 1993; 38: 345–350

25 Kotarba DD, Garner P, Perkins SL. Changes in free thyroxine, free triiodothyronine and thyroid stimulating hormone reference intervals in normal term pregnancy. J Obstet

Gynecol 1995; 15: 5–8

26 Franklyn JA, Sheppard M, Ramsden DB. Serum free thyroxine and free triiodothyronine concentrations in pregnancy. BMJ 1983; 287: 394

27 Kvetny J, Poulsen HK. Nuclear thyroxine and 3,5,3'-triiodothyronine receptors in human mononuclear blood cells during pregnancy. Acta Endocrinol 1984; 105: 19–23

28 Wiersinga WM. Serum free thyroxine during pregnancy: a meta-analysis. In: Beckers C, Reinwein D. (eds) The Thyroid and Pregnancy. Stuttgart: Schattauer, 1991; 979–994

29 Hay ID, Bayer MF, Kaplan MM et al. for the Committee on Nomenclature of the American Thyroid Association. American Thyroid Association assessment of current free thyroid hormone and thyrotrophin measurements and guidelines for future clinical assays. Clin Chem 1991; 37: 2002–2008

30 Lejeune B, Lemone M, Kinthaer J et al. The epidemiology of autoimmune and functional thyroid disorders in pregnancy. J Endocrinol Invest 1992; 15 (Suppl 2) 77

31 Klein RZ, Haddow JE, Faix JD et al. Prevalence of thyroid deficiency in pregnant women. Clin Endocrinol 1991; 35: 41–46

32 Kamijo K, Saito T, Sato M et al. Transient subclinical hypothyroidism in early pregnancy. Endocrinol Jpn 1998; 37: 397–403

33 Davis LE, Leveno KJ, Cunningham FG. Hypothyroidism complicating pregnancy. Obstet Gynecol 1988; 72: 108–112

34 Stagnaro-Green A, Roman SH, Cobin RH, et al. Detection of at-risk pregnancy by means of highly sensitive assays for thyroid autoantibodies. JAMA 1990; 264: 1422–1425

35 Toft AD. Thyroxine therapy. N Engl J Med 1994; 331: 174–180

36 Mandel SJ, Larsen PR, Seely EW, Brent GA. Increased need for thyroxine during pregnancy in women with primary hypothyroidism. N Engl J Med 1990; 323: 91–96

37 Girling JC, de Swiet M. Thyroxine dosage during pregnancy in women with primary hypothyroidism. Br J Obstet Gynaecol 1992; 99: 368–370

38 Campbell NRC, Hasinoff BB, Stalts H et al. Ferrous sulfate reduces thyroxine efficacy in patients with hypothyroidism. Ann Intern Med 1992; 117: 1010–1013

39 Liel Y, Sperber AD, Shany S. Nonspecific intestinal adsorption of levothyroxine by aluminium hydroxide. Am J Med 1994; 97: 363–365

40 Buckshee K, Kriplani A, Kapil A et al. Hypothyroidism complicating pregnancy. Aust NZ J Obstet Gynaecol 1992; 32: 240–242

41 Wasserstrum N, Anania CA. Perinatal consequences of maternal hypothyroidism in early pregnancy and inadequate replacement. Clin Endocrinol 1995; 42: 353–358

42 Leung AS, Millar LK, Koonings PP et al. Perinatal outcome in hypothyroid pregnancies. Obstet Gynecol 1993; 81: 349–353

43 Montoro M, Collea JV, Frasier SD, Mestman JH. Successful outcome of pregnancy in women with hypothyroidism. Ann Intern Med 1981; 94: 31–34

44 Dussault JH, Fisher DA. Thyroid function in mother of hypothyroid newborns. Obstet Gynecol 1999; 93: 15–20

45 Amino N. Autoimmunity and hypothyroidism. Baillière's Clin Endocrinol Metab 1988; 2: 591–617

46 Girling JC. Thyroid disease and pregnancy. Br J Hosp Med 1996; 56: 316–320

47 Amino N, Tanizawa O, Mori H et al. Aggravation of thyrotoxicosis in early pregnancy and after delivery in Graves' disease. J Clin Endocrinol Metab 1982; 55: 108–112

48 Kimura M, Amino N, Tamaki H et al. Physiologic thyroid activation in normal early pregnancy is induced by circulating hCG. Obstet Gynecol 1990; 75: 775–778

49 Jansson R, Dahlberg PA, Winsa B et al. The postpartum period constitutes an important risk for development of clinical Graves' disease in young women. Acta Endocrinol (Copenh) 1987; 116: 321–325

50 Wing DA, Millar LK, Koonings PP et al. A Comparison of propylthiouracil versus methimazole in the treatment of hyperthyroidism in pregnancy. Am J Obstet Gynecol 1994; 170: 90–95

51 Franklyn JA. The management of hyperthyroidism. N Engl J Med 1994; 330: 1731–1738

52 Burrow GN. Neonatal goitre after maternal propylthiouracil therapy. J Clin Endocrinol 1965; 25: 403–411

53 Cooper DS. Antithyroid drugs. N Engl J Med 1984; 311: 1353–1362

54 Momotani N, Ito K, Hamada N et al. Maternal hyperthyroidism and congenital malformation in the off-spring. Clin Endocrinol 1984; 20: 695–700

55 Van Dijke CP, Heydendael RJ, de Kleine MJ. Methimazole, carbimazole and congenital skin defects. Ann Intern Med 1987; 106: 60–61

56 Mandel SJ, Brent GA, Larsen PR. Review of antithyroid drug use during pregnancy and report of a case of aplasia cutis. Thyroid 1994; 4: 129–133

57 Momotani N, Noh JY, Ishikawa N, Ito K. Effects of propylthiouracil and methimazole on fetal thyroid status in mothers with Graves' hyperthyroidism. J Clin Endocrinol Metab 1997; 82: 3633–3636

58 Rosove MH. Agranulocytosis and anti-thyroid drugs. West J Med 1977; 126: 339–343

59 Amrhein JA, Kenny FM, Ross D. Granulocytopenia, lupus-like syndrome, and other complications of propylthiouracil. J Pediatr 1970; 76: 54–63

60 Okamura K, Ikenoue H, Shiroozu A et al. Re-evaluation of the effects of methylmercaptoimidazole and propylthiouracil in patients with Graves' hyperthyroidism. J Clin Endocrinol Metab 1987; 65: 719–723

61 Momotani N, Noh J, Oyanagi H et al. Antithyroid drug therapy for Graves' disease during pregnancy. Optimal regimen for fetal thyroid status. N Engl J Med 1986; 315: 24–28

62 McCarroll AM, Hutchinson M, McAuley R, Montgomery DA. Long-term assessment of children exposed in-utero to carbimazole. Arch Dis Child 1976; 51: 532–536

63 Burrow GN, Klatskin EH, Genel M. Intellectual development in children whose mothers received propylthiouracil during pregnancy. Yale J Biol Med 1978; 51: 151–156

64 Messer MP, Hauffa BP, Olbricht T. Antithyroid drug and Graves' disease in pregnancy: long term effects on somatic growth, intellectual development and thyroid function of the offspring. Acta Endocrinol 1990; 123: 311–316

65 Momotani N, Yamashita R, Yoshimoto M et al. Recovery from foetal hypothyroidism: evidence for safety of breast feeding while taking propylthiouracil. Clin Endocrinol 1989; 31: 591–595

66 Mestman JH. Hyperthyroidism in pregnancy. Clin Obstet Gynecol 1997; 40: 45–64

67 Davis LE, Lucas MJ, Hankins GDV, Cunningham FG. Thyrotoxicosis complicating pregnancy. Am J Obstet Gynecol 1989; 160: 63–70

68 Bullock JL, Harris RE, Young R. Treatment of thyrotoxicosis during pregnancy with propranolol. Am J Obstet Gynecol 1975; 121: 242–245

69 Mulder JE. Thyroid disease in women. Med Clin North Am 1998; 82: 103–125

70 Millar LK, Wing DA, Leung AS. Low birth weight and pre-eclampsia in pregnancy complicated by hyperthyroidism. Am J Obstet Gynecol 1994; 84: 946–949

71 Editorial. Dangers of iodides in pregnancy. Lancet 1970; 1: 1273–1274

72 Inzucchi SE, Comite F, Burrow GN. Graves' disease and pregnancy. Endocr Pract 1995; 1: 186–192

73 Welch CR, Franklyn JA, Whittle MJ. Fetal thyrotrophin: the best indicator of long term thyroid function after in utero exposure to iodine-131? Fetal Diagn Ther 1998; 13: 176–178

74 Brodsky JB, Cohen EN, Brown Jr BW et al. Surgery during pregnancy and fetal outcome. Am J Obstet Gynecol 1980; 138: 1165–1167

75 Furui T, Imai A, Tamaya T. Successful outcome of pregnancy complicated with thyroidectomy-induced hypoparathyroidism and sudden dyspnoea. A case report. Gynecol Obstet Invest 1993; 35: 57–59

76 Roti E, Minelli R, Gardini E, Braverman LE. Controversies in the treatment of thyrotoxicosis. Adv Endocrinol Metab 1994; 5: 429–460

77 Tan GH, Gharib H, Goellner JR. Management of thyroid nodules in pregnancy. Arch Intern Med 1996; 156: 2317–2320

78 Mazzaferri EL. Evaluation and management of common thyroid disorders in women. Am J Obstet Gynecol 1997; 176: 507–514

79 Gharib H, Goellner JR. Fine-needle aspiration biopsy of the thyroid: an appraisal. Ann Intern Med 1993; 118: 282–289

80 Mazzaferri EL. Management of a solitary thyroid nodule. N Engl J Med 1993; 328: 553–559

81 Choe W, McDougall IR. Thyroid cancer in pregnant women: diagnostic and therapeutic management. Thyroid 1994; 4: 433–435

82 Hod M, Sharony R, Friedman S, Ovadia J. Pregnancy and thyroid carcinoma: a review of incidence, course and prognosis. Obstet Gynecol Surv 1989; 44: 774–779

83 Kobayashi K, Tanaka Y, Ishiguro S, Mori T. Rapidly growing thyroid carcinoma during pregnancy. J Surg Oncol 1994; 55: 61–64

84 Gerstein HC. How common is post-partum thyroiditis: a methodologic overview of the literature. Arch Intern Med 1990; 150: 1397–1400

85 Amino N, Mori H, Iwatani Y et al. High prevalence of transient partum thyrotoxicosis and hypothyroidism. N Engl J Med 1982; 306: 849–852

86 Fung HY, Kologlu M, Collison K et al. Postpartum thyroid dysfunction in Mid Glamorgan. BMJ 1988; 296: 241–244

87 Amino N, Tada H, Hidaka Y. Autoimmune thyroid disease and pregnancy. J Endocrinol Invest 1996; 19: 59–70

88 Gerstein HC. Incidence of postpartum thyroid dysfunction in patients with type I diabetes mellitus. Ann Intern Med 1993; 118: 419–423

89 Stagnaro-Green A. Post-partum thyroiditis: prevalence, etiology, and clinical implications. Thyroid Today 1993; 16: 1–9

90 Walfish PG, Meyerson J, Provias JP et al. Prevalence and characteristics of postpartum thyroid dysfunction: results of a survey from Toronto, Canada. J Endocrinol Invest 1992; 15: 265–272

91 Jansson R, Dahlberg PA, Karlsson FA. Post-partum thyroiditis. Baillière's Clin Endocrinol Metab 1988; 2: 619–635

92 Lazarus JH, Ammari F, Oretti R, Parkes AB, Richards CJ, Harris B. Clinical aspects of recurrent postpartum thyroiditis. Br J Gen Pract 1997; 47: 305–308

93 Othman S, Phillips DI, Parkes AB et al. A long-term follow-up of post-partum thyroiditis. Clin Endocrinol 1990; 32: 559–564

94 Amino N, Tada H, Hikada Y, Crapo LM, Stagnaro-Green A. Therapeutic controversy. screening for post-partum thyroiditis. J Clin Endocrinol Metab 1999; 84: 1813–1921

95 Saddler TW. In: Gardner J. Langman's Medical Embryology, 6th edn. London: Williams & Wilkins, 1990; 312–313

96 Fisher DA, Dussault JH, Sacks J, Chopra IJ. Ontogenesis of hypothalamic-pituitary-thyroid function and metabolism in man, sheep and rat. Recent Prog Horm Res 1977; 33: 59–116

97 Shepard TH. Onset of function in the human fetal thyroid: biochemical and radioautographic studies from organ culture. J Clin Endocrinol Metab 1967; 27: 945–958

98 Thorpe-Beeston JG, Nicolaides K, Snijders JM, Felton CV, McGregor AM. Maturation of the secretion of thyroid hormone and thyroid-stimulating hormone in the fetus. N Engl J Med 1991; 324: 532–536

99 Sinha A, Prabakaran D, Godbole M et al. Thyroid hormones and human fetal brain. In: Thyroid hormones and brain maturation. Recent Advances in Developmental Neuroendocrinology, 1999: 1–14

100 Fisher DA. Endocrinology of fetal development. In: Wilson JD, Foster DW. (eds) Textbook of Endocrinology, 8th edn. Philadelphia: WB Saunders, 1992; 1049–1077

101a Theodoropoulos T, Braverman LE, Vagenakis AG. Iodide-induced hypothyroidism: a potential hazard during perinatal life. Science 1979; 205: 502–503

101b Bajora P, Peek MJ, Fisk NM. Maternal to fetal transfer of thyrotrophin-releasing hormone in-vivo. Am J Obstet Gynecol 1998; 178(2): 264–269

102 Polk DH, Reviczky A, Lam RW, Fisher DA. Thyrotrophin releasing hormone in the ovine fetus: ontogeny and effect of thyroid hormone. Am J Physiol 1991; 260: E53–E58

103 Vulsma T, Gons M, de Vijlder JM. Maternal-fetal transfer of thyroxine in congenital hypothyroidism due to a total organification defect or thyroid dysgenesis. N Engl J Med 1989; 321: 12–16

104 Thorpe-Beeston JG, Nicolaides KH, McGregor AM. Fetal thyroid function. Thyroid 1992; 2: 207–217

105 Karmarkar MG, Prabarkaran D, Godbole M. 5'-monodeiodinase activity in developing human cerebral cortex. Am J Clin Nutr 1993; 57 (Suppl 2): 291S–294S

106a Sinha AK, Pickard MR, Kim KD et al. Perturbation of thyroid hormone homeostasis in the adult and brain function. Acta Med Austriaca 1994; 21: 35–43

106b Chan S, Rathilde S, McCabe CJ et al. Early expression of thyroid hormone deiodinases and receptors in human fetal cerebral cortex. Brain Research 2002: In press

107 Visser TJ, Kaptein E, Terpstra OT, Krenning EP. Deiodination of thyroid hormone in human liver. J Clin Endocrinol Metab 1988; 67: 17–24

108 Oppenheimer JH, Schwartz HL. Molecular basis of thyroid hormone-dependent brain development. Endocr Rev 1997; 18: 462–475

109 Oppenheimer JH, Schwartz HL, Strait KA. The molecular basis of thyroid hormone actions. In: Braverman L, Utiger R. (eds) The Thyroid, 7th edn. Philadelphia: Lippincott-Raven, 1996; 162–184

110 Koenig RJ, Lazar MA, Hodin RA et al. Inhibition of thyroid hormone action by a non-hormone binding c-erbA protein generated by alternate mRNA splicing. Nature 1989; 337: 659–661

111 Lazar MA, Hodin RA, Chin WW. Human carboxy-terminal variant of α-type c-erbA inhibits transactivation by thyroid hormone receptors without binding thyroid hormone. Proc Natl Acad Sci USA 1989; 86: 7771–7774

112 Burris TP, Nawaz Z, Tsai MJ, O'Malley BW. A nuclear hormone receptor-associated protein that inhibits transactivation by thyroid hormone and retinoic acid receptors. Proc Natl Acad Sci USA 1995; 92: 9525–9529

113 Chen JD, Evans RM. A transcriptional co-repressor that interacts with nuclear hormone receptors. Nature 1995; 377: 454–457

114 Onate SA, Tsai SY, Tsai MJ, O'Malley BW. Sequence and characterisation of a co-activator for the steroid hormone receptor superfamily. Science 1995; 270: 1354–1357

115 Lazar MA. Thyroid hormone receptors: multiple forms, multiple possibilities. Endocr Rev 1993; 14: 184–193

116 Munoz A, Bernal J. Biological activities of thyroid hormone receptors. Eur J Endocrinol 1997; 137: 433–445

117 Takeda K, Sakurai A, DeGroot L, Refetoff S. Recessive inheritance of thyroid hormone resistance caused by complete deletion of the protein-encoding region of the thyroid hormone receptor-β gene. J Clin Endocrinol Metab 1992; 74: 49–55

118 Murray M, Zilz N, McCreary N et al. Isolation and characterisation of rat cDNA clones for two distinct thyroid hormone receptor. J Biol Chem 1988; 263: 12770–12777

119 Tata J. Gene expression during metamorphosis: an ideal model for post-embryonic development. Bioessays 1993; 15: 239–248

120 Chan S, Kilby MD. Thyroid hormone and central nervous system development. J Endocrinol 2000; 165: 1–8

121 Gothe S, Wang Z, Ng L et al. Mice devoid of all known thyroid hormone receptors are viable but exhibit disorders of the pituitary-thyroid axis, growth and bone maturation. Genes Development 1999; 13: 1329–1341

122 Polk DH. Diagnosis and management of altered fetal thyroid status. Fetal Drug Ther 1994; 121: 647–662

123 Sack J, Kaiserman I, Siebner R. Maternal–fetal T_4 transfer does not suffice to prevent effects of in utero hypothyroidism. Horm Res 1993; 39: 1–7

124 Legrand J. Thyroid hormone effects on growth and development. In: Henneman G. (ed) Thyroid Hormone Metabolism. New York: Marcel Dekker, 1986; 503–534

125 Rovet JF, Ehrlich RM, Sorbara DL. Neurodevelopment in infants and pre-school children with congenital hypothyroidism: etiological and treatment factors affecting outcome. J Pediatr Psychol 1992; 17: 187–213

126 Noia G, DeSantis M, Tocci A et al. Early prenatal diagnosis and therapy of fetal hypothyroid goiter. Fetal Diagn Ther 1992; 7: 138–143

127 Perelman AH, Johnson RL, Clemons RD et al. Intrauterine diagnosis and treatment of fetal goitrous hypothyroidism. J Clin Endocrinol Metab 1990; 71: 618–621

128 Fisher DA, Dussault JH, Foley Jr TP et al. Screening for congenital hypothyroidism: results of screening one million North American infants. J Pediatr 1979; 94: 700–705

129 Heyerdahl S. Intellectual development in children with congenital hypothyroidism in relation to T4 replacement. J Pediatr 1991; 118: 850–855

130 New England Congenital Collaborative. Elementary school performance of children with congenital hypothyroidism. J Pediatr 1990; 116: 27–32

131 Hetzel BZ. Progression in the prevention and control of iodine deficiency disorders. Lancet 1987; ii: 266

132 Pharoah P, Buttfield IH, Hetzel BS. Neurological damage to the fetus resulting from severe iodine deficiency during pregnancy. Lancet 1971; 1: 308–310

133 Cao XY, Jiang XM, Dou ZH et al. Timing of vulnerability of the brain to iodine deficiency in endemic cretinism. N Engl J Med 1994; 331: 1739–1744

134 Pharoah P, Connolly K, Elkins R, Harding A. Maternal thyroid hormone levels in pregnancy and the subsequent cognitive and motor performance of the children. Clin Endocrinol 1984; 21: 265–270

135 Pop VJ, Kuijpens JL, van Baar AL et al. Low maternal free thyroxine concentrations during early pregnancy are associated with impaired psychomotor development in infancy. Clin Endocrinol 1999; 50: 149–155

136 Man EB, Brown JF, Scrunian SA. Maternal hypothyroxinemia: psychoneurological deficits of progeny. Ann Clin Lab Sci 1991; 21: 227–239

137 Haddow JE, Palomaki GE, Allan WC et al. Maternal thyroid deficiency during pregnancy and subsequent neuropsychological development of the child. N Engl J Med 1999; 341: 549–555

138 Eayrs JT, Taylor SH. The effect of thyroid deficiency induced by methylthiouracil on the maturation of the central nervous system. J Anat 1951; 85: 350–358

139 Eayrs JT, Horne G. The development of cerebral cortex in hypothyroid and starved rats. Anat Rec 1955; 121: 53–61

140 Eayrs JT. The cerebral cortex of normal and hypothyroid rats. Acta Anat (Basel) 1955; 25: 160–183

141 Bernal J, Pekonen F. Ontogenesis of the nuclear 3,5,3'-triiodothyronine receptor in human fetal brain. Endocrinology 1984; 114: 677–679

142 Kilby MD, Gittoes N, McCabe C et al. Expression of thyroid receptor isoforms in the human fetal central nervous system and the effects of intrauterine growth restriction. Clin Endocrinol 2000; 53: 469–477

143 Iskaros J, Pickard M, Evans I, Sinha A, Hardiman P, Ekins R. Thyroid hormone receptor gene expression in first trimester human fetal brain. J Clin Endocrinol Metab 2000; 85: 2620–2623

144 Farsetti A, Robbins J, Nikodem V. Molecular basis of thyroid hormone regulation of myelin basic protein gene expression in rodent brain. J Biol Chem 1991; 266: 23226–23232

145 Farsetti A, Desvergne B, Hallenbeck P, Robbins J, Nokodem VM. Characterisation of myelin basic protein thyroid hormone response element and its function in the context of native and heterologous promoter. J Biol Chem 1992; 267: 15784–15788

146 de Arrieta M, Morte B, Coloma A, Bernal J. The human RC3 gene homolog, NRGN contains a thyroid hormone-responsive element located in the first intron. Endocrinology 1999; 140: 335–343

147 Strait K, Carlson D, Schwartz H, Oppenheimer JH. Transient stimulation of MBP gene expression in differentiating cultured oligodendrocytes: a model for T3-induced brain development. Endocrinology 1997; 138: 635–641

148 Strait KA, Zou L, Oppenheimer JH. β1 isoform-specific regulation of a triiodothyronine-induced gene during cerebellar development. Mol Endocrinol 1992; 6: 1874–1880

149 Hill D. Hormonal control of fetal growth. In: Rodeck CH, Hanson M, Spencer J. (eds) Fetus and Neonate, vol. 3. New York: Cambridge University Press, 1988;

150 Gaffney G. A case-controlled study of intrapartum care, cerebral palsy and perinatal death. BMJ 1994; 308: 743–750

151 Kok JH, den Ouden LA, Verloove-Vanhorick SP, Brand R. Outcome of very preterm small for gestational age infants: the first nine years. Br J Obstet Gynaecol 1998; 105: 162–168

152 Thorpe Beeston G, Nicolaides KH, Snidjers R, et al. Thyroid function in small for gestational age fetuses. Obstet Gynecol 1991; 77: 701–706

153 Klein RZ, Carlton EL, Faix JD. Thyroid function in very low birthweight infants. Clin Endocrinol 1997; 47: 419–421

154 Mallard EC, Rees S, Stringer M, Cock M, Harding R. Effects of chronic placental insufficiency on brain development in fetal sheep. Pediatr Res 1998; 43: 262–270

155 Rooman RP, DuCaju MVL, Op De Beeck L et al. Low thyroxinaemia occurs in the majority of very preterm newborns. Eur J Pediatr 1996; 155: 211–215

156 Van Wassenaer AG, Kok JH, DeVijlder JJ et al. Effects of thyroxine supplementation on neurologic development in infants born at less than 30 weeks gestation. N Engl J Med 1997; 336: 21–26

157 Ares S, Escobar-Morreale HF, Quero J et al. Neonatal hypothyroxinaemia: effects of iodine intake and premature birth. J Clin Endocrinol Metab 1997; 82: 1704–1712

158 Fisher DA. The hypothyroxinemia of prematurity [Editorial]. J Clin Endocrinol Metab 1997; 82: 1701–1703

159 Chowdry P, Scanlon JW, Auerbeck R, Abbassi V. Results of controlled double-blind study of thyroid replacement in very low birth weight premature infants with hypothyroxinaemia. Pediatrics 1984; 73: 301–305

160 Nohr S, Laurberg P. Opposite variations in maternal and neonatal thyroid function induced by iodine supplementation during pregnancy. J Clin Endocrinol Metab 2000; 85: 623–627

161 Burrow GN. The management of thyrotoxicosis in pregnancy. N Engl J Med 1985; 313: 562–565

162 Tamaki H, Amino N, Aozasa M et al. Universal predictive criteria for neonatal overt thyrotoxicosis requiring treatment. Am J Perinatol 1988; 5: 152–158

163 Zakarija M, McKenzie JM, Munro DS. Immunoglobulin G inhibitor of thyroid stimulating antibody is a cause of delay in the onset of neonatal Graves' disease. J Clin Invest 1983; 72: 1352–1356

164 Fisher DA. Neonatal thyroid disease in offspring of women with autoimmune thyroid disease. Thyroid Today 1986; 9: 1–7

165 Perelman AH, Clemons RD. The fetus in maternal hyperthyroidism. Thyroid 1992; 2: 225–228

166 Wenstrom KD, Weiner CP, Williamson RA, Grant SS. Prenatal diagnosis of fetal hyperthyroidism using funipuncture. Obstet Gynecol 1990; 76: 513–517

167 Bruinse HW, Vermeulen-Meiners C, Wit JM. Fetal treatment for thyrotoxicosis in non-thyrotoxic pregnant women. Fetal Ther 1988; 3: 152–157

168 Perreco RP, Bloch CA. Fetal blood sampling in the management of intrauterine thyrotoxicosis. Obstet Gynecol 1990; 76: 509–512

169 Mitsuda N, Tamaki H, Amino N et al. Risk factors for developmental disorders in infants born to women with Graves' disease. Obstet Gynecol 1992; 80: 359–364

170 Davidson KM, Richards DS, Schatz DA. Successful in utero treatment of fetal goiter and hypothyroidism. N Engl J Med 1991; 324: 543–546

171 Belfar HL, Foley Jr TP, Hill LM, Kislak S. Sonographic findings in maternal hyperthyroidism. Fetal hyperthyroidism/fetal goiter. J Ultrasound Med 1991; 10: 281–284

J.B. Sharma

Nutritional anaemia during pregnancy in non-industrialised countries

Anaemia is the commonest medical disorder in pregnancy and has a varied prevalence, aetiology and degree of severity in different populations, being more common in non-industrialised countries.[1] Iron deficiency anaemia is the commonest nutritional deficiency in pregnancy followed by folate deficiency anaemia. Deficiency of vitamin B_{12} is relatively less common in non-industrialised countries.[2,3]

Out of an estimated 150 million deliveries occurring annually in the world, approximately 600,000 women die from the complications of pregnancy and child birth, 35–40 million suffer serious acute complications and 15–20 million have long-term complications.[4,5] Anaemia is responsible for 40–60% of maternal deaths in non-industrialised countries.[6,7] It causes direct, as well as indirect, deaths from cardiac failure, haemorrhage, infection and pre-eclampsia.[6,7] It also increases perinatal mortality and morbidity rates consequent to preterm deliveries, intra-uterine growth retardation, low iron stores, iron deficiency anaemia and cognitive and affective dysfunction in the infant.[8,9]

PHYSIOLOGICAL CHANGES IN PREGNANCY AND ERYTHROPOIESIS

The physiological changes occurring in pregnancy are shown in Table 1.[10] The various factors required for erythropoiesis are proteins (erythropoietin), minerals (iron), trace elements (including zinc, cobalt and copper), vitamins (particularly folic acid, vitamin B_{12} [cyanocobalamin], vitamin C, pyridoxine (B_6) and riboflavin), and hormones (androgens and thyroxine).[10,11]

In addition to the common deficiencies of iron and folate, there is a growing body of evidence to implicate vitamin A (important for cell growth and differentiation, maintenance of epithelial integrity and normal immune

Dr J.B. Sharma MD DNB MRCOG MFFP MAMS, Associate Professor, Department of Obstetrics and Gynaecology, Maulana Azad Medical College, and Associated Lok Nayak Hospital, New Delhi 110002, India

Table 1 Physiological changes in blood indices during pregnancy[10]

Characteristic	Normal adult women	32–34 weeks' gestation	Increased/decreased
Plasma volume (ml)	2600	3850	1250 increase
Red cell mass (ml)	1400	1640 (without iron supplement) 1800 (with iron supplement)	
Haemoglobin (g/dl)	12–14	11–12	Decreased
Red blood cells ($10^6/mm^3$)	4–5	3-4–5	Decreased
Packed cell volume	0.36–0.44	0.32–0.36	Decreased
Mean corpuscular volume (fl)	80–97	70–95	Decreased
Mean corpuscular haemoglobin (pg)	27–33	26–31	Decreased
Mean corpuscular haemoglobin concentration (%)	32–36	30–35	Decreased
Serum iron (μg/dl)	60–175	60–75	Decreased
Total iron binding capacity (μg/100 ml)	300–350	350–400	Increased
Percentage saturation (%)	30	15	Decreased
Requirements of iron (mg/day)	1.5–2.0	4.0	Increased

Mean corpuscular haemoglobin = MCH
Mean corpuscular haemoglobin concentration = MCHC
Mean corpuscular volume = MCV
Packed cell volume = PCV
Total iron binding capacity = TIBC

function) and zinc (important in protein synthesis and nucleic acid metabolism) in nutritional anaemias.[12,13] Protein energy malnutrition can also cause anaemia.

DEFINITION OF ANAEMIA IN PREGNANCY

Anaemia is a condition of low circulating haemoglobin (Hb) in which the Hb concentration has fallen below a threshold lying at two standard deviations below the median of a healthy population of the same age, sex and stage of pregnancy.[14] This, however, is a statistical definition and is not easily understandable and practical. The WHO definition for diagnosis of anaemia in pregnancy is a Hb concentration of less than 11 g/dl (7.45 mmol/l) and a haematocrit of less than 0.33, although CDC (Centers for Disease Control, USA) proposes a cut-off point of 10.5 g/dl during the second trimester.[15]

SEVERITY OF ANAEMIA

The Indian Council of Medical Research (ICMR) uses four categories of anaemia depending upon the haemoglobin levels in their studies as summarized in Table 2 (ICMR unpublished data). Some authors use Hb levels of 9–11 g/dl in mild anaemia.

Table 2 The Indian Council of Medical Research categories of anaemia

Category	Anaemia severity	Haemoglobin level (g/dl)
1	Mild	10.0–10.9
2	Moderate	7.0–10.0
3	Severe	< 7.0
4	Very severe (decompensated)	< 4.0

PREVALENCE OF ANAEMIA IN PREGNANCY

The overall prevalence of anaemia is estimated to be about 40% of the world's population. The prevalence is 35% for non-pregnant women and 51% for pregnant women globally, and tends to be 3–4 times higher in non-industrialised than in industrialised countries.[16] Anaemia affects about 18% of women during pregnancy in industrialised countries while in non-industrialised countries prevalence varies between 35–75% with the average being 56%.[17] The prevalence of anaemia in pregnancy globally and in South-East Asian countries is shown in Table 3. The prevalence is very high in Central-Asia also, as shown by demographic and health surveys in Kazakhistan and Uzbekistan where the incidence was 80%.[18] Nearly half of the global total number of anaemic women live in the Indian sub-continent and, in India alone, the prevalence of anaemia during pregnancy may be as high as 88%.[18–21] In India, anaemia antedates pregnancy, is aggravated by increased requirements during pregnancy and blood loss at delivery, infections in the antenatal and postnatal periods, and the early advent of next pregnancy perpetuates it.[8] The prevalence of anaemia in different parts of India is shown in Table 4.[19–21] The relative prevalence of mild, moderate, and severe anaemia are 13%, 57%, and 12%, respectively, in India (ICMR unpublished data).

Table 3 Prevalence of anaemia globally and in South-East Asian countries[16,17]

Region	No. of countries Total	Included	Year	Prevalence (%)
Europe	50	4	1992	20
Americas	36	3	1992	29
Western Pacific	26	3	1992	39
Africa	46	14	1992	44
Eastern Mediterranean	22	14	1992	61
South-East Asia	11	3	1992	79
Bangladesh			1993	74
Bhutan			1995	68
India			1993	87.5
Indonesia			1995	51.0
Maldives			1995	68.0
Myanmar			1995	52.0
Nepal			1996	40.0
Sri Lanka			1995	40.0
Thailand			1995	13.4

Table 4 Prevalence of anaemia in pregnant women in different parts of India[18-21]

Place	No. of pregnant women	Normal (Hb > 11 g/dl)	Mild anaemia (Hb 10–10.9 g/dl)	Moderate anaemia (Hb 7–10 g/dl)	Severe anaemia (Hb < 7 g/dl)	Overall prevalence of anaemia
Dibrugarh (Assam)	525	45 (8.6)	52(9.9)	371 (70.7)	57 (10.8)	91.4
Gaya (Bihar)	446	71 (15.9)	21 (4.7)	267 (59.9)	87 (19.5)	84.1
Lakhimpur Kheri (U.P.)	593	122 (20.6)	88 (14.8)	325 (54.8)	58 (9.8)	79.4
Mandi (H.P.)	507	198 (39.0)	157 (31.0)	142 (28.0)	10 (2.0)	61.0
Srinagar (J&K)	498	16 (3.2)	26 (5.2)	370 (74.3)	86 (17.3)	96.8
Overall of above studies	2569	452 (17.6)	344 (13.4)	1475 (57.4)	298 (11.6)	82.4
Patiala (Punjab) (Sarin 1995)[20]	4752	661 (13.9)	1345 (28.3) Mild and moderate		2661 (56.0)	86.1
Delhi (Sharma & Malhotra, unpublished data 1999)	443	123 (27.7)	214 (48.3)	79 (17.8)	37 (6.09)	72.3
Mumbai (Brabin et al 1998)[21]	1032	440 (31.2)	197 (19.1)	352 (34.1)	33 (3.2)	79.6
Tamilnadu (Abel et al 1999)[18]	1032	440 (31.2)	197 (19.1)	352 (34.1)	33 (3.2)	68.8

Percentages in parentheses.
Prevalence of first five places: ICMR unpublished data (1996–1999).

IRON DEFICIENCY ANAEMIA

Iron deficiency anaemia (IDA) is the commonest type of anaemia in pregnancy. Iron nutritional status depends on long-term iron balance and is favoured by ingestion of adequate amounts of iron in the diet (native or fortified) or through iron supplementation as shown in Table 5.[4,7] The balance is adversely affected by the loss of iron through intestinal mucosal turnover and excretion, skin desquamation, menstruation and lactation.[4,7] The pathological causes of iron loss are mainly from excessive menstrual flow, worm infestations (hookworm and schistosomiasis), bleeding from THE gastrointestinal tract from ulcerations, haemorrhoids, diarrhoea and other occult blood losses.[22] As in a healthy state, iron loss is fairly constant; the balance is dependent on the regulation of iron absorption. Iron homeostasis is maintained in the short-term by increased absorption of iron in deficiency situations and the amount of bio-available iron present in food is important in the long-term.[23] Food iron is present in most diets in a proportion of 6 mg/1000 calories and is made of two different pools – haem and non-haem iron. The haem iron pool includes all food containing iron as haem molecules such as animal blood, flesh and viscera.[23] Its absorption in normal women is 15–30%, but it can increase to 50% in the iron deficiency state and can reduce to 5–8% with an excessive haem diet.[23] Its absorption is usually not affected by inhibitors. The non-haem iron pool is made of all other sources of iron such as cereals, seeds, vegetables, milk and eggs.[23] Its absorption can be increased by enhancers (haem, proteins, ascorbic acid and fermentation) and decreased by inhibitors (phytic acid, fibres, calcium, tannins, tea, coffee, chocolate and herbal infusion).[24] On the basis of type of food, iron bio-availability can be characterised as follows.[25]

Table 5 Factors affecting the iron status of a pregnant woman[18]

Iron absorption	Iron loss
Dietary iron (haem and non-haem)	**Physiological factors**
	Basal losses from desquamation from
Enhancers of absorption	**intestines and skin**
Haem iron	Menstruation
Proteins	Delivery
Meat	Lactation
Ascorbic acid	**Pathological factors**
Fermentation	Hookworm and other helminths
Ferrous iron	Haemorrhage from GIT
Gastric acidity	Allergies
Alcohol	Occult blood losses
Low iron stores	
Increased erythropoietic activity	
(high altitude, haemolysis, bleeding)	
Inhibitors of iron absorption	
Phytates	
Calcium	
Tannins	
Tea and coffee	
Herbal drinks	
Fortified iron supplements	

Iron bio-availability

Low bio-availability diet

This is a simple, routine diet of cereals, roots and tubers such as maize, rice, beans, whole wheat flour and sorghum with negligible amounts of meat, fish and ascorbic acid. In non-industrialised countries, a very low bio-available iron, vegetarian diet low in ascorbic acid and high in biological proteins composed almost entirely of cereals is consumed with excess of inhibitors of iron absorption (phytates); thus, absorption may be as low as 3–4%.[24]

Intermediate bio-availability diet

Diets in this category are mainly comprised of cereals, roots or tubers, but include some animal foods like meat, fish and ascorbic acid which increase the iron absorption.

High bio-availability diet

This is a varied diet rich in meat, poultry, fish and foods with a generous amount of ascorbic acid, as found in industrialised countries.

Iron requirements in pregnancy

Total iron requirements in pregnancy vary with the body weight of the mother and the size and maturity of the fetus. In an average pregnancy, the requirements are:[24] (i) basal iron, 280 mg; (ii) expansion of red cell mass, 570 mg; (iii) for transfer to the fetus, 200–350 mg; (iv) for placenta, 50–150 mg; and (v) blood loss at delivery, 100–250 mg.

After deducting iron conserved by amenorrhoea (240–480 mg), an additional 500–600 mg of iron is required in pregnancy or 4–6 mg/day of absorbed iron, which can only be achieved by mobilizing iron stores in addition to maximum iron absorption from the diet.[25] The requirements are 4 mg/day (2.5 mg/day in early pregnancy, 5.5 mg/day from weeks 20–32, and 6-8 mg/day from week 32 onwards).[5,10]

As absorption is less than 10% (3–4% in low bio-availability diets), for a minimum of 4–6 mg absorption, at least 40–60 mg of iron should be available in the diet. Diet alone can not supply such amounts of iron in non-industrialised countries making iron supplementation a necessity in all pregnant women.[10]

Causes of high prevalence of iron deficiency anaemia

Dietary habits

As discussed above, a low bio-availability diet is consumed by most pregnant women resulting in both iron and protein deficiency. Even women who are non-vegetarian eat meat sparingly due to its high cost, precluding any important source of haem iron from the diet. Poverty compounded by population explosion in non-industrialised countries, especially in the Indian subcontinent, is mainly responsible for low iron in the diet. We found a very high incidence (72.3%) of iron deficiency anaemia in our hospital catering to poor Hindu and Muslim pregnant women of Delhi. The incidence was higher in both Hindu vegetarian and Muslim (Halal meat eaters) women, while the incidence was lower in Hindu non-vegetarian women (Jhatka meat eaters).

This could be due to loss of significant amounts of haem blood from the animal in Halal meat where the animal is slaughtered by cutting its carotid artery and bled to death (Sharma and Soni 1999, unpublished data). Food fadism, in which the pregnant woman is not allowed to eat many types of food in pregnancy due to customs and rituals, is another important cause of low iron diet. Pica, a common problem, is the ingestion of various substances having no dietary value and is a manifestation of iron deficiency. These substances worsen iron deficiency by replacing iron-rich foods.[10] Pregnancy complications like hyperemesis can further reduce intake of iron.

Defective iron absorption due to intestinal infections
The prevalence of worm infestation, amoebiasis and giardiasis is up to 40% and is a significant cause of abnormal metabolism and anaemia.[26] Increased iron loss due to frequent pregnancies, menorrhagia, hookworm infestations, schistosomiasis, chronic malaria, excessive sweating and blood loss from the gut due to haemorrhoids are important causes of anaemia in pregnancy.[10,26]

Multiple pregnancies
Most women enter pregnancy with little or no iron reserve, which is further compounded by repeated and closely spaced pregnancies and prolonged periods of lactation.[8,10,18] Most deliveries in rural and tribal areas are home confinements conducted by traditional birth attendants who do not practice active management of third stage making them more prone to postpartum haemorrhage.[10]

Prevention of iron deficiency

Prevention of iron deficiency is a worth-while aim.

Prophylaxis of non-pregnant women
Girls in India are deprived of good diet from their childhood as compared to their brothers and thus enter adulthood with malnutrition, anaemia or low iron stores. As most women start their pregnancy with anaemia or low iron stores, prevention should start even before pregnancy. It is difficult to treat a severely iron deficient woman and provide for increased fetal needs through oral iron supplementation during the relatively short period of pregnancy. As a public health approach, prolonged oral supplementation beginning before the woman becomes pregnant may be a better strategy to benefit the majority of the population.[27] Iron supplementation by 30 doses administered weekly over 7 months was as effective as 90 doses consumed daily for 3 months.[27] Hence, women of child-bearing age in non-industrialised countries should receive a 2–4 months' course of 60 mg of iron daily.[25] In addition, concomitant use of folate will prevent neural tube defects in the new-born.

Iron supplementation during pregnancy
Whether routine iron supplementation be given or not is debatable in Western countries. However, there is no doubt that it has to be given to all pregnant women in non-industrialised countries.[28,29] The WHO recommended universal oral iron supplementation for pregnant women (60 mg of elemental iron and 250 µg of folic acid once or twice daily) through the primary health care system for 6 months in pregnancy in countries with a prevalence of anaemia < 40% and for an

additional 3 months post-partum in countries where the prevalence is > 40%.[25] The studies show improved maternal and perinatal outcome by routine iron supplementation during pregnancy.[30,31] As nutritional anaemia is a major heath problem, the Government of India initiated the National Nutritional Anaemia Prophylaxis Programme (NNAPP) in 1970 to provide iron and folic acid supplements to pregnant women, lactating women, family planning acceptor women and children 1–11 years old.[19] However, the problem still continued unabated. The Indian Council of Medical Research (ICMR) evaluated the programme in 1989 and found that it was not well implemented, there were more anaemic women than targeted, the actual beneficiaries were far less than shown in records, the quality of tablets was found to be very poor and there was no difference in Hb levels between beneficiary and non-beneficiary groups.[19] The Ministry of Health, Government of India has now recommended intake of 100 mg of elemental iron with 500 µg of folic acid (folifer) in the second half of pregnancy for a period of at least 100 days. Some recent studies have shown that weekly or twice-weekly iron supplements also give equally good results with better patient compliance.[32] Even two injections of iron dextran (250 mg each) given intramuscularly at 4-week intervals along with tetanus toxoid injection have been recommended for better compliance and adequate results.[33] In a recent study we found significantly higher serum ferritin levels with 3 doses of monthly 250 mg intramuscular iron dextran (Imferon) than with 100 tablets of 100 mg oral elemental iron given daily (Sharma and Jain 2002, unpublished data). However, there is no consensus about this treatment in practice.

Treatment of hookworm infestation
As worm infestation is very common and given the safety of the deworming drugs, oral antihelminthic treatment can also be given to pregnant and lactating women. Single albendazole (400 mg) or mebendazole (100 mg) doses twice daily for 3 days with iron supplementation should be given to all anaemic pregnant women in the second and third trimesters for better results.[26,34] Change in defecation habits and avoidance of walking barefooted helps in the control of hookworm infestation.

Improvement of dietary habits and improving the bio-availability of food iron
Those pregnant should eat foods rich in iron (jaggery, green leafy vegetables like spinach, mustard leaves, turnip green, cereals, and sprouted pulses) and cook their food in iron utensils.[10] They should be taught the importance of eating a nutritious diet rather than leftovers as is customary in rural areas. Avoiding tea and coffee intake also helps. Too much cooking should be avoided.

Social services
Improvement of sanitation, personal hygiene, better education and alleviation of poverty are not easy tasks and need political will also. It has been seen that, with higher female literacy rates and proper allocation of resources, Sri Lanka and Kerala state in South India have achieved some of the non-industrialised world's best rates of life expectancy, infant mortality and maternal mortality despite their low per capita income.[35,36] Female education results in improved nutritional status and higher contraceptive acceptance: 'if you educate a man you educate a person, but if you educate a woman you educate the whole family'.

Food fortification

Iron fortification of foods is a preventive measure that aims at improving and sustaining iron nutrition on a permanent basis. Many countries fortify a cereal product or fish sauce, sugar or curry powder with iron compounds like ferrous sulphate, ferrous gluconate, ferrous fumarate, ferrous succinate or chelated iron compounds such as bovine haemoglobin concentrate and Fe-Na-EDTA.[37] Even common salt, which is often fortified successfully with iodine in deficient areas, can be fortified with iron as has been successfully done in various South-East Asian and Latin American countries[37,38]. Production of iron fortified salt on a commercial scale has been approved by the Government of India and is in the process of manufacture.

Effects of anaemia on pregnancy

Maternal effects

Mild anaemia may not have any effect on pregnancy and labour except that the mother will have low iron stores and may become moderately-to-severely anaemic in subsequent pregnancies. Moderate anaemia may cause increased weakness, lack of energy, fatigue and poor work performance. Severe anaemia, however, is associated with poor outcome. The woman may have palpitations, tachycardia, breathlessness, increased cardiac output leading on to cardiac stress which can cause decompensation and cardiac failure which may be fatal.[6,10,19,26] Increased incidence of pre-term labour (28.2%), pre-eclampsia (31.2%) and sepsis have been associated with anaemia.[8,19,39]

Fetal effects

Irrespective of maternal iron stores, the fetus tends to obtain iron from maternal transferrin, which is trapped in the placenta and which, in turn, removes and actively transports iron to the fetus. Gradually, however, such fetuses tend to have decreased iron stores due to depletion of maternal stores. Adverse perinatal outcome in the form of pre-term and small-for-gestational-age babies and increased perinatal mortality rates have been observed in the neonates of anaemic mothers.[8,39] Iron supplementation to the mother during pregnancy improves perinatal outcome. Mean weight, Apgar score and haemoglobin level 3 months after birth were significantly greater in babies of the supplemented group than the placebo group.[40,41]

Clinical features of iron deficiency anaemia

Symptoms

There may be no symptoms, especially in mild and moderate anaemia. Patient may complain of feelings of weakness, exhaustion and lassitude, indigestion and loss of appetite. Palpitation, dyspnoea, giddiness, oedema and, rarely, generalised anasarca and even congestive cardiac failure can occur in severe cases.

There may be symptoms of original conditions causing anaemia-like bleeding from the rectum.

Signs

There may be no signs especially in mild anaemia. There may be pallor, glossitis and stomatitis. Patients may have oedema due to hypoproteinaemia. Soft systolic murmur can be heard in the mitral area due to hyperdynamic circulation. It must be differentiated from pathological murmur of heart diseases. There can be fine crepitations at bases of lungs due to congestion.

Diagnosis

Haemoglobin estimation is the most practical method of diagnosis as it is cost-effective and can be easily performed by a trained technician. The Taliquist's method of Hb estimation has simplicity and easy applicability, but is not very accurate. The copper sulphate method also has many drawbacks and is not reliable. Sahli's method is reliable and accurate when done by experts, and is the most commonly used method, although the cyanomethaemoglobin method appears to be the most accurate.[42] Although the WHO cut-off point of 11 g/dl Hb appears to be too high by the standard of non-industrialised world countries, it should be used by all to help in comparison of data from one centre to another.[20,42]

Peripheral blood film is another bed-side indicator for diagnosis of anaemia which will also differentiate between iron deficiency anaemia, megaloblastic anaemia and haemolytic anaemia. In iron deficiency anaemia, there is microcytosis, hypochromia, anisocytosis, poikilocytosis and target cells in the blood film.

Mean corpuscular volume (MCV < 80 fl), mean corpuscular haemoglobin (MCH < 27 pg) and mean corpuscular haemoglobin concentration (MCHC) are all low in iron deficiency anaemia. Their measurement, normal range and difference in findings in iron deficiency anaemia and thalassaemia are shown in Table 6. Modern analysers also give red cell distribution width (RDW) which is an index of anisocytosis. It is generally elevated in most nutritional anaemias. In populations with high prevalence of the beta-thalassaemia trait, RDW along with other parameters help in differentiating iron deficiency anaemia from the beta-thalassaemia trait being high in the former and normal in the latter. Iron deficiency anaemia must be differentiated from thalassaemia.[10,29]

Serum ferritin estimation gives better picture of stored iron. It is a high molecular weight glycoprotein circulating in plasma in concentrations of

Table 6 Red cell indices in iron deficiency and thalassaemia[10,11]

Characteristics	Calculation	Normal range	Iron deficiency	Thalassaemia
MCV* (fl)	PCV/RBC	75–96	Reduced	Very reduced
MCH (pg)	Hb/RBC	27–33	Reduced	Very reduced
MCHC** (g/dl)	Hb/PCV	32–35	Reduced	Normal or slightly reduced
HbF (%)	HbF/HbA × 100	< 2%	Normal	Raised
HbA$_2$ (%)	HbA$_2$/HbA × 100	2–3%	Normal or reduced	Raised
FEP (µg/dl)		< 35	> 50	Normal
Red cell width			High	Normal

*Mean corpuscular volume (MCV) is the first to get reduced and is the most sensitive indicator of iron deficiency.
**Mean corpuscular haemoglobin concentration (MCHC) is reduced in more severe cases of iron depletion.

Table 7 Categorization of women using haemoglobin and ferritin estimations[18]

Categories	Serum ferritin (μg/l)	Haemoglobin (g/dl)	Diagnosis
Category I	> 12	> 11	Normal, iron deficiency excluded
Category II	< 12	> 11	Storage iron depletion
Category III	< 12	< 11	Iron deficiency anaemia
Category IV	> 12	< 11	Other causes of anaemia

15–300 μg/l. A level below 12 μg/l is taken to indicate iron deficiency. It is stable, unaffected by recent iron intake, reflects iron stores accurately, and is the first abnormal laboratory test in iron deficiency. Hb and ferritin estimations have been used clinically to categorise the patients into normal and abnormal for iron stores as shown in Table 7.[18]

Transferrin saturation can be estimated from serum iron and total iron binding capacity (TIBC). A reduced transferrin saturation indicates a deficient iron supply to the tissues and is the second measurement to be affected in the development of iron deficiency. Serum iron varies from 60–120 μg/dl while TIBC is 300–350 μg/dl (increased to 300–400 μg/dl in pregnancy). Serum iron of less than 60 μg/dl, a TIBC of more than 350 μg/dl and transferrin saturation of less than 15% indicates deficiency of iron during pregnancy.[10,29]

Free erythrocyte protoporphyrin (FEP) is the third estimation of iron status rising with defective iron supply to the developing red cells and takes 2–3 weeks to become abnormal after depletion of iron stores. It also helps in differentiation between iron deficiency anaemia and thalassaemia (Table 6). Using Hb, ferritin, transferrin saturation and FEP, woman can be allocated to one of the following categories:[10] (i) depleted stores (decreased ferritin only); (ii) iron deficiency but no anaemia (decreased ferritin, transferrin saturation and increased FEP); or (iii) anaemia with iron depletion (decreased Hb, red cell indices, ferritin and transferrin saturation, increased TIBC and FEP).

Serum transferrin receptor appears to be a specific and sensitive marker of iron deficiency in pregnancy.[43] Its levels are increased in iron deficiency anaemia. Although it is the best indicator, its facilities are not yet routinely available.[43]

Bone marrow examination by staining with potassium ferrocyanate to see characteristic blue granules of stainable iron in erythroblasts is the most accurate method for iron stores, but is not practical in most cases as the test is invasive. Bone marrow examination is only indicated in cases where there is no response to iron therapy after 4 weeks or for diagnosis of Kala-azar or in suspected aplastic anaemia.[10,29]

As worm infestations are common causes of anaemia, stool examination for ova and cysts should be done consecutively for 3 days in all cases. In areas where schistosomiasis is prevalent, urine examination for occult blood and schistosomes should be performed. As malaria is an important cause of anaemia, peripheral blood film should be examined for malarial parasites in all the cases.[44] Significant bacteriuria should also be ruled out. If the clinical scenario demands, other tests can be done, such as sputum examination and chest X-ray for pulmonary tuberculosis (abdominal shielding should be done), renal function tests in suspected renal disease, and serum proteins in hypoproteinaemia.[10]

Table 8 Percentage and amount of iron in common iron preparations[18,25]

Preparation	Molecular iron (mg/tablet)	Percentage of iron (%)	Elemental iron (mg/tablet)
Ferrous sulphate	300	20	60
Ferrous sulphate, anhydrous	200	37	74
Ferrous sulphate, desiccated	200	30	60
Ferrous fumarate	200	33	66
Ferrous gluconate	300	12	36

Management of iron deficiency anaemia

In non-industrialised countries, it is common to see patients of moderate and severe anaemia late in pregnancy. They have had nil or inadequate antenatal care and did not take iron supplements in pregnancy. If the woman presents in mid-trimester or early third trimester, oral iron is started. Innumerable iron preparations are available on the market with each pharmaceutical company making claims of its superiority over other brands. There is no scientific evidence that any one brand is superior to others. The slow release preparations claimed to cause least side-effects are expensive and are probably not absorbed optimally. It is better to start simple preparations routinely available in the hospital. In non-industrialised countries, one must not forget the cost factor. If the woman has to buy the tablet, she will most probably not take it. One should try to prescribe, as far as possible, the iron preparation available free of cost in the local hospital and should convince the woman of the importance of taking iron preparations. The percentage and amount of iron in some commonly used iron compounds is shown in Table 8.[18,25]

Although for prophylaxis the Government of India, Ministry of Health recommends 100 mg of elemental iron with 0.5 mg folic acid, for treatment more than 180 mg of elemental iron per day is required. Three tablets of ferrous sulphate (available free of cost in most Indian hospitals) per day are required. This may cause increased incidence of side-effects and some recommend 120 mg elemental iron per day, which is more suitable for supplementation rather than treatment.[45] There is no need to give expensive preparations. One needs to change a brand only when the patient can not tolerate a particular brand of iron. Unfortunately, many patients do not take iron and compliance is thus poor.[15,18,19] Various methods have been used to increase compliance, such as giving the drug less frequently initially, followed by daily later, with increase in compliance.[42] The patient's response to 180 mg elemental iron per day is fast with significant increase in reticulocyte count within 5–10 days of start of oral therapy. Hb rises from 0.3 g to 1.0 g per week. Addition of folic acid, but not vitamin B_{12}, helps in improving the results in supervised supplementation.[46] Unsupervised supplementation did not give good results.[47] Up to 10% of women may have side-effects with oral iron in the form of gastrointestinal symptoms (such as nausea, vomiting, constipation, abdominal cramping and diarrhoea) which are dose-related. The treatment of choice is to reduce the dose or to give the tablet with meals. If this does not work, another preparation (carbonyl iron or haemoglobin preparations) may be better tolerated.

Treatment with large doses is continued until the blood parameters become normal, after which a maintenance dose of one tablet daily should be continued for at least three months after delivery. The disadvantages of oral therapy are intolerance to medication, unpredictable absorption and non-compliance. Haemoglobin concentration may be restored with the therapeutic dose, but replenishing the iron stores requires continuation of treatment for longer periods.[10,29,47] Indications of response to therapy are feeling of well-being, improved look and better appetite. Haematologically, there is reticulo-cyte response in 5–10 days with a rise in Hb concentration and haematocrit subsequently.[47,48] If there is no significant clinical or haematological improvement within 3 weeks, diagnostic re-evaluation is needed.[10,29] Reasons of failure to respond to oral therapy are inaccurate diagnosis (non-iron deficiency microcytic anaemia, such as thalassaemia, pyridoxine deficiency and lead poisoning), non-compliance, continuous loss of blood through hook worm infestation or bleeding haemorrhoids, co-existing infection, faulty iron absorption and concomitant folate deficiency.[10,29,48]

Parenteral iron therapy

It has no advantage over oral iron if the latter is well tolerated. It is rarely indicated in patients who can not absorb iron, are non-compliant or develop serious side-effects with oral iron which can not be corrected by simple means. The main advantage of parenteral therapy is the certainty of its administration to correct the Hb deficit and to build up the iron stores. The rise in Hb concentration is the same as with oral iron (up to 1 g per week). Parenteral iron is available as iron dextran (Imferon) which can be given intramuscularly or intravenously and iron sorbitol citrate (Jectofer) which can only be given intramuscularly. Jectofer plus contains folic acid and vitamin B_{12} along with elemental iron.[10,29] Iron deficit is calculated as:

Elemental iron needed (mg) =
$$\text{(Normal Hb — Patient's Hb)} \times \text{Weight (kg)} \times 2.21 + 1000 \qquad \text{Eq. 1}$$

For a woman weighing 65 kg with a Hb concentration of 7 g/dl, the iron requirement will be $(14 - 7) \times 65 \times 2.21 + 1000 = 2005$ mg. Another simple method is to give 250 mg elemental iron for each g of Hb below normal and will be $250 \times 7.0 = 1750$ mg in this example. Another 50% should be added for replenishment of iron stores. Intravenous infusion should be given in the hospital setting by a doctor to patients with no known allergy. Injection epinephrine, hydrocortisone and oxygen should be available in the event of anaphylactic reaction.[49] Iron dextran (Imferon) is diluted in normal saline or 5% dextrose and given slowly initially.[10] If there is no reaction, it can be given faster. If the calculated dose is more than 2500 mg, it should be given in 2 doses on two consecutive days.[10] One should look for any reaction in the form of chest pain, rigor, chills, fall in blood pressure, dyspnoea, haemolysis and anaphylactic reaction.[10] For any such reaction, infusion should be stopped and anti-histaminics, corticoids and epinephrine given.

The intramuscular route is more popular and is associated with less side-effects. Oral iron should be stopped before giving iron sorbitol as it is associated with toxic reactions such as headache, nausea and vomiting if given simultaneously with oral iron.[10,29,48] Initially, a test dose of 50 mg of iron dextran or iron sorbitol citrate is given followed by 100 mg daily or alternate days by deep intramuscular injection with a thick needle on the outer quadrant of the buttock using a 'Z' technique to prevent dark staining of the skin. The disadvantages of intramuscular iron include pain, skin discoloration, abscess formation, reaction in the form of nausea, vomiting, headache, fever, lymphadenopathy, allergic reactions and, rarely, anaphylaxis. There is, however, no extra risk of incurring malignancy at the injection site in man as was reported in rats.[11]

Blood transfusion is very rarely required in patients with severe anaemia beyond 36 weeks, associated infection, to replenish blood loss due to ante-partum or post-partum haemorrhage and in patients not responding to oral or parenteral iron therapy.[10,29] Packed cells are preferred for transfusion. Blood transfusion can cause transfusion reaction, precipitated preterm labour and, rarely, overloading of the heart.[10,29] Exchange transfusion is used very rarely in some centres for patients with severe anaemia.[10]

Antenatal care

The antenatal management is like any other case, but more frequent visits are required. One should be vigilant to detect and manage complications of anaemia, such as heart failure or preterm labour, as early as possible. Fetal monitoring for growth and well-being should be done as these fetuses tend to be small. Prognosis is good if anaemia is detected and treated in time. Management of a case of severe anaemia is given in Figure 1.[10]

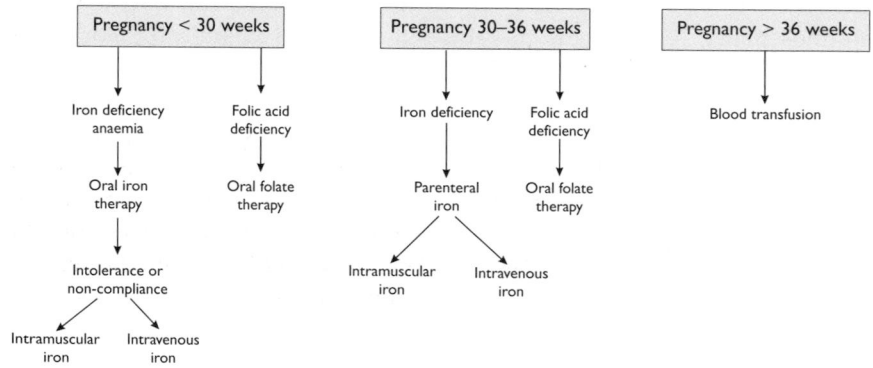

Fig. 1 Summary protocol of severe anaemia in pregnancy.[10]

Management of labour in anaemic patient

In the first stage, the patient should be in a comfortable position. Sedation and pain relief should be given. Oxygen should be kept ready and is given in dyspnoea. In cases of preterm labour, betamimetics and steroids should be given with caution to avoid the risk of pulmonary oedema. Digitalisation may be required in cardiac failure due to severe anaemia. The aim is to deliver the baby vaginally. Antibiotic prophylaxis is preferred. The second stage is the most stressful, when the patient can go into cardiac failure. A tendency for prolongation of the second stage can be curtailed by forceps. Active management of the third stage should be done except in very severe anaemia for fear of cardiac failure. However, any post-partum haemorrhage must be energetically treated as these patients tolerate bleeding very poorly.[10,29]

During puerperium, the mother should have adequate rest; iron and folate therapy should be continued for at least 3 months. Any infection must be energetically treated. Puerperal sepsis, failing lactation, subinvolution of uterus and thrombo-embolism are more common in these patients and should be carefully watched for.[10,29] Maternal mortality in severe anaemia can occur in the last trimester, during labour, immediately after delivery and during puerperium due to cardiac failure or pulmonary embolism.[10,29] The anaemic patient must use an effective method of contraception and should not conceive for at least 2 years giving time for iron stores to recover. Sterilization is preferred if the family is completed. If there is no history of menorrhagia, an intra-uterine device can be inserted. Barrier methods can be safely given, but their higher failure rate is a disadvantage[10,29]

The baby should be seen by the attending paediatrician as the baby is likely to be preterm, small for gestational age and more susceptible to infection and anaemia.[5,6] There is increased perinatal mortality and morbidity and low iron stores in such babies.[30,40]

MEGALOBLASTIC ANAEMIAS IN PREGNANCY

In megaloblastic anaemia, DNA replication is affected. There is derangement of red cell maturation with production of abnormal precursors known as megaloblasts which can be due to deficiency of folate or vitamin B_{12}.[10,11]

Folate deficiency megaloblastic anaemia

Folic acid together with iron assumes a central role in nutrition during pregnancy. It is reduced first to dihydrofolic acid and then to tetrahydrofolic acid (folinic acid) which is required for cell growth and division.[11] Its requirements are increased in pregnancy to meet the needs of the fetus, the placenta, uterine hypertrophy and expanded maternal red cell mass.[11,50,51] The prevalence of folic acid deficiency anaemia may complicate up to one-third of all pregnancies in non-industrialised countries and is more common in multiple pregnancies.[10,11,52]

Causes
Folate deficiency is mainly due to dietary lack and poverty linked to insufficient consumption of green vegetables, fruits, liver and kidney together with prolonged cooking which destroys the vitamin.[11,52] Unlike vitamin B_{12}, body reserves of folate are low. Pregnancy symptoms like nausea, vomiting and anorexia further aggravate the condition. Intake of goat's milk, which is poor in folic acid, could be the cause in rural areas. There can be poor uptake due to malabsorption syndrome and gastrointestinal diseases. Abnormally high demands are needed in multiple pregnancy, hookworm infestations, bleeding haemorrhoids, haemolytic conditions (such as chronic malaria) and other infections.[10,26,44,52] Antifolate medication such as anti-epileptic drugs (phenytoin, primidone), pyrimethamine and trimethoprim can cause deficiency.[53] Folate

requirements are increased by iron therapy in iron deficiency anaemia due to hyperplastic marrow. Hence, iron and folate should be given together for better results.[46]

Clinical features

Patients may be asymptomatic. The mother may be unwell with loss of appetite. There may be vomiting, diarrhoea or unexplained fever. There may be pallor, bleeding spots in the skin, hepatosplenomegaly and polyneuropathy.

Effects on pregnancy

There is increased incidence of abortion, growth retardation, abruptio placentae and pre-eclampsia in folate deficiency in some, but not all, studies.[11,52] Folate supplements during pregnancy have resulted in increased birth weight in cases of malnutrition.[54]

Effects on fetus

Neural tube defects can be prevented in most cases by periconceptional folic acid in dosage of 0.4 mg/day in low-risk cases and 5 mg/day in high-risk women.[55,56] Incidence of neural tube defects is very high in India and periconceptional folate supplementation is strongly recommended in all cases.[57,58] There is some evidence that the incidence of abortion, premature babies, small-for-date babies and folate deficiency in the neonates is higher in babies born to mothers with folate deficiency.[10,11,52]

Investigations

Laboratory findings consist of a fall in Hb concentration to generally <10 g/dl, MCV > 96 fl, MCH > 33 pg, and normal MCHC.[10,11] There is macrocytic anaemia with hypersegmentation of neutrophils, neutropenia and thrombocytopenia on peripheral blood film. A combination of low serum folate (< 3 ng/ml) and red cell folate (< 150 ng/ml) is diagnostic of folic acid deficiency. Serum iron is usually normal or high.[10,11] Increased formiminoglutamic acid (FIGLU) in urine following a loading dose of histidine is found in folate deficiency, but the test is rarely done these days.[11] Serum lactic dehydrogenase (LDH) and homocysteine levels are elevated in folate deficiency. The deoxyuridine suppression test helps in differentiating between folate and vitamin B_{12} deficiency. Bone marrow will show a megaloblastic picture, but is rarely required.

Prophylaxis

The WHO recommends a daily folate intake of 800 µg in the antenatal period and 600 µg during lactation.[15] However, 300–500 µg present in most iron preparations is enough for prophylaxis.[11,52] Pregnant women should eat more green vegetables (e.g. spinach and broccoli) and offal (e.g. liver and kidneys). Folate is destroyed by cooking. Even food fortification with folic acid is recommended and is already in use in Western countries.[55]

Treatment

Treatment of established folic acid deficiency is by giving 5 mg oral folate per day which should be continued for at least 4 weeks in puerperium. Response is indicated by a fall in LDH levels within 3–4 days and an increase in reticulocyte count in 5–8 days. Parenteral folate is only indicated in gastric intolerance or late in pregnancy. Vitamin C is helpful. Associated iron deficiency should be corrected by iron therapy. Blood transfusion is rarely required in severe anaemia.

Megaloblastic anaemia due to vitamin B$_{12}$ deficiency

Vitamin B$_{12}$ is synthesized by certain micro-organisms. Animals and humans are ultimately dependent on this source. It is found in meat, fish, eggs and milk but not in plants, and is not destroyed by cooking. The average daily diet contains 5–30 μg of vitamin B$_{12}$ of which 1–5 μg is absorbed.

Pernicious anaemia caused by lack of intrinsic factor resulting in lack of absorption of vitamin B$_{12}$ is rare during pregnancy as it usually causes infertility. Women with gastrectomy and ileal disease and resection can have vitamin B$_{12}$ deficiency. Acquired vitamin B$_{12}$ deficiency causing megaloblastic anaemia is also uncommon, as the daily requirement of vitamin B$_{12}$ is only 3.0 μg during pregnancy which is easily met with a normal diet.[15] Only vegans who do not eat any animal-derived substance may have a deficiency of vitamin B$_{12}$ and they should have their diet supplemented during pregnancy. Infestations with *Diphyllobothrium latum* in some countries can cause megaloblastic anaemia due to competitive utilization of ingested vitamin B$_{12}$ by the parasite. Several studies have revealed that, in the non-industrialised world, multiple nutritional deficiencies are frequent and pregnant women may manifest deficiencies of folate and vitamin B$_{12}$ in addition to iron deficiency.[59]

Investigations
Findings are the same as in folate deficiency. Vitamin B$_{12}$ levels are lower in blood (< 90 μg/l). Serum methyl malonic acid is elevated in vitamin B$_{12}$ deficiency. Serum homocysteine is elevated in both folate and vitamin B$_{12}$ deficiency. The deoxyuridine suppression test can differentiate between vitamin B$_{12}$ and folate deficiency. Schilling Test is done to diagnose pernicious anaemia.

Treatment
Parenteral cyanocobalamin (250 μg) is given intramuscularly every month.

DIMORPHIC ANAEMIA

The common picture seen in tropical countries is deficiency of both iron and folate with findings of both anaemias but dominance of one. Blood film may show macrocytic or normocytic, normochromic or hypochromic pictures. Bone marrow is usually megaloblastic. Treatment is prescription of both folic acid and iron in therapeutic doses. Women who are pregnant should eat more green vegetables and fruits and too much cooking should be avoided.

CONCLUSIONS

The control of nutritional anaemias seems a distant, but achievable goal and requires better organisation of primary health services, strengthening of the supplementation programmes, nutritional education, maternal education and development of suitable fortificants. The medical community especially the obstetricians, nutritionists, haematologists, internists, paediatricians and community medicine specialists should get actively involved in combating nutritional deficiency anaemias. Joint action is also required by governments, non-governmental organizations, WHO, UNICEF, INACG, ICMR, National Institutes of Health, medical and biomedical scientists, agriculturists and planners to channel the available resources and meticulously implementing the existing programmes to achieve the goal of safe motherhood, which is the right of every woman and a vision for the new millennium.

KEY POINTS FOR CLINICAL PRACTICE

- Nutritional deficiency anaemias during pregnancy continue to be major health problems in all non-industrialised countries, contributing significantly to high maternal and perinatal mortality and morbidity rates.

- Maternal education can decrease the incidence of anaemias by:
  (a) increasing awareness of the need for better nutritional status
  (b) offering contraceptive advice to decrease the number of pregnancies and
  (c) highlighting the benefits of increasing the spacing interval between pregnancies – as is evident from the examples of Sri Lanka and the Kerala state in India.[35,36]

ACKNOWLEDGEMENTS

I am grateful to the World Health Organization, Geneva, the Indian Council of Medical Research, New Delhi, the National Institutes of Health, Hyderabad, India, Prof. S.K. Sood, Consultant Haematologist, Sir Ganga Ram Hospital, New Delhi and Dr Sangeeta Sharma, Paediatrician and Head, LRS Institute, New Dellhi for their help in the preparation of this article.

References

1 Schwartz WJ, Thurnau GR. Iron deficiency anaemia in pregnancy. Clin Obstet Gynecol 1995; 38: 443–454
2 Diejomaeoh FME, Abdulaziz A, Adekile AD. Anemia in pregnancy. Int J Gynecol Obstet 1999; 65: 299–301
3 Kulier R, de Onis M, Gulmezoglu AM, Villar J. Nutritional interventions for the prevention of maternal morbidity. Int J Gynecol Obstet 1998; 63: 231–246
4. World Health Organization. Revised 1990 Estimates of Maternal Mortality. WHO/FRH/MSM/96.1. Geneva: WHO, 1996
5 Turmen T, AbouZahr C. Safe motherhood. Int J Gynecol Obstet 1994; 46: 145–153.
6 Bhatt R. Maternal mortality in India – FOGSI-WHO Study. J Obstet Gynecol Ind 1997; 47: 207–214
7 Viteri FE. The consequences of iron deficiency and anaemia in pregnancy. Adv Exp Med Biol 1994; 352: 127–139

8 Prema K, Neela KS, Ramalakshmi BA. Anaemia and adverse obstetric outcome. Nutr Rep Int 1981; 23: 637–643

9 Lozoff B, Jimenez E, Wolf AW. Long term developmental outcome of infants with iron deficiency. N Engl J Med 1992; 325: 687–694

10 Sharma JB. Medical complications in pregnancy. In: Sharma JB. (ed) The Obstetric Protocol, 1st edn. Delhi: Jaypee Brothers, 1998; 78–98

11 Letsky E. Blood volume, haematinics, anaemia. In: de Swiet M. (ed) Medical Disorders in Obstetric Practice, 3rd edn. Oxford: Blackwell, 1995; 33–60

12 Ross AC, Gardner EM. The function of vitamin A in cellular growth and differentiation and its role during pregnancy and lactation. Adv Exp Med Biol 1994; 352: 187–200

13 Prasad AS. Zinc deficiency in women, infants and children. J Am Coll Nutr 1996; 15: 113–120

14 WHO/UNICEF/UNU. Indicators for Assessing Iron Deficiency and Strategies for its Prevention: WHO draft. Geneva: WHO, 1996

15 World Health Organization. Report of a WHO Group of Experts on Nutritional Anaemias. Technical report series no. 503. Geneva: WHO, 1972

16 World Health Organization. The Prevalence of Anaemia in Women: A Tabulation of Available Information. Geneva: WHO, 1992

17 World Health Organization. WHO Global Database. Geneva: WHO, 1997

18 Abel R, Rajaratnam J, Sampathkumar V. Anemia in Pregnancy. Impact of Iron, Deworming and IEC, RUSHA Dept. Tamil Nadu: CMC Vellore, 1999

19 Indian Council of Medical Research. Evaluation of the National Nutritional Anaemia Prophylaxis Programme. Task Force Study. New Delhi: ICMR, 1989

20 Sarin AR. Severe anemia of pregnancy, recent experience. Int J Gynecol Obstet 1995; 50 (Suppl. 2): S45–S49

21 Brabin L, Nicholas S, Gogate A, Karande A. High prevalence of anaemia among women in Mumbai, India. Food Nutr Bull 1998; 19: 205–209

22 Bothwell TH, Charlton RW, Cook JD, Finch CA. Iron Metabolism in Man. Oxford: Blackwell, 1979

23 Hulten LE, Gramatkovski A, Gleerup A, Hallberg L. Iron absorption from the whole diet. Relation to meal composition, iron requirements and iron stores. Eur J Clin Nutr 1995; 49: 794–808

24 Hallberg L, Bjorn-Rassmussen E. Determination of iron absorption from whole diet. A new tool model using two radiation isotopes given as haem and non-haem iron. Scand J Haematol 1972; 9: 193–197

25 Stoltzfus R, Dreyfuss ML. Guidelines for the use of iron supplements to prevent and treat iron deficiency anaemia. Geneva: INACG, WHO, UNICEF, 1998

26 Sharma JB, Arora BS, Kumar S, Goel S, Dhamija A. Helminth and protozoan intestinal infections: an important cause for anaemia in pregnant women in Delhi, India. J Obstet Gynecol Ind 2001: 51(6): 58–61

27 Sloan NL, Jordan EA, Winikoff B. Does Iron Supplementation make a Difference? Mother Care Project, 15 Arlington, VA, USA. 1992

28 Milman N, Bergholt T, Byg KE, Eriksen L, Graudal N. Iron status and iron balance during pregnancy. A critical re-appraisal of iron supplementation. Acta Obstet Gynecol Scand 1999; 78: 749–757

29 Sharma JB. Iron deficiency anaemia in pregnancy-still a major cause of maternal mortality and morbidity in India. Obs Gynae Today 1999; IV: 693–701.

30 Rusia UN, Madan N, Agarwal N, Sikka M, Sood SK. Effect of maternal iron deficiency anaemia on fetal outcome. Ind J Pathol Microbiol 1995; 38: 273–279

31 Mahomed K. Routine iron supplementation during pregnancy. (Cochrane Review) The Cochrane Library, Issue 2. Oxford; Update Software, 1998

32 Ridwan E, Schultink W, Dillon D, Gross R. Effects of weekly iron supplementation on pregnant Indonesian women are similar to those of daily supplementation. Am J Clin Nutr 1996; 63: 884–890

33 Bhatt RV. Poor iron compliance – the way out. J Obstet Gynecol Ind 1997; 47: 185–190

34 Atukorala T, deSilva LD, Dechering WH, Dassenaeike TS, Perera RS. Evaluation of effectiveness of iron folate supplementation and antihelminthic therapy against anemia in pregnancy-study in the plantation sector of Sri Lanka. Am J Clin Nutr 1994; 60: 286–292

35 Franke RW, Chais BH. Kerala state, India: radical reform as development. Int J Health Serv 1992; 22: 139–156

36 Pitrof R, Johanson R. Safe motherhood-an achievable and worthwhile aim. In: Studd J. (ed) Progress in Obstetrics and Gynaecology, vol. 12. Edinburgh: Churchill Livingstone, 1996; 47–57

37 Viteri FE, Alvarez E, Batres R et al. Fortification of sugar with Na Fe EDTA improves iron status in semi-rural populations in Guatemala. Am J Clin Nutr 1995; 61: 1153–1163

38 Narasinga-Rao BS, Vijaysarthy C. Fortification of common salt with iron: effect on stability and bio-availability. Am J Clin Nutr 1975; 26: 1395–1401

39 Lops VR, Hunter LP, Dixon LR. Anemia in pregnancy. Am Fam Physician 1995; 51: 1189–1197

40 Agarwal KN, Agarwal DK, Mishra KP. Impact of anaemia prophylaxis in pregnancy on maternal haemoglobin, serum ferritin and birth weight. Ind J Med Res 1991; 94: 277–280

41 Preziosi P, Prual A, Galan P, Daouda H, Boureima H, Hereberg S. Effect of iron supplementation on the iron status of pregnant women: consequences for newborns. Am J Clin Nutr 1997; 66: 1178–1182

42 Bhatt RV. Anaemias in pregnancy: early diagnosis and treatment. J Ind Med Assoc 1995; 93: 80–82

43 Rusia U, Flowers N, Madan N, Agarwal N, Sood SK, Sikka M. Serum transferrin receptor levels in the evaluation of iron deficiency in the neonate. Acta Paediatr Jpn 1996; 38: 455–459

44 Verhoeff FH, Brabin BJ, Chimsuki L, Kazembe P, Broadhead RL. An analysis of the determinants of anaemia in pregnant women in rural Malawi – a basis for action. Ann Trop Med Parasitol 1999; 93: 119–133

45 Indian Council of Medical Research. Field Supplementation Trial in Pregnant Women with 60 mg, 120 mg and 180 mg of Iron with 500 mcg of Folic Acid. New Delhi: ICMR, 1992

46 Sood SK, Ramachandran K, Mathur M et al. WHO sponsored collaborative studies on nutritional anaemias in India. The effects of supplemental oral iron administration to pregnant women. Q J Med 1975; 44: 241–258

47 Sood SK, Madan N, Rusia U, Sharma S. Nutritional anaemia in pregnancy and its health implications with special reference to India. Ann Natl Acad Med Sci 1989; 25: 41–50

48 Prema K. Anaemia in pregnancy. In: Ratnam SS, Rao KB, Arulkumaran S. (eds) Obstetrics and Gynaecology, vol. I. Madras: Orient Longman, 1992; 42–53

49 Basu SK. Administration of iron-dextran complex by continuous intravenous infusion. J Obstet Gynaecol Br Cwlth 1965; 72: 253–258

50 Blot I, Papiernik E, Kaltwasser JP, Werner E, Techernia G. Influence of routine administration of folic acid and iron during pregnancy. Gynecol Obstet Invest 1981; 12: 294–304

51 Swain RA, St Clair L. The role of folic acid in deficiency status and prevention of disease. J Fam Pract 1997; 44: 138–144

52 Chanarin I. Folate deficiency in pregnancy. In: Chanarin I (ed). The Megaloblastic Anaemias, 3rd edn. Oxford: Blackwell, 1990: 140–148

53 Dansky LV, Rosenblatt DS, Andermann E. Mechanism of teratogenesis: folic acid and antiepileptic therapy. Neurology 1992; 42 (Suppl. 5): 32–42

54 Iyengar L. Folic acid requirements of Indian pregnant women. Am J Obstet Gynecol 1971; 111: 13–16

55 Wald N, Bower C. Folic acid and the prevention of neural tube defects. BMJ 1995; 310: 1019–1020

56 Ledward RS. Drugs in pregnancy. In Studd J. (ed) Progress in Obstetrics and Gynaecology, vol. 12. Edinburgh: Churchill Livingstone, 1996; 19–46

57 Sharma JB, Gulati N. Potential relationship between Dengue fever and neural tube defects in a northern district of India. Int J Gynecol Obstet 1992; 39: 291–294

58 Sharma JB, Newman MRB, Smith RJ. Folic acid, pernicious anaemia and prevention of neural tube defects [letter]. Lancet 1994; 343: 923

59 Basu RN, Sood SK, Ramachandran K, Mathur M, Ramalingaswami V. Etiopathogenesis of nutritional anaemia in pregnancy. A therapeutic approach. Am J. Clin Nutr 1973; 26: 591–595

Miguel Oliveira da Silva

8

Teenage sexual behaviour and pregnancy: trends and determinants

One in four girls in the world becomes a mother before the age of 19 years.[1] Every year, in excess of 14 million teenage girls give birth to a child, most of these young mothers living in non-industrialised countries. Teenage pregnancy is universal in all known cultures past and present, but it has achieved an unprecedented magnitude in some industrialised countries since the 1970s.

Teenage pregnancy, if not controlled for socio-economic pressures or when under routine prenatal care, is associated with adverse perinatal outcomes such as low birth weight, preterm delivery, and small for gestational age births.[2,3] With the exception of the very young adolescents (less than 16 years of age), in itself teenage pregnancy is not biologically harmful. Full-term teenage pregnancy may even constitute the only known primary protective factor against breast cancer.[4] Teenage pregnancy is a public health problem: high teenage pregnancy rates are linked to high levels of social exclusion and poor knowledge about, and access to, contraception.

The myth of the homogeneous family unit (as if a past, golden, and untroubled age ever did exist) is now in question: the structural diversity of present families – single parent households, blended families (never married, divorced, step-families), adopted and extended families – have social patterns that often do not match with legal definitions of the 'family'.

Adolescent motherhood, usually associated with these unorthodox families, challenges the prevailing concept of 'family' as well as the moral norms; some seeing it as another part of an on-going 'moral decay' (sex before marriage, birth out of wedlock, and divorce).

In most Western countries, teenage pregnancy rates and birth rates declined during the 1990s. This was not the case in the UK[5] and Portugal. When comparing these two countries, the UK leads the teenage mother live-birth rate

Dr Miguel Oliveira da Silva MD PhD, Departments of Obstetrics-Gynaecology & Preventive Medicine, Consultant at Hospital de Santa Maria, Professor of Lisbon Faculty of Medicine, Calçada de Palma de Baixo 4–8B, 1600 Lisboa, Portugal

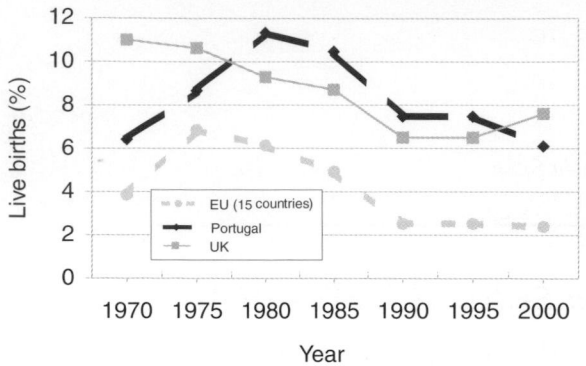

Fig. 1 Numbers of teenage mothers by area and year (data from Eurostat).

among the fifteen member states of the European Union (Fig. 1). If one considers only live-births to under 17-year-olds (the younger adolescents certainly being those at higher global risk), in 1998 Portugal had the highest EU adolescent live-birth rate (Fig. 2). Teenage pregnancy has been identified as a target for health improvement by successive British and Portuguese governments.

The reasons for the discrepancy between the UK and other European countries are complicated and exceed the remit of this article. It is likely that the main differences lie in the risk factors for early intercourse and the interaction of some of the following factors: (i) age at first intercourse; (ii) safe and successful contraceptive use; (iii) intercourse frequency and number of partners; (iv) access to emergency contraception; and (v) termination of pregnancy policy. Some of these issues are discussed below.

In the US, teenage pregnancy, abortion and birth rates are decreasing among teens of all races and ages.[6] However, in the US, the teenage birth rate is still one of the highest in the industrialised world, declining less steeply than in

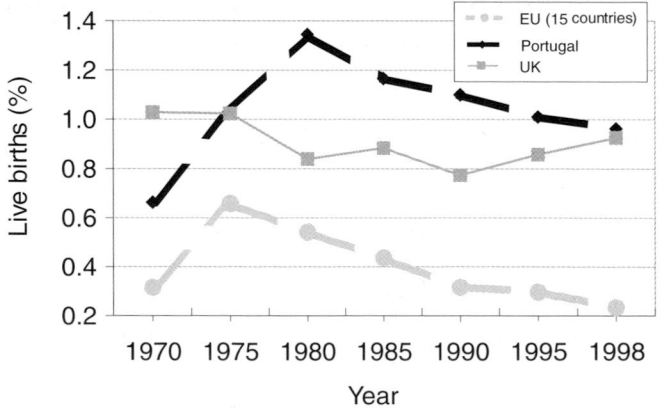

Fig. 2 Numbers of teenage mothers aged under 17 years by area and year (data from Eurostat).

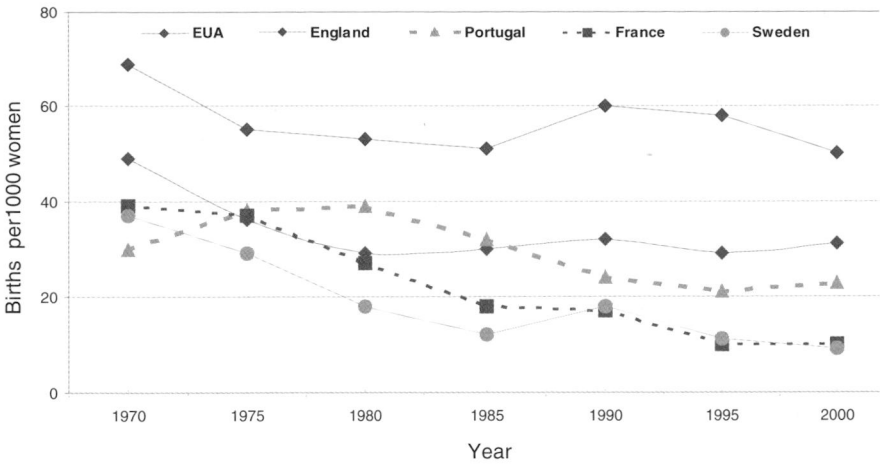

Fig. 3 Teenage birth rates in 15–19-year-old mothers.

other industrialised countries between 1970 and 2000, if Portugal and the UK are excluded.

By 2000, the teenage birth rate in the US had declined to 49 per 1000, as compared with late 1990s rates of 7 and 9 in Sweden and France, 31 in Great Britain and 23 in Portugal (Fig. 3).

The decline in teenage pregnancy in recent years may be due not only to increased and improved contraceptive use, but also to a general decrease in sexual intercourse (stabilisation of first intercourse age, less frequency and less partners). This final hypothesis needs further investigation to determine whether sexual drive and related emotions are natural, pre-cultural components of human experience, or if they are culturally produced and shaped – perhaps even susceptible to intentional change implying sexual desires can be significantly shaped by social conventions and circumstances.[7]

There are, however, some indisputable facts: in all countries, poorer and less-educated women are more likely to have a child during adolescence.[8] Indeed, from the 1980s to the 1990s, the difference in teenage pregnancy rates between more affluent and more deprived areas widened.[9]

DATA LIMITATIONS AND MISCONCEPTIONS

Age group heterogeneity and ethnic particularities

When discussing teenage sexual behaviour and pregnancy, it is important to be aware of the psychological, emotional and biological heterogeneity that exists in this age group. The sexual activity and rates of pregnancy in 15-year-old girls can not be compared with those of their 18- or 19-year-old peers. Frequently, demographic and health statistics are collected and analyzed for the entire 15–19-year-old age group rather than per age year.

Another important issue is the ethnic background of adolescent pregnant girls. Although in some countries (e.g. Portugal) it is illegal to collect such data (in order to avoid any racist discrimination), from a strictly medical and biological point of view it is desirable to know the different determinants and trends of adolescent sexuality and pregnancy rates according to their ethnic provenance.

Refining existing indicators, allowing where necessary and possible, desegregation by sex, age, urban/rural areas and specific ethnic groups is an important task for both health authorities and statisticians. For instance, if we consider two teenage pregnant girls, both 15 years old, their social and psychological burden can be different according to their socio-economic background and racial origin (see 'Planned teenage pregnancy' below).

In The Netherlands, one of the countries with the smallest relative number of teenage mothers (a teenage birth rate 9 times less than in the US), most teenage mothers come from various non-white ethnic groups (Turkey, Antilles, Surinam), reflecting cultural differences.[10] A similar trend is found in the UK, Portugal and even the US, where the most significant teenage birth rates are found amongst the Hispanics and Afro-Americans.

A reliable and robust indicator

In adolescents, several reproductive health indicators are frequently quoted when comparing the situation in different countries. Not all indicators, however, address the same issue: some are biased toward the 15–19-year-old age group, and by having more than one pregnancy, abortion or delivery per woman in that age group. Some such indicators and their definitions are given below.

Adolescent child-bearing
The proportion (percentage) of mothers (women having a child) before the age of 20 years, among all women having had children. This rate is influenced by the above mentioned factors.

Teenage pregnancies
The proportion (percentage) of births (deliveries) to women of less than 20 years among all deliveries. This measure is culture-dependent and influenced by social trends. It will be lower if the trend is towards postponing the age of having the first child, i.e. an increase in older mothers as now happens in most industrialised countries.

Teenage birth rate
The number of births to women less than 20 years of age per 1000 women aged less than 20 years. Frequently, this indicator is restricted to the 15–19-year-old sub-group, as if this sub-group was representative of the whole teenage birth rate. This is the most accurate, robust and reliable of the three indicators.

THE ACTUAL SITUATION

Age at first intercourse

Apparently, the age of first intercourse varies little in industrialised countries.[11] If this is so and assuming that sexual frequency and number of partners are not very different from country to country (see below), data on contraceptive use and termination of pregnancy are more important than data on sexual activity in explaining variations in levels of adolescent pregnancy, abortion and child-bearing among adolescents in different industrialised countries

In Britain, a recent study concluded that there appears to have been a stabilisation in the proportion of girls having first heterosexual intercourse before the age of 16 years, although a longer term study is needed to confirm this[12] – cultural changes are not linear nor unidirectional and a shift is probably now under way, the result of which is likely to be an uneasy and unpredictable synthesis.

An interaction of biological and socio-cultural pressures could explain this observation: (i) menarche anticipation (stabilised in industrialised countries for 50 years, pointing to the existence of a baseline that neither choice nor policy can alter); (ii) a more permissive and open atmosphere to discuss and talk about 'sex' and sexuality – including sexual behaviour, sexual orientation and object choice; and (iii) receiving mixed messages from an adult world in which the mass media bombards adolescents with sexual messages. The role of pornography in shaping sexuality also needs to be considered in this context.

When asking about age at first intercourse, it is important to avoid conflicting definitions, bearing in mind that the meaning of 'sex' appears to be culturally and individually determined.[13] Several authors have demonstrated the wide-spread confusion about the definition of 'having sex' or 'sexual relationships' and illustrated the need for greater specificity in future investigations of sexual behaviour.[14]

Precise knowledge of the actual sexual practices of adolescents is crucial for effective clinical practice, and awareness of the problems of ambiguity in the use of sexual terms must guide practitioners' interview procedures in order to avoid misconceptions and erroneous, biased data.

Safe use of contraceptives at first intercourse

US women report a lower proportion of contraceptive use at first intercourse (75%) than in France (89%), Great Britain (79%), Sweden (78%) and The Netherlands (75%).[10,11] However, quantitative data about contraceptive use, although necessary, are limited; in fact, such data say nothing about the adequacy, efficacy, and safety against pregnancy and sexual transmitted infections (STIs) of contraceptive use. If, as it appears, the use of the 'pill' by teenage women is lower in the US than in other industrialised countries,[11] it makes sense to question to what extent current differences in pregnancy, abortion and birth rates are associated with variations in the contraceptive quality (chosen methods, and patient satisfaction with services and practices).

This is an important and often overlooked issue. Contrary to common belief, in the UK, 91% of teenagers who become pregnant had at least one consultation in the year before pregnancy with their general practitioner (GP), 71.3% of them explicitly consulting for contraceptive advice (65% for the 'pill' and 11% for emergency contraception).[15]

Easy access to cheap and safe contraceptives (including emergency contraception) is a critical issue.

Inconsistencies in contraceptive use[16] are due to either a consultation that did not work (e.g. poor empathy between patient and doctor or patient and nurse, absence of confidentiality) or an inappropriate choice of contraceptive method. The GP needs to be aware of the complex issues that may need addressing with teenagers who consult frequently,[15] so as not to miss opportunities for correct contraceptive advice and use.

In the UK, over 70% of consultations for contraception occur in general practice, so the role of primary care services in preventing teenage pregnancies is crucial. It appears that practices with a female or young doctor had significantly lower teenage pregnancy rates than those without such doctors.[17] In some countries, adolescents are still cared for by paediatricians, although sometimes paediatricians are uncomfortable with the issues of sexuality and contraception, for which they have not been specifically trained.[18]

Compared with teenagers in other countries, US teenagers are less likely to use contraceptives, especially the more effective hormonal methods.[19] In general, in the US, the price of contraceptives is much higher than in the EU which could explain some of these differences.

Intercourse frequency and number of sexual partners

Data on intercourse frequency and multiple sexual partners (in both sexes) are usually very difficult to collect and have a low level of reliability, even in anonymous surveys. Although these two issues do not necessarily go together (in fact there is no correlation between the frequency of sex in a doubly monogamous sexual relationship and having multiple sexual partners), they are important when analysing the prevention and treatment of STIs as well as promoting safe sexual activity. Some data suggest that the higher level of multiple sexual partnerships among American teenagers may help to explain higher rates of STIs.[11]

Teenage abortion

Every year, according to the World Health Organization (WHO), an estimated 2.0–2.4 million adolescents resort to abortion.[19]. In comparison with adults, adolescents are more likely to: (i) delay the abortion; (ii) resort to unskilled persons to perform the abortion; (iii) use dangerous methods; and (iv) present late when complications arise.

Sometimes, an unplanned pregnancy is a consequence of giving up taking the 'pill': the side-effects from hormonal contraceptives can lead to poor adherence and unplanned pregnancies.[21]

A similar proportion of teenage pregnancies are resolved through abortion in the US as in other countries; however, because of their high pregnancy rate, US teenagers have the highest abortion rate.[11] In the UK, around 35% of teenage pregnancies result in a termination,[5] compared with 40% in the US and The Netherlands.[10]. In The Netherlands, when girls become pregnant against their wishes, they can decide to have an abortion which is performed confidentially and without charge.[10] In Portugal, Spain and Ireland, most abortions are illegal and, therefore, clandestine. According to a recent survey, 0.5% of high-school Portuguese teenagers have had an intentional termination of pregnancy.[22]

Finally, little is known about the role of the male partner, i.e. do differences between partners with respect to race or ethnicity increase the likelihood that a pregnancy will end in abortion or a non-marital birth?[23]

One of the more difficult areas to cover is that of those adolescents that left school before finishing their education. They are those that most need education (sexual education included), but they do not attend the school any more. The mass media could fill an enormous gap here, as the average child spends almost as much time watching television as with parents or in school.

PREVENTING STI AND UNPLANNED TEENAGE PREGNANCY

School sexual education

Sexual and reproductive health and the rights of adolescents are unquestionably part of society's values in industrialised countries. This means: (i) excellent sexual information at school; (ii) the right to discuss and have ready access to safe and successful contraceptive methods (including emergency contraception; (iii) the promotion of responsible sexual behaviour; and (iv) encouraging the adoption of health promoting values, attitudes, and norms.[24]

Some argue that the role of schools as agents of change (i.e. promoting the adoption and maintenance of behaviours that prevent pregnancy and STI) should not be exaggerated.[24] Conversely, a recent study in Britain underlined an increase in the importance of school in the sexual education of the young, particularly men.[12]

An important issue that needs particular care is the quality of sexual life, i.e. the perceived quality of emotional feelings and sexual intercourse. To know more about this and to be aware of contraception and sexual satisfaction is at least as important as knowing the contraceptive prevalence rates by age group.

According to data based on reported behaviour (and, therefore, susceptible to biases associated with recall and veracity), British women are twice as likely as men to regret their first experience of intercourse and 3 times as likely to report being the less willing partner.[12]

Sexual education deals not only with pregnancy prevention. It is essential to support teenagers when they are pregnant or after becoming mothers.

There is no reason for young mothers to be compelled to discontinue their schooling or education. A place at a day nursery has to be available at an affordable price. Flexible education arrangements should be designed for pregnant teenagers in school. Teenage mothers should be encouraged to return to education.

Abstinence promotion

Abstinence promotion is clearly a part of comprehensive sexual education, but is not synonymous with the complete sexual education.

The on-going discussion in the US about the virtue of abstinence-only education programmes, with the Bush administration intending to add $33 million to federal spending on these programmes, points to the extremely narrow definition of abstinence-only education. In the US, 35% of all local school districts that have policies on sex education require that abstinence be taught as the only appropriate option for unmarried people.[6] Abstinence-only education is now twice that originally contemplated by the 1996 law.[25]

Besides the political aspects, the ethical issues have to be considered: is it the role of a teacher or a medical practitioner to convince unmarried, young people not to have sex – and how young is young?

Some authors look at this problem as a triumph of ideology over science,[26] claiming that ideology should not interfere with science and that abstinence interventions exclusively emphasise values, attitudes and skills for postponing sexual intercourse.

The avoidance of intercourse as a means of preventing STIs and undesired pregnancy is a vital issue for public health, but any normative and repressive sexual education has to be rejected. Legal measures encouraging marriage are part of an erroneous conception that accepts that one citizen should be able to impose judgement on another, claiming to know what is good for the person.

Postponing sexual activity is not only a particular school task but mainly the natural outcome of family-life events: children whose parents talk to them about sexual matters and provide sexual education at home are more likely than others to postpone sexual activity.[27] In the US, the National Longitudinal Survey of Adolescent Health found that teenagers whose parents made it clear that they expected them not to have sex were much less likely to have had sex than their peers.[28]

Additional research on the long-term effectiveness of abstinence inter-ventions is needed to explore further the social determinants of sexuality and the social and behavioural determinants associated with postponing sexual intercourse, differentiating between those with or without previous sexual activity. Consideration is also needed of non-intercourse sexual behaviour and how this fits with moral codes.

So far, there is little evidence to suggest that abstinence-only programmes are likely to be effective in convincing many of the sexually active young to abstain from sex. Probably, these programmes may have their greatest impact on those that have not yet initiated sexual activity.[29]

PLANNED TEENAGE PREGNANCY – IS IT POSSIBLE AND ETHICAL TO PREVENT IT?

Some teenage mothers (mainly among the poorer and/or ethnic minorities) specifically want to become pregnant. They see no reason not to get pregnant as they have low expectations of employment and low self-esteem.[30] It is documented that females who later became pregnant were also more likely to have a poorer sense of personal worth – the so-called internal poverty'.[31]

On the other hand, teenage sex may reflect 'acting out' behaviour for deeper problems related to low self-esteem, poor relationships and lack of vision and goals. These are problems that endorsing safer sex cannot solve. Only major social and political modifications to every day life expectations can work here.

As recently documented in Britain, early motherhood is more strongly associated with educational level (low educational attainment) than with family background.[12]

The perceived desire of the male partner for pregnancy, particularly among low-income and ethnic groups, as well as the adolescents' ambivalence, should also be taken into consideration.[32,33] Gender differences (even if we accept them as a socially constructed category distinct from the biological 'sex') must be addressed when planning effective pregnancy prevention interventions.[34] As Stevens-Simon underlines, re-phrasing the questions used to assess childbearing intention would make teenagers' responses more useful and reliable – teenagers often become pregnant because they lack a firm commitment not to do so.[35]

KEY POINTS FOR CLINICAL PRACTICE

- Sexual abstinence programmes should be articulated (not opposed) with on-going contraception and STI prevention programmes and methods, including condom education and emergency contraception. The modern (progestogen only) emergency contraception supply in the EU changes between countries. In some countries, it is sold as an over-the-counter drug (e.g. UK and Portugal), and can be available free in some schools (UK and France), hospitals and heath centres. Practical difficulties in access still persist, however, including elevated prices in some countries (~30 ecu).

- It cannot be overstated that there is no evidence to suggest that these programmes contribute to an increased sexual activity among adolescents.[36] When comparing abstinence intervention programmes with safer-sex interventions, it is apparent that both can reduce sexual risk behaviours and unplanned pregnancies.

- Early detection and treatment of STIs as an effective prevention strategy is greatly enhanced by the advent of new, non-invasive, urinary-based testing for some of the more common bacterial STIs (i.e. chlamydia infections and gonorrhoea).[37] Due to the relatively high price of such urinary screening tests (7.5–15 ecu) further investigation is required to evaluate the cost-effectiveness of this approach.

- In public-health terms, a vulnerable group of adolescents who can get pregnant will persist, unless serious efforts and successful changes are made at the educational level. Social learning – the consequences of certain patterns of belief and conduct may turn out to be different from (and worse than) early expectations – can constitute one of the few arguments and tools to show and underline the negative long-term social outcomes of teenage mothering.

- Different cultures categorise and value things differently (leaving aside whether objective correctness is possible). Women or men, mainly from certain minorities living in areas where sexual education is not good, will not adopt dominant social roles simply because they are the prevailing ones; some behaviour patterns are resistant to social efforts to eradicate them and variability of sexual practices across and within cultures is a reality.

- Access to services by adolescents, both before and during pregnancy, has to be improved. The care of pregnant adolescents should be adjusted to their specific needs.[3,38,39]

References

1 UNFPA. World Population Report 1999. Geneva: UNFPA, 1999
2 Gortzak-Uzan L, Hallack M, Press F. Teenage pregnancy: risk factors for adverse perinatal outcome. J Matern Fetal Med 2001; 10: 393–397
3 Oliveira da Silva M, Cabral H, Zuckerman B. Adolescent pregnancy: effectiveness of continuity of care by an obstetrician. Obstet Gynecol 1993; 81: 142–147
4 Lawson A, Lawson J. Breast Cancer – can you prevent it? London: McGraw Hill, 1999
5 The Social Exclusion Unit. Teenage Pregnancy. Report No Cmnd 4342. London: Stationery Office, 1999: 1–6
6 Boonstra H. Teen pregnancy: trends and lessons learned. Fam Plann Perspect 2002; 5 :
7 Estlund DM, Nussbaum MC. Sex, Preference and Family. New York: Oxford University Press, 1997
8 Singh S. Socioeconomic disadvantage and adolescent women's sexual and reproductive behaviour: the case of five developed countries. Fam Plann Perspect 2001; 5: 7–10
9 McLeod A. Changing patterns of teenage pregnancy: population based study of small areas. BMJ 2001; 323: 199–203
10 Nisso – National Institute for Social Sexological Research, April 2000. Teenage Mothers in The Netherlands. Fact Sheet. Library@nisso.nl
11 Darroch JE, Singh S, Frost JJ. Differences in teenage pregnancy rates among five developed countries: the roles of sexual activity and contraceptive use. Fam Plann Perspect 2001; 33: 244–250
12 Wellings K, Nauphahal K, Macdowall W et al. Sexual behaviour in Britain: early heterosexual experience. Lancet 2001; 358: 1843–1854
13 Abramson PR, Pinkerton SD. With Pleasure: Thoughts on Nature of Human Sexuality. New York: Oxford University Press, 1995
14 Sanders AS, Reinisch JM. Would you say you 'had sex' if ...? JAMA 1999; 281: 275–277
15 Churchill D, Allen J, Pringle M et al. Consultation patterns and provision of contraception in general practice before teenage pregnancy: case-control study. BMJ 2000; 321: 486–489
16 Price SJ, Barreu G, Smith G et al. Use of contraception in women who present for termination of pregnancy in inner London. Public Health 1997; 11: 377–382
17 Hippisley-Cox J, Allen J, Pringle M et al. Association between teenage pregnancy rates and the age and sex of general practitioners: cross sectional survey in Trent 1994-7. BMJ 2000; 320: 842–845
18 Alvin P. Adolescents and contraception. What should the pediatrician know? Arch Pediatr 2001; 8: 1251–1259
19 Darroch JE. Teenage sexual and reproductive behaviour in developed countries: can more progress be made? Fam Plann Perspect 2001; 33: 244–250
20 Olukoya AA, Kaya A, Ferguson BJ, Abouzahr C. Unsafe abortions in adolescents. Int J Gynaecol Obstet 2001; 75: 137–147
21 Clark LP. Will the pill make me sterile? Addressing reproductive health concerns and strategies to improve adherence to hormonal contraceptive regimens in adolescent girls. J Pediatr Adolesc Gynecol 2001; 14: 153–162
22 Barros A, Correia T. Sexual knowledge and behaviour of Portuguese teenagers. 2002: In press
23 Zavodny M. The effect of partners' characteristics on teenage pregnancy and its resolution. Fam Plann Perspect 2001; 33: 192–199
24 DiClemente RJ. Development of programmes for enhancing sexual health. Lancet 2001; 358: 1828–1829
25 Dailard C. Abstinence promotion and teen family planning: the misguided drive for equal funding. The Guttmacher Report on Public Policy 2002; 5: 1–3
26 DiClemente RJ. Preventing sexually transmitted infections among adolescents: a clash of ideology and science. JAMA 1998; 279: 1574–1575
27 Sieving RE, McNeely CS, Blum RW. Maternal expectations, mother-child connectedness, and adolescent sexual debut. Arch Pediatr Adolesc Med 2000; 154: 809–816
28 Klein JD. The national longitudinal study on adolescent health: preliminary results: great expectations. JAMA 1997; 278: 864–865
29 DiClemente RJ. Reply to the editor. JAMA 1999; 281: 28
30 Mawer C. Preventing teenage pregnancies, supporting teenage mothers. BMJ 1999; 318: 1713–1714

31 Young TM, Martin SS, Young ME, Ting L. Internal poverty and teen pregnancy. Adolescence 2001; 26: 289–304

32 Crosby RA, DiClemente RJ, Wingood GM, Davies SL, Harrington K. Adolescents' ambivalence about becoming pregnant predicts infrequent contraceptive use: a prospective analysis of non pregnant African American females. Am J Obstet Gynecol 2002; 186: 251–252

33 Crosby RA, DiClemente RJ, Wingood GM et al. Correlates of adolescent females' worry about undesired pregnancy – the importance of partner desire of pregnancy. J Pediatr Adolesc Gynecol 2001; 14: 123–127

34 Watt LD. Pregnancy prevention in primary care for adolescent males. J Pediatr Health Care 2001; 15: 223–228

35 Stevens-Simon C, Beach RK, Klerman LV. To be rather than not to be – that is the problem with the questions we ask adolescents about their childbearing intentions. Arch Pediatr Adolesc Med 2001; 155: 1298–1300

36 Kaplan DW, Feinstein RA, Fisher MM et al. Condom use by adolescents. Pediatrics 2001; 107: 1463–1469

37 Orr DP, Fortenberry JD. Screening adolescents for sexually transmitted infections. JAMA 1998; 280: 564–565

38 Treffers PE, Olukoya AA, Ferguson BJ, Liljestrand J. Care of adolescent pregnancy and childbirth . Int J Obstet Gynecol 2001; 75: 111–121

39 Hancok EG, Calhoun BC, Hume RF. Adolescent pregnancy: improving outcomes through focused multidisciplinary obstetric care, In: Ransom, Domrowski, Evans, Ginsburg (eds). Contemporary Therapy in Obsterics and Gynaecology. Philadelphia:Saunders, 2002: 152–156

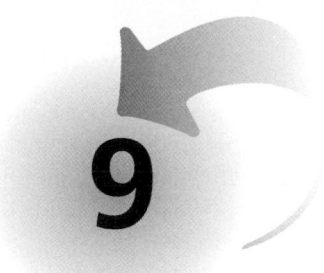

9

Charlotte Chaliha Stuart L. Stanton

Consequences of childbirth on the pelvic floor

There has been increasing recognition over the past few decades of the consequences of childbirth on the physical and psychological well-being of a woman. MacArthur et al.,[1] in a postal survey of 11,701 women 13 months to 9 years after delivery, found that 47% experienced at least one or more health problems within 3 months of delivery. These included backache, headache, haemorrhoids, depression and bowel and bladder symptoms which persisted for a minimum of 6 weeks. Glazener et al.[2] questioned 1249 women about their postnatal symptoms on three occasions after childbirth; 85% of women experienced one new symptom during the first 8 weeks and 76% reported one or more health problems persisting for up to 18 months. Sleep and Grant[3] reported that 15% of women experience dyspareunia up to 3 years after a normal vaginal delivery and up to 8% experience perineal pain 12 weeks after a normal vaginal delivery.[4] However, though health problems seem to be common after childbirth, it seems women often do not seek medical attention.[1]

Perineal trauma at the time of delivery can result in dyspareunia and perineal pain. Urinary incontinence, anal incontinence and uterovaginal prolapse are the major long-term pelvic floor sequelae of childbirth and may not manifest for many years after delivery. The epidemiological evidence to suggest that childbirth is a major aetiological factor is seen from studies showing incontinence and prolapse are less often seen in nulliparous women,[5-7] and both urinary and anal incontinence are more common in women than men.[8,9] Vaginal delivery has been shown to result in mechanical disruption of the pelvic floor and pudendal nerve injury resulting in urinary or anal incontinence or both.[10-13] There may also be women at increased predisposition to pelvic floor trauma and thus incontinence and prolapse, due to an inherent weakness of collagen within the pelvic floor.

Dr Charlotte Chaliha MB Bchir MA MD MRCOG, Specialist Registrar, East Surrey Hospital, Redmill, Surrey RH1 5RH, UK

Professor Stuart L. Stanton FRCS FRCOG, Director, Urogynaecology Unit, Department of Obstetrics and Gynaecology, Lanesborough Wing, St George's Hospital Medical School, Cranmer Terrace, London SW17 0RE, UK (for correspondence)

ANATOMY AND FUNCTION OF THE PELVIC FLOOR

The pelvic floor is a dynamic structure consisting of the levator ani muscles, the urethral and anal sphincters, the endopelvic fascia and related structures which together support the abdomino-pelvic organs and maintain continence.

The levator ani is the largest portion of the pelvic floor and consists of large amounts of type I (slow twitch) muscle fibres that are ideally suited to maintaining base-line tone as well as type II (fast twitch) muscle fibres that allow the muscle to contract quickly in response to increases in intra-abdominal pressure to maintain continence.[14] It is closely associated with both the anal and urethral sphincters mechanisms.

The anal sphincters

The anal sphincter complex is composed of the internal and external anal sphincters. The external sphincter consists of subcutaneous, superficial and deep components. The subcutaneous portion surrounds the lower-most part of the anal canal, the superficial part lying deep to this, and the deep portion surrounds the upper part of the internal anal sphincter. The internal anal sphincter is a direct continuation of the inner circular layer of rectal muscle[15] and surrounds the anal canal for 2–4 cm and is 1.5-5 mm thick.[16,17]

The anal sphincters play an essential role in the maintenance of continence both at rest and during rises in intra-abdominal pressure. The maintenance of basal tone is to a large extent an unconscious act, and continence is maintained by resting pressures that exceed rectal pressure. Peak pressures are found approximately 2 cm from the anal verge which corresponds to the site where the external sphincter overlaps the internal sphincter.[18] The external sphincter, like the internal, is continually active at rest and this activity continues during sleep and varies with posture and activity.[19-21] The internal sphincter is responsible for 50–85% of resting anal tone, while the external sphincter is responsible for the majority of squeeze pressure.[22-24] This maintenance of tone is dependent on sensory input; therefore, when sensory roots are destroyed, as in tabes dorsalis, anal tone is diminished.[25]

Rises in intra-abdominal pressure with coughing and laughing cause external sphincter contraction which protects against faecal loss. Rectal distension causes an initial contraction of the external sphincter which precedes a reflex inhibition of the internal sphincter.[26,27] This so-called 'sampling' reflex maintains continence during reflex relaxation of the internal sphincter, allowing sampling of the rectal contents. If the time for defecation is unsuitable, the external sphincter contraction continues to allow compensatory adjustments in the rectum and colon to accommodate rectal contents.

The importance of the sphincter mechanism in continence is demonstrated by finding that sphincter division during anal sphincter surgery has been associated with disturbances in continence in up to 34% of patients.[28,29]

The urethral sphincter

The striated urogenital sphincter muscle surrounds the urethra for approximately 20–60% of its length,[30] and is made up of two portions – an upper sphincteric portion (sphincter urethrae) and a lower arch-like pair of muscular bands, the compressor urethrae and urethrovaginal sphincter. These three muscles act as a functional unit and are predominately made up of slow twitch muscle fibres[31] which is ideally suited to allow them to maintain constant tone as well as to contract if required.

The urethral support mechanism is essential for continence and is dependent on the interaction of the bladder neck, pubo-urethral ligaments, urogenital diaphragm and the muscles of the pelvic diaphragm. The proximal urethra and bladder rather than being ventrally suspended by ligamentous structures are supported in a sling-like fashion by the anterior vaginal wall, which is attached bilaterally to the muscles of the pelvic diaphragm and to the arcus tendineus, the so-called 'hammock hypothesis'.[32,33] The urethra thus lies on a supportive layer of the endopelvic fascia and anterior vaginal wall. This layer gains structural stability due to its attachment to the pelvic side walls. In this scheme, a rise in intra-abdominal pressure compresses the urethra due to the downward force of abdominal pressure and the resistance of the underlying endopelvic fascia.

Nerve supply

The striated muscles of the pelvic floor are innervated by the pelvic and pudendal nerves. The pudendal nerve supplies somatic efferent pathways to the urethral sphincter as well as efferent impulses to muscles of the pelvic floor. The internal anal sphincter is both under excitatory and inhibitory autonomic control. The anal mucosa has a rich sensory nerve supply from 10–15 mm above the anal valves to the boundary with the hairy anal skin. These include Meissner's corpuscles, genital corpuscles, Golgi-Mazzoni bodies and Krause's end bulbs.[34,35] Meissner's corpuscles are sensitive to light touch, Golgi bodies and Pacinian corpuscles are sensitive to tension and pressure, and Krause's end bulbs are sensitive to temperature.

MECHANISMS OF INJURY TO THE PELVIC FLOOR

Hertz[36] suggested in 1909 that straining during childbirth may lead to atrophic damage to the pelvic floor, as seen in women suffering from chronic constipation who strain excessively to defaecate.

There are several aetiological mechanisms of pelvic floor injury – direct muscle trauma, nerve injury and connective tissue damage.

Direct perineal trauma

Direct perineal trauma may occur from perineal laceration and episiotomy and is a well-known complication of vaginal delivery. The long-term sequelae of perineal injuries include pain, dyspareunia, fistulae and anal incontinence.[12,37–40] The incidence of lacerations involving the anal sphincter has been reported as 0–6.4% when an episiotomy has not been performed, 0.2–23.9% after a midline episiotomy and 0–9% after a mediolateral episiotomy.[41]

Muscle trauma

Anatomical and functional changes to the pelvic floor may occur secondary to pelvic floor distension during descent of the fetal head and maternal expulsive efforts during the active second stage of labour. Peschers et al.[42] evaluated pelvic floor strength by means of palpation, perineometry and perineal ultrasonography and found that pelvic floor muscle strength was significantly decreased after vaginal delivery compared to caesarean section at 3–8 days postpartum. However at 6–10 weeks postpartum, there was no significant difference from antenatal values except for a lower intravaginal pressure in primiparae not multiparae. Therefore, though pelvic strength is impaired shortly after vaginal birth, it recovers in most women within 2 months.

Nerve damage

The pudendal nerve is particularly susceptible to compression and damage at the point where it curves round the ischial spine and enters the pudendal canal enclosed in a tight fibrous sheath. Nerve damage has been shown to occur in patients with a history of chronic straining on defecation who show increased pudendal nerve terminal motor latencies.[43] Childbirth-induced denervation injuries of the pubococcygeus and external sphincter muscles may occur by a similar mechanism and have been reported after 42–80% of vaginal deliveries.[10,11]

Collagen and connective tissue changes

Abnormalities of collagen have also been implicated in the development of prolapse and urinary stress incontinence.[44–48] Direct injury to the pelvic floor may result in repair with weaker collagen and so predispose to the development of prolapse and incontinence due to a weakening of the pelvic floor support mechanisms. Pregnancy may also result in alterations in collagen. Landon et al.[49] examined the tensile properties of the rectus fascia in 24 women undergoing caesarean section compared to 96 non-pregnant women having an abdominal operation, and found that the pregnant fascia had a reduced tensile strength. Lavin et al.[50] examined the biomechanical properties of the rectus fascia in pregnancy, as a model for studying the pelvic fascia, and found that pregnancy results in a reduction in total collagen content and an increase in glycosaminoglycans. This alteration in pelvic floor collagen may result in a weakening of the pelvic floor continence mechanism in pregnancy.

MORPHOLOGICAL AND PHYSIOLOGICAL CHANGES IN THE LOWER URINARY TRACT IN PREGNANCY AND AFTER DELIVERY

During pregnancy and after delivery, the urinary tract undergoes both structural and functional changes. These changes may be specific in response to pregnancy and, in some women, may be compounded by pathological changes which persist after delivery.

Dilatation of the ureter is a well-known phenomenon in pregnancy, and hydroureter is noted in approximately 90% of pregnant women by the third trimester. This dilatation is more marked on the right compared to the left side, probably related to the relative dextrorotation of the uterus. The bladder is passively drawn upwards and anteriorly as the uterus enlarges resulting in lengthening of the urethra.[51] The urethral mucosa becomes more hyperaemic and congested in pregnancy in response to the increase in circulating oestrogen levels. The detrusor muscle also hypertrophies in response to oestrogen. After delivery, cystoscopy shows changes such as mucosal congestion, submucosal haemorrhage, and capillary oozing, especially around the bladder neck, trigone and urethral orifices. These changes have been seen in association with a decrease in bladder sensation and tone[52] and are most marked in those who underwent vaginal delivery.[53]

Muellner[54] reported an increase in bladder capacity by an average of 130 ml in the third trimester. This finding was disputed later by Francis[55], who found no change in bladder capacity in the first trimester and a reduced bladder capacity in the third trimester in association with increased detrusor irritability rather than bladder hypotonia.

CHILDBIRTH AND URINARY INCONTINENCE

Incontinence is a common symptom associated with pregnancy and has been reported in up to 85% of women.[55–58] Francis[55] found that, in the first trimester of pregnancy, 16% of women complained of stress incontinence and 34% in the second half of pregnancy. Stanton et al.[59] assessed the prevalence of both stress and urge incontinence at 32 weeks' gestation and found an incidence of 36% and 13%, respectively. Both studies found that stress incontinence rarely appears for the first time postnatally without prior antenatal symptoms.

Viktrup et al.[57] interviewed 305 primiparae and found that 39% had stress incontinence before, during or after pregnancy and 7% developed de novo stress incontinence after delivery. In those with onset of stress incontinence in pregnancy, only 3% had persisting symptoms at 1 year postpartum whereas in those with onset after delivery, 24% had symptoms at 1 year postpartum. There was no relationship between obstetric risk factors and incontinence at 3 months postpartum. Wilson et al.,[60] in a postal questionnaire study of 2134 women at 3 months postpartum, found that 34.3% admitted to some degree of urinary incontinence with 3.3% having daily or more frequent leakage. The risk was significantly reduced in those women, especially primiparae, who had a caesarean section whether elective or in labour suggesting it is vaginal delivery not pregnancy that predisposes to stress incontinence. However, the prevalence of incontinence was similar in those women having three or more caesarean sections (38.9%) to those delivered vaginally (37.7%). This may be secondary to nerve damage from bladder dissection during caesarean section. This is supported by a study of women who had undergone elective caesarean section, of whom 17% reported stress incontinence, and 51% had severe symptoms that occurred for the first time in pregnancy or the puerperium.[61]

Chaliha et al.[58] interviewed 554 nulliparous women to assess the prevalence of urinary incontinence before, during and after delivery. Pregnancy and delivery resulted in a significant increase in symptoms of urinary incontinence and urgency. Stress incontinence was the most common form of incontinence and reported by 17 (3.1%), 196 (35.7%) and 68 (12.4%) women before, during and after pregnancy, respectively. The low prevalence of prepregnancy incontinence in nulliparous women agrees with previous data linking parity to incontinence.[6,9,60]

CHANGES IN THE LOWER URINARY TRACT AND PELVIC FLOOR RELATED TO STRESS INCONTINENCE

The exact aetiological mechanism of stress incontinence is unclear and probably multifactorial, related to nerve damage, and/or physiological and structural changes of the lower urinary tract.

Functional changes

Physiological studies have revealed conflicting results regarding lower urinary tract function in pregnancy and after delivery. Iosif and Ulmsten[62] compared urethral pressure profile measurements in pregnant women with stress incontinence with continent healthy women from an earlier study.[63] The women with stress incontinence showed no increase in urethral length during pregnancy and also showed a lower urethral closure pressure at rest. They concluded that an increase in urethral pressure, which was on average an increase of 12 cmH$_2$O, would compensate for a rise in intravesical pressure in pregnancy and so maintain continence. This agrees with other studies that have shown evidence of low urethral pressure in non-pregnant women with stress incontinence.[64-66]

Vaginal delivery may also affect urethral sphincter function. Tapp et al.[67] assessed two groups of women, one with competent urethral sphincter mechanisms and one group with genuine stress incontinence. Women with genuine stress incontinence showed a negative correlation between the number of vaginal deliveries and the pressure transmission ratios in the distal fourth of the urethra. An increased number of vaginal deliveries was associated with poor function of the distal urethral sphincter mechanism. As continence is thought to be maintained by the action of the proximal not distal sphincter mechanism, the authors concluded that damage to the distal sphincter mechanism may result in stress incontinence in women with impaired proximal sphincter function.

Van Geelen et al.[68] found an increase in the amplitude of vascular pulsations recorded from the urethral wall especially in the first 16 weeks of pregnancy which may be related to an increase in blood volume in pregnancy. Pregnant women with genuine stress incontinence showed a decrease in the amplitude of vascular pulsations in the periurethral plexus compared to continent women, suggesting that this affects urethral closure pressure.[69]

Urodynamic studies suggest that detrusor instability may be a cause of incontinence.[70-72] Chaliha et al.[72] performed urodynamics in the third trimester and 12 weeks' postpartum. A high prevalence of genuine stress incontinence and detrusor instability, 8.7% and 8.1% respectively, in the antenatal period and 5.0% and 6.8%, respectively, postpartum was found. The mean values for urodynamic variables in the third trimester and postpartum were lower than values defined in a non-pregnant population and not related to obstetric or neonatal variables. Urodynamic variables showed a postpartum increase in first sensation and strong sensation to void, and maximum bladder capacity. However, it was found that despite the high prevalence of symptoms, there was poor correlation between symptoms and urodynamic findings which agrees with data in non-pregnant women.[73] The authors concluded that the observed changes in bladder function were consistent with a pressure effect of a gravid uterus and not related to mode of delivery and neonatal factors.

Nerve damage

Patients with genuine stress incontinence have been shown to have abnormal conduction in the perineal branch of the pudendal nerve which innervates the periurethral striated muscle[74] and pubococcygeus muscle.[75,76] Injury to the nerve supply has also been demonstrated after childbirth. Snooks et al.[10] found prolongation of pudendal nerve terminal motor latencies 48–72 h after postpartum in 42% of those delivered vaginally, but not those delivered by caesarean section. The degree of pudendal nerve damage was greater in multiparous women and correlated with the use of forceps and a longer second stage of labour. In 60% of women with evidence of nerve damage, the pudendal nerve latency had returned to normal at 2 months' postpartum. The authors suggested that vaginal delivery results in pudendal nerve damage probably from a combination of direct and traction injury during delivery. However, this study was not prospective and included multiparous women who may have sustained prior nerve damage. Furthermore, it looked at innervation of the striated anal sphincter which may not actually reflect striated urethral sphincter innervation and there was poor correlation between abnormal latencies and symptoms. Allen et al.,[11] using concentric needle electromyography and pudendal nerve conduction tests, found evidence of denervation injury in 80% of women after delivery. Those women with a long (active) second stage of labour (> 56.7 min) and a large baby (> 3.41 kg) showed a greater degree of nerve damage.

Electromyography of the right and left pubococcygeus muscle has shown that childbirth induces both qualitative as well as quantitative changes such that sphincter weakness was due not only to loss of motor units but also asynchronous activity in those that remained.[77]

Structural changes

Gainey[78] examined 1000 women postnatally and found evidence of urethral detachment in 18% and damage to the pelvic floor muscles in 31%. Peschers et al.[79] evaluated bladder neck position and mobility using perineal ultrasound at 8 weeks' postpartum. Bladder neck position was significantly lower and bladder neck mobility increased after vaginal delivery compared with women who had an elective caesarean section and nulligravid controls. This agrees with Meyer et al.[80] who noted a significant increase in bladder neck mobility after vaginal delivery in primiparae; however, bladder neck position was only lowered after forceps delivery. Thus vaginal delivery seems to alter urethral support which may result in stress incontinence.

ANAL CANAL MORPHOLOGY DURING PREGNANCY AND AFTER DELIVERY

Sultan et al.[81] examined 20 women before and after a caesarean section and found that pregnancy did not have any significant effect on anal sphincter morphology and function.

CHILDBIRTH AND ANAL INCONTINENCE

MacArthur et al.[13] investigated the prevalence of postnatal faecal symptoms in a postal questionnaire study of 906 women, 10 months after delivery and reported that 36 women (4%) developed de novo faecal incontinence. Six of these women became incontinent after an emergency caesarean section, but none after an elective caesarean section. This estimate for faecal incontinence is conservative, as it did not enquire about incontinence of flatus which is probably more common. In another study in 349 primiparous women, 26% reported incontinence of flatus at 9 months' postpartum.[82]

Chaliha et al.[58] assessed the prevalence of anal incontinence before, during and after delivery in 554 nulliparous women. and found the prevalence of de novo faecal urgency and/or anal incontinence was 6%. Women who underwent caesarean section were significantly less likely to report faecal urgency than those who underwent vaginal delivery.

Symptoms of anal incontinence are especially common after anal sphincter rupture. The prevalence of anal incontinence in these circumstances has been estimated to be 16–47%.[83–86] Tetzschner et al.[87] assessed the long-term impact of obstetric anal sphincter rupture on the frequency of urinary and anal incontinence. At 2–4 years' postpartum, 42% of the 94 women in their study had anal incontinence, 32% had urinary incontinence and 18% had both. Despite the high number of women with incontinence, only a few had sought medical advice.

The use of episiotomy and its relationship to anal sphincter injury is unclear. Poen et al.[88] reported that the use of a mediolateral episiotomy was associated with fewer third degree tears; however, Sultan et al.,[89] in a retrospective study of women who had sustained third degree tears, reported that almost half of these women had undergone an episiotomy. The use of midline episiotomies, favoured in the US, has been strongly associated with third degree tears, with those women having midline episiotomies, 50 times more likely to sustain a third degree tear.[90] This is reflected in the 3-fold increased risk of faecal incontinence following midline episiotomy versus a spontaneous perineal laceration.[91]

Despite obvious injury to the anal sphincters, symptoms of anal incontinence may not occur for some time after delivery. Bek et al.[92] found that, in women who experienced transient anal incontinence after a complete tear, 39% had a relapse of symptoms after the next vaginal delivery. The major long-term problem seen in these women was incontinence of flatus. Fynes et al.,[93] in a study of women undergoing a second vaginal delivery with a history of occult sphincter injury or transient faecal incontinence after their first delivery, found there was a significant risk of these women having persistent faecal incontinence. Full thickness anal sphincter disruption was the most significant risk factor in the development of faecal incontinence after a second vaginal delivery.

CHANGES IN THE ANAL CANAL AND PELVIC FLOOR RELATED TO ANAL INCONTINENCE

The aetiology of postpartum anal incontinence is complex and both nerve and mechanical trauma have been implicated.

Nerve damage

Denervation injury of the pelvic floor may occur from traction and straining during vaginal delivery, similar to the mechanism of nerve damage reported in patients with chronic constipation which may result in anorectal incontinence.[94] In 80% of women with idiopathic anorectal incontinence, there is histological evidence of denervation of the striated pelvic floor muscle particularly the puborectalis and external anal sphincter muscles.[95-97] Serial measurements of pudendal nerve terminal motor latencies in patients with idiopathic anorectal incontinence show progressive damage from recurrent stretch injury during straining at stool.[98]

This mechanism of strain-induced damage may occur during vaginal delivery. Sultan et al.[99] investigated pudendal nerve function before and after delivery and found that pudendal nerve terminal motor latencies were significantly prolonged especially on the left side which the authors postulated could be due to the unequal traction from the fetal head on the two sides of the pelvic floor during descent down the birth canal. However, no relationship between abnormal neurophysiology and symptoms of anal incontinence was shown.

Sensory impairment

Much of the data regarding anal sensation in relation to pregnancy has been from studies too small to draw valid conclusions. Small and Wynne[100] measured anal sensation in 72 subjects (30 of whom were nulliparous) before delivery, 24–72 h post-delivery and again 6–8 weeks' postpartum. Anal sensation was not altered by vaginal delivery. Cornes et al.[101] measured anal pressures and sensation in 96 primiparous patients 1–10 days after delivery and again in 74 of these women who returned at 6 months' postpartum. Anal sensation was impaired in the lower, mid and upper anal canal immediately after a normal vaginal delivery and forceps delivery compared with controls or those delivered by caesarean section, but by 6 months' postpartum there were no significant differences. The authors suggested that this impairment of sensation was probably due to a combination of mucosal prolapse and pudendal neuropathy. Such prolapse of rectal mucosa would result in the less sensitive rectal mucosa being present in the anal canal and, therefore, anorectal sampling may be affected.

Chaliha et al.[102] measured anorectal sensation in 286 nulliparous women in the third trimester and again at 12 weeks' postpartum. There were no differences in anorectal sensation measurements before and after delivery nor any relationship with symptoms of anal incontinence. Thus anal sensation does not seem to be a major aetiological factor in the development of anal incontinence as deficits in anal canal sensation seem to be transient and unrelated to the development of incontinence.

Anal sphincter trauma

The use of anal endosonography has enabled accurate visualisation of the sphincters. It has provided strong direct evidence of occult anal sphincter trauma after delivery and demonstrated its importance in the pathophysiology of anal incontinence.[12,103]

Sultan et al.[12] investigated 202 pregnant women 6 weeks before delivery with anal endosonography, manometry, perineometry and pudendal nerve terminal motor latencies. These tests were repeated in 150 of these women 6 weeks after delivery and then in 32 with abnormal findings (defects on endosonography or prolonged pudendal nerve terminal motor latencies) 6 months after delivery. Antenatally, all 76 primiparae were asymptomatic; however, after delivery, 10 (13%) developed symptoms of urgency or anal incontinence. Antenatally 11 (23%) of the 48 multiparae reported symptoms dating from previous deliveries. No antenatal sphincter defects were detected in the primiparous women, but were identified in 35% postpartum. Antenatal sphincter defects were seen in 40% of multiparae and postpartum only 4% had new defects. Those women who underwent caesarean section had no evidence of new postpartum sphincter defects. The use of forceps was the single independent factor associated with anal sphincter damage and there was a strong correlation with the presence of defects and the development of symptoms. There was no correlation with abnormal latency values and the development of symptoms or anal pressures; there was, however, a significant association with abnormal nerve latencies and sphincter defects in primiparous women. The authors suggested this reflected a common traumatic cause rather than a causal relationship.

Forceps delivery results in more trauma to the anal sphincters and is associated with a higher incidence of defecatory symptoms than a ventouse delivery. Anal sphincter defects were seen in 81% of those who had a forceps delivery compared to 24% of those who had a ventouse delivery and 36% of controls.[104]

Donnelly et al.[105] performed anal vector manometry in 219 primiparae in the third trimester. Six weeks postpartum, 184 of these women returned and the bowel symptom questionnaire was completed together with anal vector manometry and pudendal nerve conduction latency. In 81 women with altered faecal incontinence or abnormal physiology, anal endosonography was performed. Instrumental vaginal delivery and a second stage of labour prolonged by the use of epidural analgesia were associated with the greatest risk of anal sphincter trauma and impaired faecal incontinence.

Chaliha et al.[103] performed anal sensation tests and manometry in 286 nulliparae in the third trimester alongside an anal symptom questionnaire. At 12 weeks postpartum, 161 of these women returned for repeat investigations and anal endosonography was also performed. Vaginal delivery, particularly instrumental, was associated with a significant decrease in maximum anal squeeze pressures. Maximum anal resting pressures were also significantly decreased in those who underwent an instrumental vaginal delivery compared to controls. Anal endosonography revealed anal sphincter defects in 38% of women and this was associated with lower anal squeeze and resting pressures. Postpartum anal sphincter trauma was associated with perineal laceration and vaginal delivery.

CHILDBIRTH AND PROLAPSE

Genital prolapse occurs as a consequence of weakness of the fibromuscular supports of the pelvic organs. There is considerable individual variability in the predisposition to prolapse, and childbirth has been implicated as a major aetiological factor. It is far commoner in parous women, with 50% of parous women having some degree of genital prolapse and, of these, 10–20% are symptomatic. In contrast, only 2% of symptomatic prolapse is found to occur in nulliparous women. The risk of prolapse is higher with increasing parity and the prevalence is 7 times higher in those who have 7 children compared to one.[106]

The mechanism of prolapse is unclear. Pathological and electro-physiological studies have shown that significant pelvic nerve denervation and re-innervation are associated with stress incontinence and prolapse; however, there are also collagenous changes in the pelvic floor which are related to ageing, childbirth, and endogenous hormone changes which may also predispose to prolapse and stress incontinence.[107–110]

During vaginal delivery, the combination of distension by the fetal head and by pressure of maternal expulsive efforts stretch the pelvic floor and this may lead to functional and anatomical alterations in the muscles, nerves and the connective tissue of the pelvic floor and anal canal. Prolapse may be a consequence of this and is more common in women after a vaginal delivery compared to after a caesarean section.[111] Trauma to the pelvic floor may also lead to repair with weaker collagen and so predispose to incontinence.

THE ROLE OF COLLAGEN IN PELVIC FLOOR DYSFUNCTION

Connective tissue defects have been implicated in the aetiology of stress incontinence and prolapse. This has been supported by reports of increased complaints of incontinence and prolapse in women with Ehlers-Danlos syndrome.[112] Alterations in the ratios of types of collagen within fascia may affect the tensile strength of collagen. An alteration in collagen types, with a reduction in the type I:III collagen ratios in women with genital prolapse[46] and in nulliparous women with stress incontinence[47] has been demonstrated.

Increased collagen degradation resulting in a reduction in both total collagen content and collagen solubility and an increase in collagen turnover has been shown in vaginal epithelial tissue of women with prolapse compared to controls.

Joint hypermobility which has been suggested to be a marker of collagen weakness is significantly greater in women with genital prolapse compared to controls.[113]

The role of collagen in the aetiology of anal incontinence is unclear. Oestrogen receptors have been identified in the anal sphincter and levator ani muscles as well as the urethra.[114] It has been shown that lack of oestrogen affects collagen cross-linkages in the skin,[115] and this may also affect the levator ani and anal sphincter resulting in alteration in function. In support of this, it has been shown that oestrogen replacement can improve or cure faecal incontinence.[116]

Alteration in collagen may occur in response to denervation as collagen biosynthesis has been shown to increase in rats with denervation injury[117] and in myogenic and neurogenic muscle diseases where there is muscle wasting, collagen accumulation, fibrosis of muscle tissue and an increase in collagen types I and II are seen.[118,119]

This alteration in collagen status may result in an alteration in mechanical strength of fascia. Ageing can further exacerbate loss of collagen, weakness of fascia and neuropathy.[120] Collagen remodelling has been shown to occur in response to pregnancy and parturition in the uterus, cervix and rectus fascia.[121,122] This may also extend to other connective tissue structures involved in pelvic floor support. A change in collagen may reduce tensile strength and so predispose to pelvic floor dysfunction during this time.

CAN WE PREDICT WHICH WOMEN ARE AT RISK OF PELVIC FLOOR DAMAGE DURING CHILDBIRTH?

Predicting which women are at risk of pelvic floor dysfunction will allow them to be counselled and preventative measures instituted, if appropriate, such as offering elective caesarean section. Identification of obstetric variables that may increase the risk of pelvic floor trauma in women with an inherent risk of incontinence, may guide decisions regarding method of delivery, e.g. caesarean section versus vaginal delivery, forceps versus ventouse delivery.

King and Freeman[123] found a significant increase in antenatal bladder neck mobility in those women who subsequently reported postnatal stress incontinence. They suggested that there may be a group of women constitutionally at greater risk of developing stress incontinence or prolapse due to defective collagen and that these women may be identified in the antenatal period.

Ulmsten et al.[45] demonstrated that women with stress urinary incontinence had 40% less total collagen in the round ligament and incisional skin compared to continent controls and suggested that this may lead to weakness in the urogenital suspensory apparatus, increased bladder neck hypermobility and thus incontinence. They also found that other markers of connective tissue defects such as abdominal hernias, varicose veins and prolapse were more common in women with stress incontinence. Patients with genital prolapse have also been reported to exhibit increased striae and joint hypermobility.[45]

If collagen abnormalities predispose to incontinence, they might be inherited defects detectable by family histories. Skoner et al.[124] compared 94 women with stress incontinence of urine with 46 controls, and found that having a mother with stress urinary incontinence was associated with a substantial increase in risk. However, these cases were obtained from private clinics and may not be representative of all women with incontinence, many of whom do not seek medical help.

Chaliha et al.[58] evaluated the role of antenatal history and physical markers suggestive of collagen weakness such as striae, hernia, varicose veins, and joint mobility in the prediction of post partum incontinence. In the third trimester, 549 nulliparous women were interviewed using a standardised urinary and bowel symptom questionnaire and a physical examination was performed to assess these markers of collagen weakness. Postnatal anal and urinary incontinence was not related to race, antenatal body-mass index, the presence of striae, hernia, varicose veins, piles or a family history of incontinence, prolapse or collagen weakness. Higher joint mobility scores were associated with incontinence of flatus, but not faecal urgency or urinary symptoms. Therefore although collagen weakness has been implicated in the pathogenesis of incontinence, physical markers of collagen weakness used in this study could not predict postpartum incontinence. It may be that these markers were not representative of collagen weakness or a larger study with longer follow-up is required.

KEY POINTS FOR CLINICAL PRACTICE

- There is much evidence to show that childbirth is implicated in the development of urinary incontinence, anal incontinence, and genital prolapse. This can result in significant deterioration in quality of life. This has led to an increase in caesarean sections that are being performed on the assumption that prevention of perineal trauma will avoid postpartum symptoms. However, caesarean section may not be wholly protective against urinary and anal incontinence and, overall, may subject a woman to greater morbidity and mortality rates.

- It has been recommended that women who experience transient or permanent anal incontinence after sphincter rupture should be offered a caesarean section as this group have been shown to be more likely to have aggravation of symptoms after a further vaginal delivery.[87,92,93] However, for asymptomatic and nulliparous women, caesarean section may not be justified. Also, though multiparous women have a higher prevalence of urinary incontinence than primiparous women, successive vaginal deliveries may not result in deterioration of incontinence.[3] A more logical approach may be to screen women to identify those at high-risk of pelvic floor dysfunction who might benefit from a caesarean section. Modification of obstetric practice to minimise perineal trauma for those who undergo vaginal delivery should also be encouraged. This includes the restricted use of the episiotomy[85] and instrumental vaginal delivery, particularly forceps.[12,125] Adequate training of the repair of perineal trauma is also important as this has been shown to be deficient,[126] and this may require improvements in education and training of doctors and midwives. Women who have recognised anal sphincter trauma should be followed with an anal symptom questionnaire, anal endosonography, and anal physiology especially if continence is impaired.

- For many women, trauma at delivery may be inevitable and research is required into the benefits of pelvic floor exercises, avoidance of excessive weight gain and constipation that may result in strain on the pelvic floor, not only in the antenatal period but also postpartum. Education regarding reduction in family size and improved nutrition will also reduce the incidence of genital prolapse.

- For those women in whom postpartum incontinence and prolapse develops, treatment strategies and follow-up should be easily available and standardised protocols developed. Not only will this encourage greater awareness of this common health problem, but it may encourage women whose quality of life may be significantly impaired by these symptoms to seek help.

References

1   MacArthur C, Lewis D, Bick D. Stress incontinence after childbirth. Br J Midwifery 1991; 1: 207–214

2   Glazener CMA, Abdalla M, Stroud P et al. Postnatal maternal morbidity: extent, causes, prevention and treatment. Br J Obstet Gynaecol 1995; 102: 282–287

3   Sleep J, Grant A. West Berkshire perineal management trial: three year follow-up. BMJ 1987; 295: 749–751

4   Sleep J, Grant A, Garcia J et al. West Berkshire perineal management trial. BMJ 1984; 289: 587–590

5   Nicholls C, Randall C. Vaginal Surgery. Baltimore, MD: Williams and Wilkins, 1976

6   Foldspang A, Lam GW, Elving L. Parity as a correlate of adult female urinary incontinence prevalence. J Epidemiol Community Health 1992; 46: 595–600

7   Milsom I, Ekelund P, Molander U, Arvidsson L, Areskoug B. The influence of age, parity, oral contraception, hysterectomy and menopause on the prevalence of urinary incontinence in women. J Urol 1993; 149: 1459–1462

8   Thomas TM, Plymat KR, Blannin J, Meade TW. Prevalence of urinary incontinence. BMJ 1980; 281: 1243–1245

9   Thomas TM, Egan M, Walgrove A, Meade TW. The prevalence of faecal and double incontinence. Community Med 1984; 6: 216–220

10 Snooks SJ, Swash M, Setchell M, Henry MM. Injury to the innervation of pelvic floor sphincter musculature in childbirth. Lancet 1984; ii: 546–550

11 Allen RE, Hosker GL, Smith ARB, Warrell DW. Pelvic floor damage and childbirth: a neurophysiological study. Br J Obstet Gynaecol 1990; 97: 770–779

12 Sultan AH, Kamm MA, Hudson CN, Thomas JM, Bartram CI. Anal sphincter disruption during vaginal delivery. N Engl J Med 1993; 329: 1905–1911

13 MacArthur C, Bick D, Keighley MRB. Faecal incontinence after childbirth. Br J Obstet Gynaecol 1997; 104: 46–50

14 Schroder HD, Reske-Nielsen E. Fiber type in the striated urethral and anal sphincters. Acta Neuropathol (Berl) 1983; 60: 278–282

15 Morgan CN, Thompson HR. Surgical anatomy of the anal canal with special reference to the surgical importance of the internal sphincter and conjoint longitudinal muscle. Ann R Coll Surg Engl 1956; 19: 88–114

16 Stonesifer Jr GL, Murphy GP, Lombardo CR. The anatomy of the anorectum. Am J Surg 1960; 100: 666–671

17 Lawson JON. Pelvic anatomy. I: Pelvic floor muscles. Ann R Coll Surg Engl 1974; 54: 244–255

18 Duthie HL. Anal continence. Gut 1971; 12, 844–852

19 Floyd WF, Walls EW. Electromyography of the sphincter ani externus in man. J Physiol (Lond) 1953; 122: 599–609

20 Kerremans R. Morphological and Physiological Aspects of Anal Incontinence and Defecation. Bruxelles: Arscia Uitgaven, 1969; 57–67

21 Melzack J, Porter NH. Studies on the reflex activity of the external sphincter ani in spinal man. Paraplegia 1964; 1: 277–296

22 Duthie HL, Watts JM. Contribution of the external anal sphincter to the pressure zone in the anal canal. Gut 1965; 51: 355–357

23 Freckner B, von Euler M. Influence of pudendal block on function of the anal sphincters. Gut 1975; 16: 482–489

24 Schweiger M. Method for determining individual contributions of voluntary and involuntary anal sphincters to resting tone. Dis Colon Rectum 1979; 22: 415–416

25 Parks AG, Porter NH, Melzack J. Experimental study of the reflex mechanism controlling the muscles of the pelvic floor. Dis Colon Rectum 1962; 5: 407–414

26 Gaston EA. The physiology of fecal continence. Surg Gynecol Obstet 1948; 87: 280–290

27 Ustach T, Tobon F, Hambrecht T, Bass DD, Schuster MM. Electrophysiological aspects of human sphincter function. J Clin Invest 1970; 49: 41–48

28 Sainio P, Husa A. Fistulo in ano. Clinical features and long term results of surgery in 199 adults. Acta Chir Scand 1985; 151: 169–176

29 Shouler PJ, Grimley RP, Keighley MR, Alexander-Williams J. Fistula in ano is usually simple to manage surgically. Int J Colorect Dis 1986; 1: 113–115

30 Gosling JA. The structure of the female lower urinary tract and pelvic floor. Urol Clin North Am 1985; 12: 207–214

31 Gosling JA, Dixon JS, Critchley HOD, Thompson SA. A comparative study of the human external sphincter and periurethral levator ani muscles. Br J Urol 1981; 53: 35–41

32 DeLancey JOL. Functional anatomy of the female lower urinary tract and pelvic floor. In: Bock G, Whelan J. (eds) The Neurobiology of Incontinence. New York: Wiley, 1991; 57–76

33 DeLancey JOL. Structural support of the urethra as it relates to stress urinary incontinence: the hammock hypothesis. Am J Obstet Gynecol 1994; 170: 1713–1723

34 Walls EW. Observations on the microscopic anatomy of the human anal canal. Br J Surg 1958; 45: 504–512

35 Duthie HL, Gairns FW. Sensory nerve endings and sensation in the anal region of man. Br J Surg 1960; 47: 585–595

36 Hertz AF. Constipation and Allied Intestinal Disorders. London: Oxford University Press, 1909

37 Madoff RD, Williams JG, Caushaj PF. Current concepts: fecal incontinence. N Engl J Med 1992; 362: 1002–1007

38 Hordnes K, Bergsjo P. Severe lacerations after childbirth. Acta Obstet Gynecol Scand 1993; 72: 413–422

39 Klein MC, Gauthier RJ, Robbins JG et al. Relationship of episiotomy to perineal trauma and morbidity, sexual dysfunction, and pelvic floor relaxation. Am J Obstet Gynecol 1994; 171: 591–598

40 Woolley RJ. Benefits and risks of episiotomy: a review of the English language literature since 1980. Obstet Gynecol Surv 1995; 50: 806–835

41 Thacker SB, Banta DH. Benefits and risks of episiotomy: an interpretative review of the English language literature, 1860–1890. Obstet Gynecol Surv 1983; 38: 322–338

42 Peschers UM, Schaer GN, DeLancey JOL, Schuessler B. Levator ani function before and after childbirth. Br J Obstet Gynaecol 1997; 104: 1004–1008

43 Kiff ES, Barnes RPH, Swash M. Evidence of pudendal neuropathy in patients with perineal descent and chronic constipation. Gut 1984; 25: 1279–1282

44 Makinen J, Soderstrom KO, Kiilolma P, Hirvonen T. Histological changes in the vaginal connective tissue of patients with and without uterine prolapse. Arch Gynecol 1986; 239: 17–20

45 Ulmsten U, Ekman G, Giertz G, Malmstrom A. Different biochemical composition of connective tissue in continent and stress incontinent women. Acta Obstet Gynecol Scand 1987; 66: 455–457

46 Norton P, Boyd C, Deak S. Collagen synthesis in women with genital prolapse or stress urinary incontinence. Neurourol Urodyn 1992; 11: 300–301

47 Keane DP, Sims TJ, Bailey AJ, Abrams P. Analysis of the pelvic floor electromyography and collagen status in premenopausal nulliparous females with genuine stress incontinence. Neurourol Urodyn 1992; 11: 308–309

48 Falconer C, Ekman G, Malmstrom A, Ulmsten U. Decreased collagen synthesis in stress-incontinent women. Obstet Gynecol 1994; 84: 583–586

49 Landon CR, Crofts CE, Smith ARB. Mechanical properties of fascia during pregnancy; a possible factor in the development of stress incontinence of urine. Contemp Rev Obstet Gynaecol 1990; 2, 40–46

50 Lavin JM, Smith ARB, Anderson J et al. The effect of the first pregnancy on the connective tissue of the rectus sheath. Neurourol Urodyn 1997; 16: 381–382

51 Lobel RW, Sand PK, Bowen LW. The urinary tract in pregnancy. In: Ostergard DR, Bent AE. (eds) Urogynaecology and Urodynamics, 4th edn. Baltimore, MD: Williams & Wilkins, 1996; 323

52 Bennetts FA, Judd GE. Studies of the postpartum bladder. Am J Obstet Gynecol 1941; 42: 419

53 Seski AG, Duprey WM. Postpartum intravesical photography. Obstet Gynecol 1961; 18: 548–556

54 Muellner SR. Physiological bladder changes during pregnancy and the puerperium. J Urol 1939; 41: 691–692

55 Francis WJA. Disturbances of bladder function in relation to pregnancy. J Obstet Gynaecol Br Empire 1960; 67: 353–366

56   Francis WJA. The onset of stress incontinence. J Obstet Gynaecol Br Empire 1960; 67: 899–903

57   Viktrup L, Lose G, Rolff M, Barfoed K. The symptom of stress incontinence caused by pregnancy or delivery in primiparas. Obstet Gynecol 1992; 79: 945–949

58   Chaliha C, Kalia V, Stanton SL, Monga A, Sultan AH. Antenatal prediction of postpartum urinary and fecal incontinence. Obstet Gynecol 1999; 94: 689–694

59   Stanton SL, Kerr-Wilson R, Harris GV. The incidence of urological symptoms in normal pregnancy. Br J Obstet Gynaecol 1980; 87: 897–900

60   Wilson PD, Herbison RM, Herbison GP. Obstetric practice and the prevalence of urinary incontinence three months after delivery. Br J Obstet Gynaecol 1996; 103: 154–161

61   Iosif S, Ingermarsson I. Prevalence of stress incontinence among women delivered by elective caesarean section. Int J Gynaecol Obstet 1982; 20: 87–89

62   Iosif S, Ulmsten U. Comparative urodynamic studies of continent and stress incontinent women in pregnancy and the puerperium. Am J Obstet Gynecol 1981; 140: 645–650

63   Iosif S, Ingermarsson I, Ulmsten U. Urodynamic studies in normal pregnancy and the puerperium. Am J Obstet Gynecol 1980; 137: 696–700

64   Toews H. Intraurethral pressure in normal and stress incontinent women. Obstet Gynecol 1967; 29: 613–624

65   Edwards L, Malvern J. The urethral pressure profile: theoretical considerations and clinical application. Br J Urol 1974; 46: 325–335

66   Bunne G, Obrink A. Urethral closure pressure in stress – a comparison between stress incontinent and continent women. Urol Res 1977; 6: 127–134

67   Tapp A, Cardozo L, Versi E, Montgomery J, Studd J. The effect of vaginal delivery on the urethral sphincter. Br J Obstet Gynaecol 1988; 95: 142–146

68   Van Geelen JM, Lemmens WAJG, Eskes TKAB, Martin Jr CB. The urethral pressure profile in pregnancy and after delivery in healthy nulliparous women. Am J Obstet Gynecol 1982; 144: 636–649

69   Schultze H, Wolansky D. Urethral wall pulsation in pregnant patients, continent and stress incontinent females. Zentralbl Gynakol 1990; 112: 19–22

70   Cutner A. The lower urinary tract in pregnancy. London: MD Thesis, University of London, 1993

71   Cutner A, Cardozo LD. The association between pregnancy and abnormal detrusor activity. J Obstet Gynaecol 1996; 16: 143–145

72   Chaliha C, Kalia V, Monga A, Sultan AH, Stanton SL. Pregnancy, childbirth and delivery: a urodynamic viewpoint. Br J Obstet Gynaecol 2000; 107: 1354–1359

73   Benness CJ, Barnick CG, Cardozo L. Normal urodynamic findings in symptomatic women – who to believe, the patient or the test? Int Urogynecol J 1990; 1: 173–174

74   Snooks SJ, Badenoch DF, Tiptaft RC, Swash M. Perineal nerve damage in genuine stress incontinence. An electrophysiological study. Br J Urol 1985; 57: 422–426

75   Smith ARB, Hosker G, Warrell DW. The role of partial denervation on the pelvic floor in the aetiology of genitourinary prolapse and stress incontinence of urine: a neurophysiological study. Br J Obstet Gynaecol 1989; 96: 24–28

76   Smith ARB, Hosker GL, Warrell DW. The role of pudendal nerve damage in the aetiology of genuine stress incontinence in women. Br J Obstet Gynaecol 1989; 96: 29–32

77   Deindl FM, Vodusek DB, Hesse U, Schussler B. Pelvic floor activity patterns: comparison of nulliparous continent and parous urinary stress incontinent women. Br J Urol 1994; 73: 413–417

78   Gainey HL. Postpartum observation of pelvic tissue damage. Am J Obstet Gynecol 1943; 45: 457–466

79   Peschers U, Schaer G, Anthuber C, Delancey JOL, Schuessler B. Changes in vesical neck mobility following vaginal delivery. Obstet Gynecol 1996; 88: 1001–1006

80   Meyer S, Schreyer A, De Grandi P, Hohlfeld P. The effects of birth on urinary continence mechanisms and other pelvic floor characteristics. Obstet Gynecol 1998; 92: 613–618

81   Sultan AH, Kamm MA, Hudson CN, Bartram CI. Effect of pregnancy on anal sphincter morphology and function. Int J Colorect Dis 1993; 8: 206–209

82 Zetterstrom JP, Lopez A, Anzen B et al. Anal incontinence after vaginal delivery: a prospective study in primiparous women. Br J Obstet Gynaecol 1999; 106: 324–330

83 Combs CA, Robertson PA, Laros RK. Risk factors for third-degree and fourth degree perineal lacerations in forceps and vacuum deliveries. Am J Obstet Gynecol 1990; 163: 100–104

84 Walker M, Farine D, Robin S, Ritchie J. Epidural analgesia, episiotomy and obstetric laceration. Obstet Gynecol 1991; 77: 668–671

85 Henriksen TB, Bek KM, Hedegaard M, Secher NJ. Episiotomy and perineal lesions in spontaneous vaginal deliveries. Br J Obstet Gynaecol 1992; 99: 950–954

86 Crawford LA, Quint EH, Pearl ML, Delancey JO. Incontinence following rupture of the anal sphincter during delivery. Obstet Gynecol 1993; 82: 527–531

87 Tetzschner T, Sorensen M, Lose G, Christiansen J. Anal and urinary incontinence in women with obstetric anal sphincter rupture. Br J Obstet Gynaecol 1996; 103: 1034–1040

88 Poen AC, Felt-Bersma RJF, Dekker GA, Deville W, Cuesta MA, Muewissen SGM. Third degree obstetric perineal tears: risk factors and the preventative role of mediolateral episiotomy. Br J Obstet Gynaecol 1997; 104: 563–566

89 Sultan AH, Kamm MA, Hudson CN, Bartram CI. Third degree obstetric anal sphincter tears: risk factors and outcome of primary repair. BMJ 1994; 308: 887–891

90 Shiono P, Klebanoff MA, Carey JC. Midline episiotomies: more harm then good? Obstet Gynecol 1990; 75: 765–770

91 Signorello L, Harlo LB, Chekos AK, Repke JT. Midline episiotomy and anal incontinence: a retrospective cohort study. BMJ 2000; 320: 86–90

92 Bek KM, Laurberg S. Risks of anal incontinence from subsequent vaginal delivery after a complete obstetric anal sphincter tear. Br J Obstet Gynaecol 1992; 99: 724–726

93 Fynes M, Donnelly V, O'Connell PR, O'Herlihy C. Cesarean delivery and anal sphincter injury. Obstet Gynecol 1998; 92: 496–500

94 Snooks SJ, Barnes PRH, Swash M, Henry MM. Damage to the innervation of the pelvic floor musculature in chronic constipation. Gastroenterology 1985; 89: 977–981

95 Parks AG, Swash M, Urich H. Sphincter denervation in anorectal incontinence and rectal prolapse. Gut 1977; 18: 656–665

96 Parks AG, Swash M. Denervation of the anal sphincter causing idiopathic ano-rectal incontinence. J R Coll Surg Edinb 1979; 24: 94–96

97 Beersiek F, Parks AG, Swash AM. Pathogenesis of anorectal incontinence: a histometric study of anal sphincter musculature. J Neurol Sci 1979; 42: 111–127

98 Lubowski DZ, Swash M, Nicholls RJ, Henry MM. Increase in pudendal nerve terminal motor latency with defaecation straining. Br J Surg 1988; 75: 786–788

99 Sultan AH, Kamm MA, Bartram CI, Hudson CN. Pudendal nerve damage during labour: prospective study before and after childbirth. Br J Obstet Gynaecol 1994; 101: 22–28

100 Small KA, Wynne JM. Evaluating the pelvic floor in obstetric patients. Aust N Z J Obstet Gynaecol 1990; 30: 41–45

101 Cornes H, Bartolo DCC, Stirrat GM. Changes in anal canal sensation after childbirth. Br J Surg 1991; 78: 74–77

102 Chaliha C, Kalia V, Sultan AH, Monga AK, Stanton SL. Anal function: effect of pregnancy and delivery. Am J Obstet Gynecol 2001; 185: 427–432

103 Sultan AH, Kamm MA, Talbot IC, Nicholls RJ, Bartram CI. Anal endosonography for identifying external sphincter defects confirmed histologically. Br J Surg 1994; 81: 463–465

104 Sultan AH, Kamm MA, Bartram CI, Hudson CN. Anal sphincter trauma during instrumental delivery. A comparison between forceps and vacuum extraction. Int J Gynecol Obstet 1993; 43: 263–270

105 Donnelly V, Fynes M, Campbell D et al. Obstetric events leading to anal sphincter damage. Obstet Gynecol 1998; 92: 955–961

106 WHO Population Report. Healthier Mothers and Children through Family Planning Programmes. Geneva: Geneva, 1984; J677

107 Hayflick L. Theories of biological aging. Exp Gerontol 1985; 20: 145–159

108 Yamauchi M, Woodley DT, Mechanic GL. Aging and crosslinking of skin collagen. Biochem Biophys Res Commun 1988; 152: 898–903

109 Norton PA. Pelvic floor disorders: the role of fascia and ligaments. Clin Obstet Gynecol 1993; 36: 926–938

110 Morley R, Cumming J, Weller R. Morphology and neuropathology of the pelvic floor in patients with stress incontinence. Int Urogynecol J 1966; 7: 3–12

111 De Gregorio G, Hillemans HG, Quaas L, Mentzel J. Late morbidity following cesarian section: a neglected factor. Geburtshilfe Frauenheilkd 1988; 48: 16–19

112 McIntosh LJ, Mallett VT, Frahm J, Richardson DA. Ehlers-Danlos syndrome and gynaecologic disorders. Int Urogynecol J 1993; 4: 394

113 Norton PA, Baker JE, Sharp HC, Warenski JC. Genitourinary prolapse and joint hypermobility in women. Obstet Gynecol 1995; 85: 225–228

114 Haadem K, Ling L, Ferno M, Graffner H. Estrogen receptors in the external anal sphincter. Obstet Gynecol 1991; 164: 609–610

115 Brincat M. Skin collagen content and thickness and their relationship to bone in untreated and oestrogen treated postmenopausal women. London: PhD Thesis, University of London, 1985

116 Donnelly V, O'Connell PR, O'Herlihy C. The influence of oestrogen replacement on faecal incontinence in postmenopausal women. Br J Obstet Gynaecol 1997; 104: 311–315

116 Savolainen J, Myllyla V, Myllyla R et al. Effects of denervation and immobilisation on collagen biosynthesis in rat skeletal muscle and tendon. Am J Physiol 1988; 254: R897–R902

118 Peltonen L, Myllyla U, Tolenen U, Myllya V. Changes in collagen metabolism in diseased muscles. II. Immunhistochemical studies. Arch Neurol 1982; 39: 756–759

119 Stephens HR, Duance VC, Dunn MJ, Bailey AJ, Dubowitz V. Collagen types in neuromuscular diseases. J Neurosci 1982; 53: 45–62

120 Laurberg S, Swash M. Effects of aging on the anorectal sphincters and their innervation. Dis Colon Rectum 1989; 32: 737–742

121 Uldbjerg N, Ekman G, Malmstrom A, Olsson K, Ulmsten U. Ripening of the human uterine cervix related to changes in collagen, glycosaminoglycans and collagenolytic activity. Am J Obstet Gynecol 1983; 147: 662–666

122 Granstrom L, Ekman G, Ulmsten U, Barchan K, Malmstrom A. Proteoglycan metabolism in the connective tissue of corpus and cervix uteri during ripening and term labour in term pregnancy. Br J Obstet Gynaecol 1989; 96: 1198–1202

123 King JK Freeman RM. Is antenatal bladder neck mobility a risk factor for postpartum stress incontinence? Br J Obstet Gynaecol 1998; 105: 1300–1307

124 Skoner M, Thompson WD, Caron VA. Factors associated with risk of stress urinary incontinence in women. Nurs Res 1994; 43: 301–306

125 Johanson RB, Rice C, Doyle M et al. A randomised prospective study comparing the new vacuum extractor policy with forceps delivery. Br J Obstet Gynaecol 1993; 100: 524–530

126 Sultan AH, Kamm MA, Hudson CN. Obstetric perineal tears: an audit of training. J Obstet Gynecol 1995; 15: 19–23

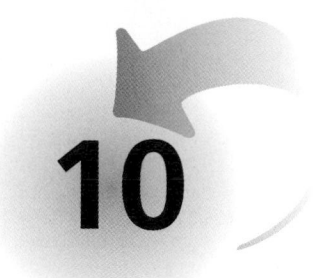

Colin G. Fink

Diagnostic molecular microbiology for the gynaecologist

The last 15 years have seen a quiet revolution in the technical and clinical possibilities for rapid diagnosis of infectious disease. So-called molecular techniques which amplify organism- or genus-specific fragments of DNA or RNA have enabled an unparalleled sensitivity and specificity in testing for the presence of pathogens in clinical material.[1,2] These techniques may be applied to many diagnostic problems arising with a presentation of clinical infection. The same techniques have revolutionised genetic studies and have been central to the analysis within the human genome project.[3]

An ability to amplify and recognise specific DNA and RNA of organisms[1,2] is central to these new laboratory diagnostic techniques which are now increasingly available as an adjunct to existing laboratory facilities. Many traditional micro biologists see themselves threatened by this technical change, so it is worth stating that molecular technology is not intended nor yet seen as a wholesale replacement of traditional laboratory microbiology. The newer techniques are used to ask very specific diagnostic questions of the clinical samples within the laboratory (see below) These new methods may be integrated into the laboratory repertoire, so forming an improved diagnostic service for clinical use. We have an opportunity with this nucleic acid technology to make real progress in improving the speed and accuracy of clinical diagnosis. This advance is applicable in both the field of infection and in human genetic studies. These two areas are not especially different as we recognise that it is the genetic characteristics of the organism which confers virulence and which is a part of any host/parasite relationship.[4] It does seem likely that, in the very near future, the same molecular diagnostic techniques will also impinge on clinical biochemical studies and in pharmaceutical interventions; tailoring drugs to the individual's genetic biochemical profile.[3,5]

In problems of infection, there is an obvious and attractive economy for clinical activity including a rapid diagnosis so that earlier treatment in a

Dr Colin G. Fink BSc MB ChB PhD FRCPath, Micropathology Ltd, University of Warwick Science Park, Barclays Venture Centre, Sir William Lyons Road, Coventry CV4 7EZ, UK.   www.micropathology.com

A double strand of DNA separating at 94°C

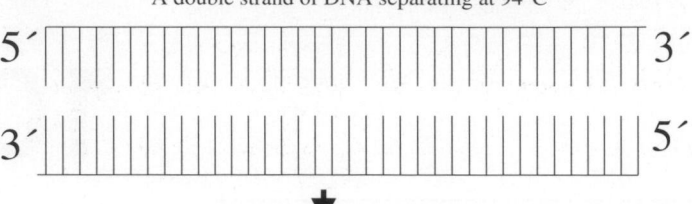

Extension of new strands of DNA with Taq enzyme adding nucleotide triphosphates

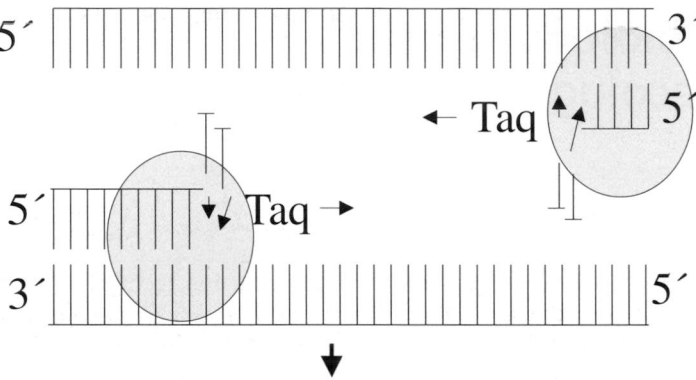

Two double strands of DNA after replication. The process is repeated for 20–40 cycles

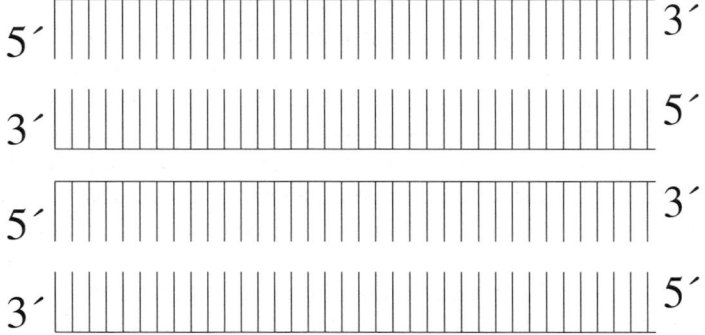

Fig. 1 DNA amplification – an illustration of the principle.[1,2] DNA is normally double-stranded. Heating to 94°C will disassociate the strands. If there are short lengths of matching 'primers' within the reaction tube, these will adhere as the temperature drops, to the single strands, if exactly complementary sequences are present. An enzyme derived from a hot vent organism (*Thermophylus aquaticus*, Taq polymerase) will adhere to the internal 3'-end of the primer and encourage nucleotides from the reaction mixture to extend a new complementary DNA strand. If the heating and cooling cycle is repeated on a so-called 'thermocycler', the reaction will take place again and again and an 'amplification' of specific DNA may take place within the reaction tube. In the case of RNA-containing organisms, an extra enzyme step at the beginning of the reaction will convert any RNA to complementary DNA (cDNA) by using an enzyme called reverse transcriptase (RT). The amplified DNA may be identified and visualised by running it on an agarose gel. It will migrate under the influence of an electric current at a rate dictated by its molecular size. It is the prediction of the DNA product size which will define the organism.

Table 1 Specimens for diagnosing infection

Source of material	Suitable specimens
Organism within blood or white cells	EDTA blood specimen at room temperature
Endocervical organisms	Endocervical swab sent dry/cytoplasmic cell suspension
Amniotic fluid	Amniotic fluid in EDTA blood bottle or sterile tube
Urinary or urethral material	Urine sent in a sterile universal container. Refrigerate at 4°C and send overnight; kept cool, swab sent dry
Vaginal organisms	Vaginal swab sent dry in sterile container
Faeces	Send in a sterile universal container; keep cool
Throat swab	Send dry for DNA-containing organisms. For RNA-containing organisms use viral transport medium

Remember that contamination of a specimen will invalidate the test result. Use scrupulously sterile techniques to obtain any specimen for molecular diagnostic testing.

If in doubt telephone the microbiologist/virologist for advice.

disease cycle is made possible. This chapter will review the traditional and newer laboratory approaches that are available to the clinician to diagnose infection. Using examples relevant to gynaecological practice, some advantages of the newer, rapid techniques will be demonstrated to show how they may contribute to the gynaecologist's ability to make early clinical diagnosis and provide timely and effective treatment. The clinician armed with this information can create a demand on the diagnostic laboratory to provide these rapid diagnostic techniques.

Molecular DNA/RNA amplification techniques (Fig. 1) are exquisitely sensitive and, to avoid contamination risks, they require scrupulously clean laboratory facilities with absolute separation of clinical material from reagent areas and high stringency in all procedures. This is one reason that provision and development of these tests may be more appropriate from within specialist reference laboratories (Table 1). Organisms which may be detected in 2002 within the author's laboratory using molecular techniques for DNA and RNA characterisation during 2002 are listed in Table 2.

COMBINED CLINICAL AND LABORATORY APPROACHES TO DIAGNOSING INFECTION

The search for an organism or organism-unique material

The theory which is applied for a confident diagnosis of infection in an individual patient is always dependent on the demonstration of an organism

Table 2 Organisms in the year 2002 which may be detected in the author's laboratory using molecular techniques for DNA and RNA analysis

Organisms (alphabetically)
- Adenovirus (T)
- *Aspergillus* genus
- *Borrelia burgdorferi*
- *Brucella* genus
- *Candida/Cryptococcus*
- *Chlamydia pneumoniae*
- *Chlamydia psittaci*
- *Chlamydia trachomatis*
- Coronavirus
- Cytomegalovirus
- Epstein Barr virus
- *Haemophilus influenzae*
- *Haemophilus parainfluenzae*
- Hepatitis B (genotyping & resistance detection)
- Hepatitis C (genotyping available)
- Hepatitis D
- Hepatitis G
- Human herpes virus 6 (HHV6)
- Human herpes virus 7 (HHV7)
- Human herpes virus 8 (HHV8)
- Influenza viruses A & B
- *Leptospira* genus (T)
- *Listeria monocytogenes*
- Measles virus
- Mumps virus
- *Mycobacterium* genus (T)
- *Mycoplasma* genus (T)
- *Mycoplasma pneumoniae*
- *Neisseria gonorrhoeae*
- *Neisseria meningitides* (T)
- Papillomavirus (T)
- Parainfluenza viruses 1, 2, 3
- Parvovirus B19
- Polyoma virus (JC & BK)
- Respiratory syncytial virus
- Retrovirus genus
- Rhinovirus
- Rubella virus
- *Propionibacterium/Actinomyces*
- *Staphylococcus* genus
- *Streptococcus pneumoniae*
- *Toxoplasma gondii*

Organism specific genes
- HIV-1 env gene including type O
- HIV-1 gag gene
- HIV-1 pol gene
- 16S rRNA bacterial gene
- 18S rRNA fungal gene

Cerebrospinal fluid (multiplex) viral screen
- Enterovirus
- Herpes simplex virus types 1 & 2
- Varicella zoster virus

Quantitative assays for viral load
- Hepatitis B virus (T)
- Hepatitis C virus (T)
- HIV-1
- Cytomegalovirus
- Epstein Barr virus
- Polyoma BK virus

(T) Sequencing of a genome enables typing and speciation of an organism. The gynaecologist should always seek advice from the clinician in charge of the laboratory to ensure that the most appropriate samples are sent for each test requested.

known to cause disease in association with the clinical picture of the disease (Koch's postulates).[6] This may be the scientific ideal but it is, of course, not our experience in clinical life and the astute gynaecologist will look for infection before it causes disease (for example, and see later, *Chlamydia trachomatis*[7] or papillomavirus[8] infection in the endocervix, *Toxoplasma gondii*[9] or HIV in the pregnant woman[10]).

In contrast, when trying to diagnose the cause of a specific clinical picture such as fever and associated miscarriage, it is good practice to formulate a differential diagnosis and to look for a range of organisms that may be responsible for an infectious event. Defining the cause of a miscarriage apparently associated with infection may be difficult and require both antibody studies (see below) and a search for an organism or organism-derived toxin. Nonetheless, a firm diagnosis in this event is always a worthwhile exercise as it may provide both the patient and physician with an understanding and reassure to allow planning for a future pregnancy (see below).

The host response to infection

Sometimes, in concert with a search for the organism or in the absence of an organism and as an alternative, a laboratory may be able to demonstrate a host antibody response as specific IgM seen as an early response to infection. It may be possible to demonstrate immunoglobulin as IgG with an improving 'fit' to the antigen[11,12] as further evidence of recent infection with that organism. Although strictly these antibody investigations might be considered to be the province of the immunologist, this interest has always been within the microbiologist's and, more particularly, the virologist's laboratory and there is good reason to have the diagnostic exercise for one patient under one roof.

A search for a specific immunoglobulin also may be used by the clinician as a re-assurance of relative immunity and reduced risk in the newly pregnant patient, for example of rubella,[13] varicella zoster (chicken pox)[14] or *T. gondii*[15] antibodies. An antibody screen may also be used as a precautionary investigation, to plan treatment, or to provide a continuing review ('screening') of infection exposure during a pregnancy, for example monitoring for hepatitis B carrier status,[16] syphilis serology, and *T. gondii* antibody production in the non-immune pregnancy.[17]

In later pregnancy, antibody studies may provide information of benefit to both mother and baby, for example the presence of parvovirus IgM in a pregnant woman who suffers a rash during pregnancy.[18] This will alert the obstetrician and paediatrician of a risk of anaemia and hydropic disease in the fetus as late as 11 weeks after a transient rash in the mother (also see below).

If we monitor for the presence HIV antibodies in the pregnant patient,[19] in the mother found to be sero-positive steps may be taken to intervene for a caesarean delivery and also to prevent breast feeding. Both these interventions reduce the risk of transmission of virus from mother to the new-born.[19]

A population review of infection

If an investigator reports an increased incidence of a clinical problem in a population,[20] any investigation of an individual patient with symptoms, within that population, looking for either the organism or a host response, will be guided by this recent epidemiological information. Information derived by wide-spread and continuing survey on the pattern of disease and populations involved is essential in a medically responsible society for economic and focused individual disease investigation. An example of this informed clinical investigation was seen in our laboratory, where a high fever and associated miscarriage of a precious pregnancy was determined in retrospect to be due to the influenza A virus circulating 5 weeks before the time of the fetal loss. The investigation required both antibody and an organism search on stored antenatal blood and blood taken during the fever. The UK *Communicable Disease Reports* (CDR) published weekly by the Public Health Laboratory and the *Morbidity and Mortality Weekly Report* (MMWR) published by the Centers for Disease Control in Atlanta, Georgia, USA are an example of this disease guidance from population surveillance. Rapid molecular diagnostic systems are now contributing to this surveillance work both to define the organism, monitor the prevalence of infection in the clinically unaffected population and provide information on the natural history of the organism.

A landmark population investigation of this nature was seen during the rubella outbreaks in Australia[20] and the US[21] with high numbers of fetal abnormalities noted months later. It is this disease surveillance which is central to epidemic monitoring, and to a formulation of governments' vaccination policy. In the case of congenital rubella, this epidemiological information was reason to develop a vaccine and encourage wide-spread uptake of the vaccine to remove wild-type rubella virus from the population.

TRADITIONAL LABORATORY MICROBIOLOGY AND VIROLOGY

In acute illness diagnosis, the defined swab or body fluid for examination is sent to the laboratory in appropriate preserving or transport medium and should be accompanied by clinical information. Traditionally, the microbiologist is a specialist 'gardener' who may first examine the clinical material by staining for organisms seen with the light microscope and then 'planting' the clinical samples on or within an agar plate or culture medium or, in the case of suspected viral disease, onto a permissive continuous human or animal cell line. Growth of the organisms is awaited. In this way the microbiologist asks the basic question: what organisms are within this material? The question concerning the likely organisms is focused by what is known of the clinical presentation and exposure history. This enquiry is also guided by a vast microbiology information resource developed over the last 100 years which enables the microbiologist to have narrowed the selection of growth media for encouraging the clinically-likely organisms to grow within the laboratory.[22] Although the question asked must be kept broad enough to be inclusive of all likely pathogens, it is narrowed by combined clinical and laboratory experience and knowing what organisms are within the local community. The colonies of bacterial organisms that grow in the laboratory may be identified by appearance and further speciated by the colony biochemical reaction to laboratory fermentation assays.[22] In cases of virus growth from clinical specimens placed in laboratory tissue culture, these growths may first be identified by characteristic cytopathic effects in cell culture,[23] and then further identified in some cases by looking at the inhibition of virus growth in cell culture by specific antisera.

Other methods for defining a virus use immunological techniques which may include immunofluorescence using monoclonal antibodies[24] from infected laboratory cultured cells, placental biopsy or ulcer material or fetal cells or any source of exfoliated cells. These techniques look for viral protein which fluoresce having bound specific fluorescent tagged antisera. They may be seen under the light microscope as a marker for viruses which themselves are too small to be seen under these conditions, but which may be seen under the electron microscope. This organism identification procedure is often supplemented, in a diagnostic exercise, by investigation of the maternal antibody responses (see above). In the fetus, the presence of an antibody response indicative of viral infection is dependent on actual infection within fetal tissue and the maturity of the developing fetus at the time of infection. IgM response in the fetus is not usual before 28–33 weeks' gestation and fetal IgG production to intra-uterine infection is not at all certain until near term. After birth, the new-born shows increasing competence to produce IgG to new infection and cell-mediated responses to infection develop steadily after birth.[25] It is the presence of maternal, passively-acquired IgG, from placental transfer and colostrum, which provides some passive protection for the new-born whilst immune competence develops.

The clinical relevance of a laboratory diagnostic service

Microbiological laboratory diagnostic systems have steadily improved over the last 100 years. In scientific terms, the procedures work reasonably well, helped by an enquiring microbiologist, but the limiting step which is obvious to any clinician is the time required for the laboratory to produce a diagnosis. In some cases, the patient may be clinical deteriorating too rapidly for directed and effective treatment to await a laboratory-defined diagnosis. In these circumstances, there is pressure on a clinician to act and treat without the pathogen being defined. Culture and identification of some organisms may take days and other organisms are too fastidious to grow within the standard laboratory facilities. It is still a problem that an unusual clinical presentation may not be recognised to be associated with a particular organism or the pathogen may be, with increased international travel, an imported zoonosis which is not permissive (it will not grow) or may it be unsafe for the local laboratory facilities.

Virological laboratory investigations have always attracted justified criticism by clinical staff that the result arrived after the clinical event. It is in this diagnostic area where a transformation is now possible with an immediate and rapid molecular diagnosis providing real clinical value. It is perhaps fortuitous that this rapid diagnostic facility has appeared contemporaneously with the recent developments of effective antiviral drug therapy. The obstetrician and gynaecologist now see a burgeoning population of immunosuppressed and transplant patients. It is especially valuable and relevant that rapid diagnostic methods for infection are now available for this susceptible cohort.

HOW DOES RAPID MOLECULAR DIAGNOSIS IMPROVE PRESENT MICROBIOLOGY SERVICES?

The molecular microbiologist or scientist asks very specific questions and searches for specific organisms. This makes the clinical information supplied to the laboratory of great importance. At best, 'multiplexing' allows a search for up to three organisms in one test, or primers may be genus specific only so that, for example all serovars of *Chlamydia trachomatis* will be detected or all *Mycobacteria* detected. This is in marked contrast to the traditional microbiologist who 'plants' the clinical sample and awaits growth. If more than three sets of organism-specific 'primers' are combined in one test, the sensitivity of the test may be adversely affected by DNA interference.

A major advantage of molecular diagnostic techniques is that no viable organisms are required to reach the laboratory in order to make the diagnosis. These newer methods rely only on the presence of DNA or RNA unique to the organism which may be preserved in a clinical specimen. (see Table 1 for best preservation methods for specimens and Table 2 for organism-available assays). DNA is remarkably tough and travels in relatively sterile material without deterioration. RNA is more labile, but there is good evidence that EDTA in blood bottles stops blood-borne RNA viruses deteriorating, and any clinical sample containing patient's cells with intracellular organisms seems to be relatively resilient with good organism preservation, even when transported at room temperatures. It is in this critical area of best specimen preservation that the specialist laboratory will always advise the clinician. If the specimen is suboptimal or contaminated to start with, then any improvement in techniques for diagnosis will be of limited value.

EXAMPLES OF RAPID CLINICAL DIAGNOSIS AND PROSPECTIVE TREATMENT

There are within this section examples of rapid diagnostic services for the obstetrician and gynaecologist. This is not an exhaustive review and new developments extend the range of organisms that may be identified using rapid diagnostic techniques. The best advice is to contact the laboratory that specialises in these techniques, to find out the most up-to-date information on what testing is available. When a clinical demand indicates a diagnostic need, the specialist molecular laboratory may quite quickly design and have available a suitable assay. This is a great attraction and supporting argument for specialist molecular diagnostic laboratories.

Infection in the sexually active woman

An example of clinical pressure to act prospectively is seen with a young, sexually active patient presenting with exquisitely tender genital ulcers of recent onset of just hours or days duration. Meningism may be seen in association with this presentation and may be sufficient for an acute hospital admission. Sometimes, there is a sudden onset and semi-intentional urinary retention to avoid an acute burning pain associated with micturition. These observations alone would support a clinical diagnosis of herpes genitalis.

Confusingly, in some cases, meningism without clinical genital ulceration may be the only clinical presentation (Mollaret's meningitis[26]) which may warrant acute medical admission and examination of the cerebrospinal fluid (CSF) for pathogens.[27] On clinical diagnosis, this florid case will be acute genital herpes virus infection, but good practice requires a rapid laboratory confirmation:[28] sometimes this is important, because although a clinical diagnosis may seem to be obvious, it may still be wrong.[29] In a clinical presentation of this clarity, most authorities would support treatment even before a laboratory confirmation was available, with at least high dose oral acyclovir or i.v. treatment may be indicated for severe systemic involvement. One of the longer acting and orally better absorbed acyclovir derivatives may be considered.

There is evidence that this treatment will shorten the duration of the lesions and reduce morbidity. There is, therefore, an economy of purpose to be gained by a rapid and definitive diagnosis. DNA amplification of material from the lesions will define the organism in a matter of hours, whereas culture of the organism ,if possible, may take 2–6 days. The rapid diagnostic methods improve both the speed and test sensitivity for the detection of these organisms and do not require any residual viability of the organism in the specimen arriving at the laboratory. As herpes genitalis is a latent and persistent infection, laboratory diagnosis and virus typing is also valuable information for the management of any future pregnancy and to advise the patient. Typing the virus (herpes virus type 1 or type 2) is clinically valuable as the two types have quite different expectation of recrudescent genital disease.

In less florid clinical cases of genital inflammation with or without ulceration, a molecular search for organisms with similar presentation may include *Chlamydia trachomatis* including serovars responsible for lymphogranuloma venereum, *Neisseria gonnorhoeae*, and also to consider other organisms common in tropical countries to which travellers may be exposed. These may include canchroid (*Haomophyluo duoroyn*), and with anaesthetic rather than painful ulcers – syphilis yaws and pinta.[30] The risk of HIV and hepatitis B should not be overlooked in those that have been sexually exposed and have contracted any STD.

Rapid diagnosis of infection in the pregnant woman

Any disease in the pregnant mother is always a dilemma because two lives are at risk. Modern methods of rapid diagnosis may provide a timely answer for both the patient and clinician, reduce a period of anxiety from weeks to hours and allow appropriate therapeutic intervention.

Parvovirus B19 infection

This is believed to be the only parvovirus to infect the human host, although there are many parvoviruses that infect mammals.[18] This virus replicates preferentially within the normoblasts (red cell precursors) in the marrow and will cause a transient loss of reticulocytes in the normal infected adult or child. In childhood infection, 'slapped cheek' exanthem may be seen and in adults a rash, malaise and also a degree of transient arthropathy. Infection with this virus is associated with sickle cell crises in the homozygous or heterozygous carriers of sickle cell anaemia and this alone may jeopardise the viability of a pregnancy. Unfortunately, the virus easily crosses the placenta as it is associated with a profound viraemia even in the relatively asymptomatic adult and the resulting infection of the fetus may take place up to 11 weeks after the maternal infection. Further diagnostic difficulties may be encountered in that maternal infection may be a transient rash and virtually asymptomatic. Fetal infection is recognised as severe hydropic disease as a result of a loss of fetal red cells secondary to normoblast loss and the profound anaemia is associated with high output cardiac failure. This is one of the main causes of non-immune hydropic loss of pregnancies. The hydrops may sometimes resolve without intervention. Parvovirus B19 is a once-only infection in contrast to rubella with which it may be clinically confused. Rubella may re-infect even in the presence of maternal antibody.[31] In a Spring outbreak of parvovirus infection, the presence of parvovirus IgG in the pregnant mother may be re-assuring providing that there has been no recent illness and no IgM is present. Rapid DNA amplification may be used to demonstrate parvovirus DNA in the serum of a pregnant woman with a rash. This is a defining diagnostic exercise and the absence of DNA and parvovirus IgM at the time of the rash excludes this infection. Rapid diagnostic techniques may also be applied to the same presenting patient to look for rubella virus and also enterovirus which are other common causes of similar exanthems in pregnancy. If there is hydropic disease in the late second or third trimester, amniotic fluid may be tapped and the presence of parvovirus DNA will confirm the nature of the problem and prevent further unnecessary diagnostic investigation of hydropic disease. In such a case, fetal transfusion may save the pregnancy. There is evidence that, if the fetus survives the hydropic crises, no long-term developmental sequelae are associated with the infection.[18]

Toxoplasma gondii infection

T. gondii is a hugely successful protozoan parasite in temperate regions and infects all mammalian species and many birds. Many infections in the human host are from eating undercooked meat (lamb and pork) containing cysts. Deep frozen, UK-imported New Zealand lamb appears to have a lower infection risk probably because the *Toxoplasma* tissue cysts do not survive the colder temperatures associated with sea transportation of meat. Barbecue meat and French-style pink meat, lightly cooked, are the sources of infection which may also come from unwashed vegetables. In Paris, > 70% of fertile women aged 25 years are already immune.[32] In the UK, less then 20% are immune at the same age.[33] The source for sheep and pig infection and also some human infection is the *Toxoplasma* oocysts excreted by all cats when they first hunt and become infected from eating small mammals which themselves carry encysted *Toxoplasma* in their flesh. The cat is the definitive host and a sexual life-cycle in the cat's gut produces thousands of oocysts, for a few weeks only, in the faeces. The excreted oocysts survive for up to 18 months in damp soil. The distribution of these soil oocysts is wide-spread in all areas of urban and farm activity in temperate regions. Keeping domestic cats does not increase the risk if simple hygiene precautions are observed when their litter trays and faeces are handled. The organism when ingested may cause 'flu-like' symptoms in the human host and also a lymphadenopathy. The disease is self-limiting in the immunocompetent and the parasitaemia lasts for a few weeks.

Problems of interest to the obstetrician arise if a primary infection occurs during pregnancy or 3–6 months before conception. A persistent parasitaemia may pose a risk to the fetus. The infection may be virtually asymptomatic in pregnancy; the risk of infection for the fetus increases as pregnancy progresses and the placental vascular bed increases. Paradoxically, the degree of fetal damage, which may be catastrophic, is likely to be greatest during the first and second trimesters when the risk of transplacental infection is lower. If infection is suspected, testing for *Toxoplasma* IgM and IgG may be helpful. The IgM may persist for at least a year after infection, which may have occurred many months before conception, and this IgM persists well after any risk of parasitaemia. In this event, the IgG may be tested for 'fit' or adherence which is a measure of its avidity to the parasite antigen. This gives a measure of the time since first infection and thus the relative risk to the pregnancy. Maternal blood may be checked for parasite DNA using rapid amplification techniques. If fetal infection is suspected, amniotic fluid may also be sampled after 13–16 weeks of gestation looking for parasite DNA by rapid molecular testing. All these test results should be carefully considered together and in conjunction with a microbiologist who has a special interest in this parasite. The aim is to diagnose infection early and ensure adequate treatment to protect the fetus if recent maternal infection is shown. No one test in this situation should be definitive and it is the combination of tests which will provide the most information for the obstetrician to plan adequate treatment to minimise fetal risk. The most recent addition of DNA testing for the parasite has improved the positive predictive value of the combined test results.

Rubella infection

Unfortunately, although previous wild-type infection or vaccination will provide the pregnant mother with antibodies and a degree of protection, re-infection with rubella may still take place. This is one of the main arguments for ensuring complete population vaccine uptake so that wild-type rubella does not circulate within a community. In the event of a rubelliform rash or exanthem, the obstetrician, the GP and the patient will all seek re-assurance about the nature of the infection. Other organisms which may present in this way include parvovirus B19 infection and also many of the 70+ enterovirus infections. Rapid molecular diagnosis, looking at throat swabs, EDTA blood samples and faeces (enteroviruses show faecal/oral transfer and they replicate within the gut wall as well as invading the blood stream) may allow a rapid diagnosis for any of these organisms.

Traditionally, two sera one when the rash is noted and the other 4 weeks later may be checked for a rise in rubella antibodies. In contrast, the appropriate use of rapid molecular diagnostic techniques together with the right specimens may define the organism and allay the anxiety in hours.

Farming risks

In the aftermath of foot and mouth disease in the UK in 2001, many farmers are trying to rebuild their animal flocks. There are, however, specific risks for the pregnant patient.

Chlamydia psittici infection

If a pregnant farmer's wife, who has been delivering lambs some of which have suffered ovine abortion, presents with a high fever, in the UK one would suspect *Chlamydia psittici* infection.[34] Prospective treatment in this case is i.v. high-dose antibiotic and delivery of the pregnancy to preserve the mother's life and maybe to preserve the fetus. The exposure to infected lamb placenta provides an aerosol derived from up to 10^5 organisms/g of placental tissue, so infection of the attendant pregnant farmer's wife is with a huge organism load which is inhaled. DNA detection methods for this organism would include sampling of the ovine material and also sputum and blood from the fevered woman. A diagnosis is possible within hours. Semi-quantitative DNA methods would also allow a considered view on the organism load within the patient.

Toxoplasma gondii infection

Another cause of ovine abortion is *T. gondii*. In this event, the placental tissues and aborted lamb fetus will be heavily contaminated with the organisms. All the clothing used for this lambing procedure must be handled with gloves and should not be allowed to contaminate kitchen work-surfaces or food-stuffs. Great care is essential for the non-immune pregnant women involved in these procedures.

In any fever in a pregnant women, the clinician must consider her exposure and risks very fully. Rapid diagnostic techniques may provide a timely diagnosis and offer the chance of early re-assurance or appropriate intervention. The fever alone, which is a host response to infection, is enough to precipitate miscarriage.

INFECTION OF THE NEW-BORN

Children born with any of the collection of hepatosplenomegaly, jaundice, failure to thrive, anaemia or congenital anomaly present a dilemma to the attendant obstetrician and paediatrician. If there is an infectious or genetic process, then this must be discovered with all speed to (i) limit organism activity, if possible; (ii) determine the true cause of the fetal disease; and (iii) offer optimal clinical support.

Congenital rubella infection

In cases of suspected infection, maternal blood and new-born urine, stool and blood may be sent to the laboratory The presence of specific IgM in the new-born is diagnostic of congenital rubella syndrome and molecular diagnostic techniques may be used to demonstrate the RNA of the virus in the new-born. The congenitally infected infant will excrete the virus for many weeks.

Congenital cytomegalovirus infection

Cytomegalovirus is one of the persistent herpes virus group. Recrudescence in pregnancy and a corresponding placental transfer and fetal infection is always a risk.[35,36] In the case of suspected congenital cytomegalovirus infection, the diagnosis may be more difficult if not undertaken within 7 days from birth. A rapid demonstration of virus in the body fluids with the possibility of a quantitation of the viral load of the new-born before 7 days of age is required to define and separate true congenital disease caused by this virus, in contrast to a congenitally abnormal child for other reasons that may be infected with cytomegalovirus during birth. Many women carry the organism within their cervical tissues and infection, which may rapidly disseminate in the new-born without necessarily causing overt problems, may be an infection acquired at birth and not true congenital infection.

In this infection, the advent of rapid diagnostic testing providing evidence for the presence of virus in blood and urine from the new-born will confirm congenital infection and allow antiviral treatment, if clinically appropriate, to reduce the viral load. This infection has gained a rather greater significance in the HIV-infected population.

Congenital *Toxoplasma gondii* infection

There are estimated to be 750–1500 congenitally infected births in the UK each year.[37] In suspected congenital *T. gondii* infection, the organism may be demonstrated in the buffy coat cells of the new-born, and this together with a high level of maternal antibody may allow a rapid diagnosis and appropriate antibiotic therapy to limit the continuing damage to the new-born from the parasite.

New-born virus infection: herpes or enterovirus infection?

Two of the most common virus infections to present with rapidly fatal consequences in the new-born are infections with herpes simplex virus 1 and 2 and any of the enteroviruses. Enteroviruses in the new-born are also a constant fear within premature baby units and also any mother and baby unit where infection may travel through the residents with alarming speed. Rapid molecular techniques will detect which virus is in any body fluid and allow isolation of infected individuals. Whilst good antiviral therapy is available (acyclovir) for herpes virus infection with a sound safety record in the new-born, effective antiviral (pleconaril) treatments for Enterovirus infection are still being tested.[38,39]

Human immunodeficiency virus infection

Rapid quantitative diagnostic techniques for HIV in conjunction with antiviral treatment for the pregnant women facilitates well-timed antiviral treatment to lower the maternal viral load towards the time of delivery. This treatment together with consideration of Caesarean section for delivery and, where possible, no breast-feeding of the infant, may dramatically cut the rate of mother-to-child transmission of infection with the virus. This is perhaps the best known example where rapid DNA/RNA diagnostic methods have revolutionised treatment and outcome for the infant.[40]

New-born *Chlamydia trachomatis*, *Gonococcus* or other bacterial infection

The infant presenting with sticky eyes (ophthalmia neonatorum) within 2–3 weeks of birth presents the paediatrician with a diagnostic dilemma. Rapid molecular diagnostic techniques may rapidly resolve this and, on a good conjunctival specimen, will differentiate between *Gonococcus*, *C. trachomatis* and staphylococcal infection. This rapid diagnosis may also provide the obstetrician with valuable information for discrete and humane treatment for a mother at a post-natal clinic who has no knowledge or clinical evidence of her infection.

KEY POINTS FOR CLINICAL PRACTICE

- Molecular diagnostic methods have revolutionised the speed, sensitivity. and specificity of diagnosis in infection

- The techniques are continuously being adapted to include more organisms for which a rapid diagnostic service is available

- Clinical information is critically important to the molecular microbiologist/virologist, because the detection of organisms is primer specific and the search must be carefully directed

- This technology enables the O&G specialist to ask for a one-swab or one-cytocell endocervical sample diagnosis covering *Chlamydia trachomatis*, *Gonococcus*, human papillomavirus and may include a cytological smear screening exercise all at one clinic visit with infection results ready in hours and the organisms genetically typed

- The sensitivity of the tests are so good that the clinician must be sure to use scrupulous techniques to avoid contamination of the sample

- The clinical relevance of the presence of residual organism DNA after treatment may require discussion with the microbiologist

- One can identify a nucleic acid and also quantitate an organism 'load' or infectious burden. A diagnosis may be secured in hours and treatment may be tailored to viral 'load'

- Molecular diagnosis is entirely compatible and may be integrated with more traditional microbiology. This integration requires good-will from the traditional service providers

---

References

1 Baumforth KRN, Nelson PN, Digby JE et al. The polymerase chain reaction. J Clin Pathol Mol 1999; 52: 1–10
2 Saiki RK, Gelfand DH, Stoltel S et al. Primer directed enzymatic amplification of DNA with a thermostable DNA polymerase. Science 1988; 239: 487–491
3 Ganguly NK, Bano R, Seth SD. Human genome project: pharmacogenomics and drug development. Indian J Exp Biol 2001; 39: 955–961
4 Mims CA, Playfair JHL, Roitt IM et al. Host/parasite relationship. In: Medical Microbiology. London: Mosby, 1993; 2.1–2.10
5 Danzon P, Towse A. The economics of gene therapy and of pharmacogenetics. Value Health 2002; 5: 5–13
6 Falkow S. Molecular Koch's postulates applied to microbiological pathogenicity. Rev Infect Dis 1988; 10 (Suppl): 274–276
7 Centres for Disease Control and Prevention. Recommendations for the prevention and management of *Chlamydia trachomatis* infection. MMWR 1993; 42: 1–39

8 Kurman RJ, Henson DE, Herbst AL et al. Interim guidelines for the management of abnormal cervical cytology. JAMA 1994; 271: 1866–1869

9 Chatterton JMW. Pregnancy. In: Ho-Yen DO, Joss AWL. (eds) Human Toxoplasmosis. Oxford: Oxford University Press, 1992; 144–183

10 Mandelbrot L. Vertical transmission of viral infections. Curr Opin Obstet Gynecol 1998; 10: 123–128

11 Davidson MM. New techniques. In: Ho-Yen DO, Joss AWL. (eds) Human Toxoplasmosis. Oxford: Oxford University Press, 1992; 144–183

12 Thomas HI, Morgan-Capner P. Rubella specific IgG avidity: a comparison of methods. J Virol Methods 1991; 31: 219–228

13 Skendzel LP. Rubella immunity – defining the level of protective antibody. Am J Clin Pathol 1996; 106: 170–174

14 Hanshaw JB, Dudgeon JA, Marshal JC. Varicella zoster infections, Ch.7. In: Viral Diseases of the Fetus and Newborn. Philadelphia: WB Saunders 1985; 161–174

15 Gilbert RE, Tookey PA, Cubitt WD et al. Prevalence of *Toxoplasma gondii* IgG among pregnant women in west London according to country of birth and ethnic group. BMJ 1993; 306: 185

16 Boxall E. Antenatal screening for carriers of hepatitis B. BMJ 1995; 331: 1178–1179

17 Horizon M, Thoumsin H, Senterre J et al. 20 years of screening for toxoplasmosis in pregnant women. The Liège experience in 20,000 pregnancies. Rev Med Liège 1990; 45: 492–297

18 Pattison JR. Human parvoviruses. In: Zuckerman AJ, Banatvala JE, Pattison JR. (eds) Principles and Practice of Clinical Virology, 4th edn. Chichester: Wiley, 2000; 645–558

19 Connor EM, Sperling RS, Gelber R. Reduction of maternal infant transmission of human immunodeficiency virus type 1 with zidovudine treatment. N Engl J Med 1994; 331: 1173–1180

20 Gregg N McA. Congenital cataract following German measles in mother. Trans Ophthal Soc Aust 1941; 3: 35–46

21 Cooper LZ. Congenital rubella in the United States. Prog Clin Biol Res 1975; 3: 1–21

22 Thomas CGA. Cultivation of organisms. In: Thomas CGA. Medical Microbiology, 3rd edn. London: Ballière Tindall, 1973; 37–46

23 Versteeg J. Cell culture techniques. In: A Colour Atlas of Virology. London: Wolfe Medical, 1985; 98–131

24 Fox AJ. Monoclonal antibodies as immunofluorescence agents. In: Caul EO. (ed) Immunofluorescence – antigen detection techniques in diagnostic microbiology. London: PHLS Colindale, 1992; 15–20

25 Roitt I. The immune response – further aspects. In: Roitt I. Essential Immunology. Oxford: Blackwell, 1980; 87–119

26 Mollaret P. La meningite endothelio-leucocytaire multireccurente benigne: syndrome nouveau ou maladie nouvelle? Rev Neurol (Paris) 1944; 76: 57–76

27 Read SJ, Kurtz JB. Laboratory diagnosis of common viral infections of the CNS using a single multiplex PCR screening assay. J Clin Microbiol 1999; 37: 1352–1355

28 Scoular A, Gillespie G, Carmen WE. Polymerase chain reaction for diagnosis of genital herpes in a genito-urinary clinic. Sex Transm Infect 2002; 78: 21–25

29 Willet M. Bechet's syndrome presenting as acute genital ulcers. BMJ 2002; 324: 746

30 Mims CA, Playfair JHL, Roitt IM et al. Sexually transmitted disease. In: Medical Microbiology. London: Mosby, 1993; 24.1–24.22

31 Best JM, Banatvala JE, Morgan-Capner P et al. Fetal infection after maternal re-infection with rubella. Criteria for defining infection. BMJ 1989; 299: 773–775

32 Desmouts G, Couvreur J, Alison F et al. Etude epidemiologique sur la toxoplasmose: d'influence de la cuisson des viandes de boucherie sur la frequence de l'infection humaine. Rev Franc Etud Clin Biol 1965; 10: 952–958

33 Beverley JKA, Beattie CP, Roseman C. Human *Toxoplasma* infection. J Hygiene 1954; 52: 37–46

34 Helm CW, Smart GE, Cumming AD et al. Sheep acquired severe *Chlamydia psittici* infection in pregnancy. Int J Gynaecol Obstet 1989; 28: 369–372

35 Daley AJ, Gilbert GL. Cytomegalovirus infections in pregnancy. J Paediatr Child Health 2001 37: 589–591

36 Gouarin S, Palmer P, Cointe D et al. Congenital HCMV infection: a collaborative and comparative study of virus detection in amniotic fluid by culture and PCR. J Clin Virol 2001; 21: 47–55

37 Joss AW, Chatterton JM, Ho-Yen DO. Congenital toxoplasmosis: to screen or not to screen? Public Health 1990; 104: 9–20

38 Sawyer MH. Enteroviral infections: diagnosis and treatment. Curr Opin Pediatr 2001; 13: 65–69

39 Aradottir E, Alonso EM, Shulman ST. Severe neonatal enteroviral hepatitis treated with pleconaril. Pediatr Infect Dis 2001; 20: 457–459

40 Gottlieb S. Drug therapy reduces birth rate of HIV infected babies from 19% to 3%. BMJ 2002; 324: 381

11

Wilhelm H. Cronje A.P. Hawkins John W.W. Studd

Premenstrual syndrome

A good working definition for the premenstrual syndrome (PMS) is: 'distressing physical, psychological and behavioural symptoms, not caused by organic disease, which regularly occur during the same phase of the menstrual (ovarian) cycle, and which significantly regress or disappear during the remainder of the cycle'.[1] This definition describes a complex condition that is poorly understood and it is estimated to affect up to 95% of women to some degree. Of these symptomatic women, 5% will be affected severely enough to cause disruption of their daily activities and social interactions.[2] Women are affected during the luteal phase of the menstrual cycle and the syndrome includes virtually all symptoms that affect any system in a cyclical manner. The fact that no biological marker has yet been identified only adds to our lack of understanding. No one has as yet provided a universal definition of PMS as so many symptoms have been associated with the condition, but there is no doubt that it does not occur prior to puberty, after the menopause, or during pregnancy. It is not dependent on the presence of monthly bleeds, as women who have undergone hysterectomy without bilateral salpingo-oophorectomy could still suffer cyclical symptoms.[3] This condition, best-called 'the ovarian cycle syndrome',[4] is usually not recognised to be hormonal in aetiology, as there is no reference point of menstruation. The basic pathogenesis of PMS was summarised best by Studd:

Mr Wilhelm H. Cronje MB ChB, Research Fellow, Academic Department of Obstetrics and Gynaecology, Chelsea and Westminster Hospital, 369 Fulham Road, London SW10 9NH, UK (for correspondence)

Ms A.P. Hawkins BSc MRCOG DFFP, Research Fellow, Academic Department of Obstetrics and Gynaecology, Chelsea and Westminster Hospital, 369 Fulham Road, London SW10 9NH, UK

Prof. John W.W. Studd DSc MD FRCOG, Professor of Gynaecology and Consultant Gynaecologist, Academic Department of Obstetrics and Gynaecology, Chelsea and Westminster Hospital, 369 Fulham Road, London SW10 9NH, UK

Table 1 Proposed theories for premenstrual syndrome

Biological

	Female sex hormones	Oestrogen excess
		Progesterone deficiency
		Oestrogen/progesterone ratio
		Oestrogen/progesterone withdrawal
	Neurotransmitters	Serotonin
		Catecholamines
		Cholinergic
	Fluid retention	Sex hormones
		Renin-angiotensin-aldosterone axis
		Prolactin
		Vasopressin
		Dietary factors
	Glucocorticoids	
	Androgens	
	Prolactin	
	Antidiuretic hormone	
	Vitamin deficiency	A,
		B6
	Reactive hypoglaecaemia	
	Endogenous hormone allergy	
	Prostaglandins	Excess
		Deficiency
	Endogenous opiate peptides	Mid-luteal increase
		Premenstrual withdrawal
	Menstrual toxin	
	Magnesium deficiency	
	Melatonin	

Psychological

Social and evolutionary

Genetic

'whatever the details of the hormone imbalance, and no doubt they vary from case to case, the ultimate cause of premenstrual tension must be a **change** in plasma hormone values from the time of ovulation. The symptoms for this common condition can usually be relieved by ablating these hormone changes.' In other words, premenstrual syndrome does not occur if there is no ovarian function.[5]

HISTORICAL BACKGROUND

Hippocrates[6] mentioned the condition as early as the fourth century BC, but it only became a medical epidemic in the nineteenth century. Physicians in Victorian times were aware of menstrual madness, hysteria, chlorosis, ovarian mania, as well as the commonplace neurasthenia. The psychiatrist Maudsley[7] wrote in the 1870s: 'The monthly activity of the ovaries which marks the advent of puberty in women has a notable effect upon the mind and body; wherefore it may become an important cause of mental and physical derangement'. Frank was the first to introduce the phrase 'premenstrual tension' in 1931,[8] when he described 15 women with the typical symptoms of PMS as we know it. Greene and Dalton extended the definition to 'premenstrual syndrome' in 1953,[9] recognising the wider range of symptoms.

AETIOLOGY

The exact cause of PMS is uncertain, as the range of symptoms are so wide. As Magos[10] showed there are an abundance of theories (Table 1). The contradictory theories, sometimes even direct opposites, merely underlines the complexity and ignorance surrounding this condition. It is a complex combination of some of these mechanisms that underlies the cause to the premenstrual syndrome, but fluctuating levels of ovarian hormones, particularly progesterone, would seem to be a fundamental factor.

SYMPTOMS

More than 160 symptoms have been associated with the menstrual cycle.[8] It could probably be stated that virtually any symptom affecting any system in

Table 2 The six most common premenstrual syndrome symptoms as categorised into clusters by Moos[11]

1	Pain	Headache
		Cramps
		Muscle stiffness
		Backache
		Fatigue
		General aches and pains
2	Concentration	Difficulty concentrating
		Accidents
		Forgetfulness
		Insomnia
		Confusion
		Lowered judgement
		Lowered motor co-ordination
		Distractable
3	Behavioural change	Avoid social activities
		Lowered work or school performance
		Stay in bed
		Stay at home
		Decreased efficiency
4	Autonomic reaction	Dizziness, faintness
		Cold sweats
		Nausea vomiting
		Hot flushes
5	Water retention	Breast tenderness
		Bloating
		Weight gain
		Skin disorders
6	Negative affect	Depression
		Mood swings
		Irritability
		Restlessness
		Anxiety
		Tension
		Loneliness
		Crying

the body can fluctuate and cause distress during the ovarian cycle. The most common symptoms were categorised into eight symptom clusters, with six being more important, by Moos (Table 2).[11] It is, however, almost impossible to list specific symptoms as this would place unnecessary limitations on the diagnosis of premenstrual syndrome. A broader classification would, therefore, include physical, psychological and behavioural symptoms.

Physical symptoms

These are common symptoms, present more often than not. The most common manifestations are breast tenderness and swelling, bloating, oedema and weight gain. Other frequent complaints include pelvic discomfort, headaches or migraine, changes in bowel habit and reduced co-ordination.

Psychological symptoms

Depression, tension, irritability, anxiety and tiredness seem to the most common complaints. Libido, sleeping, and eating patterns could also be affected. Even though doubts have been expressed with regards to including premenstrual depression in the diagnosis,[12] there can be no doubt that psychological symptoms are the most important aspect of morbidity in PMS.

Behavioural changes

Many activities are reported to change during the menstrual cycle. Criminal behaviour, suicide attempts, hospital admissions, absenteeism from work, decrease in cognitive function, reports of minor illness in children, and increased proneness to accidents have all been associated with the menstrual cycle. These are, however, less common occurrences and therefore not so easy to include in any definition of this complex condition.

Other medical conditions

There are many medical problems that deteriorate in the week before the menstrual period. These include asthma, depression, epilepsy, rheumatoid arthritis, migraine and many others.[13] The severity of these medical conditions are also responsive to hormonal manipulation.

TREATMENT

General

It is still too common to find women suffering from PMS claiming that their symptoms are not taken seriously, either by family and friends or the family physician. In a study of 100 women questioned at a specialist PMS clinic, Leather and co-workers[14] found that 40% of these women had not been referred by their own general practitioner. This would make it more likely that these practitioners were not understanding or sympathetic. Often a sympathetic ear and a good explanation will be enough in milder forms of this condition. Re-assurance that many women suffer from PMS to a certain degree could also be all a woman needs in certain cases. A healthy life-style should be the first step in conquering the condition and gaining self-confidence. Regular exercise and relaxation will allow the release of natural endorphins. It is also helpful if important events are scheduled for the symptom-free period. A general healthy low-fat, high-fibre diet with adequate vitamins and minerals and avoiding long periods without food could be beneficial, as would reduced salt, alcohol, sugar and caffeine intake.

Vitamins

Vitamin B6 is an important co-factor in the synthesis of neurotransmitters serotonin and dopamine. With a serotonin deficiency being described as one of the possible mechanisms involved in PMS, vitamin B6 has been suggested as a possible treatment. A review of 12 trials by Kleijnen and co-workers[15] found that there was no definite evidence for any benefit. There is a risk of peripheral neuropathy with excessive ingestion of vitamin B6[16] and care should be taken in recommending it as treatment if no definite benefit has been shown. A systematic review by Wyatt et al.[17] found 25 published studies of which only 9 were suitable for meta-analysis. Even the included studies were of poor quality, but they conclude that daily doses of 100 mg (and possibly 50 mg) of vitamin B6 are likely to be beneficial in the treatment of PMS. They also found no conclusive evidence of neurological side-effects with these doses in the 940 women included in the review.

Vitamins A and E have also been used as treatment even though there is very little evidence of benefit. The recommended doses of vitamin A are high[18] and may lead to potentially toxic serum levels. It is thought to be most effective in treating the symptoms of bloating, weight gain, and breast tenderness. Vitamin E is believed to be most beneficial for symptoms such as anxiety and irritability, but evidence is lacking.

Essential fatty acids

Evening primrose oil (EPO) is a widely known and often used remedy, which has been used by women over the years. It contains the polyunsaturated essential fatty acids linoleic and γ-linolenic acids which are the precursors of prostaglandins PGE_1 and PGE_2. Although Massil and O'Brien[19] showed benefit over placebo for some symptoms, particularly breast tenderness, Collins and colleagues[20] failed to show a difference when comparing the drug to placebo. Similarly, a meta-analysis of the use of EPO in the treatment of PMS failed to show any significant benefit.[21] There is, however, anecdotal evidence that it helps in milder forms of PMS and with no side-effects it could sometimes prove useful.

Minerals

There is some evidence to suggest that disturbances of calcium regulation may play a role in the pathophysiological development of PMS.[22] Studies such as these showed benefit of calcium supplementation on symptoms including irritability, depression, anxiety, social withdrawal, headache and cramps, but sample populations were small. Thys-Jacobs and colleagues[23] conducted a randomised, double-blind, placebo-controlled multicentre trial and showed major reduction in overall luteal phase symptoms in 466 eligible women. They used a dose of 1200 mg of calcium carbonate over three menstrual cycles.

Low levels of red cell magnesium have been found in women suffering from PMS.[24] Magnesium is a co-factor in many enzymatic reactions and this has lead to the suggestion that a deficiency in magnesium could be responsible for the cyclical symptoms of PMS. Fachinetti et al.[25] showed an improvement in symptoms over 2 months in a double-blind, placebo-controlled study of 32 women and they also showed an improvement in menstrual migraine.[26] In another randomised, double-blind, placebo-controlled, crossover study Walker et al.[27] demonstrated a beneficial effect of 200 mg of magnesium on the symptoms of fluid retention (weight gain, swelling of extremities, breast tenderness, and abdominal bloating). Again, the study lasted only 2 months.

Another theory of a possible cause for premenstrual symptomatology is a deficiency of iron, zinc and manganese.[28] Evidence of benefit of treatment is lacking.

Complementary therapies

Exercise techniques (like yoga) and behavioural therapies (such as acupuncture and hypnosis) have all been reported as having a beneficial effect when used in the treatment of PMS. No controlled trials are available to substantiate this.

One prospective, randomised, placebo-controlled, cross-over trial[29] demonstrated benefit in patients receiving high-velocity, low-amplitude spinal manipulation and soft tissue therapy 2–3 times a week before menses for 3 cycles. There was some question as to the effect of placebo response. Hernandez-Reif et al.[30] showed decreases in anxiety, depressed mood and pain immediately after the first and last massage sessions. Longer term (5 week) benefits included a reduction in pain, water retention and overall menstrual distress, but no long-term changes in activity level or mood. These forms of therapy may be adjunctive therapy when treating premenstrual syndrome, but care should be taken as it is very difficult to establish the effect of the one-to-one personal attention that methods such as these entail.

Some women prefer to use 'natural' medication as opposed to conventional treatments used for PMS and herbal medicines have long been used to treat conditions particular to women including premenstrual syndrome and menstrual disorders. Hardy[31] reviewed the efficacy and safety of specific herbal preparations, traditionally used by women. Evening primrose oil and chaste tree berry were found to have benefits for some sufferers of PMS and dong quai used in traditional Chinese multiple-herb formulas also proved to be effective in some. A recent study by Schellenberg[32] demonstrated a significant benefit of the extract of agnus castus fruit (*Vitex agnus castus*) over placebo in 170 women suffering from PMS. The trial was prospective, randomised and placebo-controlled over three menstrual cycles and very few side-effects were encountered. A pilot study[33] on the effects of *Hypericum perforatum* (St John's Wort One-A-Day; Kira Limited, Lichtwer Pharma AG, Berlin, Germany) demonstrated a 51% improvement of overall premenstrual symptoms over two cycles, but there was no placebo arm in this study. To be certain of benefit, there

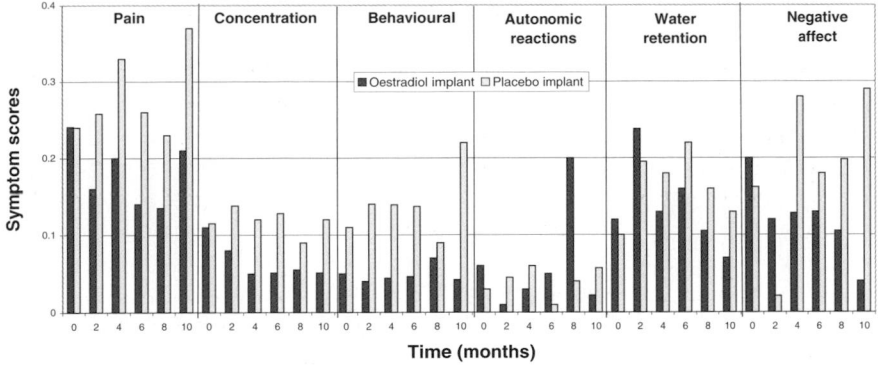

Fig. 1 This diagram shows oestradiol implants superior to placebo implants in all the symptom clusters of PMS. Adapted from Magos et al.[37]

need to be more trials over longer periods with larger sample sizes and these trials should be placebo-controlled. Other herbal formulations used include cayenne, ginseng, pulsatilla, raspberry leaves and wild yam.

Drug treatment

Diuretics

Women who experience true water retention as one of their symptoms may benefit from small doses of diuretics. Long-term use is not advocated,[34] and side-effects include potassium depletion, except when spironolactone is used. Before use, oedema should be demonstrated clearly and weight should be confirmed by weighing patients. It should not be used purely for the symptom of bloating. Wang et al.[35] used 100 mg spironolactone in a double-blind, placebo-controlled, cross over study and showed beneficial effects over placebo on negative mood changes and somatic symptoms.

Hormones

Oestrogens

Perhaps the most important hormone used in the treatment of severe PMS. The first study to show the anovulatory effects of oestradiol implants was by Greenblatt et al. for the use of contraception,[36] and the first study for its use in PMS was by Magos et al.[37] using 100 mg oestradiol implants. This showed an improvement with placebo implants but the improvements of every symptom group was greater in the active oestradiol group (Fig. 1). In addition, the placebo effect waned after a few months with continued response to oestradiol.

These patients were also given 7–13 days of oral progestogen per month to prevent endometrial hyperplasia and irregular bleeding.[38] Subsequently, a placebo-controlled trial of cyclical norethisterone in hysterectomised women reproduced the typical symptoms of PMS (Figs 2–4).[39]

We believe that cyclical oral progestogen in the oestrogen primed woman is the model for PMS. It is also significant that progestogen intolerance is one of the principal reasons why older, post-menopausal women stop taking HRT.[41] It is

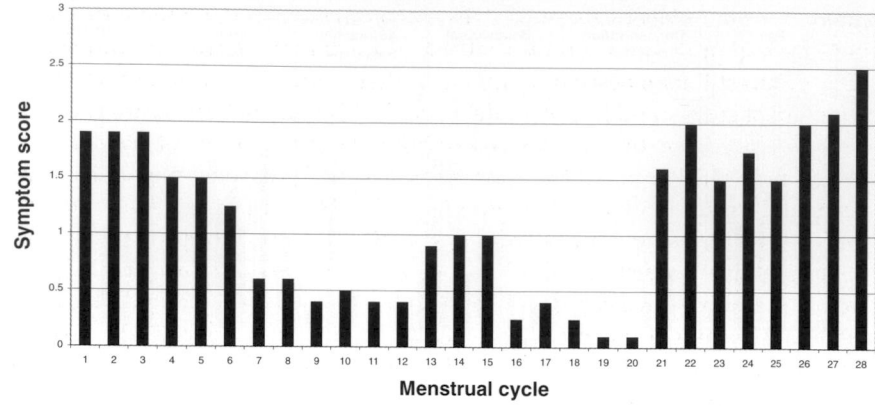

Fig. 2 Symptom scores for premenstrual syndrome during menstrual cycle. Adapted from Watson et al.[40]

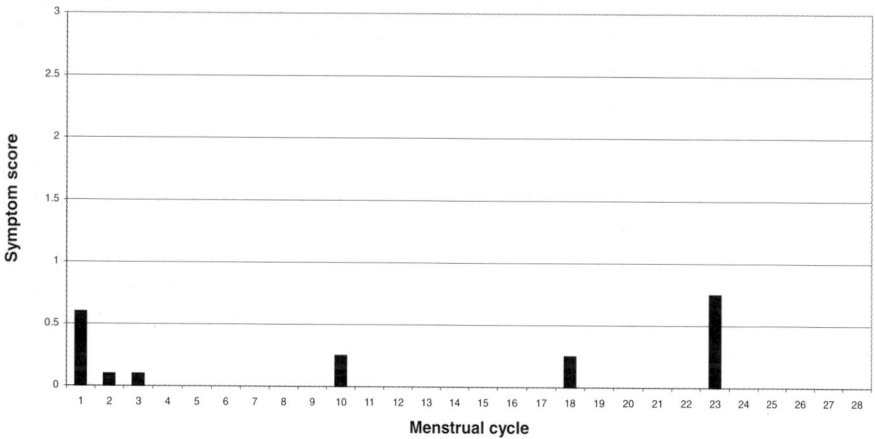

Fig. 3 Symptom scores for premenstrual syndrome after oestradiol treatment during menstrual cycle. Adapted from Watson et al.[40]

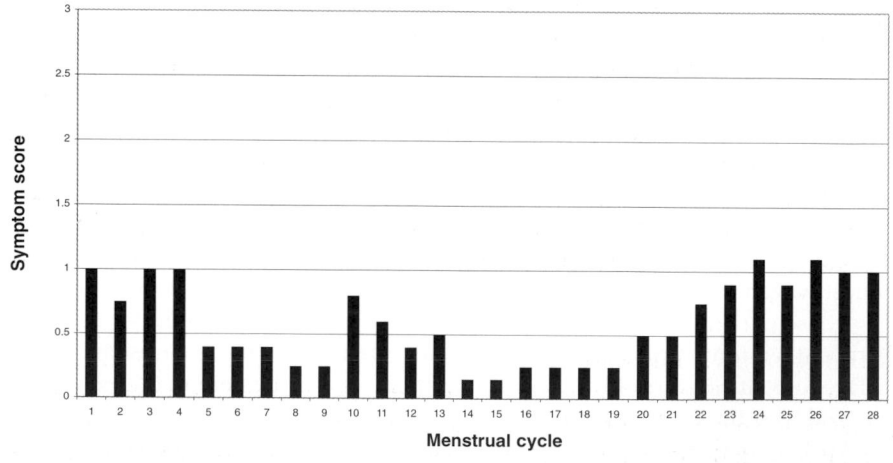

Fig. 4 Symptoms of PMS recur almost daily when norethisterone is added to treatment after almost disappearing with oestradiol treatment. Adapted from Watson et al.[40]

common for progestogens to cause PMS-like symptoms; in the same way, endogenous cyclical progesterone is the probable cause of premenstrual syndrome.

Our group still uses oestradiol implants, often with the addition of testosterone for loss of energy and loss of libido, in our PMS clinics but the oestradiol dose has been reduced. Treatment never starts with 100 mg, but pellets of oestradiol 50 mg or 75 mg with 100 mg of testosterone are inserted. These women must have endometrial protection by oral progestogen or a Mirena (Schering Healthcare) levonorgestrel-releasing intra-uterine system (LNG IUS). These women with PMS respond well to oestrogens but are often intolerant to progestogens and it is, therefore, common-place to reduce the orthodox 13-day course of progestogen to 10 or 7 days starting, for convenience, on the first day of every calendar month. Thus, the menstrual cycle is reset. The Mirena IUS could also play a vital role in preventing PMS-like symptoms as it performs its role of protecting the endometrium without systemic absorption. In a recent study,[42] we have shown a 50% decrease in hysterectomies in our practice since the introduction of the Mirena IUS in 1995. With its profound effect on menorrhagia and the possibility of less progestogenic side-effects, Mirena looks a very promising component of PMS treatment in the future and we are currently performing a study to compare Mirena with oral progestogens in the treatment of PMS.

Hormone implants are not licensed in all countries and are unsuitable for women who may wish to easily discontinue treatment in order to become pregnant. Oestradiol patches are an alternative and our original double-blind cross-over study used 200 mcg of oestradiol patch twice weekly.[43] This produced plasma oestradiol levels of 800 pmol/l and suppressed luteal phase progesterone and ovulation. Once again, this treatment was better than placebo in every symptom cluster of PMS. Figures 5–7 show the changes that occurred in three symptom clusters.

When active treatment was substituted by placebo, there was deterioration in response, whereas there was continued improvement when placebo was replaced by active treatment. Subsequently, an uncontrolled observational study from our PMS clinic indicated that PMS sufferers could have the same response to 100 mcg patches with fewer symptoms of breast discomfort and bloating with less anxiety about high-dose oestrogen therapy.[44]

The original studies outlined in this chapter are all scientifically valid, placebo-controlled trials showing a considerable improvement in PMS symptoms with oestrogens. Although this treatment is used by many gynaecologists in the UK, it has not been used by psychiatrists anywhere in the world. We believe that the benefit of this therapy in severe PMS is due to its inhibition of ovulation, but there is probably also a central mental tonic effect. Klaiber et al.[45] using very high doses of premarin showed this and our other psycho-endocrine studies of climacteric depression and post-natal depression have shown the benefit of high dose transdermal oestrogens for these conditions.[46]

Combined oral contraceptive pill

In theory, the combined oral contraceptive pill should treat PMS as it functions by suppressing ovulation. This effect is, however not always seen in practice[47] and this could be due to the daily administration of progestogen. There is also the possibility of breakthrough symptoms during the pill-free interval when hormone levels drop.

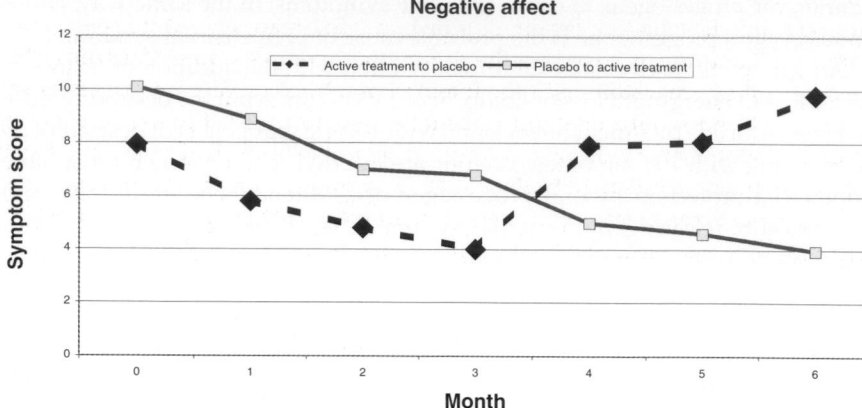

Fig. 5 After crossover at 3 months, it is clear that oestradiol patches are superior to placebo in the treatment of the PMS symptom negative affect. Adapted from Watson et al.[43]

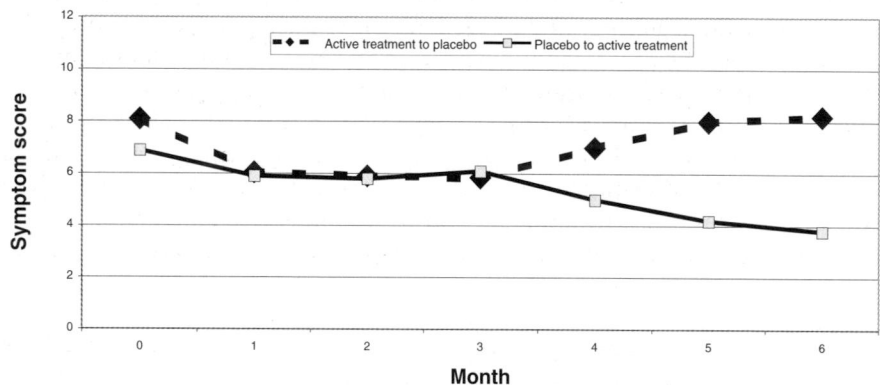

Fig. 6 After crossover at 3 months, it is clear that oestradiol patches are superior to placebo in the treatment of the PMS symptom pain. Adapted from Watson et al.[43]

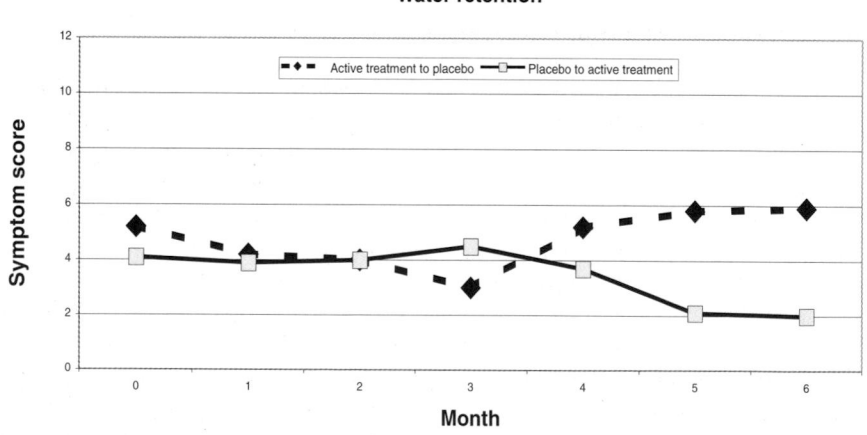

Fig. 7 After crossover at 3 months, it is clear that oestradiol patches are superior to placebo in the treatment of the PMS symptom water retention. Adapted from Watson et al.[43]

Progesterone

Progesterone has had a lot of support in the treatment of premenstrual syndrome[48] and this is based on the theory that women who suffer from PMS are deficient of progesterone in the luteal phase. Most studies on progesterone were not placebo-controlled and this makes it very difficult to assess efficacy. A recent meta-analysis of all randomised, placebo-controlled trials by Wyatt and co-workers included 10 trials where progesterone was used and four trials where progestogens were used. They concluded that there was no evidence to support the use of either hormones in the management of PMS.

GnRH analogues

Leather et al.[49] have demonstrated that 3 months of Zoladex therapy cures all of the symptom groups of PMS. The use of these and other GnRH analogues achieves a medical oophorectomy. These women will experience hot flushes and sweats, but such side-effects are usually far preferable to the debilitating symptoms that they had previously experienced. Long-term therapy with GnRH analogues will lead to bone demineralisation, but the above group showed that 'add-back' with a product containing 2 mg of oestradiol valerate and cyclical levonorgestrel (Nuvelle, Schering Health) maintained the bone density at both the spine and the hip.[50] Most of the PMS symptoms remain improved with this 'add-back', but bloating, tension and irritability recur – probably due to the cyclical progestogen. These can largely be avoided by using another form of effective 'add-back' therapy like tibolone. Sundstrom and colleagues used low-dose GnRH analogues (100 μg buserelin) with good results on the symptoms of PMS, but the treatment still caused anovulation in as many as 56% of patients.[51]

Danazol

Danazol is a further hormonal option for the treatment of PMS.[52] It acts by inhibiting pituitary gonadotrophins, but it can have severe masculinising side-effects. The fear also exists of masculinising a fetus in an unplanned pregnancy. When used in the luteal phase only,[53] it only relieved mastalgia and not the general symptoms of PMS even though side-effects were minimal.

Hysterectomy and bilateral oophorectomy

It is well recognised that in some women all treatment options will fail or side-effects may be unbearable. Some women are unlikely to want to continue with treatment that needs to be taken for many years until the menopause or in some cases concomitant pathology may co-exist. In all of these instances, it may be necessary to perform a hysterectomy and bilateral salpingo-oophorectomy (TAH/BSO). It is important to stress that the bilateral oophorectomy is the essential part of the surgery as this would remove all ovarian function. By removing the uterus at the same time, it would be unnecessary to administer progestogens postoperatively and thus potential side-effects are avoided. In a study by our group (not yet published), we have shown more than 95% of women who needed this surgery appeared to be satisfied with the outcome. When this route is embarked upon, it is extremely important to provide these women with effective, long-term hormone replacement therapy. Not only do they need to receive oestrogen – it is also extremely important to replace their androgens as the ovaries secrete up to 50% of the body's androgens after the menopause.

Selective serotonin re-uptake inhibitors (SSRIs)

It has been shown that women suffering from PMS have lower levels of serotonin than controls in the luteal phase of the menstrual cycle.[54] This has lead to the introduction of SSRIs in the treatment of PMS. In a double-blind, placebo-controlled trial,[55] fluoxetine at 20 mg/day was significantly superior to placebo in the treatment of PMS. Steiner and colleagues[56] had similar results when comparing fluoxetine in doses of 20 mg and 60 mg daily to placebo, but side-effects were much higher in the 60 mg group. Certain women are reluctant to be treated with an anti-depressant for what they consider a gynaecological problem, but intermittent dosing of fluoxetine can overcome this obstacle. Another study by Steiner et al.[57] showed that 20 mg of fluoxetine during the luteal phase was no less effective than daily fluoxetine with less side-effects. Onset of action with intermittent dosing usually occurs during the first cycle, in contrast with 3–6 weeks normally experienced in the treatment of depression. This implies a possible different mechanism of action in women with PMS as opposed to women with mood disorders.

A recent meta-analysis[58] of all published clinical trials of SSRIs in the treatment of PMS identified 29 trials and found 15 randomised placebo-controlled trials suitable for analysis. Fluoxetine and sertraline were studied the most and fluoxetine was found to be the most effective. The positive effects of SSRIs were seen on both physical and behavioural symptoms, but the authors did make the point that the majority of trials included (13/15) had enrolled patients with predominantly behavioural symptoms. They conclude that it is not possible to extrapolate the effectiveness of SSRIs to patients who suffer predominantly from physical symptoms. Steiner et al.[59] did, however, show fluoxetine to be superior to placebo in the treatment of physical symptoms of PMS in a randomised, double-blind, placebo-controlled, parallel study. In this study, 320 women were randomised to 20 mg or 60 mg fluoxetine or placebo, and there were no significant differences between the two doses of fluoxetine.

The most common side-effects of SSRIs were insomnia, gastrointestinal disturbances, and fatigue. There were less sexual side-effects (decreased libido and anorgasmia) than normally found when treating depression,[60] but the authors warn that this finding should be treated with caution. Side-effects can be reduced by using intermittent dosing regimens.

KEY POINTS FOR CLINICAL PRACTICE

- We have attempted to discuss the most common and relevant options for the woman with severe PMS. It is almost impossible to cover all the options available for the treatment of premenstrual syndrome, as one reviewer suggested as many as 327 different treatment options.[61]

- With severe PMS, it is likely that only hormonal treatment and SSRIs will be of help, but there is certainly no harm in attempting any of the other treatments for milder forms of premenstrual syndrome.

References

1 Magos AL, Studd JWW. The premenstrual syndrome. In: Studd JWW. (ed) Progress in Obstetrics and Gynaecology, vol 4. Edinburgh: Churchill Livingstone, 1984, 334–350

2 O'Brien PMS. Helping women with premenstrual syndrome. BMJ 1993; 307:1471–1475

3 Backstrom T, Boyle H, Baird DT. Persistence of symptoms of premenstrual tension in hysterectomised women. Br J Obstet Gynaecol 1981; 88: 530–536

4 Studd JWW. Prophylactic oophorectomy at hysterectomy. Br J Obstet Gynaecol 1989; 96: 506–509

5 Studd JWW. Premenstrual tension syndrome. BMJ 1979; i: 410

6 Chadwick J, Mann WN. The Medical Works of Hippocrates. Oxford: Blackwell, 1950; 267–268

7 Maudsley H. Sex in mind and education. Fortnightly Review, 1874

8 Frank RT. The hormonal basis of premenstrual tension. Arch Neurol Psychiatr 1931; 26: 1053–1057

9 Greene R, Dalton K. The premenstrual syndrome. BMJ 1953; i: 1007–1014

10 Magos AL. Premenstrual syndrome. Contemp Rev Obstet Gynaecol 1988; 1: 80–92

11 Moos RH. Typology of menstrual cycle symptoms. Am J Obstet Gynecol 1969; 103: 390–402

12 Haskett RF, Steiner M, Osmun JN et al. Severe premenstrual syndrome: delineation of the syndrome. Biol Psychiatr 1980; 15: 121–139

13 Magos A, Studd J. Effects of the menstrual cycle on medical disorders. Br J Hosp Med 1985; 33: 68–77

14 Leather AT, Holland EFN, Studd JWW et al. A study of the referral patterns and therapeutic experiences of 100 women attending a specialist premenstrual syndrome clinic. J R Soc Med 1993; 86: 191–201

15 Kleijnen J, Ter riet G, Knipschild P. Vitamin B6 in the treatment of the premenstrual syndrome: a review. Br J Obstet Gynaecol 1990; 97: 847–852

16 Berger AR, Schaumburg HR, Schroeder C et al. Dose response, coasting, and differential fibre vulnerability in human toxic neuropathy: a prospective study of pyridoxine neurotoxicity. Neurology 1992; 42: 1367–1370

17 Wyatt KM, Dimmock PW, Jones PW et al. Efficacy of vitamin B-6 in the treatment of premenstrual syndrome: systematic review. BMJ 1999; 318: 1375–1381

18 Block E. The use of vitamin A in premenstrual syndrome. Acta Obstet Gynecol Scand 1960; 39: 586

19 Massil H, O'Brien PMS. Clinical algorithms; premenstrual syndrome. BMJ 1986; 293: 1298–1302

20 Collins A, Cerin A, Coleman G et al. Essential fatty acids in the treatment of premenstrual syndrome. Obstet Gynecol 1993; 81: 93–98

21 Budeiri D, Li Wan Po A, Dornan JC. Is evening primrose oil of value in the treatment of premenstrual syndrome? Control Clin Trials 1996; 17: 60–68

22 Penland JG, Johnson PE. Dietary calcium and manganese effects on menstrual cycle symptoms. Am J Obstet Gynecol 1993; 168: 1417–1423

23 Thys-Jacobs S, Starkey P, Bernstein D et al. Calcium carbonate and the premenstrual syndrome: effects on premenstrual and menstrual symptoms. Am J Obstet Gynecol 1998; 179: 444–452

24 Abraham GE, Lubran MM. Serum and red cell magnesium levels in patients with premenstrual tension. Am J Clin Nutr 1981; 34: 2364

25 Fachinetti F, Borella P, Sances G et al. Oral magnesium successfully relieves premenstrual mood changes. Obstet Gynecol 1991; 78: 177–181

26 Fachinetti F, Sances G, Borella P et al. Magnesium prophylaxis of menstrual migraine: effects on intracellular magnesium. Headache 1991; 31: 298–301

27 Walker AF, De Souza MC, Vickers MF et al. Magnesium supplementation alleviates premenstrual symptoms of fluid retention. J Womens Health 1998; 7: 1157–1165

28 Abraham GE, Rumley RE. Role of nutrition in the premenstrual syndrome. J Reprod Med 1987; 32: 405–422

29 Walsh MJ, Polus BI. A randomised, placebo-controlled clinical trial on the efficacy of chiropractic therapy on premenstrual syndrome. J Manipulative Physiol Ther 1999; 22: 582–585

30 Hernandez-Reif M, Martinez A, Field T et al. Premenstrual symptoms are relieved by massage therapy. J Psychosom Obstet Gynaecol 2000; 21: 9–15

31 Hardy ML. Herbs of special interest to women. J Am Pharm Assoc 2000; 40: 327–329

32 Schellenberg R. Treatment for the premenstrual syndrome with agnus castus fruit extract: prospective, randomised, placebo controlled study. BMJ 2001; 322: 134–137

33 Stevinson C, Ernst E. A pilot study of *Hypericum perforatum* for the treatment of premenstrual syndrome. Br J Obstet Gynaecol 2000; 107: 870–876

34 Barnhart KT, Freeman EW, Sondheimer SJ. A clinician's guide to premenstrual syndrome. Med Clin North Am 1995; 79: 1457–1472

35 Wang M, Hammarback S, Lindhe BA et al. Treatment of premenstrual syndrome by spironolactone: a double-blind, placebo-controlled study. Acta Obstet Gynecol Scand 1995; 74: 803–808

36 Greenblatt RB, Asch RH, Mahesh VB, Bryner JR. Implantation of pure crystalline pellets of estradiol for conception control. Am J Obstet Gynecol 1977; 127: 520–527

37 Magos AL, Brincat M, Studd JWW. Treatment of the premenstrual syndrome by subcutaneous oestradiol implants and cyclical oral norethisterone: placebo controlled study. BMJ 1986; 292: 1629–1633

38 Studd JWW, Thom MH. Oestrogens and endometrial cancer. In: Studd JWW. (ed) Progress in Obstetrics and Gynaecology, vol 1. Edinburgh, Churchill Livingstone, 1981; 182–198

39 Magos AL, Brewster E, Singh R, O'Dowd T, Brincat M, Studd JWW. The effects of norethisterone in postmenopausal women on oestrogen replacement therapy: a model for the premenstrual syndrome. Br J Obstet Gynaecol 1986; 93: 1290–1296

40 Watson NR, Studd JWW. Use of oestrogen in treatment of the premenstrual syndrome: a comparison of the routes of administration. Contemp Rev Obstet Gynaecol 1990; 2: 117–123

41 Bjorn I, Backstrom T. Drug related negative side-effects is a common reason for poor compliance in hormone replacement therapy. Maturitas 1999; 32: 77–86

42 Studd JWW, Domoney C, Khastgir G. The place of hysterectomy in the treatment of menstrual disorders. In: O'Brien PMS, Cameron I, MacLean A(eds). Disorders of the Menstrual Cycle, vol 29. London: RCOG Press, 2000; 313–323

43 Watson NR, Studd JWW, Savvas M, Garnett T, Baber RJ. Treatment of severe premenstrual syndrome with oestradiol patches and cyclical oral norethisterone. Lancet 1989; ii: 730–734

44 Smith RNJ, Studd JWW, Zamblera D, Holland EFN. A randomised comparison over 8 months of 100 mcgs and 200 mcgs twice weekly doses of transdermal oestradiol in the treatment of severe premenstrual syndrome. Br J Obstet Gynaecol 1995; 102: 475–484

45 Klaiber EL, Broverman DM, Vogel W, Kobayashi Y. Estrogen therapy for severe persistent depressions in women. Arch Gen Psychiatry 1979; 36: 550–559

46 Gregoire AJP, Kumar R, Everitt B, Henderson A, Studd JWW. Transdermal oestrogen for treatment of severe postnatal depression. Lancet 1996; 347: 930–933

47 Watson NR, Studd JWW. Use of oestrogen in treatment of the premenstrual syndrome: a comparison of the routes of administration. Contemp Rev Obstet Gynaecol 1990; 2: 117–123

48 Dalton K. The Premenstrual Syndrome and Progesterone Therapy, 2nd edn. London: Heinemann, 1984

49 Leather AT, Studd JWW, Watson NR, Holland EFN. The treatment of severe premenstrual syndrome with goserelin with and without 'add-back' estrogen therapy: a placebo-controlled study. Gynecol Endocrinol 1999; 13: 48–55

50 Holland EF, Leather AT, Studd JW, Garnett TJ. The effect of a new sequential oestradiol valerate and levonorgestrel preparation on the bone mineral density of postmenopausal women. Br J Obstet Gynaecol 1993; 100: 966–967

51 Sundstrom I, Nyberg S, Bixo M, Hammarback S, Backstrom T. Treatment of premenstrual syndrome with gonadotropin-releasing hormone agonist in a low dose regimen. Acta Obstet Gynecol Scand 1999; 78: 891–899

52 Halbriech U, Rojansky N, Palter S. Elimination of ovulation and menstrual cyclicity (with danazol) improves dysphoric premenstrual syndromes. Fertil Steril 1991; 56: 1066–1069

53 O'Brien PM, Abukhalil IE. Randomized controlled trial of the management of premenstrual syndrome and premenstrual mastalgia using luteal phase-only danazol. Am J Obstet Gynecol 1999; 180: 18–23

54 Rapkin AJ, Edelmuth E, Chang LC et al. Whole-blood serotonin in premenstrual syndrome. Obstet Gynecol 1987; 70: 533–537

55 Ozeren S, Coracki A, Yucesoy I et al. Fluoxetine in the treatment of premenstrual syndrome. Eur J Obstet Gynecol Reprod Biol 1997; 73: 167–170

56 Steiner M, Steinberg S, Stewart D et al. Fluoxetine in the treatment of premenstrual dysphoria. N Engl J Med 1995; 332: 1529–1534

57 Steiner M, Korzewka M, Lamont J et al. Intermittent fluoxetine dosing in the treatment of women with premenstrual dysphoria. Psychopharmacol Bull 1997; 33: 771–774

58 Dimmock PW, Wyatt KM, Jones PW et al: Efficacy of selective serotonin-reuptake inhibitors in premenstrual syndrome: a systematic review. Lancet 2000; 356: 1131–1136

59 Steiner M, Romano SJ, Babcock S et al. The efficacy of fluoxetine in improving physical symptoms associated with premenstrual dysphoric disorder. Br J Obstet Gynaecol 2001; 108: 462–468

60 Shen WW, Hsu JH. Female sexual side effects associated with selective serotonin reuptake inhibitors: a descriptive clinical study of 33 patients. Int J Psychiatry Med 1995; 25: 239–248

61 Chakmakjian ZH. A critical assessment of therapy for the premenstrual tension syndrome. J Reprod Med 1983; 28: 532–538

12

Deborah C.M. Boyle Paul E. Adinkra
Ronnie F. Lamont

Bacterial vaginosis

Abnormal vaginal bacterial flora is an important cause of obstetric and gynaecological adverse sequelae. In obstetrics, bacterial vaginosis (BV) and its related organisms have been implicated in higher rates of late miscarriage, preterm prelabour rupture of membranes (PPROM), chorio-amnionitis, spontaneous preterm labour (SPTL), preterm birth (PTB) and postpartum endometritis. BV has also been associated with conditions in gynaecology such as early miscarriage, pelvic inflammatory disease (PID), cervical intra-epithelial neoplasia (CIN) and post-hysterectomy vaginal cuff infection. This chapter aims to be a comprehensive review of the definition, epidemiology, aetiology, diagnosis and treatment of BV as well as exploring some of the evidence pertaining to its adverse sequelae.

NOMENCLATURE

The term 'bacterial vaginosis' has evolved over more than a century. The discovery of *Lactobacillus* spp. in vaginal secretions by Albert Döderlein in 1892 marked the beginning of extensive research into the detailed composition of the vaginal flora. Following his findings, normal vaginal flora was regarded as homogeneous, consisting only of Gram-positive rods, mainly of the *Lactobacillus* spp. Any individual with a more heterogeneous pattern was regarded as unhealthy and women with this pattern were described as having an infection known then as non-specific vaginitis. In 1954, Gardner and Dukes[1] discovered a

Dr Deborah C.M. Boyle MD MRCOG DFFP, Specialist Registrar in Obsterics and Gynaecology, Hillingdon Hospital, Pield Health Road, Uxbridge, Middlesex UB8 3NN, UK

Dr Paul E. Adinkra DFFP Department of Obstetrics and Gynaecology, Norwick Park Hospital, Watford Road, Harrow, Middlesex HA1 3UJ, UK

Mr Ronnie F. Lamont BSc MD FRCOG, Consultant in Obstetrics and Gynaecology, Norwick Park Hospital, Watford Road, Harrow, Middlesex HA1 3UJ, UK

new micro-organism, which was named *Haemophilus vaginalis,* and was thought to be the sole organism responsible for non-specific vaginitis.[2] As identification techniques improved with time, this organism was then categorized into the genus *Corynebacterium,* and thus became known as *Corynebacterium vaginalis.*[3] Further identification revealed this to be a new genus and, in honour of the work carried out by Gardner in this field, it was renamed *Gardnerella vaginalis* and the condition became known as *Gardnerella* vaginitis.

Since *G. vaginalis* can be cultured from at least 50% of women without signs or symptoms of vaginitis,[4,5] it has become clear that many micro-organisms other than *G. vaginalis* are associated with the condition. In the early 1980s, various anaerobic bacteria were implicated in causing the characteristic fishy malodour produced by volatile amines in vaginal secretions. This led to the term 'anaerobic vaginosis' being adopted until, in 1984,[6] the term bacterial vaginosis was adopted to reflect the polymicrobial alteration in vaginal flora causing an increase in vaginal pH, sometimes associated with an homogeneous discharge, but in the absence of a demonstrable inflammatory response.[7]

EPIDEMIOLOGY AND RISK FACTORS

BV is the commonest cause of abnormal vaginal discharge in young women of reproductive age. Inappropriate treatment through failure to diagnose the cause can result in prolonged morbidity and complications resulting directly from persistent or recurrent infection. The incidence of BV varies according to the population studied (Table 1).

There are several proposed risk factors for BV, some of which are still disputed. The trigger for the change from *Lactobacillus*-dominated flora to BV-associated flora has been linked to many possible factors including age at first sexual intercourse,[14,15] change in sexual partners,[16,17] greater number of life-time sexual partners,[14,18] and concurrent sexually transmitted diseases.[14] Cigarette smoking[14,19] and the use of an intra-uterine contraceptive device[20] are both linked to an increased risk of acquiring BV. Vaginal douching[17,19,21] has

Table 1 Incidence rates of bacterial vaginosis		
Year of study	Population studied	Incidence of bacterial vaginosis
Embree et al. (1984)[8]	Women attending an STD clinic, USA	64%
Eschenbach et al. (1988)[7]	Asymptomatic college students, USA	4%
Bump et al. (1988)[9]	Group of virginal post-menarchal girls, USA	12%
Hay et al. (1992)[10]	Low-risk gynaecology clinic, Harrow, UK	11%
Blackwell et al. (1993)[11]	Group of women undergoing termination of pregnancy, USA	28%
Hay et al (1994)[12]	A routine antenatal clinic, Harrow, UK	15%
Lamont et al. (2000)[13]	Group of asymptomatic women attending general practitioner for cervical cytology, UK	9%

also been implicated as a risk factor for BV, by aiding the ascent of micro-organisms into the upper genital tract. There is also evidence of racial disparity of BV, which is seen to occur more frequently in women of Afro-Caribbean origin living in the UK compared to Caucasian women.[19] Other research has also shown that black women have a higher prevalence of BV compared to white women. Royce et al.[22] found differences in vaginal flora between black women and white women in pregnancy. They demonstrated a 2.6-fold increase in BV in over 300 black women in their third trimester of pregnancy compared to a similar number of white women even after adjustment for confounding factors. There were higher levels of each BV-related micro-organism in the black group compared to the white women. There have also been studies that have identified a link to lesbian activity,[23–25] one showing a prevalence of over 50% in a group of lesbians attending a genito-urinary medicine clinic. This figure appeared to be related to the life-time number of female sexual partners rather than the frequency of sexual activity. The higher prevalence found in the lesbian population when compared to heterosexual women poses the question as to whether there is the possibility of sexual transmission between women.

AETIOLOGY

Even after many years of research, the underlying pathogenesis of BV is still unknown. Apart from the links drawn from studies involving factors such as smoking, sexual history and race, the underlying reason for the alteration in flora is unclear. Several studies have attempted to ascertain whether changes in vaginal bacterial flora are related to the menstrual cycle.

In studies where a relationship between the menstrual cycle and BV could be demonstrated, changes in microbial flora were found to occur more often during the follicular phase of the cycle at a time when oestrogen concentration was relatively high compared to progesterone. Relative oestrogen dominance favours *Candida* colonisation of the vagina and infection[26,27] which has led to speculation that sex hormones, whether by virtue of absolute levels or by change of relative concentrations, may influence the development of BV.[28] Studies using rodent models, although not primarily designed to investigate BV, add further evidence to the argument that BV is in some way endocrine-related.[29–32] These studies show that the administration of oestrogen results in increased susceptibility to infection by *Mycoplasma hominis*[29] and *Neisseria gonorrhoeae*[31] to which mice are not ordinarily susceptible, and that there was a large increase in the number of organisms in the genital tract.[32] This change was accompanied by the appearance of vaginal epithelial cells with many adherent organisms, described as 'clue' cells. The prevalence of BV decreases as pregnancy progresses and, although the concentrations of oestrogens is elevated throughout, the relative concentrations of oestrogens and progesterone alter as pregnancy progresses.[33] If an endocrine change is the cause of BV, the mechanism is unclear. One theory suggests that a change in endocrine status encourages the growth of endogenous bacteria, normally present in small numbers and that these overwhelm the *Lactobacilli* by sheer numbers, or it may be that this change favours disappearance of *Lactobacilli* which allows unopposed growth of other organisms. Evidence against sexual transmission comes from studies that have demonstrated no benefit in treating male partners[34-36] and the detection of BV in 12% of girls who are *virgo intacta* post-menarche.[9]

Other theories propose an enzymatic role in the pathogenesis of BV. Mucinase and sialidase levels measured in samples of vaginal fluid in women with BV were found to be significantly elevated compared to women with normal vaginal flora and it may be possible that they allow the entry of pathogens by promoting the breakdown of the mucosal barrier.[37]

More recently, there has been evidence to suggest a role for phage viruses in the aetiology of BV. A phage or bacteriophage in this context, is a virus that infects bacteria. They are capable of lysing bacteria and releasing further phages into the environment, or they can co-exist within the bacteria as parasites and exert their effect. Phages that affect *Lactobacilli* strains have been found in dairy products and in meat-processing factories, where, in *Lactobacilli* starter cultures used in meat-processing, their action is known to delay acid production and reduce *Lactobacilli* numbers, slowing down ripening. This process, if applied to vaginal *Lactobacilli*, could result in the inhibition of acid production and decreased numbers of these bacteria and an overgrowth of anaerobes. It has been proven that phages can be isolated from vaginal *Lactobacilli* and in vitro experiments show that these phages have the potential to infect vaginal *Lactobacilli* of other women.[38] In an analysis of products containing *Lactobacillus* strains such as yoghurts, Tao et al. found 43 different types of *Lactobacilli*. Phages were detected in 11 of these strains, 7 of which were found to inhibit vaginal *Lactobacilli*.[39]

Despite intense research, the underlying aetiology for BV remains unclear.

MICROBIOLOGY

The normal vaginal flora is dominated by *Lactobacillus* spp. which play a major part in maintaining the dynamic ecosystem in the vagina. By metabolising glycogen in the vagina, *Lactobacilli* produce lactic acid which lowers the vaginal pH to below 4.5. This creates a hostile environment which deters the growth of potentially pathogenic bacteria, particularly *G. vaginalis* and anaerobes.[40] The low pH generated by the production of lactic acid also reduces the adherence of bacteria to the vaginal epithelium. Other compounds produced by the *Lactobacilli* such as lactacin B,[41] acidolin[42] and hydrogen peroxide[43] inhibit the growth of other bacteria. Certain *Lactobacilli* are capable of producing hydrogen peroxide (H_2O_2) and have been shown to reduce BV and Trichomoniasis[44] and have a bactericidal effect on *G. vaginalis* and *Prevotella bivia* in vitro.[45] *Lactobacillus crispatus* and *Lactobacillus jensenii* both produce H_2O_2 and the presence of increased numbers of these species is linked to a lower prevalence of BV.[46] *Mobiluncus* spp. and *Bacteroides* spp. produce the keto-acid, succinate, as a major biochemical metabolite and this is found in elevated concentrations in women with bacterial vaginosis.[4] The absence of lactic acid and the production of succinate, which also raises vaginal pH, has been postulated to blunt the chemotactic response of polymorphonuclear leukocytes and to reduce their killing ability. This may explain why BV produces no cellular inflammatory response despite the presence of high numbers of potentially pathogenic micro-organisms.[47]

Other aerobic and anaerobic bacteria are also present as part of the normal flora. Gram-negative anaerobic bacteria such as *Bacteroides* spp., *Prevotella* spp.

and *Porphyromonas* spp. can be found in over 50% of healthy women.[48] However, these obligate anaerobes are also important pathogens and are strongly linked to BV. Common yeasts such as *Candida albicans* may also be seen in healthy women. Genital mycoplasmas such as *Mycoplasma hominis* and *Ureaplasma urealyticum* can be part of the flora in healthy women, but may also be involved in genital tract infection. Potential pathogens such as *Klebsiella* spp., *Staphylococcus aureus* and *Escherichia coli* can also be present. The presence of *Mobiluncus* spp., an anaerobic fastidious curved rod, has been shown to be highly specific for BV.

While 5–15 species of bacteria may be cultured from normal vaginal secretions,[49] the total bacterial count of normal flora is $< 10^6$ organisms/ml,[50] whereas women with BV have up to 10^9 organisms/ml. The normal microbial balance is upset when there is a dramatic rise in anaerobes and other organisms and a decrease in *Lactobacilli*, resulting in the polymicrobial pattern characteristic of bacterial vaginosis. Anaerobic bacterial numbers increase 1000-fold[48,51] and BV-related organisms such as *G. vaginalis*, *Bacteroides spp.*, *Mobiluncus spp.* and *M. hominis* dominate the flora with a reduction in the quantity and quality of *Lactobacilli*. *G. vaginalis* and other anaerobes are capable of producing volatile amines and organic acids other than lactic acid,[52] which may be responsible for the fishy odour of BV. Other exogenous micro-organisms such as *N. gonorrhoeae*, *Chlamydia trachomatis* and *Trichomonas vaginalis* are sometimes detected in the flora, but these are pathogens that have been sexually acquired.

In pregnancy, there is a rise in the overall numbers of vaginal flora compared to the non-pregnant state due mainly to an increase in *Lactobacilli* by approximately 10-fold. There is a concurrent reduction in anaerobes but relative stability of aerobes. With increasing gestation, the flora tend to become more benign, mainly due to the increasing numbers of *Lactobacilli* such that, at term, the vaginal flora is dominated by organisms of low virulence which pose no threat to the fetus. Any alteration in this balance such as occurs in BV, can result in any of the adverse sequelae discussed later in the chapter.

DIAGNOSIS

Clinical features

Up to half the women diagnosed with BV are asymptomatic. If symptoms are present, they will usually be described as an increased vaginal discharge which is malodourous. Pruritus and vulvovaginitis are uncommon symptoms and another cause should be sought if these are present. On examination, there may be the characteristic vaginal discharge of BV which is whitish-grey, thin, homogeneous and adherent to the vaginal walls and in addition, a fishy smell may be noted.

Composite clinical criteria

There has been the tendency in the clinical setting to misdiagnose BV due to the lack of simple laboratory testing. Various methods exist for the clinical diagnosis of BV. In 1983, Amsel[15] developed a set of composite clinical criteria which are still widely used both in clinical practice and in research. The diagnosis is made by finding three of the following four signs: (i) a homogeneous vaginal discharge; (ii) an elevated vaginal pH > 4.5; (iii) a positive 'whiff' test on addition of a solution of 10% potassium hydroxide (KOH) to a sample of vaginal secretions; and (iv) the presence of 'clue cells' on microscopic examination of a wet preparation of vaginal secretions.

The presence of at least three out of four of these criteria is regarded as diagnostic of BV. The assessment of vaginal discharge is the most subjective of these, but still correlates better with the presence of BV than the patient's own impression of whether or not she has an abnormal vaginal discharge.[10] However, it is important to realise that the absence of discharge does not imply the absence of BV. It is not accepted as a reliable indicator on its own as it is neither sensitive nor specific to BV.

Vaginal pH is measured using narrow-range pH paper and assessing the colour change produced by a sample of vaginal secretion taken from the posterior fornix. A low pH virtually excludes BV. An elevated pH is the most sensitive, but least specific of the criteria used for the diagnosis of BV, as an increase can also be associated with menstruation, recent sexual intercourse or infection with *T. vaginalis*. The 'whiff' test involves the addition of a drop of 10% KOH to a sample of vaginal secretions which produces a characteristic fishy odour in the presence of bacterial vaginosis. It has been demonstrated that some BV micro-organisms such as *Mobiluncus* spp. produce trimethylamine, a substance linked to the smell of rotting fish which may explains the characteristic malodour of BV.[53] As a single entity, the 'whiff' test has a positive predictive value of 90% and a specificity of 70%.[54]

'Clue cells' are desquamated vaginal epithelial cells that are densely coated in adherent bacteria such that their borders are indistinct. The detection of clue cells on direct microscopy is the single most sensitive and specific criterion for BV, but is operator-dependent.[55] Debris and degenerated cells may be mistaken for clue cells and *Lactobacilli* may adhere to epithelial cells in low numbers.[55] Clue cells can be identified on a Gram stain or a 'wet preparation' (small sample of vaginal secretions to which a drop of saline has been added) and are regarded as pathognomonic of BV. It is not necessary to see clue cells to make the diagnosis of BV, as the key feature is the reduced or absent Gram-positive large rods or *Lactobacilli*, and their replacement by Gram-variable or Gram-negative rods. The grading of the microbial flora seen on Gram-stained slides provides a cheap, simple, reproducible and objective method of diagnosing BV. It has been demonstrated that Gram stain diagnosis alone corresponds well to the use of composite criteria[56–58] and to the presence of the associated bacteria.[56]

The advantages of the Gram stain alone, particularly for research purposes, are that it provides a more objective method of diagnosis. The slide can also be stored for future reference and patient-collected 'blind' vaginal swabs have been demonstrated to be as accurate as swabs taken using a speculum.[59] This provides a valuable tool for longitudinal studies as patients can collect specimens at home and air-dry them thus avoiding the need for multiple clinic visits. Gram stains are the only method of diagnosing an intermediate category of vaginal flora which is not as dramatic as BV but is still abnormal.

The main difficulty for obstetricians and gynaecologists is the lack of instant access to direct microscopy which, as discussed above, is the most reliable method of diagnosing BV. This should not deter us from seeking to diagnose the condition. A roll of narrow range pH paper is cheap and a normal vaginal pH virtually excludes BV. The whiff test is also cheap and easy to do with high sensitivity and good specificity. Women can be referred to the local genito-urinary medicine clinic where microscopy is available alongside screening for other important potential pathogens. New rapid tests for BV have been developed which measure metabolic products from anaerobic bacteria such as proline aminopeptidase or are based on DNA probes, for example 'Affirm VPIII' which probes for *G. vaginalis* genes.[60,61] If a simple but accurate test similar to urine pregnancy tests could be developed for the diagnosis of BV in the 'office gynaecology' or antenatal clinic setting, this would be an enormous advance in the clinical setting.

OBSTETRIC COMPLICATIONS ASSOCIATED WITH BACTERIAL VAGINOSIS

Spontaneous preterm labour (SPTL) and preterm birth (PTB)

In the industrialised world, PTB accounts for 8–10% of all births and is the major cause of perinatal morbidity, mortality and subsequent neurodevelopmental problems such as cerebral palsy.[62] The aetiology of PTB is multifactorial, but there is now well-accepted evidence to implicate infection as a cause in up to 40% of cases.[12,62–71] Abnormal genital tract colonisation has been found to be associated with PTB.[72,73] The total numbers of vaginal microbial flora increase as pregnancy progresses, with the concentration of *Lactobacilli* increasing 10-fold. The concentration of anaerobes decreases while the number of aerobes remains constant. With increasing gestation, the vaginal flora becomes more benign and, at term, the microbiological make-up of the vagina generally poses no significant threat to the fetus with the exception of Group B *Streptococcus*. However, if there is a disturbance in vaginal flora, this constitutes a potential danger to the pregnancy. There is evidence now that suggests that the earlier in pregnancy that BV is detected, the greater the risk of PTB (Table 2). Even if BV resolves spontaneously, the risk of PTB is not reduced. In a follow-up study of 92 pregnant women with BV, the vaginal flora spontaneously reverted to normal in 50% of cases but the risk of PTB was unaltered.[74] Whether very early screening and intervention with treatment in pregnancy, even in 'low-risk' pregnancies would make an appreciable difference in the risk of PTB attributable to BV is unknown.

Table 2 Relationship of abnormal colonisation to preterm delivery or preterm labour according to gestational age at screening

Study	Maximum gestational age at screening	Relative risk	Confidence interval
Gravett et al. (1986)[156]	32	2.0	1.1–3.5
McDonald et al. (1992)[157]	28	1.8	1.0–3.2
Hillier et al. (1995)[158]	26	1.4	1.2–1.8
Krohn et al. (1995)[159]	26	1.5	1.1–2.2
Hillier et al. (1995)[160]	26	1.5	0.8–3.0
McGregor et al (1990)[161]	24	2.0	1.1–6.5
Riduan et al. (1993)[162]	20	2.0	1.0–3.9
Hay et al. (1994)[163]	20	5.5	2.3–13.30
Kurki et al (1992)[164]	17	6.9	2.5–19

The mechanism by which BV can induce PTB is linked to ascending genital tract infection, with an immune response resulting in the production of pro-inflammatory cytokines such as interleukin-1α (IL-1α), interleukin 1β (IL-1β) and tumour necrosis factor-α (TNF-α).[75–80] Cytokines are proteins secreted during inflammatory processes with an immunological basis and play a role in intercellular signalling. They are present during the process of normal labour, but higher concentrations have been found in the amniotic fluid of women in SPTL due to infection, which sets off a cascade resulting in the recruitment of inflammatory mediators such as prostaglandins. This eventually leads to cervical ripening and uterine contractions that may result in preterm labour. Phospholipase A$_2$ (PLA$_2$) and phospholipase C (PLC) are enzymes responsible for cleaving arachidonic acid, the obligate precursor for prostaglandin synthesis, from glycerophospholipids in the cell membrane and have been found to be elevated in the lower genital tract of women with BV.[81,82] Another important development has been the link between an increased cytokine level associated with preterm labour and the additional finding of intra-amniotic bacterial colonisation.[83–86] The prediction of infection in the amniotic fluid by measurement of cytokines is now at the forefront of research. More recently, studies have been carried out into the role and regulation of maternal and fetal tissues in determining the cellular source of cytokines. The contributions of these tissues appear to be differentially regulated. Animal experiments suggest that the main source of IL-1, IL-6 and TNF-α appears to be the uterus, whereas the fetus and placenta were the main sites for the anti-inflammatory cytokine IL-1 receptor antagonist (IL-1ra).[87] This cytokine modulates expression of IL-1 by competitive inhibition, and prevents damage to the host by the potent IL-1. Another recent study showed that, in preterm labour in the absence of chorio-amnionitis, cytokine activity (IL-1β and IL-6) was concentrated in fetal endothelial cells within trophoblastic villi, whereas in preterm labour with confirmed chorio-amnionitis, activity was low in the placental tissue but highest within polymorphonuclear cells infiltrating the amniochorionic membranes.[88] Evidence from human and animal studies suggests that the development and growth of oligodendrocytes in the fetal brain are impaired by IL-6 and TNF-α.[89,90] If there is a cytokine-mediated/immune response-related neurodevelopmental disturbance, this may explain why there is a high incidence of cerebral palsy in babies delivered by women with evidence of perinatal infection[91–93] and provides an indirect link between BV and cerebral palsy. Several recent studies have examined the positive relationship between ante-/intra-partum infection, production of inflammatory cytokines, periventricular leukomalacia and subsequent development of cerebral palsy (CP) in babies delivered preterm.[92,94,95] An increased incidence of neurodevelopmental disorders in babies of 2.5 kg or more has suggested that PTB alone does not account for the excess numbers of babies affected by neurodevelopmental disorders.[93] Methods to block the action of cytokines by the use of cytokine-binding-proteins such as anticytokine antibodies are being developed in conditions such as rheumatoid arthritis. This approach could potentially be applied to other cytokine-dependent conditions,[96] such as SPTL and PTB. Inflammation of the choriodecidual space causes release of fibronectin. Detection of fibronectin in cervicovaginal secretions after 22 weeks' gestation is predictive of preterm delivery and associated with BV.[97] Phosphorylated insulin-like growth factor binding protein is produced by inflamed decidua and can be detected as early as 8 weeks' gestation and may, therefore, be a better marker for adverse pregnancy outcome.[98]

Approximately 15–20% of all pregnant women will have BV[4,12] and these women are up to 4 times more likely to have a PTB than women without BV.[12,70,99] In a longitudinal study, Hillier et al.[70] demonstrated that women with BV are 40% more likely to deliver a preterm, low birthweight infant than women without BV.

The earlier in pregnancy that BV is detected the greater the risk of PTB (Table 2). Hillier et al.[56] showed that pregnant women predominantly have one of two primary vaginal flora patterns – either normal or BV – and a few women will have an intermediate pattern. Women with BV in the second trimester tended to remain BV positive in the third trimester and those women with intermediate flora had a significant chance of progressing to BV. In a longitudinal study by Hay et al.,[33] the Gram-stained vaginal smears of 718 pregnant women were examined for BV until 36 weeks' gestation. The results showed that, of those women who initially had normal flora at their first antenatal visit, only 2.4% had developed BV by 36 weeks' gestation. Of 32 women who had BV initially, half had abnormal vaginal flora by 36 weeks.

A number of intervention studies have been undertaken to assess the benefit of treating BV in an attempt to reduce the incidence of PTB. The treatment of high-risk, BV-positive pregnant women has resulted in reduction of PTB by 37–50%,[100–102] which could be construed as an argument for the treatment of BV in all women with a high-risk pregnancy. However, with a reported prevalence of BV in high-risk pregnant women of, at maximum, 45% this would result in many women being treated unnecessarily. The details of treatment trials carried out in pregnancy are described later in the chapter.

In summary, the evidence associating abnormal vaginal flora with PTB is strong, but does not amount to a definitive causal relationship. There may be other associated factors which predispose some, but not all, women with BV to PTB as most women with BV carry their pregnancies to term. Cervical length, strength of inflammatory response to an infective stimulus or enzymatic activity resulting from micro-organisms may all have a role. There is evidence that the stage of pregnancy at which BV is detected is also of importance.

Late miscarriage

The incidence of late miscarriage (13–23 weeks' gestation) has been demonstrated to be significantly higher in women who have BV than those who do not,[12,19,100] and to be independent of other risk factors as in PTB. Since late miscarriage is on a continuum with extremely early PTB, the mechanisms by which BV is associated with late miscarriage are assumed to be similar to those outlined for PTB.

Postpartum endometritis

Postpartum endometritis is a relatively common obstetric complication and, although the incidence is higher in women undergoing Caesarean section, it may also occur following a vaginal delivery. Risk factors include prolonged rupture of membranes, prolonged labour and increased number of vaginal examinations. Postpartum endometritis following a Caesarean section tends to develop within 2 days and is described as early endometritis. This is most likely to be due to the introduction of bacteria into the endometrial cavity at delivery. Women who have a vaginal delivery usually develop late endometritis, which can occur up to 6 weeks post-natally. This delayed infection tends to result from ascending infection over a course of time. Facultative anaerobes linked to BV are commonly isolated in cases of endometritis. One study demonstrated that, in women diagnosed with early endometritis, the majority were found to have bacteria such as *Peptostreptococcus* spp. and *G. vaginalis* as predominant isolates. In a study which examined the rate of postpartum endometritis in women delivered by caesarean section, those women with BV were nearly 6 times more likely to develop the condition than women without BV despite antibiotic prophylaxis.[103] In another study, which looked at women delivered both vaginally and by caesarean section, BV was the strongest predictor of postpartum endometritis irrespective of mode of delivery.[104] This led the authors to conclude that women should be screened and treated for BV in late pregnancy. The effective use of antibiotic regimens, especially in women undergoing an elective or emergency caesarean section, reduces post-partum complications.

GYNAECOLOGICAL COMPLICATIONS ASSOCIATED WITH BACTERIAL VAGINOSIS

Bacterial vaginosis and cervical intra-epithelial neoplasia (CIN)

A possible association between BV and CIN has been explored by various studies over many years. Platz-Christensen et al., in a large retrospective study, found a relative risk of 5.0 (95% CI 2.2–11.6) of having CIN III/carcinoma *in situ* in women with BV when compared to women without BV.[105] Further research has shown that the presence of large numbers of vaginal anaerobes was associated with women having CIN or invasive cervical carcinoma.[106] The relationship between BV and cervical dysplasia/carcinoma is inconsistent, as other studies have found no relationship between BV and CIN/cervical carcinoma.[14,107] The main criticism of previous studies investigating the possible role of BV in the aetiology of CIN is failure to control for sexually transmitted infections, particularly oncogenic human papilloma virus (HPV) infection – a known risk factor for cervical neoplasia.

It has been suggested that some vaginal flora, such as the anaerobes associated with BV, are capable of producing carcinogenic substances called nitrosamines.[108] Evidence regarding production of nitrosamines by BV organisms is conflicting and the proposed mechanism of action by which nitrosamines may act has also been ill-defined although thought to be by exerting an influence via enhanced replication of oncogenic HPV.

In the only study to date which examined the relationship between BV and CIN whilst adequately controlling for HPV and other sexually transmitted diseases, BV has not been shown to be associated with higher rates of CIN and nor has it been demonstrated to produce higher levels of nitrosamines in the vagina of women with the condition than in women who do not have BV (Boyle DCM et al., in press).

Pelvic inflammatory disease (PID)

Acute PID remains a serious cause of morbidity in young women and is usually polymicrobial in nature. The sequelae of PID such as tubal damage leading to infertility and ectopic pregnancy create further problems for both patient and clinician. In the past, PID was commonly caused by *Chlamydia trachomatis* or *N. gonorrhoeae*, but current attention is focused on the effects of BV-related micro-organisms. Cervicovaginal fluids can be sucked through the cervix into the uterus and beyond during spontaneous hormone-mediated uterine contractions at mid-cycle.[109] This may explain, at least in part, the finding of BV-related micro-organisms in the endometrium of women with PID. These organisms tend to be found less frequently in the fallopian tubes[110,111] and, occasionally, within abscesses associated with PID.[112] Due to the polymicrobial nature of BV, it is difficult to attribute BV-associated PID to any one organism. One study found that *M. hominis* was isolated from the endometrium and uterine tubes of 10% of women diagnosed by laparoscopy as having PID[113] and the role of BV is further corroborated by the fact that specific antibody responses occur to this organism.[114] The evidence available appears to implicate *M. hominis* as a cause of PID and the organism rarely occurs in large numbers except in BV.

Infertility and first trimester loss

Several studies have examined the possible relationships between BV and infertility.[115–117]. Although in one study,[115] a higher prevalence of BV was found in women undergoing in vitro fertilisation (IVF) than in the general population, other studies have not found this to be the case, except in women whose infertility was attributable to tubal disease.[116,117] A recent UK study found that there was a high prevalence of BV in women undergoing IVF and that women with BV had a higher rate of first trimester miscarriage than those with normal vaginal flora. Most of these losses were in 'chemical' pregnancies with a non-significant trend towards greater loss rates of clinical pregnancies in the BV group.[118] Recurrent first trimester miscarriage has not been demonstrated to be associated with BV.[19]

There is speculation that BV-related bacteria may have an adverse effect on sperm deposited in the vagina and thus reduce fertility,[119] although this has been disputed.[115,116]

Post-hysterectomy vaginal cuff infection

In two separate studies, post-abdominal hysterectomy vaginal cuff infection occurred 3–4 times more commonly in women with BV than in those without.[120,121] Neither study group received antibiotics prior to the hysterectomy, but screening for BV took place beforehand. In one of these studies by Larsson et al., the presence of clue cells on air-dried smears of vaginal secretions was used as a diagnostic basis for BV. Of women who had clue cells, 35% developed postoperative infection. Only 8% of women without clue cells developed an infection. The second study involved the analysis of vaginal secretions prior to surgery in order to detect BV and Trichomoniasis.

The patients who had these two conditions diagnosed were 3 times more likely to develop postoperative vaginal cuff cellulitis compared to the control group. This suggests that there is a place for the pre-operative assessment of vaginal flora and administration of appropriate treatment if necessary. The use of prophylactic antibiotics is now generally accepted practice, but wide-spread use of different antibiotics may not result in eradicating BV and its related organisms but lead to greater resistance. The identification of the most suitable prophylactic treatment regimen to target BV organisms will prevent adverse outcomes.

Postabortal sepsis

First trimester surgical termination of pregnancy remains a common procedure in gynaecological practice. Postoperative infection, such as endometritis, occurs at rates between 4–12%. Pelvic infection following termination of pregnancy may be due to vaginal infections particularly with *N. gonorrhoeae*, *C. trachomatis* and BV-related organisms. In one study, a 2.4-fold increased risk of postabortal infection was reported if women had clue cells in their vaginal secretions[122] compared to women with normal vaginal flora. In a later study, the same authors reported a 3.8-fold reduction in the risk of postabortal infection in women with BV who were randomised to receive treatment with metronidazole compared to the group who received no treatment.[123] One double-blind trial recently was carried out in over 1000 women undergoing a termination of pregnancy randomised to receive 2% clindamycin cream or placebo prior to the procedure.[124] Their results showed that pre-operative treatment with clindamycin cream significantly reduced the risk of postabortal infection (RR 4.2, 95% CI 1.2–15.9) among women with BV but less so in women who had normal pre-operative flora. The use of antibiotic prophylaxis before surgical termination of pregnancy demonstrates a protective effect. There is strong evidence to suggest that women should preferably be screened and treated for BV as well as other infections, such as *C. trachomatis*, prior to termination of pregnancy or given appropriate prophylactic antibiotics.

Urethral syndrome

Urethral syndrome can be defined as dysuria in women that cannot be explained by the bacteria that normally cause urinary tract infection. *C. trachomatis* has been implicated in some cases.[125] The role of *Lactobacilli* in maintaining urinary tract health is disputed,[125,126] but speculation has arisen that if *Lactobacilli* are important in the prevention of urethral syndrome, and BV is associated with a reduction or an absence of such bacteria, then BV may be implicated in the aetiology of urethral syndrome.[119] This theory needs further investigation.

BV and sexual acquisition of human immunodeficiency virus (HIV)

Several studies have demonstrated the possibility of an association between BV and the transmission of HIV.[22,45,127] Klebanoff et al. showed that the presence of hydrogen-peroxide-producing *Lactobacilli* in the vagina results in a more acidic environment which is not only toxic to BV-associated flora but also to HIV.[45] They postulated that a lower vaginal pH may, therefore, block the production of CD4 lymphocytes whereas a higher, more alkaline pH associated with BV, may enhance HIV survival. Cohen et al. demonstrated that BV is linked to the increased detection of the anti-inflammatory cytokine, IL-10 in endocervical secretions, which in turn increases macrophage susceptibility to HIV-1 infection.[128]

It has been shown that BV micro-organisms, especially *M. hominis*, are able to increase the activity of a soluble HIV-inducing factor (HIF) and, therefore, increase HIV-1 expression.[129] Genital tract infection with *G. vaginalis*, which is commonly isolated in BV, has been shown to be able to stimulate HIV-1 production and hence increase the likelihood of sexual transmission.[130] One cross-sectional study in Thailand was carried out on 144 commercial sex workers and results showed that 47% of women infected with HIV had BV compared to 24% who were not infected with HIV.[131] Using the clinical criteria for diagnosis of BV, there was a significant, but independent, association between BV and HIV seropositivity. Results from another study in rural Uganda demonstrated that HIV-1 frequency in young women with normal vaginal flora was half that of women with severe BV.[132] HIV may promote abnormal flora in the vagina or BV may enhance the acquisition of HIV through sexual transmission. The evidence available supports a causal relationship between BV and HIV and BV may be an independent risk factor or a cofactor for transmission of HIV infection. A better understanding of the pathogenesis of BV and methods to reduce the risk of BV-related transmission are required.

THERAPY

Drug treatment

The polymicrobial nature of BV poses a problem to clinicians in attempting to find the most appropriate drug therapy. There is a need for drug therapy that is both sufficiently broad spectrum, but targeted against the bacteria involved in BV. Many trials have suggested different antibiotics with varying doses and treatment regimens. Currently, treatment recommendations world-wide advocate that BV may be treated with either metronidazole or clindamycin, given either orally or vaginally. Oral metronidazole is generally well-tolerated, but may give rise to nausea and a metallic taste in the mouth. Alcohol can exacerbate this effect as well as causing a disulfiram-like reaction so should be avoided. Despite this, allergy to metronidazole is rare, the drug is inexpensive and also *Lactobacilli*-sparing. Metronidazole vaginal gel produces systemic levels of drug far below those of the oral preparation, spares *Lactobacilli* but costs approximately 8 times that of the same drug given orally. Clindamycin cream is the most expensive of the treatments and has been shown to delay return of *Lactobacilli* to the vagina compared to metronidazole. Both oral and vaginal preparations of clindamycin have been linked to the development of pseudomembranous colitis.[133] However, clindamycin 2% vaginal cream is associated with few side-effects and only a very small fraction is absorbed systemically. It is licensed for use in pregnancy and can also be used by women who wish to drink alcohol. The efficacy of oral clindamycin compared to other recommended regimens needs further evaluation.

Clindamycin has good activity against organisms such as *Mobiluncus* spp. and *G. vaginalis* and metronidazole is effective against most anaerobes. Metronidazole is not harmful to *Lactobacilli* and thus it may encourage the rapid restoration of normal vaginal flora compared to clindamycin. Various treatment regimens exist for both drugs and one important factor in administering therapy is whether the woman is pregnant or not.

The current National Guidelines recommend that, in the non-pregnant woman, clindamycin may be used as an intravaginal cream (2%; 5 g once daily for 7 days) or may be given orally (300 mg twice daily for 7 days).[134] Metronidazole may be given orally (400–500 mg twice daily for 5-7 days), or as a vaginal gel (0.75%) once daily for 5 days, and occasionally as a suppository. It is often used prophylactically prior to gynaecological surgery (1 g *per rectum*). Most of these treatment regimens achieve cure rates between 70–80% after 4 weeks, as shown in trials comparing them to oral metronidazole.[135] Cure rates for symptomatic women with BV have been found to be only slightly different for oral metronidazole and intravaginal clindamycin cream immediately and one month after treatment (Table 3).136–140 Only one trial using oral clindamycin (300 mg twice daily for 7 days) compared to oral metronidazole (500 mg twice daily for 7 days) has been performed and both drugs showed high efficacy rates of 94% and 96%, respectively,[141] but further research into the efficacy of oral clindamycin is needed. These differences in cure rates even after evaluation at 4 weeks after completion were not found to be statistically significant. Other treatment studies comparing metronidazole vaginal gel and clindamycin cream have demonstrated similar cure rates.[142-144] The definition of 'cure' and 'relapse' varies between studies making comparison of regimens difficult. In practical terms, the efficacy of the various treatments for the cure of BV in non-pregnant women can be regarded as similar and decisions regarding the choice of drug and route of administration can be based on side-effect profile, patient preference and cost factors.

Treatment of BV in pregnancy

There is a great deal of experience of the inadvertent use of metronidazole in the first trimester of pregnancy because of unknown pregnancy status at the time of treatment. The possible teratogenic effect of metronidazole in early pregnancy is still disputed. A few cases of facial defects in the first trimester following a course of treatment have been reported,[145,146] although a more recent study has not demonstrated any mutagenicity following the use of metronidazole in the first trimester of pregnancy.[146] Mutagenicity in animals with long-term use has not been reflected in humans. Metronidazole and clindamycin can be secreted in breast milk; therefore, it is recommended that high doses of metronidazole are avoided if breast feeding, although standard treatment doses are not harmful. A vaginal preparation of clindamycin may be used as an alternative.

High-risk pregnancies
The strongest predictor of preterm birth is a history of a previous similar episode, but studies examining this have each had their methodological flaws.

Table 3 Comparison of studies comparing oral metronidazole (500 mg b.d. for 7 days), clindamycin vaginal cream 2% (5 g b.d. for 7 nights) and metronidazole vaginal gel 0.75% (5 g b.d. for 5 days) in the treatment of non-pregnant women

Study	Study design and number of subjects	Inclusion criteria	Definition of cure	Follow-up visit	Treatment	Cure rate (%)
Schmitt et al. (1992)[136]	RDBCT, 61 symptomatic women	AO, ≥ 20% CC, pH > 4.5	No symptoms and ≥ 2 of: pH > 4.5, AO, and ≥ 20% CC	5–8 days	Oral met	87
					CVC	72
				4 weeks	Oral met	61
					CVC	61
Andres et al. 1992)[137]	RDBCT, 60 symptomatic women	AO, CC, GS, pH > 4.5	Absence of 3 of: AO, CC and pH > 4.5	5–10 days	Oral met	83
					CVC	96
				4 weeks	Oral met	94
					CVC	89
Fishbach et al. (1993)[138]	RDBCT, 407 women	HD, AO, CC, GS, pH > 4.5	Absence of 3 of: AO, CC and pH > 4.5	5–10 days	Oral met	87
					CVC	85
				25–39 days	Oral met	81
					CVC	84
Ferris et al. (1995)[139]	RCT, 101 symptomatic women	CC and 2 of: AO, HD, pH > 4.5	Absence of ≥ 3 of: AO, HD, CC and pH > 4.5	7–10 days	Oral met	84
					CVC	86
					Met gel	75
McGregor et al. (1995)[140]	RSBCT, 112 women	≥ 20% CC and 2 of: AO, HD, pH ≥ 4.7	< 20% CC and absence of ≥ 2 of: AO, HD, pH ≥ 4.7	1 week	Oral met	85
					Met gel	84
				4 weeks	Oral met	71
					Met gel	71

RDBCT, randomised double-blind controlled trial; RCT, randomised controlled trial; RSBCT, randomised single-blind controlled trial; AO, amine odour; CC, clue cells; HD, homogeneous discharge; GS, Gram stain positive; met, metronidazole; CVC, clindamycin vaginal cream.

Treatment of BV in high-risk pregnancies has suggested that the risk of preterm delivery and infectious morbidity can be reduced.[100–102] Morales et al. randomised 80 women with BV and a history of either PTB or PPROM at 13–20 weeks' gestation to take oral metronidazole 250 mg TDS or placebo for 7 days. Women in the treatment arm had significantly fewer admissions for preterm labour, PTB and PPROM compared to women in the placebo arm.[102]

Hauth[101] randomised 624 women at risk of PTB due to a previous PTB or a low maternal weight (less than 50 kg) to take both erythromycin and metronidazole or placebo. The mean gestational age of treatment was 23 weeks. In the women with BV, there was a demonstrable decrease in the rate of PTB which was not seen in women who did not have BV. It is not clear which of the two drugs in the treatment arm was effective and the beneficial effect of treating BV was derived from subgroup analysis. Small study size and discrepant ethnic populations caused further criticism of these studies.

Unselected pregnancies

In a study which examined the impact of treatment of women with BV on rates of PTB, 1138 women were studied from 20 weeks' gestation onwards. The initial phase of the study was observational and only symptomatic women were treated for BV. All women were screened and treated as appropriate for *Chlamydia*, gonorrhoea and syphilis. BV treatment was oral clindamycin 300 mg twice daily for 7 days. During the treatment phase of the study, all women were screened for BV and treated regardless of symptoms with the same treatment regimen. There was a 50% reduction in the rates of PTB between the observational and treatment phases of the study. The methodology of this study can be criticised in that the population under study had high prevalences of BV, STDs and the results would have been more robust had it been a randomised double-blind placebo controlled trial.[100]

Lamont et al.[147,148] performed a study using a 3-day regimen of clindamycin 2% intravaginal cream (CVC) in pregnancy in comparison to the usual 7-day course. Over 400 pregnant women with BV diagnosed by Gram-stain were randomised to receive treatment or placebo at their first antenatal clinic visit at 13–20 weeks' gestation. The cure rates in the CVC group were statistically significantly superior to placebo and clindamycin appeared to be safe to use in pregnancy and well-tolerated. There was a statistically significant decrease in preterm birth in the treatment group (4.1%) compared to the placebo group (10%, P = 0.02), reflected by a higher mean birthweight of babies in the treated women. As part of this multicentre study, it was shown that pregnancy outcome was related to the degree of change in vaginal flora.[149] In women with grade III BV flora, the difference in the rate of preterm birth in women was close to statistical significance dependent on whether they received placebo or CVC. This subgroup with grade III flora may, therefore, benefit most from treatment with CVC.

In a large multicentre, randomised, placebo-controlled study of the impact of treatment of asymptomatic women with BV, no reduction in rates of PTD was found in the treatment arm compared to the placebo arm.[150] There are a number of criticisms of this study. Following exclusions for a variety of reasons, less than 10% of the original number or recruits was eligible (1953/29,625). An important potential confounding factor was that women complaining of vaginal symptoms were excluded which means that women with symptomatic BV were not studied. The treatment regimen was unusual in that it was a single 2 g dose of oral metronidazole repeated 2 days later and again after a 4 week interval. Treatment was often administered late, at 20 weeks' gestation and beyond. It is arguable that giving this particular treatment at the stated doses and intervals is inadequate to treat upper genital tract infection and to have sufficient activity against the spectrum of organisms involved in the development of BV-related chorio-amnionitis. Furthermore, intervention at a relatively late stage in pregnancy may have missed the optimum intervention time to reduce adverse sequelae.

It has been suggested that a combination of systemic and vaginal therapy may help to reduce BV – a large intravaginal dose of treatment to eradicate BV-related organisms locally and a smaller systemic dose to eliminate any ascending micro-organisms.

Current guidelines from the Centers for Disease Control and Prevention based in Atlanta, GA, USA recommend that there is ample evidence that pregnant women presenting with symptoms of BV can benefit from antibiotic treatment and women deemed to be at high-risk of adverse sequelae in pregnancy should be screened and treated.[135]

Self-help

The avoidance of washing the genital area with soap, shower gel or other alkaline detergents will help prevent BV. Women often state that they use 'pH balanced' products for washing, but these are still considerably more alkaline than the vagina and may, therefore, promote the emergence of bacterial overgrowth. The practice of douching should be discouraged, but may have roots in ethnic practice and is passed on from generation to generation. It is twice as common in black women compared to white women. In some small studies, the use of natural yoghurt or *Lactobacillus acidophilus* has only provided short-term relief,[151] but others have reported anecdotally that the use of natural yoghurt intravaginally following a drug treatment course appears to produce symptomatic relief. Products sold to the general public containing *Lactobacillus* spp. are widely available and are used in an attempt to restore normal flora. Hughes,[152] however, showed that of 16 products available on the market containing *Lactobacilli*, most did not actually contain the species advertised and of those species present, there was doubt as to the benefit in restoring normal flora. Hillier[46] demonstrated the effectiveness of a vaginal capsule containing *Lactobacillus crispatus* for colonisation in 90 sexually active adolescent young women. Capsules contained either 10^6 or 10^8 *L. crispatus* and were inserted twice daily for 3 days; assessment carried out weekly for one month. In the women who had significantly reduced numbers of hydrogen peroxide-producing *Lactobacilli* prior to use of the capsule, 76–85% of follow-up visits showed sustained colonisation at assessment. There appears, therefore, to be some potential value in the use of exogenous strains of some *Lactobacilli*.

Treatment of male partners

There is still some debate about whether the treatment of male sexual partners of women affected by BV is necessary. A study by Keane et al.[153] showed an association between non-gonococcal urethritis in men and BV in their female partners. This was thought to result from the large number of BV-associated vaginal flora in affected women leading to colonisation of the urethra of men following a sexual relationship. In the past, the isolation of BV-associated flora in male partners and the association of BV with an increased number of sexual partners provided a basis for the possibility of sexual transmission of BV, but this theory is strongly disputed. Most trials involving treatment of the male partner for BV have not resulted in any improvement in the cure rate in the female.[34,35] A recent appraisal of six trials assessing the treatment of the male sexual partner of women with BV suggests that there appears to be no benefit in doing so.[154] This may be open to debate as some of the trials involved small numbers, had large drop-out rates and differing methods of diagnosis. The general consensus currently appears to be that there is no justification in treating the male partner of a woman with BV.

Recurrent bacterial vaginosis

Some women have frequent episodes of BV, which are probably new episodes rather than treatment failures. The reason why some women have these relapses is not fully understood because the underlying factors involved in the pathogenesis of BV are not clear. One small study involving 30 women with symptomatic recurrent BV demonstrated the effectiveness of hydrogen peroxide 3% vaginally as an agent in treatment.[155] In the 23 women who completed the study, all had a negative amine test at re-assessment after 3 weeks, as well as the absence of clue cells and the absence of the mixed anaerobes which were present prior to treatment. In practice, some approaches to management of recurrent BV involve repeated antibiotic treatment, occasionally with antifungal agents. The evidence to support the use of prophylactic treatment is limited and its wide-spread use is not recommended, as this can result in drug resistance and repeated treatment may not be acceptable to the individual concerned. The use of *Lactobacillus* strains cultured under laboratory conditions to replace the vaginal flora is still being investigated.

CONCLUSIONS

Bacterial vaginosis is common and may affect the majority of women at some point in their lives. Whilst it may be asymptomatic, it can cause distressing vaginal discharge and malodour and is an important cause of pathology in both obstetric and gynaecological practice. There is good evidence that BV is associated with preterm labour and delivery, late miscarriage, postpartum endometritis, pelvic inflammatory disease, post-hysterectomy vaginal cuff infection and postabortal sepsis.

Obstetricians and gynaecologists should be aware of the potentially serious adverse sequelae of BV and familiarise themselves with its diagnosis and treatment.

KEY POINTS FOR CLINICAL PRACTICE

- Bacterial vaginosis is the commonest cause of vaginal discharge in women of reproductive age

- The precise aetiology of bacterial vaginosis is uncertain

- Bacterial vaginosis involves replacement of normal *Lactobacilli*-dominated vaginal bacteria with anaerobes and other organisms

- Classically, bacterial vaginosis produces a thin, homogeneous fishy-smelling discharge although up to 50% women with bacterial vaginosis may be asymptomatic

- Direct microscopy of a Gram-stained preparation of vaginal secretions is the ideal method of diagnosis, although other techniques more suited to the general gynaecologist in the office setting may also be used

- Bacterial vaginosis is associated with preterm labour and delivery, late miscarriage and postpartum endometritis

- Gynaecological complications associated with bacterial vaginosis include pelvic inflammatory disease, post-hysterectomy vaginal cuff infection and postabortal sepsis. Complications for which there is less convincing evidence of the role of bacterial vaginosis are urethral syndrome and infertility/early pregnancy loss

References

1 Gardner HL, Dukes CD. New etiologic agent in non-specific bacterial vaginosis. Science 1954; 120: 853

2 Gardner HL, Dukes CD. *Haemophilus vaginalis* vaginitis: a newly defined specific infection previously classified 'non-specific' vaginitis. Am J Obstet Gynecol 1955; 69: 962–976

3 Zinneman K, Turner GC. The taxonomic position of *Haemophilus vaginalis* (*Corynebacterium vaginale*). J Pathol Bacteriol 1963; 85: 213–219

4 Spiegel CA, Amsel R, Eschenbach DA et al. Anaerobic bacteria in non-specific vaginitis. N Engl J Med 1980; 303: 601–606

5 Totten P, Amsel R, Hale J et al. Selective differential human blood bilayer media for isolation of *Gardnerella vaginalis*. J Clin Microbiol 1982; 15: 141–147

6 Blackwell A, Barlow D. Clinical diagnosis of anaerobic vaginosis: a practical guide. Br J Vener Dis 1982; 58: 387–393

7 Eschenbach DA, Hillier SL, Critchlow CW et al. Diagnosis and clinical manifestations of bacterial vaginosis. Am J Obstet Gynecol 1988; 158: 819–828

8 Embree J, Caliando JJ, McCormack WM. Non-specific vaginitis among women attending a sexually transmitted diseases clinic. Sex Transm Dis 1984; 11: 81–84

9 Bump RC, Buesching WJ. Bacterial vaginosis in virginal and sexually active adolescent females: evidence against exclusive sexual transmission. Obstet Gynecol 1988; 158: 935–939

10 Hay PE, Taylor-Robinson D, Lamont RF. Diagnosis of bacterial vaginosis in a gynaecology clinic. Br J Obstet Gynaecol 1992; 99: 63–66

11 Blackwell A, Thomas PD, Wareham K et al. Health gains from screening for infection of the lower genital tract in women attending for termination of pregnancy. Lancet 1993; 342: 206–210

12   Hay PE, Lamont RF, Taylor-Robinson D, Morgan DJ, Ison CA, Pearson J. Abnormal colonisation of the genital tract and subsequent preterm delivery and late miscarriage. BMJ 1994; 308: 295–298

13   Lamont RF, Morgan DJ, Wilden S, Taylor-Robinson D. Prevalence of bacterial vaginosis in women attending one of three general practices for routine cervical cytology. Int J STD AIDS 2000; 11(8); 495–501

14   Peters N, van Leeuvan AM, Peters W. Bacterial vaginosis is not important in the etiology of cervical neoplasia: a survey on women with dyskaryotic smears. Sex Transm Dis 1995; 22: 296–302

15   Amsel R, Totten P, Spiegel CA, Chen KC, Eschenbach DA, Holmes KK. Non-specific vaginitis: diagnostic criteria and microbial and epidemiological associations. Am J Med 1983; 74: 14–22

16   Hillier SL, Holmes KK. Bacterial vaginosis. In: Holmes KK, Mardh P-A, Sparling PF et al. (eds) Sexually Transmitted Diseases. New York: McGraw Hill, 1990; 547–560

17   Klebanoff SJ, Hillier SL, Eschenbach DA, Waltersdorf AM. Control of the microbial flora of the vagina by H_2O_2-generating *Lactobacilli*. J Infect Dis 1991; 164: 94–100

18   Taylor E, Blackwell AL, Barlow D, Phillips I. *G. vaginalis*, anaerobes and vaginal discharge. Lancet 1982; 1: 1376–1379

19   Llahi-Camp JM, Rai R, Ison C, Regan L, Taylor-Robinson D. Association of bacterial vaginosis with a history of second trimester miscarriage. Hum Reprod 1996; 11: 1575–1578

20   Avonts D, Sercu M, Heyrick P, Vandermeerden I, Meheus A, Piot P. Incidence of uncomplicated genital tract infections in women using oral contraception or an intrauterine device: a prospective study. Sex Transm Dis 1990; 17: 23–29

21   Hawes SE, Hillier SL, Benedetti J et al. Hydrogen-peroxide producing *Lactobacilli* and acquisition of vaginal infections. J Infect Dis 1996; 174: 1058–1063

22   Royce RA, Jackson TP, Thorp Jr J et al. Race/ethnicity, vaginal flora patterns and pH during pregnancy. Sex Transm Dis 1999; 26: 96–102

23   Berger BJ, Kolton S, Zenilman JM, Cummings C, Feldman J, McCormack WM. Bacterial vaginosis in lesbians: a sexually transmitted disease. Clin Infect Dis 1995; 21: 1402–1405

24   Skinner CJ, Stokes J, Kirlew Y, Kavanagh J, Forster GE. A case-controlled study of the sexual health needs of lesbians. Genitourin Med 1996; 72: 277–280

25   McCaffrey M, Varney PA, Evans B, Taylor-Robinson D. A study of bacterial vaginosis in lesbians. Int J STD AIDS 1997; 8: 11

26   Larsen B, Galask RP. Influence of estrogen and normal flora on vaginal candidiasis in the rat. J Reprod Med 1984; 29: 863–868

27   Kinsman OS, Pitblado K, Coulson CJ. Effect of mammalian steroid hormones on the germination of *Candida albicans* and implications for vaginal candidiasis. Mycosis 1988; 31: 617–626

28   Taylor-Robinson D, Hay PE. The pathogenesis of the clinical signs of bacterial vaginosis and possible reasons for its occurrence. Int J STD AIDS 1998; 8: 13–16

29   Furr PM, Taylor-Robinson D. Oestradiol-induced infection of the genital tract of female mice by *Mycoplasma hominis*. J Gen Microbiol 1989; 135: 2743–2749

30   Furr PM, Taylor-Robinson D. The establishment and persistence of *Ureaplasma urealyticum* in oestradiol treated mice. J Med Microbiol 1989; 29: 111–114

31   Taylor-Robinson D, Furr PM, Hetherington CM. *Neisseria gonorrhoeae* colonises the genital tract of oestradiol-treated germ-free female mice. Microb Pathog 1990; 9: 369–374

32   Furr PM, Taylor-Robinson D. The influence of hormones on the bacterial flora of the murine vagina and implications for human disease. Microb Ecol Health Dis 1991; 4: 141–148

33   Hay PE, Morgan DJ, Ison CA et al. A longitudinal study of bacterial vaginosis during pregnancy. Br J Obstet Gynaecol 1994; 101: 1048–1053

34   Vejtorp M, Bollerup AC, Vejtorp L et al. Bacterial vaginosis: a double-blind randomised trial of the effect of treatment of the sexual partner. Br J Obstet Gynaecol 1988; 95: 920–926

35   Moi H, Erkkola R, Jerve F et al. Should male partners of women with bacterial vaginosis be treated? Genitourin Med 1989; 65: 263–268

36 Colli E, Landoni M, Parazzini F. Treatment of male partners and recurrence of bacterial vaginosis: a randomised trial. Genitourin Med 1997; 73: 267–270

37 Howe L, Wiggins R, Soothill PW, Millar MR, Horner PJ, Coorfield AP. Mucinase and sialidase activity of the vaginal microflora: implications in the pathogenesis of preterm labour. Int J STD AIDS 1999; 10: 442–447

38 Pavlova S, Kilic AO, Mou SM et al. Phage infection in vaginal Lactobacilli: an in vitro study. Infect Dis Obstet Gynecol 1997; 5: 36–44

39 Tao L, Pavlova S, Mou SM et al. Analysis of Lactobacilli products for phages and bacteriocins that inhibit vaginal Lactobacilli. Infect Dis Obstet Gynecol 1997; 5: 244–251

40 Skarin A, Sylwan F. Vaginal Lactobacilli inhibiting growth of G. vaginalis, Mobiluncus and other bacterial species cultured from vaginal content of women with bacterial vaginosis. Acta Pathol Microbiol Immunol Scand 1987; 94: 399–403

41 Barefood SF, Klaenhammer TR. Detection and activity of lactacin B, a bacteriocin produced by Lactobacillus acidophilus. Appl Environ Microbiol 1983; 45: 1808–1815

42 Hamden IY, Mikolajcik EM. Acidolin: an antibiotic produced by Lactobacillus acidophilus. J Antibiot (Tokyo) 1974; 27: 632–636

43 Eschenbach DA, Davick PR, William BL et al. Prevalence of hydrogen peroxide-producing Lactobacilli in normal women and women with bacterial vaginosis. J Clin Microbiol 1989; 27: 251–256

44 Hillier SL, Krohn M, Klebanoff SJ, Eschenbach DA. The relationship of hydrogen-peroxide producing Lactobacilli to bacterial vaginosis and genital microflora in pregnant women. Obstet Gynecol 1992; 79: 369–373

45 Klebanoff SJ, Coombs RW. Viricidal effects of L. acidophilus on human immunodeficiency virus type-1: possible role in heterosexual transmission. J Exp Med 1991; 174: 289–292

46 Hillier SL, Krohn M, Meyn L et al. Recolonisation of the vagina with an exogenous strain of Lactobacillus crispatus. Conference Proceeding of International Bacterial Vaginitis Conference, Aspen, Colorado, USA, September 1998

47 Rotstein OD, Pruett TL, Fiegel VD, Nelson RD, Simmons RL. Succinic acid, a metabolic byproduct of Bacteroides species inhibits polymorphonuclear leukocyte function. Infect Immun 1985; 48: 402–408

48 Hill GB, Eschenbach DA, Holmes KK. Bacteriology of the vagina. Scand J Urol Nephrol 1984; 86: 23–29

49 McCue JD. Evaluation and management of vaginitis. Arch Intern Med 1989; 149: 565–568

50 Masfari AN, Duerden BI, Kinghorn GI. Quantitative studies of vaginal bacteria. Genitourin Med 1986; 62: 256–263

51 Piot P, Van Dyke E, Godts P, Vanderheyden J. The vaginal microbial flora in non-specific vaginitis. Eur J Clin Microbiol 1982; 1: 301–306

52 Chen KC, Forsyth PS, Buchanan TM, Holmes KK. Amine content of vaginal fluid from untreated and treated patients with non-specific vaginitis. J Clin Invest 1979; 63: 828–835

53 Brand JM, Galask RP. Trimethylamine: the substance mainly responsible for the fishy odour often associated with bacterial vaginosis. Obstet Gynecol 1986; 63: 682–695

54 Erkkola R, Jarvinen H, Terho P et al. Microbiological flora in women showing symptoms of non-specific vaginosis: applicability of KOH test for diagnosis. Scand J Infect Dis 1983; 40: 59–63

55 Easmon CS, Hay PE, Ison CA. Bacterial vaginosis: a diagnostic approach. Genitourin Med 1992; 68: 134–138

56 Hillier SL, Krohn MA, Nugent RP, Gibbs RS. Characteristics of three vaginal flora patterns assessed by Gram stain among pregnant women. Am J Obstet Gynecol 1992; 166: 938–944

57 Schwebke JR, Hillier SL, Sobel JD, McGregor JA, Sweet RL. Validity of the vaginal Gram stain for the diagnosis of bacterial vaginosis. Obstet Gynecol 1996; 88: 573–576

58 Platz-Christensen JJ, Larsson PG, Sundstrom E, Wiqvist N. Detection of bacterial vaginosis in wet mount, Papanicolaou stained vaginal smears and in Gram stained smears. Acta Obstet Gynecol Scand 1995; 74: 67–70

59 Morgan DJ, Aboud CJ, Bhide SA, McCaffrey M, Lamont RF, Taylor-Robinson D. Comparison of Gram-stained smears from blind vaginal swabs with those obtained at

speculum examination for the assessment of vaginal flora. Br J Obstet Gynaecol 1996; 103: 1105–1108

60 Thomason JL, Gelbart SM, Wilcoski LM, Peterson AK, Jilly BJ, Hamilton PR. Proline aminopeptidase activity as a rapid diagnostic test to confirm bacterial vaginosis. Obstet Gynecol 1988; 71: 607–611

61 O'Dowd TC, West RR, Winterburn PJ, Hewlins MJ. Evaluation of a rapid diagnostic test for bacterial vaginosis. Br J Obstet Gynaecol 1996; 103: 366–370

62 Andrews WW, Goldenberg RL, Hauth JC. Preterm labour: emerging role of genital tract infections. Infect Agents Dis 1995; 4: 196–211

63 Owen P, Patel N. Prevention of preterm birth. Baillière's Clin Obstet Gynaecol 1995; 9: 465–479

64 McGregor JA, French JI, Lawellin D et al. Preterm birth and infection: pathogenic possibilities. Am J Reprod Immunol Microbiol 1988; 16: 123–132

65 Romero R, Mazor M, Wu YK et al. Infection in the pathogenesis of preterm labour. Semin Pathol 1988; 12: 262–279

66 Mazor M, Chaim W, Horowitz S et al. The biomolecular mechanisms of preterm labour in women with intrauterine infection. Isr J Med Sci 1994; 30: 317–322

67 Gibbs RS, Romero R, Hillier SL et al. A review of premature birth and subclinical infection. Am J Obstet Gynecol 1992; 166: 1515–1528

68 Goepfert AR, Goldenberg RL. Prediction of prematurity. Curr Opin Obstet Gynecol 1996; 8: 417–427

69 Lamont RF, Fisk NM. The role of infection in preterm birth. In: Studd J. (ed) Progress in Obstetrics and Gynaecology. Edinburgh: Churchill Livingstone, 1993; 135–158

70 Hillier SL, Nugent RP. Association between bacterial vaginosis and preterm delivery of a low birth weight infant. N Engl J Med 1995; 333: 1737–1742

71 Gibbs RS. Chorioamnionitis and bacterial vaginosis. Am J Obstet Gynecol 1993; 169: 460–462

72 Lamont RF, Taylor-Robinson D, Newman M et al. Spontaneous early preterm labour associated with abnormal genital bacterial colonisation. Br J Obstet Gynaecol 1986; 93: 804–810

73 McDonald HM, O'Loughlin JA, Jolley PT et al. Changes in vaginal flora during pregnancy and association with preterm birth. J Infect Dis 1994; 170: 724–728

74 Gratacos E, Figueras F, Barranco M et al. Spontaneous recovery of bacterial vaginosis during pregnancy is not associated with an improved perinatal outcome. Acta Obstet Gynecol Scand 1998; 77: 37–40

75 Romero R, Brody D, Oyarzun F et al. Infection and labor: III. Interleukin-1: a signal for the initiation of parturition. Am J Obstet Gynecol 1989; 160: 1117–1123

76 Romero R, Mazor M, Sepulveda W, Avila C, Copeland D, Williams J. Tumor necrosis factor in preterm and term labor. Am J Obstet Gynecol 1992; 166: 1576–1587

77 Romero R, Avila C, Santhanam U, Sehgal P. Amniotic fluid interleukin-6 in preterm labor. J Clin Invest 1990; 85: 1392–1400

78 Liechty K, Koennig J, Mitchell M, Romero R, Christensen R. Production of interleukin-6 by fetal and maternal cells in vitro after stimulation with interleukin-1. Paediatr Res 1991; 29: 1–4

79 Hillier SL, Witkin S, Krohn M, Watts D, Kiviat N, Eschenbach DA. The relationship of amniotic fluid cytokines and preterm delivery, amniotic fluid infection, histologic chorioamnionitis and chorioamnion infection. Obstet Gynecol 1993; 81: 941–948

80 Mitchell M, Dudely DJ, Edwin SS, Schiller SL. Interleukin-6 stimulated prostaglandin production by human amnion and decidual cells. Eur J Pharmacol 1991; 192: 189–191

81 McGregor JA, French JI, Jones W, Parker R, Patterson E, Draper D. Association of cervicovaginal infections with increased vaginal fluid phospholipase A_2 activity. Am J Obstet Gynecol 1992; 167: 1588–1594

82 McGregor JA, Lawellin D, Franco-Buff A, Todd J. Phospholipase C activity in microorganisms associated with reproductive tract infection. Am J Obstet Gynecol 1991; 164: 682–686

83 Romero R, Manogue KR, Mitchell M et al. Infection and labor IV: cachectin-tumor necrosis factor in the amniotic fluid of women with intra-amniotic infection and preterm labor. Am J Obstet Gynecol 1989; 161: 336–341

84 Coultrip LL, Lien JM, Gomez R et al. The value of amniotic fluid interleukin-6 determination in patients with preterm labor and intact membranes in the detection of microbial invasion of the amniotic cavity. Am J Obstet Gynecol 1994; 171: 901–911

85 Byrne MA, Turner MJ, Griffiths M. Evidence that patients presenting with dyskaryotic cervical smears should be screened for genital tract infections other than human papilloma virus infection. Eur J Obstet Gynaecol Reprod Biol 1991; 41: 129–133

86 McNichol P, Paraskevas M, Guijon F. Variability of polymerase chain reaction based detection of human papilloma virus DNA is associated with the composition of vaginal microbial flora. J Med Virol 1994; 43: 194–200

87 Hirsch E, Blanchard R, Mehta P. Differential fetal and maternal contributions to the cytokine milieu in a murine model of infection-induced preterm birth. Obstet Gynecol 1999; 180: 429–434

88 Steinborn A, Niederhut A, Solbach C, Hildenbrand R, et al. Cytokine release from placental endothelial cells: a process associated with preterm labor in the absence of intrauterine infection. Cytokine 1999; 11: 66–73

89 Kahn M, De Vellis J. Regulation of an oligodendrocyte progenitor cell line by the interleukin-6 family of cytokines. Glia 1994; 12: 87–98

90 Robbins D, Shirazi Y, Drysdale B, Lieberman A, Shin M. Production of cytotoxic factor for oligodendrocytes by stimulated astrocytes. J Immunol 1987; 139: 2593–2597

91 Murphy DJ, Hope DL, Johnson A. Neonatal risk factors for cerebral palsy in very preterm babies: case-control-study. BMJ 1997; 314: 404–408

92 Murphy DJ, Sellers S, Mackenzie IZ, Yudkin PL, Johnson AM. Case-control-study of antenatal and intrapartum risk factors in very preterm singleton babies. Lancet 1995; 346: 1449–1454

93 Grether JK, Nelson KB. Maternal infection and cerebral palsy in infants of normal birth weight. JAMA 1997; 278: 207–211

94 Perlman JM, Risser R, Broyles RS. Bilateral cystic periventricular leukomalacia in the premature infant: associated risk factors. Pediatrics 1996; 97: 822–827

95 Zupan V, Gonzales P, Lacaze-Masmonteil T et al. Periventricular leukomalacia: risk factors revisited. Dev Med Child Neurol 1996; 38: 1061–1067

96 Montero-Julian FA, Klein B, Gautherot E, Brailly H. Pharmacokinetic study of anti-interleukin-6 (IL-6) therapy with monoclonal antibodies: enhancement of IL-6 clearance by cocktails of anti-IL-6 antibodies. Blood 2000; 85: 917–924

97 Goldenberg RL, Mercer BM, Meis PJ, Copper RL, Das A, McNellis D. The preterm prediction study: fetal fibronectin testing and spontaneous preterm birth. Obstet Gynecol 1996; 87: 643–648

98 Kekki M, Kurki T, Paavonen J, Rutanen EM. Insulin-like growth factor binding protein-1 in the cervix as a marker of infectious complications in pregnant women with bacterial vaginosis [Letter]. Lancet 1999; 353: 1494

99 McGregor JA, French JI, Jones W et al. Bacterial vaginosis is associated with prematurity and vaginal fluid mucinase and sialidase: results of a controlled trial of topical clindamycin cream. Am J Obstet Gynecol 1994; 170: 1048–1059

100 McGregor JA, French JI, Parker R et al. Prevention of premature birth by screening and treatment of common genital tract infections: results of a prospective controlled trial. Am J Obstet Gynecol 1995; 157–167

101 Hauth JC, Goldenberg RL, Andrews WW, DuBard MB, Copper RL. Reduced incidence of preterm delivery with metronidazole and erythromycin in women with bacterial vaginosis. N Engl J Med 1995; 333: 1732–1736

102 Morales WJ, Schorr S, Albritton J. Effect of metronidazole in patients with preterm birth in preceding pregnancy and bacterial vaginosis: a placebo-controlled, double-blind study. Am J Obstet Gynecol 1994; 171: 345–349

103 Watts D, Krohn MA, Hillier SL, Eschenbach DA. Bacterial vaginosis as a risk factor for post cesarean endometritis. Obstet Gynecol 1990; 75: 52–58

104 Newton ER, Prihoda TJ, Gibbs RS. A clinical and microbiologic analysis of risk factors for puerperal endometritis. Obstet Gynecol 1990; 75: 402–406

105 Platz-Christensen JJ, Sundstrom E, Larsson PG. Bacterial vaginosis and cervical intraepithelial neoplasia. Acta Obstet Gynecol Scand 1994; 73: 586–588

106 Mead PA. Cervical-vaginal flora of women with invasive cervical cancer. JAMA 1978; 52: 601–604

107 Frega A, Stentella P, Spera G et al. Cervical intraepithelial neoplasia and bacterial vaginosis: correlation or risk factor ? Eur J Gynaecol Oncol 1997; 18: 76–77

108 Pavic N. Is there a local production of nitrosamines by the vaginal microflora in anaerobic vaginosis/trichomoniasis? Med Hypotheses 1982; 15: 433–436

109 Parsons A, McGregor JA. Pathogens on the move: active uterine transport of cervico-vaginal fluid into the uterus and fallopian tubes at ovarian mid-cycle. Int J STD AIDS 1997; 8: 22–22

110 Paavonen J, Teisala K, Heinonen PK et al. Microbiological and histopathological findings in acute pelvic inflammatory disease. Br J Obstet Gynaecol 1987; 94: 454–460

111 Sweet RL. Pelvic inflammatory disease and infertility in women. Infect Dis Clin North Am 1987; 1: 99–125

112 Eschenbach DA. Bacterial vaginosis: emphasis on upper genital tract complications. Obstet Gynecol Clin North Am 1989; 16: 593–610

113 Mardh P-A, Westrom L. Tubal and cervical cultures in acute salpingitis with special reference to *Mycoplasma hominis* and T-strain Mycoplasmas. Br J Vener Dis 1970; 46: 179–186

114 Mardh P-A, Westrom L. Antibodies to *Mycoplasma hominis* in patients with genital infections and in healthy controls. Br J Vener Dis 1970; 46: 390–397

115 McCaffrey M, Cottell E, Keane D et al. Bacterial vaginosis and infertility. Int J STD AIDS 1997; 8: 25

116 Llahi-Camp JM, Ison CA, Regan L, Taylor-Robinson D. The association between bacterial vaginosis and infertility. Int J STD AIDS 1997; 8: 23–24

117 Morgan DJ, Wong SJ, Trueman G et al. Can bacterial vaginosis influence fertility? Its increased prevalence in a subfertile population. Int J STD AIDS 1997; 8: 19–20

118 Ralph SG, Rutherford AJ, WilsonJD. Influence of bacterial vaginosis on conception and miscarriage in the first trimester: cohort study. BMJ 1999; 319: 220–223

119 Taylor-Robinson D. Non-pregnancy complications: an introduction. Int J STD AIDS 1997; 8: 17–18

120 Soper DE, Bump RC, Hurt WG. Bacterial vaginosis and *Trichomoniasis vaginitis* are risk factors for cuff cellulitis after abdominal hysterectomy. Am J Obstet Gynecol 1990; 163: 1016–1023

121 Larsson PG, Platz-Christensen JJ, Forsum U, Pahlson C. Clue cells in predicting infections after abdominal hysterectomy. Obstet Gynecol 1991; 77: 450–453

122 Larsson PG, Bergman B, Forsum H, Platz-Christensen JJ, Pahlson C. Mobiluncus and clue cells as predictors of PID after first trimester abortion. Acta Obstet Gynecol Scand 1989; 68: 217–220

123 Larsson PG, Platz-Christensen JJ, Thejls H, Forsum U, Pahlson C. Incidence of pelvic inflammatory disease after first trimester legal abortion in women with bacterial vaginosis after treatment with metronidazole: a double blind randomised study. Am J Obstet Gynecol 1992; 166: 100–103

124 Larsson PG, Platz-Christensen JJ, Dalaker K et al. Treatment with 2% clindamycin vaginal cream prior to first trimester surgical abortion to reduce signs of postoperative infection: a prospective, double-blinded, placebo-controlled multicenter study. Acta Obstet Gynecol Scand 2000; 79: 390–396

125 Stamm WE, Wagner KF, Amsel R et al. Causes of the acute urethral syndrome in women. N Engl J Med 1980; 303: 409–415

126 Maskell R. Are fastidious organisms an important cause of dysuria and frequency? The case for. In: Asscher AW, Brumfitt W. (eds) Microbial Diseases in Nephrology. Chichester: Wiley, 1986; 19–30

127 Taha T, Gray R, Kumwenda N, Hoover D et al. HIV infection and disturbances of vaginal flora during pregnancy. J Acquir Immune Defic Syndr Hum Retrovirol 1999; 20: 52–59

128 Cohen CR, Plummer FA, Mugo N et al. Increased interleukin-10 in the endocervical secretions of women with non-ulcerative sexually transmitted diseases: a mechanism for enhanced HIV-1 transmission? AIDS 1999; 13: 327–332

129 Al-Harthi L, Roebuck KA, Olinger GG et al. Bacterial vaginosis-associated microflora isolated from the female genital tract activates HIV-1 expression. J Acquir Immune Defic Syndr Hum Retrovirol 1999; 21: 194–202

130 Hashemi FB, Ghassemi M, Roebuck KA, Spear GT. Activation of human immuno-deficiency virus type 1 expression by *Gardnerella vaginalis*. J Infect Dis 2000; 179: 924–930

131 Cohen CR, Duerr A, Pruthithada N et al. Bacterial vaginosis and HIV seroprevalence among commercial female sex workers in Chiang Mai, Thailand. AIDS 1995; 9: 1093–1097

132 Sewankambo N, Gray R, Wawer M et al. HIV infection associated with abnormal vaginal flora morphology and bacterial vaginosis. Lancet 1997; 350: 546–549

133 Trexler MF, Fraser TG, Jones MP. Fulminant pseudomembranous colitis caused by clindamycin phosphate vaginal cream. Am J Gastroenterol 1997; 92: 2112–2113

134 Hay PE. National guidelines for the management of bacterial vaginosis. Sex Transm Dis 1999; 75: S16–S18

135 CDC. Guidelines for the treatment of sexually transmitted diseases. MMWR 1998; 47: 1–118

136 Schmitt C, Sobel JD, Meriwether C. Bacterial vaginosis: treatment with clindamycin cream versus oral metronidazole. Obstet Gynecol 1992; 79: 1020–1030

137 Andres FJ, Parker R, Hosein I, Benrubi GI. Clindamycin vaginal cream versus oral metronidazole in the treatment of bacterial vaginosis: a prospective double-blind clinical trial. Southern Med J 1992; 85: 1077–1080

138 Fischbach F, Peterson EE, Weissenbacher ER et al. Efficacy of clindamycin vaginal cream versus oral metronidazole in the treatment of bacterial vaginosis. Obstet Gynecol 1993; 82: 405–410

139 Ferris DG, Litaker MS, Woodward L, Heindrich J. Treatment of bacterial vaginosis: a comparison of oral metronidazole, metronidazole vaginal gel and clindamycin vaginal cream. J Fam Pract 1995; 41: 443–449

140 McGregor JA, Hillier SL, Eschenbach DA et al. Efficacy of metrogel-vaginal versus oral metronidazole for the treatment of bacterial vaginosis: a randomised single-blind parallel comparison. Presented at 11th International Meeting of the ISSVD, New Orleans. 1995. 1995

141 Greaves WL, Chungafung J, Morris B, Haile A, Townsend JL. Clindamycin versus metronidazole in the treatment of bacterial vaginosis. Obstet Gynecol 1988; 72: 799–802

142 Hillier SL, Lipinski C, Briselden AM, Eschenbach DA. Efficacy of intravaginal 0.75% metronidazole gel for the treatment of bacterial vaginosis. Obstet Gynecol 1993; 81: 963–967

143 Livengood III C, McGregor JA, Soper DE, Newton E, Thomason JL. Bacterial vaginosis: efficacy and safety of intravaginal metronidazole treatment. Am J Obstet Gynecol 1994; 170: 759–764

144 Sobel JD, Cairn W, Thomason JL et al. Comparative study of intravaginal metronidazole and triple-sulfa cream for bacterial vaginosis. Int J Obstet Gynecol 1996; 4: 66–70

145 Cantu JM, Garcia-Cruz D. Midline facial defect as a teratogenic effect of metronidazole. Birth Defects 1982; 18: 85–88

146 Greenberg F. Possible metronidazole teratogenicity and clefting. Am J Med Genet 1985; 22: 825

147 Lamont RF, Sheehan M, Morgan DJ, Duncan S, Mandal D. Safety and efficacy of clindamycin intravaginal cream for the treatment of bacterial vaginosis in pregnancy. A randomised double-blind, placebo-controlled, multicentre study. Gynaecol Obstet 1999; 67: S45

148 Lamont RF, Morgan DJ, Sheehan M, Duncan S, Mandal D. The outcome of pregnancy following the use of clindamycin intravaginal cream for the treatment of abnormal bacterial colonisation: a prospective, randomised, double-blind, placebo-controlled multicentre study. Int J Obstet Gynecol 2000; 67: S42

149 Rosenstein IJ, Morgan DJ, Lamont RF et al. Effect of vaginally applied clindamycin on vaginal microbial flora and outcome of pregnancy in women with bacterial vaginosis. Infect Dis Obstet Gynecol 2000; 8: 158–165

150 Carey JC, Klebanoff SJ, Hauth JC et al. Metronidazole to prevent preterm delivery in pregnant women with asymptomatic bacterial vaginosis. N Engl J Med 2000; 342: 534–540

151 Larsson PG. Treatment of bacterial vaginosis. Int J STD AIDS 1992; 3: 239–247

152 Hughes VL, Hillier SL. Microbiologic characteristics of *Lactobacillus* products used for colonisation of the vagina. Obstet Gynecol 1990; 75: 244–248

153 Keane F, Thomas B, Renton A, Whitaker L, Taylor-Robinson D. An investigation into a possible causal role of bacterial vaginosis in non-gonococcal urethritis. Genitourin Med 1997; 73: 373–377

154 Potter J. Should sexual partners of women with bacterial vaginosis receive treatment? Br J Gen Pract 1999; 49: 913–918

155 Wincelaus SJ, Calver G. Recurrent bacterial vaginosis: an old approach to a new problem. Int J STD AIDS 2000; 8: 210

156 Gravett MG. Causes of preterm delivery. Semin Perinatal 1984; 8: 246–257

157 McDonald H, O'Loughlin JA, Jolley PT, Vigneswaran R, McDonald PJ. Prenatal microbiological risk factors associated with preterm birth. Br J Obstet Gynaecol 1992; 99: 190–195

158 Hillier SL, Nugent RP. Association between bacterial vaginosis and preterm delivery of a low birth weight infant. N Engl J Med 1995; 333: 1737–1742

159 Krohn M, Hillier SL, Nugent RP et al. The genital flora of women with intra-amniotic infection. Vaginal Infection and Prematurity Study Group. J Infect Dis 1995; 171: 1475–1480

160 Hillier SL, Krohn M, Cassen E, Easterling TR, Rabe LK, Eschenbach DA. The role of bacterial vaginosis and vaginal bacteria in amniotic fluid infection in women in preterm labour with intact fetal membranes. Clin Infect Dis 1995; 20: S276–S278

161 McGregor JA, French JI, Richter R et al. Antenatal microbiologic and maternal risk factors associated with prematurity. Am J Obstet Gynaecol 1991; 163: 1465–1473

162 RiduanJM, Hillier SL, Utomo B, Wiknjosastro G, Linnan M, Kandun N. Bacterial vaginosis and prematurity in Indonesia: association in early and late pregnancy. Am J Obstet Gynecol 1993; 169: 175–178

163 Hay PE, Morgan DJ, Ison CA et al. A longitudinal study of bacterial vaginosis during pregnancy. Br J Obstet Gynaecol 1994; 101: 1048–1053

164 Kurki T, Sivonen A, Renkovan OV, Savita E, Ylikorkala O. Bacterial vaginosis in early pregnancy and pregnancy outcome. Obstet Gynaecol 1992; 80: 173–177

David Nunns Steven Dobbs

Vulval pain syndromes

The vulval pain syndromes (vulval vestibulitis and dysaesthetic vulvodynia) are enigmatic causes of vulval pain and incorporate a heterogeneous group of women who are invariably difficult to manage. Although not new conditions, only since the mid-1980s have the clinical descriptions of these women, who complain of pain rather than itching, been standardised. In 1991, the term vulvodynia and its subsets were introduced by the International Society for the Study of Vulval Diseases (ISSVD) to describe women with 'chronic vulval discomfort characterised by burning, stinging, rawness or irritation'.[1] The terminology is potentially confusing, as vulvodynia was originally described as having subsets including both infective and dermatological diagnoses. These included vulval dermatoses (e.g. lichen sclerosus), vulval vestibulitis, vestibular papillomatosis, dysaesthetic (formerly essential vulvodynia) and cyclical vulvitis. Vulval vestibulitis, a cause of introital dyspareunia among women of reproductive age, and dysaesthetic vulvodynia, where constant, localised vulval pain is experienced, together form the vulval pain syndromes as these relate to vulval pain when infection and organic causes have been excluded. It should be emphasised that a diagnosis of vulval dermatoses (e.g. lichen sclerosis), vestibular papillomatosis or cyclical vulvitis do not fit into a diagnosis of vulval pain syndrome. Vestibular papillomatosis where filamentous projections of epithelium are found within the vestibule and inner labia minora is now considered a variant of normal.[2] Its inclusion in the original definition of vulvodynia subsets relates to work from the 1980s which implicated human papilloma virus (HPV) infection with pain. Recent work using DNA hybridization techniques has now discounted this association and any link with

Mr David Nunns MD MRCOG, Consultant Gynaecological Oncologist, Nottingham City Hospital, Hucknall Road, Nottingham NG5 1PB, UK (for correspondence)

Mr Steven Dobbs MD MRCOG, Consultant Gynaecologist and Gynaecological Oncologist, Belfast City Hospital, Lisburn Road, Belfast BT9 7AB, UK

HPV is likely to be coincidental.[2] Cyclical vulvitis causes intermittent swelling and pain of the labia usually prior to menstruation, which resolves soon after. The cause remains elusive; however, many women respond to maintenance treatment with antifungals.[3] Recent interest in these pain syndromes probably relates to an increasing number of patients attending vulval clinics, patients' demands and general increased awareness amongst women and health professionals.

HISTORY

Reports of unexplained vulval pain have been recorded in the medical literature for more than a century.[4] One of the first accounts was by Skene in 1888 who writes of vulval hyperaesthesia:[4]

Pruritus is absent, and on examination of the parts affected no redness or other external manifestation of the disease is visible. When, however, the examining finger comes in contact with the hyperaesthetic part, the patient complains of pain, which is sometimes as great as to cause her to cry out. Indeed, the sensitiveness is occasionally so exaggerated as to keep the patient from consulting her physician until it becomes absolutely unbearable.

Kelly in 1928 also described 'exquisitely, sensitive, deep red spots in the mucosa of the hymenal ring as a fruitful cause of dyspareunia.[5] Despite these initial observations, there have been few references in the literature over the last 40 years, even in major gynaecological textbooks.[6] The reasons for this remain unclear. In the 1970s as revival of interest took place, many loose, ambiguous definitions were introduced. The terms, focal vulvitis, erythematous vulvitis en plaque, burning vulva syndrome and vestibular adenitis were introduced, all probably describing the same condition.[7-10] In 1985, a specific task force was instituted by the ISSVD to deal with the problem of recognition and therapy for these patients. The task force consisted of gynaecologists, dermatologists and venereologists all interested in managing women with vulval diseases. Lynch introduced the term 'vulvodynia' in 1985 and, in 1991, McKay on behalf of the ISSVD defined several distinct subsets of vulvodynia, which have now been adopted for general clinical use.[1,3]

DIAGNOSIS AND CLINICAL FINDINGS

Vulval vestibulitis and dysaesthetic vulvodynia are separate conditions (Fig. 1); however, there are many clinical and aetiological overlaps.[11] Many studies wrongly use vulval vestibulitis and vulvodynia synonymously, as the clinical aspects and the management options of these two groups can differ considerably. Of the two conditions, vulval vestibulitis has received the most attention, yet women with dysaesthetic vulvodynia remain under-researched and pose difficulties in management.

Vulval vestibulitis

Vulval vestibulitis is diagnosed clinically on history and examination. Friedrich, in 1987, defined the condition and included three criteria for

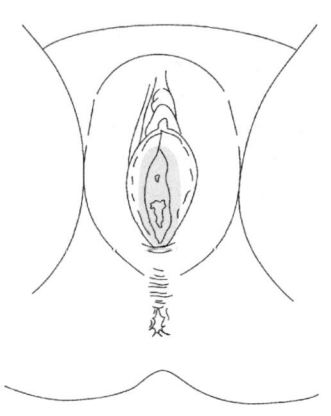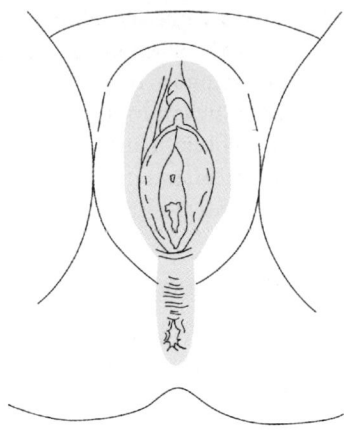

Fig. 1 Vulval pain syndromes – shaded areas indicate location of pain.

diagnosis: (i) severe pain on vestibular touch or attempted vaginal entry; (ii) tenderness to pressure localised within the vestibule; and (iii) the physical findings of erythema confined to the vestibule.[12] Although these useful criteria are widely quoted, it is the second criterion, which is specific to vulval vestibulitis. The swab test was introduced by Friedrich as a useful way of demonstrating tenderness within the vestibule. A cotton tipped swab is applied gently to normal skin as a control and then around different areas of the external genitalia. In vulval vestibulitis, pain on light touch is elicited typically in the vestibule area – so-called 'allodynia' where innocuous stimuli cause pain. This hyperaesthesia can be generalised throughout the vestibule or can be more focal involving the opening of the ducts of the major vestibular glands (focal vestibulitis) or the posterior fourchette.[7] Apart from demonstrating tenderness, the swab test does quantify the tenderness elicited and is not a reproducible method of assessment as it is completely operator-dependent. A more objective way of measuring hyperaesthesia has been developed by Curnow, using a hand-probe applied to the skin which gives variable degrees of pressure producing a recorded numerical result with the degree of symptoms correlating with the numerical result.[13,14] This vulval algesiometer is not, however, routinely available. The other criteria for diagnosing vulval vestibulitis are not specific and may occur with other vulval conditions. Pain on touching the vestibule can occur with a variety of inflammatory or infective vulval conditions which exclude a diagnosis of vulval vestibulitis. Vestibular erythema is a subjective finding often present on normal examination; however, if it is associated with vulval vestibulitis, the degree of erythema does not correlate with symptoms.[15] The application of diluted acetic acid to the vulva does not assist in making a diagnosis.[16]

Typically, women with vulval vestibulitis are Caucasian, aged 20–40 years and present with a history of provoked pain such as superficial dyspareunia, tampon intolerance and pain during gynaecological examinations.[10,12,18–21] Women may have had pain from their first attempt at sexual intercourse or there may have been a period of normal sexual activity with the development of pain subsequently.[18,19] There is often a delay from the onset of symptoms to receiving a diagnosis, which varies from months to years. Arbitrarily, a 6-month period of time has been suggested from the onset of symptoms to making a diagnosis of vulval vestibulitis so to exclude women recovering from acute vulval inflammation from other causes.[7,13] Many women have been seen by various specialists and often give a history of using multiple, inappropriate topical medications.[11,12,17] Hence, when an accurate diagnosis has been made, fear, anger and frustration are commonly encountered among these women.

Dysaesthetic vulvodynia

Dysaesthetic vulvodynia is a cutaneous dysaesthesia causing non-localised vulval pain. Unlike vulval vestibulitis where pain is provoked, women with dysaesthetic vulvodynia have more constant neuralgic type pain in the region of the vulva occasionally involving the perianal area.[20,22] The nature of the pain is often described as burning or aching and is often analogous to other neuralgic pain syndromes such as post-herpetic neuralgia.[11] Clinical examination of the vulva is normal and allodynia seen with vulval vestibulitis is not commonly present.[18,20] Erythema if present may represent normal anatomical variations as mentioned previously. Women with dysaesthetic vulvodynia are typically peri- or post-menopausal and, as with women with vulval vestibulitis, can present with a long history of multiple, inappropriate use of topical agents prior to a diagnosis.[20,22] Superficial dyspareunia is not consistently reported, as many women are less sexually active.[12] In addition, many experience rectal, perineal and urethral discomfort and there may be an overlap with other perineal pain syndromes.[22] There can be a history of other chronic pain syndromes (e.g. glossodynia and chronic low backache).

Psychological morbidity is significantly higher in women with vulval pain syndromes compared to asymptomatic women; however, the data are conflicting when women with vulval pain syndromes are compared to women with other chronic vulval diseases.[21,23–26] Stewart et al. found that women with dysaesthetic vulvodynia had the greatest levels of psychological distress compared to other subsets of vulvodynia and to other vulval diseases in general.[24] Jadresic et al., however, found no difference between women with vulval pain syndromes and other attenders to their London vulval clinic.[25] Many studies demonstrate high degrees of anxiety, depressive symptoms, somantization disorders and hypochondrical symptoms.[21,23,24] Schover et al.[21] reported marital conflict to be common and Stewart et al.[24] noticed that women were highly aware of their body image and were more likely to consult their doctors over other symptoms.

Sexual dysfunction is common and frequently reported.[21,24] Most studies focus on vulval vestibulitis where superficial dyspareunia is the presenting feature. Reduced sexual arousal, more negative feelings and less spontaneous interest in sex (not elicited by a partner) have all been described. Meana et al.[26] found that women with vulval vestibulitis were more erotophobic than controls and had more conservative attitudes to sex. These are all risk factors for significant psychosexual dysfunction such as vaginismus and anorgasmia.

ASSESSMENT

It is important to exclude other causes of pain before giving a diagnosis of vulval pain syndrome. Inflammatory vulval diseases such as lichen sclerosis and eczema can cause vulval pain and soreness through excoriation, splitting and fissuring of the vulval skin as well as itching.[27] Some conditions may not be manifest at the time of examination such as a tight posterior fourchette and the fragile fissured vulval syndrome.[28] Symptomatic dermographism is a rare cause of vulval pain, but this may be suggested by dermographism evident at other body sites.[29,30] Other less common causes of vulval pain are worth considering including apthous ulceration, erosive lichen planus, bullous disorders and herpes simplex infections. Although sacral meningeal cysts are a rare cause of chronic perineal pain, the routine investigation of patients with vulvodynia using magnetic resonance imaging has not been shown to be of value.[31] Rarely, vulval pain may be the presenting feature of the pudendal canal syndrome in which diminished electromyographic activity in the external anal and urethral sphincter and levator muscles are characteristic features.[32]

PREVALENCE

Little is known of the prevalence of the vulval pain syndromes. A much quoted paper by Goetsch suggested that 15% of patients attending a general gynaecological out-patient department fulfilled Friedrich's criteria for vulval vestibulitis; however, this was a biased group of women seen in private practice in the US.[18] In a recent study in the UK, the prevalence of vulval vestibulitis was 1.3% of women attending a central London genito-urinary medicine clinic.[33] This conflicts with a study by Nunns et al., where a postal survey of consultant of genito-urinary medicine physicians in the UK suggested that 48% saw greater than one patient a month with vulvodynia and 10.5% saw more than five patients a month.[34] There may have been a potential bias in this survey where, of the consultants who saw more than one patient a month, 41% expressed an interest in managing vulval diseases. The prevalence of vulval pain syndromes within general gynaecology settings remains unknown.

There is little doubt as more vulval clinics become established in the UK an increasing proportion of referrals to these clinics will be with women with vulval pain syndromes. In some instances up to a third of new referrals will be patients either vulval vestibulitis or dysaesthetic vulvodynia.[35]

AETIOLOGY

As with other chronic pain syndromes, finding a specific cause for symptoms remains elusive and has little value when faced with managing patients. Difficulty in determining an exact cause relates to a long history of symptoms prior to an accurate diagnosis and other factors which may have protracted symptoms such as physical agents (e.g. inappropriate medications), psychological and psychosexual factors. Women with vulval pain syndromes form a heterogeneous group and the cause of symptoms is probably multifactorial. In the literature, there is a heavy bias towards vulval vestibulitis whilst dysaesthetic vulvodynia remains under-researched.

A history of vulvovaginal candidiasis is the single most consistently reported feature reported by women with vulval vestibulitis.[1,12,17,20,36] Many women recall an acute attack with the onset of symptoms and many complain of repeated attacks of thrush prior to an accurate diagnosis; however, many studies rely on self-reporting and confirmatory microbiology is rarely documented. The use of multiple inappropriate topical antifungals may also have contributed to symptoms.[36] Animal studies have suggested that the antigens of *Candida albicans* are cross-reactive with certain tissue antigens in genetically susceptible women and an effective immune response against the organism is thereby aborted.[37] With repeated infections, the immune system becomes hyper-reactive against cross-reactive antigens and with defective local immunity, self-reactive cells triggered by exogenous factors (e.g. hormonal changes) initiate the inflammatory response. Hence the symptoms of vulval pain could be evident without active infection. Follow-up studies, however, have not been carried out. Colonisation rates of *Candida* in women with vulval vestibulitis are not increased compared to controls.[38]

Iatrogenic factors must be considered as a possible cause for initiating and protracting symptoms.[3] Multiple use of topical agents on the skin of women with vulval pain syndromes is common, including prescription based treatments (e.g. antifungals), over-the-counter preparations, soaps, bubble-baths and scented hygiene sprays.[1,17,20] Irritancy from topical medications is commoner on the vulva compared to skin elsewhere as the stratum corneum of the vulval skin functions less efficiently as a protective barrier.[39,40] Many women admit to excessive skin sensitivity at extragenital sites, particularly face and hands, to highly perfumed soaps and cosmetics. Irritant dermatitis usually causes vulvitis and settles once the irritant is removed. Although irritancy is unlikely to be responsible for initiating symptoms, it may possibly protract symptoms against a background of vulval pain. Many women complain of being allergic to many products and there is an increased background incidence of atopy within the group as a whole.[17] Unlike other chronic vulval conditions, however, the incidence of sensitisation to allergens in not increased and there is no evidence histologically to confirm or refute an allergic contact dermatitis response.[41,42]

As mentioned previously, psychological and psychosexual morbidity are significant in women with vulval pain syndromes, but it remains debatable as to whether these factors could be responsible for the onset of symptoms. Nunns et al. found that certain personality traits of women with vulval vestibulitis suggested a proneness to stress and anxiety, which may ultimately influence pain perception and symptoms.[23] Many patients will volunteer excessive concerns over other aspects of their health. Irritable bowel syndrome, migraine and back problems have all been commonly reported.[1] Schover et al. found that in some women the onset of pain with vulval vestibulitis was linked to a stressful period in the women's life such as marital disharmony and suggested that poor arousal could result in reduced lubrication during sexual intercourse leading to vulvovaginal irritation and a cycle of irritative vulval symptoms producing the syndrome of vulval vestibulitis.[21] Several studies have failed to show high rates of previous unpleasant sexual experiences or sexual and physical abuse compared to controls.[43] The partners of women with vulval vestibulitis have been studied and do not appear to have any significant psychosexual dysfunction.[44,45]

A genetic predisposition to vulval pain syndromes has been suggested as many studies indicate that the condition affects predominantly Caucasians with few cases reported in black or Asian populations.[18,46] Whether there is a true underlying genetic tendency or whether sociodemographic factors are involved remains debatable. Vulval vestibulitis has been reported to be more common among first-degree relatives.[18] In Goetsch's series, one-third of women with vulval vestibulitis knew of a relative with 'dyspareunia' or 'tampon intolerance'; however, no matched controls were present to support this association.[18]

Dietary factors have been suggested as a cause of vulvovaginal pain.[47] Most attention has focused on urinary oxalates, which are breakdown products in the diet.[48] Solomons et al. proposed that oxalate crystals when in combination with calcium cause vulvovaginal burning by direct contact with tissues and episodes of hyperoxaluria coincided with pain. Hence, a low-oxalate diet and treatment with calcium citrate which completes with oxalic acid for calcium has been suggested.[48] The diet has received much media attention in the US by its promotion through patients' support groups and the media; however, the original data are based on only case report of a women with vulval vestibulitis who was symptom-free after 3 months with this treatment. One controlled study, however, failed to show this treatment as effective.[49] In this study, 24-hourly oxalate levels were not higher than controls and periodical hyperoxaluria was not evident as previously reported. It is unlikely that urinary oxalates are instigators of vulval pain syndromes; however, they may act as non-specific irritants, which aggravate an already chronic condition. In a study by Poole et al.,[50] 31 patients with vulval vestibulitis had urinary oxalate levels within normal limits; however, 6 out of 16 patients who followed the low oxalate diet noticed an improvement in symptoms suggesting the possible placebo effect of this dietary intervention.

A hormonal basis for symptoms has been suggested but the data from the literature are conflicting. Certainly, hormonal factors may be contributory to symptoms as many women notice symptoms worse at the time of menstruation.[7,21] A low level of serum oestrogen has been found in women with vulval vestibulitis and it has been reported to develop postnatally (a time of relative oestrogen deficiency) even when caesarean sections were carried out.[18,51] Taking the oral contraceptive pill has also been linked to an increased relative risk of developing vulval pain with an 11-fold increased relative risk if the pill was started before the age of 17 years.[38] The role of hormonal factors requires further evaluation. There are no controlled studies to suggest that oestrogen replacement either topically or orally is of benefit.

Infection with the human papilloma virus (HPV) was suggested in the 1980s to be a possible cause of vulval pain syndromes and the term 'HPV vulvitis' was introduced.[52–54] This heralded a number of interventions aimed to eradicate the virus including treatment with local or systemic interferon, which in the long-term has not shown to be effective.[55–61] Many studies failed to have controls samples and HPV was probably over-diagnosed both clinically and histologically.[62] With the advent of sensitive DNA hybridisation and amplification techniques, the association between vulval pain syndromes and HPV is now thought to be coincidental with rates of infection not significantly higher than controls.[2,63,64] This relationship seems logical, as HPV is not a neurotropic virus.

Recent interest has focused on the pelvic floor muscles of patients with vulval vestibulitis.[65–67] Tension in the levator ani muscles when the vulval/vestibular area is touched is common and is often seen as a protective guarding response.

White et al. noticed that using pelvic floor muscle electromyography with a surface skin sensor, the majority of patients with vulval vestibulitis demonstrated levator ani instability, poor muscle recovery after a contraction and elevated resting baseline tension when there was no attempt to provoke pain.[65] Whether pelvic floor muscle tension is responsible for the perpetuation of symptoms remains to be answered, but treatment with biofeedback therapy to overcome levator hypertonia does have promising results.[66]

A COMPLEX REGIONAL PAIN SYNDROME?

Histopathological reviews of vestibulectomy specimens taken from women undergoing surgery for vulval vestibulitis have failed to find any specific diagnostic features.[42,67–69] Most studies point to a chronic, non-specific inflammatory process present in the lamina propria and periglandular tissues. This has recently been challenged in a well-controlled study where inflammatory cells were commonly found in control as well as study specimens.[60] A variety of other non-specific findings have been reported including squamous metaplasia, parakeratosis and non-specific complement and fibrin deposition.[42,71] Recent interest has focused on vulval pain syndromes as being analogous to other chronic pain syndromes.[11,46,72] Although there have been few recent improvements in the clinical management of pain, there have been significant improvements in understanding its pathophysiology.[73] Allodynia and hyperalgesia, both seen with vulval pain syndromes and other complex regional pain syndromes, can possibly be explained by both central and peripheral nervous system adaptations. Animal studies have suggested that repeated activation of skin nociceptors (C-fibres) leads to changes both within the peripheral and central nervous system.[74] Normally, afferent fibres from nociceptor synapse within the grey horn of the spinal cord in an area reserved for pain stimuli (laminae II), before synapsing with higher cortical areas giving the perception of pain.[74] In chronic pain, afferent fibres responsible for innocuous stimuli (A-beta fibres) sprout into the laminae of the grey horn where pain fibres normally end. Stimuli such as touch and pressure, therefore, elicit pain at a cortical level through these changes within the grey horn of the central nervous system, so-called 'central sensitization'. Changes in the peripheral nervous system may also be involved.[75] Cutaneous hyperalgesia is a protective response allowing damaged tissues to heal and is mediated though an increase in sensitivity of the skin nociceptors through various inflammatory mediators and cytokine release (e.g. substance P and calcitonin gene regulatory peptide). Their release leads to increased sensitivity of cutaneous nociceptors called 'peripheral sensitization', which has been demonstrated among women with vulval vestibulitis, where substance P levels have been shown to be higher within the vestibule than controls.[76] These neuropeptides have pro-inflammatory effects and may reinforce the inflammatory process seen histologically. Thus central and peripheral sensitisation may be responsible for the perpetuation of symptoms once the original tissue 'trauma' has resolved and also explain why tricyclic antidepressants, which influence pain perception centrally, help alleviate symptoms in women with dysaesthetic vulvodynia (see below).[22]

Some studies have shown an increase in the intra-epithelial nerve fibre density among women with vulval vestibulitis.[77,78] Although there is little neurophysiological evidence to confirm these nerve fibres as nociceptors, this is an interesting development as neural hyperplasia is seen in bladder biopsies of women with interstitial cystitis.[79] As the bladder trigone, urethra and vestibule all originate embryologically from the urogenital sinus, the term urogenital syndrome has been coined to describe women who have both conditions.[80–82] In practice, women with the urogenital syndrome represent a small proportion of patients with vulval pain syndromes.

TREATMENT

The natural history of the condition remains unknown, but up to 30% of women with vulval vestibulitis may experience resolution of their symptoms without treatment.[7] Peckham et al. found that approximately 30% of patients had a spontaneous remission of symptoms and in 50% of these resolution occurred within 12 months.[7] This has to be considered when interpreting studies which lack a control arm. There is often a sense of relief for the woman when a diagnosis has been given. Explaining the condition, allaying any fears and re-assuring her that the condition is not infectious or related to cancer is essential. Providing women with patient information sheets is often helpful and are available from the Vulval Pain Society, an information and support network for patients.[83] Patients should be encouraged to practice strict vulval hygiene measures when being treated, using water to clean the vulval area only, avoiding any scented products and antiseptics as vulval irritancy is common.[41] Minimising this by reducing exposure to contact irritants from everyday products will help.

It is important to recognise the concept of a pain-syndrome and that factors other than physical agents may be responsible for symptoms. The vulval pain syndromes incorporate a heterogeneous group of women and involve physical, sensory, behavioural and psychosexual factors. It is a mistake to consider the condition as a 'skin problem'. There is a heavy bias in the literature towards physical treatments such as interferon and surgery, which oversimplify the condition without taking into consideration a more holistic view. Ultimately, the treatment best suited for the women will depend on an accurate assessment based on a detailed history and clinical examination. It is up to the lead clinician to decide which treatment should be employed and what other health professionals would be of benefit. A multidisciplinary approach to these women using clinical psychologists, physiotherapists and psychosexual counsellors is the likely way forward for many patients.[11,46]

There is a dearth of good quality research relating to vulval pain syndromes in the literature and many studies are poorly controlled, have small numbers, and fail to give adequate follow-up. Most research focuses on vulval vestibulitis with infrequent mention of dysaesthetic vulvodynia. The benefits and disadvantages of various treatments for vulval vestibulitis and dysaesthetic vulvodynia are summarised in Table 1.

Medical treatments

It is naive to think that topical agents will cure the majority of women. Although topical agents are commonly given to women with vulval pain syndromes, they

Table 1 Benefits and disadvantages of treatments for vulval vestibulitis and dysaesthetic vulvodynia

	Benefits of treatment		Disadvantages
	Vulval vestibulitis	Dysaesthetic vulvodynia	
Topical lignocaine	Useful prior to sex, penetrative sex possible	Less benefit as effects are short lived	Potential sensitiser, can irritate vulval skin
Amitryptyline	Usually of benefit for continuous pain, but can be used	Controls pain centrally – useful for constant pain	Side-effect profile, other tricyclics may be of benefit
Steroid creams	Commonly used but results variable	None	Potential sensitiser, can cause skin atrophy and secondary infections
Surgery (modified vestibulectomy)	Successful in well-selected patients	None	Postoperative pain and rarely scarring
Laser vaporisation of vulva	None	None	Prolonged postoperative healing and scarring
Interferon injections	Some short-term benefit, but most relapse, now not routinely used	None	Extremely painful on injecting into vulva
Emollients	Short-term soothing of skin, can be used as a soap substitute	As for vulval vestibulitis	Rarely irritancy
Pain control skills (e.g. pain-gate theory)	Not usually of benefit as pain is on provocation	Useful for patients where pain controls life-style	Requires structured sessions usually with clinical psychologist
Biofeedback	Overcomes pelvic floor muscle hypertonia	Unknown	Not routinely available, main studies included patients on amitryptyline
Dietary manipulations (e.g. low oxalate diet)	Likely high placebo benefits, patients very keen to try	As for vulval vestibulitis	Scientific basis not substantiated
Acupuncture	Unknown	Will help a minority of patients	Procedure-related only
Complimentary creams (e.g. aloe vera, calendula)	Unknown, patients often keen to try	As for vulval vestibulitis	Irritancy can occur

are rarely mentioned in the literature and few controlled studies exist to determine which are the most effective. Local anaesthetic jellies and emollients are worthy of mention as first-line treatments. Topical lignocaine gel/ointments can be used in women with vulval vestibulitis making penetrative sex possible as well as acting as a lubricant.[72,84] Lignocaine is preferred as it has a lower incidence of sensitisation. It is generally advised that the application is 15–20 min prior to sex and patients need to be warned of irritancy. Emollients such as aqueous cream BP or emulsifying ointment BP are soothing and fragrance-free and can be used liberally on the vulval area and as a soap substitute.[72] The role of steroid creams remains to be defined. In theory, the anti-inflammatory effects reverse the inflammatory process present with vulval vestibulitis; however, results are unpredictable and contact allergy is potential problem.[85] Steroids are not successful in women with dysaesthetic vulvodynia where the skin is essentially normal. Many other topical agents have been suggested including capsaisin cream, ketoconazole cream and interferon gel.[6,8,11,87–89]. Results are variable and proper controlled trials are required. What should be discouraged in the long-term is the empirical prescribing of topical medicaments. This invariably results in disappointment when it fails and places the woman at unnecessary risk of irritancy and contact allergy.

Tricyclic antidepressants are useful in other chronic pain syndromes (e.g. post-herpetic neuralgia) and have a role in managing dysaesthetic vulvodynia where the pain is more constant in nature.[22,72] The response among patients with vulval vestibulitis is variable.[72] Amitryptyline, the best studied tricyclic, addresses both the central and peripheral components of pain and works by enhancing the activity of the descending inhibitory tracts within the central nervous system and so modifying activity within the dorsal horn of the spinal cord.[90] A dose of 10 mg/day increasing every week until the pain is controlled has been suggested.[22] The average dosage is 60 mg/day, although up to 150 mg/day can be used. Imipramine, dothiepin and nortryptyline are alternative drugs, although no controlled studies exist to suggest benefits over amitryptyline.[92] Side-effects are commonly reported including dry mouth, weight gain and sedation and patients should be warned of the 'hangover' effects during treatment. Conversely many women notice improved sleep quality and, therefore, are potentially more receptive to other pain management strategies during the day. The duration of treatment is debatable, but 3–6 months has been suggested.[22]

Interferon therapy was popularised in the 1980s as a treatment for vulval pain thought to be attributed to HPV. A total of 8 studies have been reported using interferon either systemically or locally injected into the vestibule.[54–61] Despite short-term success, long-term follow-up studies have failed to produce significant results. In the longest follow-up study, Bornstein's series of 19 patients treated with systemic interferon, only 21% of patients remained in full remission after 3 years.[58]

Biofeedback therapy has been used successfully to help overcome pelvic floor muscle dysfunction in women with vulval vestibulitis.[65,66] In a series of 33 patients, Kegels exercises were carried out by using portable home biofeedback machines with a special vaginal skin sensor. After 16 weeks of therapy, 22 out of 28 patients with apareunia had resumed penetrative sex and there was an objective improvement in the EMG reading of the pelvic floor; however, many of these patients were also treated with amitryptyline and were likely to benefits from the intensive follow-up that they received as a part of this long study.[66]

Surgery

Although surgery should only be rarely used as a last resort for patients with vulval vestibulitis, many large studies relate to merits of removing vulval skin to relieve symptoms. Surgery maybe of benefit in selected patients once all other treatment options should have been exhausted.[93–100] The procedure that yields the best result is the modified vestibulectomy where a horseshoe-shaped area of the vestibule and inner labial fold is excised followed by dissection of the posterior vaginal wall.[93–96]. The vaginal tissue is then advanced to cover the skin defect. Postoperative complications are uncommon and there is evidence that women who respond to lignocaine gel prior to sex have a more successful outcome.[93] In Kehoe's series of 37 patients with vulval vestibulitis, 59% had a complete response, 30% had a partial response and 11% had no response. The median follow-up was 10 months.[93] Other authors suggest greater excision of the vestibular tissue including close to the urethral meatus and clitoris.[96] The vestibuloplasty, where the vestibule is excised then replaced so to sever the nerve supply to the skin is not an effective procedure.[97]

Many studies are flawed by low numbers, short-term follow-up, a lack of controls and a failure to define accurately a successful outcome. In addition, most studies fail to account for concurrent treatments or factors that may also be responsible for the improvement of symptoms. The variable success rates may in part reflect the selection of patients for surgery. Many earlier studies not only included patients with vulval vestibulitis, but others without vestibular hyperaesthesia suggestive of dysaesthetic vulvodynia in whom surgery is invariably unsuccessful.[7,101]

The success rates of surgery can be improved with adjuvant therapy to help rehabilitate the patient postoperatively.[21,102] In her series of 32 patients with vulval vestibulitis, Schover et al found that pre-operative psychological assessment and postoperative sex therapy increased the success rates of surgery.[21] Patients willing to undergo psychological assessment prior to surgery had higher success rates than those who refused such an assessment, the latter group being less willing to take an active step in their own pain rehabilitation. Patients did better even with one session of psychosexual counselling to help overcome pelvic floor muscle hypertonia and poor vaginal lubrication. Vaginal dilators have also been suggested postoperatively.[102] Only one study showed no benefit of a surgical approach to women with vulval vestibulitis and advocated a behavioural approach. In Weijmer's series, patients with vulvar vestibulitis were randomised to surgery or a behavioural approach using pain management strategies, sex education, partner therapy and pelvic floor exercises.[101] Both groups achieved similar results and patients preferred the behavioural approach in preference to surgery.

Laser vaporisation of the vestibule for vulval vestibulitis was introduced in the mid-1980s in an attempt to destroy hyperaesthetic skin. Initial experience with the carbon dioxide laser in treating patients with vulval vestibulitis produced a remission rate of 61%; however, this was overshadowed by the onset of exquisitely painful vestibular hyperaemia in 25% of women after treatment.[103] Following treatment healing of the area often took as long as 6 months and the procedure and its complications were considered unacceptable. This technique has largely been abandoned.

THE MULTIDISCIPLINARY APPROACH

A multidisciplinary approach employing a variety of health professionals including clinical psychologists, pain management teams, psychosexual counsellors and physiotherapists will be of benefit to many. For all women with vulval pain syndromes, a cognitive-behavioural assessment has been suggested to complement the physical treatments.[11,72] Over a series of sessions a clinical psychologist can teach patients coping mechanisms, pain management strategies such as the pain-gate theory and can address the patient's expectations of treatment which might not necessarily be a cure for pain, but the ability to have penetrative sex.[104] Melzack and Wall's pain-gate theory has been widely used in pain management and is useful for women with constant pain. In its simplest form, the theory states the spinal cord has a series of gates into which incoming pain messages pass from all over the body. The kind of messages which emerge from the gates to reach the brain eventually depends on social and psychological factors in the woman's life. With stress, tension and anxiety, more gates are more open, more pain messages pass through to the brain and the person experience high levels of pain. Factors which close the gates and prevent pain messages getting through including relaxation, exercise and mobility. This technique enables many women to take charge of their pain and self-rehabilitate.[104] For many women with vulval vestibulitis, sexual rehabilitation may be required and this can be structured over several sessions with a psychosexual counsellor preferably with the woman's partner. Improving physical non-coital sexual contact, helping to overcome pelvic floor muscle hypertonia using sensate focus therapy and addressing secondary psychosexual dysfunction such as low libido and anorgasmia will be of help to many.[21,105] Placing a ban on penetrative sex during the initial phase of treatment is often helpful as this takes away pressure on the woman to 'perform' that may be present in the relationship. Sex is commonly associated with pain and vaginismus is common among women with vulval vestibulitis which often need addressing in addition to the medical treatments. Physiotherapists are ideally suited to provide biofeedback therapy. Several women report mixed success with complimentary treatments which they have investigated themselves usually through a failure to respond to conventional treatments. One recent trial of acupuncture for women with dysaesthetic vulvodynia showed resolution of symptoms in a minority of patients who had failed to respond to conventional treatment.[106]

The increasing volume of patients with vulval pain syndromes attending clinics who are difficult to manage who give long histories of pain and misdiagnosis emphasises the need to develop more effective management strategies. Efforts should focus on good quality research and raising awareness of this condition as an important aspect of women's' health. Vulval pain is isolating for many women and several vulval clinics within the UK have set-up support groups to allow women with chronic symptoms to share their experiences, overcome the isolation associated with pain and to extend support to others.[107] This informal support is vital to the many women in whom vulval pain is chronic and becomes a way of life.

KEY POINTS FOR CLINICAL PRACTICE

- A detailed history and clinical examination is necessary to make a diagnosis and distinguish between the two subgroups.

- Surgery should only be considered for patients with vulval vestibulitis.

- Tricyclic antidepressants are the first line treatment for dysaesthetic vulvodynia.

- A mtultidisciplinary approach may be beneficial for chronic parients.

References

1   Lynch PJ. Report of the ISSVD Committee on Vulvodynia. Vulvar vestibulitis and vestibular papillomatosis. J Reprod Med 1991; 36: 413–415

2   Bergeron C, Moyal-Barraco M, Pelisse M, Lewin P. Vulvar vestibulitis: lack of evidence for a human papillomavirus aetiology. J Reprod Med 1994; 39: 936–940

3   McKay M. Vulvodynia diagnostic patterns. Dermatol Clin 1992; 10: 423–433

4   Skene AJC. Treatise on the Diseases of Women. New York: Appelton and Company, 1888

5   Kelly HA. Medical Gynecology. Philadelphia: WB Saunders, 1928

6   Nunns D. Unexplained disorders of the vulva J Reprod Med 1996; 41: 779–780

7   Peckham BM, Mak DG, Patterson JJ. Focal vulvitis: a characteristic syndrome and a cause of dyspareunia. Am J Obstet Gynecol 1986; 154: 855–864

8   Pelisse M, Hewitt J. Erythematous vulvitis an plaque. In: Proceedings of the Third Congress of the International Society for the Study of Vulval Disease, Coccyoc, Mexico. Milwaukee. International Society for the Study of Vulvar Disease, 1976; 35–36

9   Young AW. Burning vulvar syndrome: a report on the ISSVD task force. J Reprod Med 1984; 29: 457–458

10   Woodruff JD, Parmerley TH. Infection of the minor vestibular gland. Obstet Gynecol 1983; 62: 609–612

11   Ridley CM. Vulvodynia. Theory and management. Sex Trans Dis 1998; 16: 775–778

12   Friedrich EG. Vulvar vestibulitis syndrome. J Reprod Med 1987; 32: 110–114

13   Curnow JSH, Barron L, Morrison G, Sergeant P. Vulval algesiometer. Med Biol Eng Comput 1996; 34: 266–269

14   Eva L, Reid WM, MacLean AB, Morrison GD. Assessment of response to treatment in vulvar vestibulitis syndrome by means of the vulvar algesiometer. Am J Obstet Gynecol 1999; 181: 99–102

15   Van Beurden W, van der Vange N, de Craen AJM et al. Normal findings in vulvar examination and vulvoscopy. Br J Obstet Gynaecol 1997; 104: 320–324

16   Sonni L, Cattaneo A, De Marco A et al. Idiopathic vulvodynia: clinical evaluation of the pain threshold with acetic acid solutions. J Reprod Med 1995; 40: 337–341

17   Marinnoff SC, Turner MLC. Vulvar vestibulitis syndrome: an overview. Am J Obstet Gynecol 1991; 165: 1228–1233

18   Goetsch MF. Vulval vestibulitis: prevalence and historic features in a general gynecologic private. Am J Obstet Gynecol 1991; 164: 1606–1611

19   Bazin S, Bouchard C, Brisson J et al. Vulvar vestibulitis syndrome: an exploratory case-controlled study. Obstet Gynecol 1994; 83: 43–50

20   McKay M. Subsets of vulvodynia. J Reprod Med 1987; 32: 110–114

21   Schover LR, Youngs DD, Cannata RN. Psychosexual aspects of the evaluation and management of vulval vestibulitis. Am J Obstet Gynecol 1991; 167: 630–636

22   McKay M. Dysaesthetic vulvodynia. J Reprod Med 1993; 38: 9–13

23   Nunns D, Mandal D. Psychological and psychosexual aspects of vulval vestibulitis. Genitourin Med 1997; 73: 541–544

24   Stewart D Reicher A, Gerulath AH, Boydall K. Vulvodynia and psychological distress. Obstet Gynecol 1994; 84: 587–590

25   Jadresic D, Barton S, Neill S et al. Psychiatric morbidity in women attending a clinic for vulval problems – is there a higher rate in vulvodynia? Int J STD AIDS 1993; 4: 587–590

26   Meana M, Binik YM, Khalife S, Cohen DR. Deconstructing Dyspareunia: Description, Classification and Biopsychosocial Correlates of a Pain Disorder [Thesis]. Montreal, Canada: McGill University, 1995

27   Wakelin SH, Marren P. Lichen sclerosis in women. Clin Dermatol 1997; 15: 155–169

28   Harrington C. Presidential address. In: Proceedings of the British Society for the Study of Vulval Disease Biennial Meeting, Oxford, UK, 1999

29   Lambiris A, Greaves MW. Urticaria: increasingly recognised but not adequately highlighted cause of dyspareunia and vulvodynia. Acta Derm Venereol (Stockh) 1996; 77: 160–116

30   Pernicaiaro C, Bustamante A, Gutierrez M. Two cases of vulvodynia with unusual causes. Acta Derm Venereol 1993; 73: 227–228

31   Lewis F, Harrington CI. Use of magnetic resonance imaging in vulvodynia. J Reprod Med 1997; 42: 169

32   Shafik A. Pudendal canal syndrome as a cause of vulvodynia and its treatment by pudendal nerve decompression. Eur J Obstet Gynaecol 1998; 80: 215–220

33   Denbow ML, Byrne MA. Prevalence, causes and outcome of vulval pain in a genitourinary medicine clinic population Int J STD AIDS 1998; 9: 88–91

34   Nunns D, Higgins SP, Mandal D. National vulvodynia questionnaire. Int J STD AIDS 1995; 6: 366–367

35   Wojnarowska F. Personal communication

36   Marrinoff SC, Turner MLC. Hypersensitivity to vaginal candidiasis or treatment vehicles in the pathogenesis of minor vestibular gland syndrome. J Reprod Med 1986; 31: 796–799

37   Ashman R, Ott A. Autoimmunity as a factor in recurrent vaginal candidiasis ad the minor vestibular gland syndrome. J Reprod Med 1989; 34: 264–266

38   Sjoberg I, Nylander Lundqvist E. Vulvar vestibulitis in the North of Sweden. J Reprod Med 1991; 42: 166–168

39   Elsner P, Wilhelm D, Maibach HI. Multiple parameter assessment of vulval irritant contact dermatitis. Contact Dermatitis 1990; 23: 20–26

40   Britz MB, Maibach HL. Human cutaneous vulval reactivity to irritants. Contact Dermatitis 1979; 5: 375–377

41   Nunns D, Ferguson J, Beck M et al. Vulval vestibulitis: is testing for contact allergy necessary? Contact Dermatitis 1997; 37: 88–89

42   Pyka RE, Wilkinson EJ, Friedrich EG, Croker BP. The histopathology of vulvar vestibulitis syndrome. Int J Gynaecol Pathol 1988; 7: 249–257

43   Edwards L, Mason M, Phillips M et al. Childhood sexual and physical abuse: incidence in patients with vulvodynia. J Reprod Med 1997; 42: 135–139

44   Van Lankfeld JDM, Weijenborg PM, Ter Kuile MM. Psychologic profiles of and sexual dysfunction in women with vulval vestibulitis and their partners. Obstet Gynecol 1996; 88: 65–70

45   Jarvis R. The psychosexual profiles of partners of women with vulvar vestibulitis. In: Proceedings of the British Society for the Study of Vulval Disease, Oxford, UK:

International Society for the Study of Vulvar Disease, 1998

46 Bergeron S, Binik YM, Khalife S et al. Vulvar vestibulitis syndrome: a critical review. Clin J Pain 1997; 13: 27–43

47 Poole S, Munday P. Low oxalate diets for vestibulitis – are they effective? In: Proceedings of the British Society for the Study of Vulval Disease, Plymouth 1996

48 Solomons CC, Melmed MH, Heitler SM. Calcium citrate for vulval vestibulitis: a case report. J Reprod Med 1991; 36: 879–882

49 Baggish MS, Sze EH, Johnson R. Urinary oxalate excretion and its role in vulval pain syndromes. Am J Obstet Gynecol 1997; 177: 507–511

50 Poole S, Ravenhill G, Munday PE. A pilot study of the use of a low oxalate diet in the treatment of vulval vestibulitis. J Obstet Gynaecol 1999; 19: 271–272

51 Eva L, MacClean A. Oestrogen levels and vulval vestibulitis. In: Proceedings British Congress of Obstetrics and Gynaecology, Harrogate, 1997

52 Dennerstein GJ, Scurry JP, Garland SM et al. Human papillomavirus vulvitis: a new disease or an unfortunate mistake? Br J Obstet Gynaecol 1994: 101: 992-998

53 Turner MLC, Marrinoff S. Association of human papillomavirus with vulvodynia and the vulvar vestibulitis syndrome. J Reprod Med 1988; 33: 533–537

54 Umpierre SA, Kaufman RH, Adam E et al. Human papilloma virus DNA in tissue biopsy specimens of vulvar vestibulitis patients treated with interferon. Obstet Gynecol 1991; 78: 693–696

55 Kent HL, Wisniewski PM. Interferon for vulval vestibulitis. J Reprod Med 1990; 35: 1138

56 Walzman M, Wade AAH. Intradermal interferon treatment for vulvar vestibulitis due to occult human papilloma virus infection. J Obstet Gynaecol 1991; 11: 145–147

57 Bornstein Pascal B, Abraovici H. Treatment of a patient with vulvar vestibulitis by intramuscular interferon beta: a case report. Eur J Obstet Gynaecol Reprod Biol 1991; 42: 237–239

58 Bornstein Pascal B, Abraovici H. Intramuscular interferon beta treatment for vulvar vestibulitis. J Reprod Med 1993; 38: 118–119

59 Bornstein Pascal B, Abraovici H. Long-term follow-up of patients treated for severe vulvar vestibulitis by intramuscular interferon beta. Israel J Obstet Gynaecol 1994; 5: 146–148

60 Marrinoff SC, Turner M, Hircsch RP, Richard G. Intralesional alpha interferon: cost-effective therapy for vulvar vestibulitis syndrome. J Reprod Med 1993; 38: 19–24

61 Larsen J, Peters K, Petersen CS et al. Interferon alpha treatment of symptomatic vulvodynia with koilocytosis. Acta Derm Venereol (Stockh) 1993; 73: 385–387

62 DiPaola GR, Rueda NG. Deceptive papillomavirus infection. J Reprod Med 1986; 31: 966–970

63 Wilkinson E, Guerrero E, Daniel R et al. Vulvar vestibulitis is rarely associated with human papilloma virus infection types 6, 11, 16, or 18. Int J Gynaecol Pathol 1993; 12: 344–349

64 Prayson R, Stoler M, Hart WR. Vulvar vestibulitis: a histopathologic study of 36 cases, including human papillomavirus in situ hybridisation analysis. Am J Surg Pathol 1995; 19: 154–160

65 White G, Jantos M, Glazer H. Establishing the diagnosis of vulvar vestibulitis. J Reprod Med 1997; 42: 157–161

66 Glazer HI. Treatment of vulval vestibulitis syndrome with electromyographic biofeedback of pelvic floor musculature. J Reprod Med 1995; 40: 283–290

67 Chaim W, Meriwether C, Gonik B et al. Vulvar vestibulitis subjects undergoing surgical intervention: a descriptive analysis and histopathological correlates. Eur J Obstet Gynaecol Reprod Biol 1996; 68: 165–168

68 Chadva S, Gianotten WL, Drogendijk A et al. Histopathologic feature of vulvar vestibulitis. Int J Gynaecol Pathol 1998; 17: 7–11

69 Furlonge CB, Thin RN, Evans BE, McKee PH. Vulvar vestibulitis syndrome: a clinic-pathological study. Br J Obstet Gynaecol 1991; 98: 703–706

70 Lundqvist EL, Hofer R, Olofsson JI, Sjoberg I. Is vulvar vestibulitis an inflammatory condition? A comparison of histological findings in affected and healthy women. Acta Derm Venereol 1997; 77: 319–322

71 Warner TF, Tomic S, Chang CK. Neuroendocrine cell-axonal complexes in the minor vestibular gland. J Reprod Med 1996; 41; 397–402

72 Edwards A, Wojnarowska F. The vulval pain syndromes. Int J STD AIDS 1998; 9: 74–79

73 Woolf C, Doubell TP. The pathophysiology of chronic pain-increased sensitivity to low threshold A-beta fibres inputs. Curr Opin Neurobiol 1990; 4: 525–534

74 Treede RD, Meyr RA, Raja SN et al. Peripheral and central mechanisms of cutaneous hyperalgesia. Prog Neurobiol 1992; 38: 397–421

75 Suigiura Y, Lee CL, Perl ER. Central projections of identified unmyelinated (c) afferent fibres innervating mammalian skin. Science 1986; 234: 358–361

76 Warner T, Tomic S, Chang M. Neuroendocrine cell-axonal complexes in the minor vestibular gland. J Reprod Med 1996; 41: 397–402

77 Westrom LV, Willen R. Vestibular nerve fibre proliferation in vulvar vestibulitis syndrome. Obstet Gynecol 1998; 91: 572–575

78 Bohm-Starke N, Hilliges M, Falconer C, Rylander E. Increased innervation in women with vulvar vestibulitis syndrome. Gynaecol Obstet Invest 1998; 46: 256–260

79 Lundeberg T. Interstitial cystitis: correlation with nerve fibres, mast cells and histamine. Br J Urol 1993; 71: 427–432

80 Stewart EG, Berger BM. Parallel pathologies? Vulvar vestibulitis and interstitial cystitis. J Reprod Med 1997; 42: 131–134

81 Foster D, Robinson JC, Davis KM. Urethral pressure variability in women with vulvar vestibulitis syndrome. Am J Obstet Gynecol 1993; 169: 107–112

82 Fitzpatrick CC, DeLancey JO, Elkins TE, McGuire E. Vulvar vestibulitis and interstitial cystitis: a disorder of urogenital sinus-derived epithelium? Obstet Gynecol 1993; 81: 860–861

83 The Vulval Pain Society, PO Box 514, Slough, Berks SL1 2BP, UK (send a SAE)

84 Turner MLC, Marrinoff SC. General principles in the management of vulvar diseases. Dermatol Clin 1992; 10: 275–281

85 Wilkinson SM, English JSC. Hydrocortisone sensitivity: clinical feature of fifty-nine cases. J Am Acad Dermatol 1992; 27: 683–687

86 Friedrich EG. Therapeutic studies on vulvar vestibulitis. J Reprod Med 1988; 33: 514–517

87 Morrison GD, Adams SJ, Curnow JS et al. A preliminary study of topical ketoconazole in vulvar vestibulitis syndrome. J Dermatol Treat 1996; 7: 219–221

88 Mann MS, Kaufman R Brown D, Adam E. Vulvar vestibulitis: significant clinical variables and treatment outcome. Obstet Gynecol 1992; 79: 122–125

89 Michlewtiz H, Kennison RD, Turksoy RN, Ferritta LC. Vulvar vestibulitis-subgroup with bartholin gland duct inflammation. Obstet Gynecol 1989; 73: 410–413

90 Diamond AW, Coniam SW. Neurogenic pain. In: Diamond AW, Coniam SW. (eds) The Management of Chronic Pain. Oxford: Blackwells, 1997

91 Charlton E. Neuropathic pain. Prescribers J 1993; 33: 244–247

92 McQuay H, Carroll D, Jadad AR et al. Anticonvulsant drugs for management of pain: a systematic review. BMJ 1995; 311: 1047–1052

93 Kehoe S, Leusley D. An evaluation of modified vestibulectomy in the treatment of vulvar vestibulitis: preliminary results. Acta Obstet Gynecol Scand 1996; 75: 676–677

94 Davis GD. The surgical treatment of vulval vestibulitis. Proceedings of the ISSVD Post-congress Postgraduate Course 19–20 September 1997; 46–49

95 Goestsch M. Simplified vestibulectomy for the treatment of vulvar vestibulitis. Am J Obstet Gynecol 1996; 174: 1701–1707

96 Woodruff JD, Friedrich EG. The vestibule. Clin Obstet Gynecol 1985; 28: 134–141

97 Bornstein J, Zarfeati D, Goldik Z et al. Perineoplasty compared to vestibuloplasty for severe vulval vestibulitis. Br J Obstet Gynaecol 1995; 102: 652–655

98   Bergeron S, Bouchard C, Fortier M et al. The surgical treatment of vulvar vestibulitis syndrome: a follow-up study. J Sex Marital Ther 1997; 23: 317–325

99   Barbero M, Micheletti L, Valentino MCZ et al. Membranous hypertrophy of the posterior fourchette as a cause of dyspareunia and vulvodynia. J Reprod Med 1994; 39: 949–952

100   Weijmar SWC, Gianotten WL, van der Meijden et al. Behavioural approach with or without surgical intervention to the vulvar vestibulitis syndrome: a prospective randomised and non-randomised study. J Psychosom Obstet Gynecol 1996; 17: 143–148

101   Reid R, Omoto KH, Precop RN et al. Flashlamp-excited laser therapy of idiopathic vulvodynia is safe and efficacious. Am J Obstet Gynecol 1995; 172: 1684–1701

102   Abramov L, Wolman I, David MP. Vaginismus: an important factor in the evaluation and management of vulvar vestibulitis syndrome. Gynaecol Obstet Invest 1994; 38: 194–197

103   Reid, R. Laser surgery of the vulva. Obstet Gynecol Clin North Am 1991; 18: 491–510

104   Melzack R. Pain theory: exception to the rule. Behav Brain Sci 1980; 2: 313

105   Kielme G. The psychosexual counsellor's approach to vulval pain syndromes. J Obstet Gynaecol 1999; 19: 566–585

107   Maloney L. The role of support groups in vulval pain syndromes. J Obstet Gynaecol 1999; 19: 566–568

106   Wojnarowska F. Use of acupuncture in the management of vulvodynia. In: Proceeding of the British Society for the Study of Vulval Disease Meeting, Oxford, UK, 1998

Barry O'Reilly   Peter L. Dwyer

14

The overactive bladder syndrome in the female

The term 'overactive bladder (OAB) syndrome' refers to a spectrum of lower urinary tract symptoms, namely frequency (eight or more voids in a day), urgency (the complaint of a sudden compelling desire to pass urine which is difficult to defer), nocturia (waking more than once during the night to void) and often incontinence as a result of urgency. This symptom complex is not a diagnosis and can be caused by a number of conditions. The OAB syndrome is a functional disorder of the lower urinary tract where other local pathologies such as infection, malignancy, calculi, and interstitial cystitis have been excluded. These symptoms can also occur in women with urethral sphincter incompetence, which can be excluded by clinical assessment and urodynamic studies. Polydypsia and polyuria from whatever cause can also result in frequency and nocturia and are diagnosed from a voiding diary.

Detrusor instability, however, is a diagnosis made by cystometry, that results in the symptom complex of OAB syndrome. It is one of the most important causes of urinary incontinence (UI), and yet its aetiology is not clearly understood. The unstable detrusor is one that is shown objectively to contract, spontaneously or on provocation, during the filling phase of cystometry whilst the patient is attempting to inhibit micturition.[1] Detrusor contractions may be either phasic, or systolic where they mimic the normal voiding reflex, or the bladder may demonstrate low compliance. Detrusor instability can be caused by urinary outflow obstruction or as a result of upper motor neuron lesions (neuropathic) or of unknown cause (idiopathic). Idiopathic detrusor instability is a common urodynamic diagnosis that is found in 10% of men and 29% of women undergoing conventional urodynamic investigation.[2] Women usually

Dr Barry O'Reilly MD MRCOG, Fellow in Urogynaecology and Pelvic Floor Reconstructive Surgery, The Royal Women's Hospital and Mercy Hospital for Women, Melbourne, Victoria, Australia (for correspondence)

Dr Peter L. Dwyer MB BS FRCOG FRACOG CU, Head, Department of Urogynaecology, The Royal Women's Hospital and Mercy Hospital for Women, Melbourne, Victoria, Australia

present with multiple symptoms, most commonly urgency, urge incontinence, frequency and nocturia.

UI is a major health issue, a fact that was highlighted by the 1st International Consultation on Incontinence sponsored by the World Health Organization (WHO) in 1998.[3] Many sufferers feel that urinary incontinence is a natural part of ageing and childbirth and as such this condition is a 'taboo subject' both for those affected and the health professionals. However, the scale of this problem is illustrated by the fact that there are over 200 million people world-wide who experience problems associated with UI, and estimates of between 50–100 million people suffering from OAB syndrome.[4] The impact of UI is on both health resources and on the sufferer's quality-of-life. In the UK alone, over £80 million is spent on containables (e.g. pads and catheters) and over £18 million on drug treatments of incontinence per annum. In 1997, the NIH published direct costs in terms of 'burden to society' in the US, of various diseases concluding that $17.5 billion was spent on urinary incontinence ($12.7 billion on overactive bladder) compared with $13.8 billion on osteoarthritis and $11.1 billion on gynaecological and breast carcinoma. This has resulted in a greater emphasis on cost effectiveness of management and treatments of incontinence.

A recent review quoted an overall figure of 16% of adults having one or more symptoms of the OAB syndrome in a European population-based study.[5] In the US, the National Overactive Bladder Evaluation (NOBLE) study was undertaken to help better understand and define the prevalence and burden of OAB and this has recently concluded similar results to the European study with an overall prevalence in the community of 16.6%, which increases with advancing age. Interestingly, the most commonly reported symptoms in NOBLE were nocturia (29%), urgency (22%), frequency (15%), and urge incontinence (6%).[6] Although incontinence was the major problem associated with OAB, recent evidence suggests that frequency, urgency and nocturia are more prevalent and significantly affect quality-of-life. Incontinence is not necessary, as roughly one-half of patients with overactive bladder do not experience incontinence but are, nonetheless, severely affected by the symptoms of urgency and frequency.[4] The epidemiological studies have encountered difficulties because of the lack of consensus on definitions but this issue is being addressed by the International Continence Society.

In this chapter, the physiology of bladder contraction is briefly discussed followed by diagnosis of the OAB. The clinical evaluation of OAB has been reviewed to provide the clinician with a clear picture of the appropriate assessment with history and examination followed by a discussion on the indications, value and limitations of investigations as well as the treatment options available.

BLADDER PHYSIOLOGY

The main function of the bladder is to convert the steady stream of urine produced by the kidney into a convenient intermittent process of storage and evacuation. Therefore, the bladder must first act as a stable reservoir holding 500 ml of urine with comfort and second as an intermittent voluntary excretory organ, conforming to socially acceptable restraints to allow voiding. This requires a complex neurological network, which co-ordinates sensory afferent input and motor efferent output in a reciprocal fashion. In order to understand the drug therapies in common use, it is necessary to understand the complex neurological control of the bladder. Connections of the lower urinary tract to the CNS are extraordinarily complex and many discrete centres with influences on micturition have been identified which will not be discussed since most drugs in clinical use are believed to act peripherally.

Involuntary leakage of urine can only occur if the intravesical pressure exceeds the urethral closure pressure. Urethral sphincter contraction and detrusor relaxation are achieved by different mechanisms and so no simple drug therapy effectively achieves both.

Motor innervation of the bladder

The autonomic innervation of the human bladder is thought to be principally parasympathetic cholinergic. Efferent sympathetic and parasympathetic fibres are conveyed to the bladder and urethra via the hypogastric and pelvic splanchnic nerves, respectively. These nerves (as well as the somatic pudendal nerves) convey afferent (sensory) fibres to the spinal cord. Preganglionic parasympathetic fibres originate in the second, third, and fourth sacral segments of the spinal cord (the nervi erigentes or pelvic splanchnics). They then enter the pelvic plexus and synapse in ganglia situated in the adventitia and between the bundles of smooth muscle of the bladder wall.[7,8] Therefore, damage to these neurons at the time of radical pelvic surgery such as Wertheims' hysterectomy results in a hypertonic and poorly compliant bladder.[9]

Neurones have axonal varicosities, which contain the granules associated with cholinergic nerve terminals. Each muscle cell has at least one associated varicosity and the stimulation of the nerve initiates release of acetylcholine from the vesicles within it to cause bladder contraction via muscarinic receptors.[10] Sympathetic supply to the detrusor is extremely sparse acting through noradrenergic nerves found within the detrusor[11,12] close to the vascular supply of the muscle.

It must be acknowledged that there may be other neurotransmitters and neuromodulators in the bladder. These include ATP, serotonin, dopamine, GABA, prostaglandins, VIP and substance P.[13] The 'changing face of autonomic neurotransmission'[14-16] which encompasses the concepts of multiple transmitters and co-transmission, makes this an increasingly complex field and it is likely that some or all of these compounds have a modulatory activity on neurotransmission.

Sensory innervation of the bladder

Afferent impulses arising from sensory nerve endings in the wall of the bladder pass to the spinal cord via the pelvic splanchnics and hypogastric nerves[17] with their cell bodies residing in dorsal root ganglia lumbosacral segments. The afferent path of the micturition reflex is carried in the pelvic splanchnics, together with the nociceptive nerves. The sensory nerves supplying the bladder are either thin myelinated Aδ or unmyelinated C fibres. Aδ bladder afferents appear to be low threshold mechanoreceptors,[18] whereas C bladder afferents are generally mechano-insensitive ('silent C fibres').[19] Some of these silent C fibres may be nociceptive which respond to inflammatory mediators such as ischaemia and temperature, and can be sensitised by intravesical administration of chemicals like capsaicin or resiniferatoxin.

However, it has been suggested that chemicals released by the bladder as a result of stretch (e.g. prostaglandins,[20] nitric oxide or ATP[21]) may influence sensory neurotransmission. The sensory nerves that supply the bladder have been shown to display plasticity as a result of inflammation,[22] nerve injury[23] or bladder hypertrophy in animals.[24,25] More recently, this plasticity has been demonstrated in human diseased bladder states such as detrusor instability.[26] ATP and NO are also released by afferent nerves and may modulate afferent excitability.[27]

CLINICAL ASSESSMENT

Assessment of presenting symptoms should provide a clinical diagnosis and indication of the severity and duration of the urinary incontinence. A large cross-sectional epidemiological survey[28] of 1546 interviewed women aged 15–97 years found 20.8% of women had symptoms of stress incontinence alone, 2.9% urge incontinence alone, and 11.6% mixed incontinence.

Results of previous medical and surgical treatment should be obtained and other lower urinary tract symptoms such as voiding difficulty, haematuria, pain or recurrent infections must be excluded. Important information includes neurological conditions and the use of medications particularly those with diuretic, anticholinergic, antidepressant, psychotropic or alpha blockade effect. Women with urinary incontinence frequently have other problems of pelvic floor dysfunction, including urogenital prolapse and faecal incontinence and so one should enquire about sexual and bowel dysfunction. Women with an overactive bladder have a high incidence of irritable bowel symptoms with some authors suggesting that both conditions may have a common aetiology.

Some factors may have a profound effect on OAB symptoms and are often reversible such as diet (e.g. spicy food or caffeine), high fluid intake and output and psychological problems such as stress or personality disorders. Polyuria or polydypsia, if no obvious cause is apparent, should be further investigated with serum creatinine, urea and glucose measurements to exclude underlying renal disease or diabetes mellitus. Poor patient mobility or disability from any cause will aggravate urge symptoms and may precipitate urge incontinence.

A complete physical examination for any co-existing disease is an essential part of the evaluation process, although sometimes neglected.[29] The abdomen should be examined for a palpable pelvic mass or distended bladder. Vaginal examination should be performed to assess pelvic organ prolapse, oestrogen status, presence of infection or a pelvic mass. An assessment of pelvic floor strength using digital examination or a perineometer during voluntary contraction of the levator muscle is important, particularly in pelvic floor re-education. The clinical sign of stress incontinence, demonstrated in the supine or standing position with the patient coughing or straining is a reliable guide to the urodynamic diagnosis of genuine stress incontinence with a positive predictive value of 91%.[30] However, 40% of these patients will have an additional urodynamic diagnosis of detrusor instability, hypersensitive bladder or voiding dysfunction.

Neurological assessment of the vulval and perianal skin sensation as well as lower limb reflexes, motor strength and sensation can determine damage to the sacral spinal cord segments S2–4.

BLADDER DIARY

A urinary diary records the times of micturitions and voided volumes, incontinence episodes, pad usage and other information such as fluid intake, the degree of urgency and the degree of incontinence. It is an essential assessment tool in any women with urge symptoms and should be recorded by the patient for 2–7 days.

In addition to providing information on bladder behaviour and severity of incontinence, the urinary diary may suggest the particular type of urinary disorder, reveal excessive fluid intake and serve as a useful baseline for on-going treatment. Women with detrusor instability and hypersensitive bladders have frequent small volumes of micturition with a low maximum voided volume. Women with interstitial cystitis may have extreme frequency, urgency and bladder pain with volumes of less than 100 ml and these women frequently markedly decrease their fluid intake to minimise their symptoms. The bladder diary is becoming the method of choice in the evaluation of both conservative and surgical treatments for incontinence.

ANALYSIS OF URINE

Urine should be examined for the presence of bacteriuria, pyuria and hematuria in women with urge symptoms. Bacteriuria of $> 10^5$ uropathogens per ml of voided midstream urine has traditionally been the accepted criterion for urinary tract infection, although levels of 10^3 organisms per ml are now being used to diagnose symptomatic acute cystitis.[31] Significant haematuria particularly of non-glomerular origin may be an early sign of urinary tract pathology and should be fully investigated by cystourethroscopy to exclude malignancy or calculi.

Commercial dipstick tests are cheap and can rapidly analyse urine for the presence of nitrate, leukocyte esterase, blood and protein. The leukocyte esterase test is a more sensitive indicator of infection compared to the nitrate test and detects the presence of 10–12 leukocytes per high power field.[32]

PAD TESTING

Perineal pad testing is a simple non-invasive method of confirmation and quantification of urine leakage and is used to evaluate treatment outcomes.[33] Pad testing can be of short (20–120 min) or longer duration (24–48 h). Perineal pads are weighed before and after the test period. Evaporation even in warmer climates is minimal if weighed within 72 h of completion. The test/retest variability of the short-term pad test is considerable (up to 150%) while the long-term test has a test/retest variability of 7%.[34]

QUALITY-OF-LIFE QUESTIONNAIRES

Objective measurements of UI such as voiding diaries, pad tests, and urodynamic studies are used in the evaluation of the severity of the condition.

However, they neglect the importance upon women's quality of life of urinary incontinence. Quality-of-life is a multidimensional concept combining patient-assessed measures of health, including physical function, role function, social function, emotional or mental state burden of symptoms, and sense of well-being.

Lower urinary tract symptoms alone have been shown to be a disappointing correlator with diagnosis in both men and women with incontinence[35] and different symptoms clearly affect patients in different ways.[36] It is, therefore, inappropriate for symptoms alone to be used as outcome measures of treatment. Objective measurement of improvement in incontinence, coupled with the quality-of-life benefits of treatments offered to patients is thus important in the assessment of treatment outcome. It is for this reason that the ICS has recommended that quality-of-life assessment be included in all clinical trials in continence care and a number of different quality-of-life questionnaires have evolved to fulfil this role.[37]

The Kings Health Questionnaire (KHQ)[38] was developed at a tertiary referral centre for urogynaecology in London over a 3-year period and involved over 1000 patients in its development. This questionnaire has now been translated into over 22 different linguistic validated versions, which makes it the most widely translated of its kind yet developed. In addition, the KHQ has been shown to be easy to use and sensitive to clinical change in clinical trials.

ESTIMATION OF RESIDUAL URINE VOLUME

A residual urine greater than 30 ml measured by ultrasonography 1 min after a normal void of 200 ml or more, and confirmed on more than one occasion occurs in only 5% of the normal female population and 13% of symptomatic women.[39] This was described also as the level of chronic residual urine above which recurrent urinary tract infection occurs.[40]

Therefore, the measurement of post-void urine residual (PVR) should be an important early investigation in women with urge symptoms especially the elderly, women with previous pelvic surgery, or neurogenic conditions who are at higher risk.

Urethral catheterisation is the traditional method of PVR urine measurement and also allows a clean specimen of urine to be obtained for microscopy and culture; it does, however, carry a 1–2% risk of urinary tract infection. Ultrasound measurement of PVR is non-invasive, will provide information about bladder capacity and may detect pathology such as calculi, bladder diverticulae or carcinoma. It is less accurate than urethral catheterisation and under-estimates PVR particularly at higher volumes.[41]

URODYNAMIC EVALUATION

Urodynamic studies provide an objective assessment of lower urinary tract function and will aid the clinician in understanding the pathophysiology of urge symptoms and incontinence, as frequently there is more than one cause to consider.

The standard urodynamic evaluation comprises uroflowmetry and measurement of post-void residual urine, filling cystometry and pressure flow study. Cystometry is used to study both the storage and voiding phases of micturition in order to make a diagnosis. The pressure–volume relationship of the bladder is measured by instilling fluid at medium-fill rates of 10–100 ml/min. The volume of first sensation, urgency, bladder capacity and the volume at which the first rise in detrusor pressure occurs are important indices in assessment as well as the presence of unstable detrusor contractions or low bladder compliance during filling. Additional tests include video-urodynamics, urethral pressure studies, sphincter electromyography and pharmacological testing. Neurophysiological studies assessing the neural and muscular components of the lower urinary tract and pelvic floor have played an important part in helping us understand the pathophysiology of urinary incontinence. Electromyographic recording of urethral sphincter activity performed during urodynamic assessment may aid the diagnosis of detrusor–sphincter dyssynergia secondary to neurological disease. Nerve conduction studies using motor and sensory evoked potentials test the integrity of the sacral reflex and pudendal nerves. The routine use of these tests in the assessment of the overactive bladder is still debatable.[42]

The urodynamic assessment aims to answer the following questions: (i) is the bladder normal or overactive; (ii) is the urethral sphincter competent during filling and provocation; and (iii) does the lower urinary tract empty normally and completely?

Urodynamic findings during bladder filling in women with OAB symptoms can vary from: (i) unstable phasic contractions (detrusor instability);[43] (ii) a tonic rise in pressure (reduced bladder compliance); (iii) a stable but low capacity (hypersensitive bladder); or (iv) the bladder may have a normal function (stable, normal compliance and capacity). The filling cystometry can be made more provocative by increasing the filling speed, changing the posture from supine to standing, ice-water filling and hand-washing to increase the incidence of unstable contractions.

Bladder compliance describes the relationship between the change in bladder pressure for a given change in volume. Reduced bladder compliance can be secondary to bladder injury resulting in a loss of its musculo-elastic properties. Idiopathic reduced compliance is probably a variant of detrusor instability, as most low compliance patterns on routine cystometric testing change into phasic contractions on ambulatory testing.

Uroflowmetry (measurement of urinary flow rate) and PVR estimation assess voiding function and are routinely performed during urodynamic assessment. The flow curve is normally bell-shaped with a maximum of at least 20 ml/s. Women with voiding dysfunction have prolonged voiding and lower urinary flow rates (< 15 ml/s) and can be diagnosed using nomograms and centile charts of flow rates against voided volumes.[39,44]

The measurement of bladder pressure during voiding (pressure-flow study) is also helpful in distinguishing between hypotonic bladder and outlet obstruction as the cause of the voiding dysfunction. Intermittent flow can occur in neurogenic patients with detrusor-sphincter dyssynergia, which is diagnosed with simultaneous urethral sphincter EMG and pressure flow studies.

Urodynamic evaluation is recommended in women with mixed symptomatology when conservative treatment with anticholinergic medication, behavioural modification and pelvic floor re-education has failed, if the patient is suspected or known to be suffering from a neurological disorder or prior to incontinence surgery.

Assessment prior to surgery for genito-urinary prolapse will detect occult stress incontinence and any co-existing detrusor instability or voiding dysfunction.

AMBULATORY URODYNAMICS

In order to assess lower urinary tract function under more normal conditions, long-term monitoring using portable pressure transducers and electric pads (ambulatory urodynamics) have been developed.[45] Unstable detrusor contractions were present during ambulatory urodynamics 50% more often when compared to conventional filling cystometry[46] and also in 10–30% of women with urge symptoms who had negative standard cystometry. Unstable detrusor contractions have been found in 60% of asymptomatic volunteers,[47] raising the question of whether these contractions are real or artefactual. The incidence of detrusor instability in healthy volunteers using standard filling cystometry has been reported to occur in 10–20% of cases.[47] Salvatore and colleagues, using a symptom diary and two bladder transducers during ambulatory urodynamics, reduced by two-thirds the number of asymptomatic artefactual pressure rises previously diagnosed as bladder overactivity. In this study, unstable contractions were identified in 10% of asymptomatic volunteers, which is similar to that of conventional cystometry.[48]

IMAGING OF THE URINARY TRACT

Videocystourethrography is a more complex cystometric investigation in which bladder filling is performed using a contrast medium enabling the clinician to screen the lower urinary tract. Bladder pathology such as calculi, tumours or intravesical sutures may be visualised. In addition, the mobility and opening of the urethra and bladder neck and the presence of incontinence can be assessed. In the patient with co-existing stress incontinence, an anatomic classification of stress incontinence has been suggested based on the appearance at fluoroscopic urodynamics.[49] Urethrocystography is indicated in the investigation of urinary tract fistula, vesico-ureteric reflux, bladder and urethral diverticulae.

Ultrasound or IVP assessment of the upper urinary tract is recommended where there is co-existing loin pain, severe prolapse, recurrent urinary tract infection, suspected extra-urethral incontinence from a fistula or ectopic ureter, and neurogenic detrusor instability. Patients with neurogenic bladder need to have regular radiological assessment as they are at increased risk of upper tract deterioration.[51] Ultrasound assessment of bladder wall thickness has been used in a research setting to predict detrusor instability.[50]

CYSTOURETHROSCOPY

Visualisation of the lower urinary tract by endoscopy is the most reliable and direct method of excluding bladder pathology in women with irritable bladder symptoms and can easily be performed in the out-patient setting for a large proportion of patients. Women with severe sensory urgency, bladder pain and low functional bladder capacity may be better assessed under general or regional anaesthesia especially if a biopsy is to be considered. Clinical

Table 1 Clinical presentations for which early endoscopic assessment is recommended

Microscopic haematuria to exclude urinary malignancy

A past history of stress incontinence or pelvic surgery. Non-absorbable permanent intravesical sutures can be present following suture misplacement or erosion. This should be suspected if pain, recurrent UTI or irritable bladder symptoms occur after surgery[52]

Bladder pain and severe urge symptoms to exclude interstitial cystitis and other pathologies (e.g. calculi)

Women with suspected urinary tract fistula, urethral diverticulum or urinary tract malformation

---

presentations for which early endoscopic assessment is recommended are summarised in Table 1.

Bladder hydrodistention is an important part of the diagnostic process for interstitial cystitis and provides short-term symptomatic relief in a third of women with sensory urgency. Interstitial cystitis is diagnosed in women with symptoms of bladder pain, frequency or urgency; evidence of low bladder capacity in a bladder diary or urodynamic assessment and cystoscopic findings of petechial haemorrhage and mucosal tearing during cysto-distension.

MEDICAL AND CONSERVATIVE THERAPY

Drugs currently in use for overactive bladder syndrome fall into four categories: (i) drugs whose major action is to reduce detrusor contractility; (ii) drugs that affect sensory nerves; (iii) drugs that alter outlet resistance; and (iv) drugs that decrease urine production.[53]

The muscarinic actions of acetylcholine can be selectively blocked by atropine. Tertiary ammonium analogues of atropine are often used for their effects on the eye or CNS and smooth muscle. Many antihistaminic, anti-psychotic and antidepressant drugs have similar structures and, predictably, significant antimuscarinic effects. Quaternary ammonium antimuscarinic agents (e.g. trospium chloride) have been developed to produce more peripheral effects with decreased CNS adverse effects which have proven efficacy in the treatment of overactive bladder.[54] Because acetylcholine is the best-known excitatory transmitter in human detrusor muscle, muscarinic antagonists have been used in patients suffering from irritable or unstable bladders. Pure antimuscarinic drugs such as propantheline or darifenacin reduce unstable contractions and increase functional bladder capacity by targeting the M_2 and M_3 muscarinic receptor subtypes in the bladder. These drugs, along with oxybutynin, have a degree of selectivity for these receptor subtypes but tolterodine is more selective for the bladder than for the salivary glands in comparison. Once daily or extended release formulations of both oxybutynin and tolterodine have been developed to lower adverse effects and to improve compliance by avoiding the peaks serum levels of the short duration drugs.[55,56]

As unstable detrusor contractions can only be partially blocked by atropine, pharmacologists have sought drugs with alternative mechanisms of action. Many of the drugs in clinical practice have multiple modes of action and illustrate the different ways in which detrusor contraction can be reduced.

Oxybutynin has a direct smooth muscle relaxant action on the bladder in addition to its antimuscarinic action. Propiverine hydrochloride is a bladder spasmolytic and has antimuscarinic and Ca^{2+} blocking properties.

Flavoxate is a tertiary amine with a papiverine-like effect on smooth muscle. It inhibits phosphodiesterase, resulting in raised levels of cAMP, which leads to muscle relaxation. It also has analgesic and local anaesthetic properties.

Tricyclic antidepressants (e.g. imipramine hydrochloride) have a complex pharmacological action. Very high doses of imipramine have local anaesthetic and sedative properties. When combined with diclofenac sodium, a prostaglandin synthesis inhibitor, imipramine has been used to treat primary nocturnal enuresis.

Potassium channel opening drugs are currently in experimental use in treating bladder instability reducing detrusor contractility by hyperpolarizing the smooth muscle membrane. Cromokalim is one such drug that opens the K_{ATP} channels, causing detrusor relaxation but also causes significant hypotension. However, this adverse effect may be minimised by the development of bladder specific compounds.

In women with neuropathic bladder (detrusor hyperreflexia), central control is lost and micturition is completely under control of the micturition reflex arc. The sensory afferents in the reflex are a combination of fast conducting myelinated Aδ fibres and the slower conducting unmyelinated C fibres. Detrusor hyperreflexia can result in overactive bladder symptoms and urinary incontinence. Detrusor-sphincter dyssynergia is a result of similar disruption to central control in which voiding detrusor contractions are unsustained and uncoordinated with sphincter overactivity resulting in voiding dysfunction and overflow incontinence. However, the C-fibres can be blocked by the intravesical administration of capsaicin or a similar substance called resiniferatoxin, which initially causes the destruction of the sensory nerve terminals removing the afferent limb of the reflex arc and stabilizing the bladder. Capsaicin has been used with moderate success to treat patients with spinal cord disease.[57]

Oestrogen may be of benefit to postmenopausal patients with sensory urgency by correcting atrophic genital changes and increasing urethral resistance by a direct effect on sensory nerves and α-adrenergic receptors in urethral smooth muscle.

Drugs, which decrease urine production, are useful in the treatment of nocturia and nocturnal enuresis, which are common symptoms of bladder overactivity. Endogenous antidiuretic hormone, vasopressin, increases at night resulting in a decreased production of urine. 1-Desamino-8-D-arginine vaso-pressin (DDAVP), an octapeptide hormone, is a synthetic analogue of vaso-pressin. It increases permeability in the distal convoluted tubule and collecting ducts of the kidney but, unlike vasopressin, has no effect on blood pressure. DDAVP acts by reducing urine output during sleep. It must be used with care amongst elderly patients with heart or renal failure who normally diurese to a greater extent at night.

Bladder retraining involves a programme of scheduled voiding with progressive increases in the interval between each void and is also known as bladder drill. The treatment assumes that the patient consciously suppresses sensory stimulation to the bladder thus emphasizing cortical control over an uninhibited bladder. This was first described in 1966 as 'bladder discipline' by Jeffcoate and Francis.[58] Subsequent studies have shown this type of management is effective in up to 80% of patients.[59]

Biofeedback techniques use the principle of increasing patient awareness of the normally unconscious physiological process to stabilise detrusor pressure in detrusor instability during cystometry. Using an audible signal and visual input of the cystometry trace, the patient attempts to inhibit the unstable detrusor contractions while the bladder is repeatedly filled. This technique requires a highly motivated patient, but subjective and objective cure rates of up to 80% have been noted.[60]

Neuromodulation using peripheral electrical stimulation of the afferent limb of the pudendal reflex arc with vaginal or anal plugs will result in increased pelvic floor and striated muscle contractility as well as reflex inhibition of detrusor contractility. Early studies showed that during elevated bladder pressure, intravaginal electrical stimulation resulted in abolition of the spontaneous efferent activity of the pelvic nerves.[61,62] Alternative methods, involve transcutaneous nerve stimulation over the S3 dermatome, posterior tibial nerve stimulation and direct stimulation of sacral nerves through the S3 foramen with implantable electrodes have shown early promise.[63]

TREATMENT OVERVIEW

The above assessment of overactive bladder symptoms will allow an accurate diagnosis of causation, severity, and their effect on quality-of-life and exclude possible pathology. Women with mild symptoms may only require re-assurance or conservative measures such as decreased fluid intake, abstinence from caffeine drinks and alcohol, a change in voiding habit, and alteration of medications (e.g. diuretics). However, the mainstay of treatment if symptoms are incapacitating is drug therapy and bladder drill. We believe the main purpose of drug therapy is to overcome the initial symptoms so that simple measures like bladder re-training have a greater impact in the long-term. We would not always advocate long-term drug therapy and, although this may be required, it is interesting that many patients use the drug treatments on an 'as required' basis. We would advise 'practical prescribing' in the drug treatment of incontinence. This involves advice on conservative measures in the first instance; the choice of a suitable therapy for relief of predominant symptoms; starting with low doses with the aim of a balance achieved between symptom improvement and inevitable side-effects; patient information sheets on side-effects; encouraging persistence with treatment; and the benefits of 'social' usage – medication taken as and when needed if continuous usage is difficult due to side-effects. Obviously, follow-up and re-assurance of these patients is vital.

CONCLUSION

More research is needed to discover new, more effective and safer agents to overcome the overactive bladder syndrome. One such area of research into the aetiology of OAB is that of alternative routes of bladder innervation and neurotransmission and the role that these may play in the unstable bladder. Recent work,[64,65] for example, has investigated the role of ATP as a neurotransmitter in the bladder and this has opened up an exciting area, which may give options for future pharmacological manipulations of the unstable bladder.

KEY POINTS FOR CLINICAL PRACTICE

- Most women with OAB symptoms can be successfully treated by conservative measures and re-assurance following simple clinical evaluation with history, physical examination and a few basic investigations.

- There is a place for treatment in the primary care setting on the basis of urinary symptoms provided there is no contra-indication to treatment and that referral for further investigation is made if the treatment is not successful. We would not advocate empirical drug treatment in the presence of the following symptoms: UTI; haematuria; neuropathy; uropathology; voiding difficulty; previous surgery; and if uncertainty of the cause of the urinary symptoms exists.

- Once the diagnosis of detrusor instability has been made, the various treatment modalities should be considered starting with simple conservative measures and bladder re-training. In prescribing drug therapies, consideration should be given to effectiveness, adverse effect profile and cost. Whilst urinary incontinence cannot always be cured, the symptoms can usually be significantly improved for the vast majority of women.

References

1   Abrams P, Blaivas JG, Stanton SL, Andersen JT. The standardisation of terminology of lower urinary tract function. Scand J Urol Nephrol 1988; Suppl. 114: 5–19

2   Moore KH, Richmond DH, Parys BT. Sex distribution of adult idiopathic detrusor instability in relation to childhood bedwetting. Br J Urol 1991; 68: 479–482

3   1st International Consultation on Incontinence. Incontinence. Plymouth: Plymbridge Distributors Ltd, 1999

4   Abrams P, Wein AJ. Introduction: overactive bladder and its treatments. Urology 2000; 55: 1–3

5   Milsom I, Abrams P, Cardozo L, Roberts RG, Thuroff J, Wein AJ. How widespread are the symptoms of an overactive bladder and how are they managed? A population based prevalence study. Br J Urol Int 2001; 87: 760–766

6   Stewart W, Herzog R, Wein AJ et al. Prevalence of overactive bladder in the US: results from the NOBLE program. Poster presented at the WHO International Consultation on Incontinence, Paris, France, 2001

7   Gosling JA. Lower urinary tract: structure of bladder and urethra. In: Mundy AR, Stephenson TP, Wein AJ. (eds). Urodynamics, Principles, Practise and Application. Edinburgh: Churchill Livingstone, 1984

8 Mundy AR. Clinical physiology of the bladder, urethra and pelvic floor. In: Mundy AR, Stephenson TP, Wein AJ. (eds). Urodynamics, Principles, Practise and Application. Edinburgh: Churchill Livingstone, 1984

9 O'Callaghan DJ, Dwyer PL. Clinical and urodynamic follow-up of women with established urinary dysfunction after radical hysterectomy. Aust N Z J Obstet Gynaecol 1994; 34: 557–561

10 Kluck P. The autonomic innervation of the urinary bladder, bladder neck and urethra: a histochemical study. Anat Rec 1980; 198: 439–443

11 Ek A, Alm P, Andersson KE, Persson CGA. Adrenergic and cholinergic nerves of the human urinary bladder. A histochemical study. Acta Physiol Scand 1977; 99: 345–351

12 Benson GS, McConnell JA, Wood JG. Adrenergic innervation of the human bladder body. Invest Urol 1979; 122: 189–191

13 Andersson KE. Clinical relevance of some findings in neuroanatomy and neurophysiology of the lower urinary tract. Clin Sci 1986; 70: 21s–32s

14 Burnstock G. Neurotransmitters and trophic factors in the autonomic nervous system. J Physiol 1981; 313: 1–35

15 Burnstock G. Purinergic nerves and receptors. Prog Biochem Pharmacol 1980; 16: 141–154

16 Burnstock G. The cotransmitter hypothesis with special reference to the storage and release of ATP with noradrenaline and acetylcholine. In: Cuello AC. (ed) Cotransmission. London: MacMillan, 1982

17 Vaughan CW, Satchell PM. Urine storage mechanisms. Prog Neurobiol 1995; 46: 215–237

18 Habler HJ, Janig W, Koltzenburg M. Myelinated primary afferents of the sacral spinal cord responding to slow filling and distension of the cat urinary bladder. J Physiol 1993; 463: 449–460

19 Habler HJ, Janig W, Koltzenburg M. Activation of unmyelinated afferent fibres by mechanical stimuli and inflammation of the urinary bladder in the cat. J Physiol 1990, 425: 545–562

20 Maggi CA, Meli A. The sensory-efferent function of capsaicin-sensitive sensory neurons. Gen Pharmacol 1988; 19: 1–63

21 Ferguson DR, Kennedy I, Burton TJ. ATP is released from rabbit urinary bladder epithelial cells by hydrostatic pressure changes- a possible sensory mechanism? J Physiol 1997; 505: 503–511

22 Dupont M, Steers WD, Albo M, Nataluk E. Neural plasticity and alterations in nerve growth factor and norepinephrine in response to bladder inflammation. J Urol 1994; 151: 284

23 Tuttle JB, Steers WD, Albo M, Nataluk E. Neural input regulates tissue NGF and growth of the adult rat urinary bladder. J Auton Nerv Syst 1994; 49: 147–158

24 Steers WD, Ciambotti J, Etzel B, Erdman S, De Groat WC. Alterations in afferent pathways from the urinary bladder of the rat in response to partial urethral obstruction. J Comp Neurol 1991; 310: 401–410

25 Steers WD, Creedon DJ, Tuttle JB. Immunity to nerve growth factor prevents afferent plasticity following urinary bladder hypertrophy. J Urol 1996; 155: 379–385

26 Smet PJ, Moore KH, Jonavicius J. Distribution and colocalization of calcitonin gene-related peptide, tachykinins, and vasoactive intestinal peptide in normal and idiopathic unstable human urinary bladder. Lab Invest 1997; 77: 37–49

27 Dmitrieva NBG, McMahon SB. ATP and 2-methyl thio ATP activate bladder reflexes and induce discharge of bladder sensory neurones. Soc Neurosci Abstr 1998; 24: 2088

28 MacLennan AH, Taylor AW, Wilson DH, Wilson D. The prevalence of pelvic floor disorders and relationship to gender, age, parity and mode of delivery. Br J Obstet Gynaecol 2000; 107: 1460–1470

29 Brocklehurst JC. Urinary incontinence in the community-analysis of the MORI-poll. BMJ 1993; 306: 832–834

30 Carey MP, Dwyer PL, Glenning PP. The sign of stress incontinence – should we believe what we see? Aust N Z J Obstet Gynaecol 1997; 37: 436–445

31 Hooton TM. Epidemiology. In: Stanton SL, Dwyer PL. (eds) Urinary Tract Infection in the Female. London: Martin Dunitz, 2000; 2–18

32 Johnson JR, Stamm WE. Urinary tract infections in women; diagnosis and treatment. Am J Intern Med 1989; 111: 906–917

33 Sutherst J, Brown M, Shawer M. Assessing the severity of urinary incontinence by weighing perineal pads. Lancet 1981; 1: 1128–1130

34 Versi E, Orrego G, Hardy E, Seddon G, Smith P, Anand D. Evaluation of the home pad test in the investigation of female urinary incontinence. Br J Obstet Gynaecol 1996; 103: 162–165

35 De La Rossette JJMCH, Witjes WPJ, Schafer W. Relationships between lower urinary tract symptoms and bladder outlet obstruction: results from the ICS-BPH study. Neurourol Urodyn 1998; 17: 99–108

36 Jarvis GJ, Hall S, Stamp S, Millar DR, Johnson A. An assessment of urodynamic examination in incontinent women. Br J Obstet Gynaecol 1980; 87: 893–896

37 Hu T. Impact of urinary incontinence on health care costs. J Am Geriatr Soc 1990; 38: 292–295

38 Kelleher CJ, Cardozo LD, Khullar V, Salvatore S. A new questionnaire to assess the quality of life of urinary incontinent women. Br J Obstet Gynaecol 1997; 104: 1374–1379

39 Haylen BT, Law MG, Frazer M et al. Urine flow rates and residual urine volumes in urogynaecology patients. Int Urogynecol J 1999; 10: 378–383

40 O'Grady F, Cattell WR. Kinetics of urinary tract infection. The bladder. Br J Urol 1966; 38: 156–162

41 Alnaif B, Drutz HP. The accuracy of portable abdominal ultrasound equipment in measuring postvoid residual urine. Int Urogynecol J 1999; 10: 215–218

42 Vodusek DB, Bemelmans B, Chancellor M et al. Clinical neurophysiology, In: Abrams P, Khowry S, Wein AJ eds. Incontinence, Monaco June 28–July 1, 1998. Plymouth,UK: Health Publications Ltd, 1999: 157–193

43 Abrams P, Blaivas JG, Stanton SL et al. The standardisation of terminology of lower urinary tract function. Br J Obstet Gynaecol 1990; 97: 1–16

44 Haylen BT, Ashby D, Sutherst JR, Frazer MI, West CR. Maximum and average urine flow rates in normal male and female populations – the Liverpool nomograms. Br J Urol 1989; 64: 30–38

45 van Waalwijk van Doorn ES, Remmers A, Janknegt RA. Extramural ambulatory urodynamic monitoring during natural filling and normal daily activity: evaluation of 100 patients. J Urol 1991; 146: 124–131

46 Kulseng-Hanssen S, Klevmark B. Ambulatory urethrocystorectometry, a new technique. Neurourol Urodyn 1988; 7: 119–130

47 Heslington K, Hilton P. Ambulatory monitoring and conventional cystometry in asymptomatic female volunteers. Br J Obstet Gynaecol 1996; 103: 434–441

48 Salvatore S, Khullar V, Cardozo L, Anders K, Zocchi J, Soligo M. Evaluating ambulatory urodynamics: a prospective study in asymptomatic women. Br J Obstet Gynaecol 2001; 108: 107–111

49 Blaivas JG, Olsson CA. Stress incontinence: classification and surgical approach. J Urol 1988; 139: 727–731

50 Khullar V, Cardozo L, Salvatore S et al. Ultrasound: a non-invasive screening test for detrusor instability. Br J Obstet Gynaecol 1996; 103: 904–908

51 McGuire EJ, Woodside JR, Borden TA et al. Prognostic value of urodynamic testing in myelodysplastic patients. J Urol 1981; 126: 205–209

52 Dwyer PL, Carey MP, Rosamilia A. Suture injury to the urinary tract in urethral suspension procedures for stress incontinence. Int Urogynecol J 1999; 10: 15–21

53 Ferguson DR, Christopher N. Urinary bladder function and drug development. Trends

Pharmacol Sci 1996; 17: 161–165

54 Cardozo L, Chapple CR, Toozs-Hobson P et al. Efficacy of trospium chloride in patients with detrusor instability: a placebo-controlled, randomised, double-blind, multicentre clinical trial. Br J Urol Int 2000; 85: 659–664

55 Van Kerrebroek P, Kreder K, Jonas U, Zinner N, Wein AJ. Tolterodine once-daily: superior efficacy and tolerability in the treatment of the overactive bladder. Urology 2001; 57: 414–421

56 Gleason DM, Susset J, White C, Munoz DR, Sand PK. Evaluation of a new once-daily formulation of oxybutynin for the treatment of urinary urge incontinence. Urology 1999; 54: 420–423

57 Fowler CJ, Jewkes D, McDonald WI, Lynn B, De Groat WC. Intravesical capsaicin for neurogenic bladder dysfunction. Lancet 1992; 339: 1239

58 Jeffcoate TNA, Francis WJA. Urgency incontinence in the female. Am J Obstet Gynecol 1966; 94: 604–618

59 Fantl JA, Hurt WG, Dunn LJ. Detrusor instability syndrome: the use of bladder re-training drills with and without anticholinergics. Am J Obstet Gynecol 1981; 140: 885–889

60 Cardozo LD, Stanton SL, Hafner J et al. Biofeedback in the treatment of detrusor instability. Br J Urol 1978; 50: 250–256

61 Lindstrom S, Fall M, Carlsson CA, Erlandson BE. The neurophysiological basis of bladder inhibition in response to intravaginal electrical stimulation. J Urol 1983; 129: 405–410

62 Wise BG, Cardozo LD, Cutner A, Kelleher CJ, Burton G. Maximal electrical stimulation: an acceptable alternative to anticholinergic therapy. Int Urogynecol J 1992; 3: 270

63 Webb RJ, Powell PH. Transcutaneous electrical nerve stimulation in patients with idiopathic detrusor instability. Neurourol Urodyn 1992; 11: 327–328

64 Cockayne D, Hamilton SG, Zhu Q-M et al. Urinary bladder hyporeflexia and reduced nocifensive behaviour in P2X$_3$ receptor-deficient mice. Nature 2000; 407: 1011–1015

65 O'Reilly BA, Kosaka AH, Knight GF et al. P2X receptors and their role in female idiopathic detrusor instability. J Urol 2002; 167: 157–164

Mann J, Truswell S, editors.
44. Gardner L, Langvad K, Olausson K. Exercise-induced asthma. Clinical features and their reproducibility ... ... clinical study in man, 9th ed. 1981: 39–56 ... ...
45. ... Savoiardo G, Pozzoli ... Bonsi M, Monti G. Intracellular magnesium ... magnesium ... ... myocardium with ... in the presence of ischemia ... ... 1988; 8(6): 9–17.
46. ... Reese Williams, Watts DH, Seeds DR. Transient cardiac arrhythmias ... ... vol. 346 in Rhône de Mende 1986.

Catherine L. Minto Gerard Conway Sarah Creighton

The XY female

Throughout history there have been individuals who are intersex, that is neither clearly male nor clearly female. Historically, interest centred around hermaphrodites, i.e. individuals who displayed features of both male and female anatomy. One of the earliest descriptions of surgery for hermaphroditism was by the famous physician from the 7th century, Paul of Aegina.[1] His writings acknowledge the ancient Greeks as detailing the genital surgical techniques he described. As abdominal surgery became more widely performed and anatomical knowledge of the gonads improved, a new category of pseudo-hermaphrodites was added to include individuals with unambiguous genital anatomy but discordance internally, e.g. females with testes or males with ovaries. These intersex conditions occur in all cultures around the world. Queen Elizabeth I was rumoured to have been a famous example of an XY female.[2]

It is important for gynaecologists to have an understanding of these conditions as they may present in a variety of ways. Intersex conditions are relatively rare, and can be difficult to diagnose accurately and manage appropriately. Some have other associated anomalies or particular malignancy risks, and, because of all these factors, all suspected intersex cases should be referred to a specialist unit with multidisciplinary expertise. There are many controversies and different theories in the medical management of intersex cases. In the past, traditional medical care, while well-intentioned, has often led to great secrecy, stigmatism and psychological trauma for intersex people.

Dr Catherine L. Minto MB ChB, Specialist registrar and Clinical Research Fellow, Academic Department of Obstetrics and Gynaecology, University College London, 86–96 Chenies Mews, London WC1E 6AU, UK (for correspondence)

Dr Gerard Conway MD FRCP, Consultant Endocrinologist, Department of Endocrinology, Middlesex Hospital, Mortimer Street, London W1N 8AA, UK

Ms Sarah Creighton MD FRCOG, Consultant Gynaecologist, Department of Obstetrics and Gynaecology, University College London Hospitals, Huntley Street, London WC1E 6AU, UK

New understandings of the underlying aetiology and developmental mechanisms are stimulating a rethink of traditional treatment models. This chapter presents a contemporary view of the intersex conditions in which a female will have a 46 XY karyotype.

SEXUAL DIFFERENTIATION *IN UTERO*

Genetic sex is decided at the time of conception. However, it is not until 6 weeks later that sexual determination begins. The first step in the pathway to a male or female phenotype is dependent on the SRY gene (sex determining region of the Y chromosome). This gene, and probably other as yet unidentified genes, causes the gonad to begin development into a testis.[3] First, Sertoli cells develop and produce AMH (anti-Mullerian hormone) which promotes the regression of Mullerian structures. Then Leydig cells appear and, at around 8 weeks under the stimulation of hCG, start to secrete testosterone.[4] This causes development of the Woolfian structures (the vas deferens, seminal vesicles and epididymis) and peripheral conversion of testosterone to dihydrotestosterone (DHT) virilises the external genitalia.[5] At 12 weeks, the fetus is recognisably male and masculinisation of the genitalia is said to be complete by 14 weeks.[4] The penis, similar in size to the clitoris at 14 weeks, then enlarges from around 20 weeks until birth.

Ovarian differentiation requires the absence of SRY and probably the functioning of other ovarian-determining genes.[6] The ovarian cortex develops at 12 weeks and by 13.5 weeks primordial follicles are present.[7] As AMH is not produced, the Mullerian ducts develop into the uterus, fallopian tubes and upper portion of the vagina. Without androgens, the urogenital sinus develops into the female external genitalia, forming the clitoris, labia and lower vagina. The Woolfian structures regress at around 10 weeks due to the absence of testosterone.[5] By 15 weeks, the urogenital and Mullerian parts of the vagina meet and fuse and this 'vaginal plate' develops a lumen at around 20 weeks,[8]

Ovarian differentiation is not a requirement for the development of female genitalia, and so this pathway is also known as the 'default route'.[9] It is the absence of testicular androgen (or AMH production), or an inability of the body to respond to these hormones that causes the female phenotype to occur in XY females.[10] Other errors in this complex process can also cause ambiguous genitalia or a male phenotype with a 46XX karyotype.

DEVELOPMENT OF GENDER IDENTITY, GENDER ROLE AND SEXUALITY

Just as an individual's hormones and genes guide the fetal anatomical development of their genitalia, so they also play an important role in the developing fetal brain.[11] While we still have much to learn about the development of human gender identity, gender role and sexuality, it is likely that sex steroids, along with other important factors including genetic, social and environmental influences will have both pre- and postnatal determining effects on these functions.[12]

Knowledge in this area is vital when considering gender assignment for intersexed infants.[13] Males born with a micropenis (i.e. a small but normally

Table 1 Presentation of XY females

CVS/amniocentesis karyotype different to ultrasound observed fetal sex
Ambiguous genitalia at birth
Childhood inguinal hernias (containing testes)
Primary amenorrhoea
Virilisation at puberty
Infertility
Sexual problems related to vaginal hypoplasia
Gonadal tumour
Diagnosis in family member
Part of a syndrome with other anomalies, e.g. Wilms tumours

structured penis, testes and a 46 XY karyotype) have previously been assigned a female gender and accordingly had feminising surgery and medication.[14] Several case reports of such sex-reassigned infants have revealed that long-term outcomes are poor, and there is now a growing awareness that, although gender identity in humans may be surprisingly flexible, consideration of these other influences is as vital a factor as genital size in advising sex of rearing.[15]

CLINICAL PRESENTATION

Intersex conditions present in a wide variety of ways (Table 1). The incidence is believed to be around 1 in 2000 births. Each intersex condition may have variable physical signs and this wide spectrum of phenotypes combined with the often complex endocrine profile can lead easily to diagnostic error. Each different condition requires varied and expert management, with careful multidisciplinary evaluation of aetiology and surgical therapy. In some cases, gonadal tissue may be preserved, and fertility may even be possible in true hermaphrodites. If gonadal tissue is to be removed, an accurate diagnosis must be decided prior to irreversible surgery, with cryopreservation of gonadal material where appropriate. Hence referral to specialist centres possessing multidisciplinary teams is essential.

CAUSES

Classifying the causes of XY females is difficult; however, we have used a simple approach based on the basic area of the underlying anomaly (Table 2). Not considered in this classification are transsexuals, i.e. those adults that have chosen to have surgery to change their phenotype from male to female to match their gender identity.

END ORGAN INSENSITIVITY TO ANDROGENS

Complete androgen insensitivity syndrome (CAIS)

Until recently, this condition was called testicular feminisation syndrome (TFS); however, this name is both stigmatising and inaccurate (the testes do not

Table 2 Causes of XY females

End organ insensitivity to androgens
        Complete androgen insensitivity syndrome
        Partial androgen insensitivity syndrome
Enzyme errors in androgen production
        5α-Reductase deficiency
        17β-Hydroxysteroid dehydrogenase deficiency
        3β-Hydroxysteroid dehydrogenase deficiency
        Congenital lipoid adrenal hyperplasia or STAR deficiency
        17α-Hydroxylase deficiency
Structural abnormalities in the testes
        Complete XY gonadal dysgenesis
        Mixed gonadal dysgenesis
        True hermaphrodite
        Drash syndrome
        Campomelic dysplasia
        Frasier syndrome
Leydig cell dysfunction
        Leydig cell hypoplasia
Miscellaneous conditions
        Ambiguous genitalia of unknown aetiology
        Cloacal and bladder extrophy
        Urogenital sinus anomalies
        Micropenis
        Penile agenesis
        Traumatic loss of the penis

produce feminising factors). The preferred name, androgen insensitivity syndrome (AIS), reflects the underlying aetiology and is more acceptable to women who have the condition. Complete AIS (CAIS) occurs when there is no response to androgens, and partial androgen insensitivity syndrome (PAIS) occurs when the androgen receptor can partially respond to androgen stimulation (see below). Other synonyms used in the past include Goldberg-Maxwell syndrome (early textbooks), Morris syndrome (Morris first described and coined the phrase TFS in 1953),[16] androgen resistance syndrome and androgen receptor deficiency syndrome.

The cause of CAIS is an abnormality of the androgen receptor (AR).[17] In the fetus with CAIS, testes form normally due to the action of the SRY gene. At the appropriate time, these testes secrete anti-Mullerian hormone (AMH) leading to the regression of the Mullerian ducts. Hence, CAIS women do not have a uterus. Testosterone is also produced at the appropriate time; however, due to the complete inability of the androgen receptor to respond, the external genitalia do not virilise and instead undergo female development. Other areas where testosterone may have important fetal effects, such as the brain, will also develop along the female path. The result is a female (both physically and psychologically)[18] with no uterus, and testes found at some point in their line of descent through the abdomen from the pelvis to the inguinal canal. During puberty, breast development will be normal; however, the effects of androgens will not be seen, so pubic and axillary hair growth will be minimal. Normal

Table 3 Clinical features of CAIS

Female external genitalia
46 XY karyotype
Primary amenorrhoea
Absent uterus
Intra-abdominal or inguinal testes
Reduced or absent sexual hair (pubic and axillary)
Normal breast development
Vaginal hypoplasia

adult pubic hair, hirsutism and any clitoromegaly or labial fusion rules out the diagnosis of CAIS. The clinical features of CAIS are summarised in Table 3.

The androgen receptor was cloned and sequenced in 1988.[19] A year later, the androgen receptor gene was found to lie on the long arm of the X chromosome (Xq 11-12).[20] Around two-thirds of women with CAIS have inherited the androgen receptor gene mutation from their mother (i.e. X-linked inheritance) with the remaining one-third thought to be new mutations.[21] Incidence is probably around 1 in 40,000–60,000 births.[22]

The areas to consider in management are: (i) making the correct diagnosis (endocrine evaluation, karyotype to rule out mosaicism, hCG test, androgen binding studies, etc.); (ii) communicating the diagnosis to the patient along with expert psychological support; (iii) considering the indications for gonadectomy and hormone replacement therapy; and (iv) treatment for vaginal hypoplasia and on-going psychological support. It is worth emphasising again the need for referral to a suitably experienced centre, which can offer treatment in all the above areas. Before any treatment is considered, especially any form of genital or gonadal surgery, it is vital to have made the correct diagnosis from suitable investigations.

Gonadectomy is often advised in CAIS due to the risk of gonadal malignancy. This malignancy risk is poorly defined (possibly 5–10%[23] in childhood rising to 30% by the age of 50 years[24]) and thought to be due to the intra-abdominal position of the testes.[23] Timing of gonadectomy is controversial. Some clinicians advocate early (i.e. childhood) gonadectomy due to the malignant potential with subsequent HRT to induce puberty.[25] Others prefer to delay gonadectomy until after puberty to allow: (i) the endogenous gonadal hormones to work throughout puberty; (ii) the patient the opportunity to balance the pros and cons of surgery; and (iii) if chosen, the patient time to give fully informed consent to gonadectomy.[26] Hormone replacement therapy is essential after gonadectomy for many aspects of health and well-being. One of these is the maintenance of bone mineral density (BMD).[27] Some studies on bone density in CAIS suggest that patients may be osteopenic despite HRT,[28] perhaps due to inadequate HRT, previous oestrogen deficiency, or possibly reflecting an essential function of androgen on bone.

The majority of women with CAIS will have a shortened vagina, when compared with the population average length of 10–12 cm. This occurs due to the embryological development of the vagina, with the upper portion developing with the Mullerian ducts and the lower portion derived from the urogenital sinus.

Anti-Mullerian hormone (AMH) production from the testes causes regression of the Mullerian duct part of the vagina, leaving just the part derived from the urogenital sinus. In reality, there is a wide variation in vaginal sizes, from 2-10 cm length, with no way of identifying those that will be in the shorter end of the spectrum. Hence, in early adolescence, all CAIS girls should be offered an assessment of the vagina by an experienced gynaecologist, often by EUA and vaginoscopy. If the vagina is hypoplastic, the options for treatment need to be discussed. The two main options for vaginal enlargement are vaginoplasty surgery or manual vaginal dilatation. Vaginal dilatation is usually the first-line treatment, and can be very successful when provided with the appropriate support, information and setting. If surgery is required, vaginal dilatation is often also required as an integral part of the treatment postoperatively. Unfortunately, there is little information currently available on the outcomes of these different methods of vaginal enlargement, especially with regard to long-term sexual function.[29]

Psychological input from a suitably trained professional who has clinical experience with intersex conditions is a vital part of management.[30] Initially in childhood, the emphasis will be on preparing the way for a truthful and fully informed explanation of the diagnosis later on and also providing support for the parents.[31] Later, in adolescence and adulthood, there are many varied issues that may arise, and psychological support needs to be expert and easy to access as required.

The management of intersex conditions is undergoing a renaissance, with society becoming more aware of their existence and more willing to discuss these issues. This was highlighted recently by the case of Joella Holliday (a 46 XY girl due to a cloacal anomaly) who was registered as a male on her birth certificate and has publicly fought to have her birth certificate changed.[32] Her case is remarkable in that at the age of 10 years she is fully informed about her XY genetics and seems openly accepted as an XY female within her community.[33] Although our society still expects a gender to be assigned that is either male or female, we are moving slowly towards an acceptance of the occurrence of variations within these rigid bounds.

There are now well-informed patient support groups in many countries for people with AIS and other intersex conditions.[34] In the UK, they are working with the medical profession to research long-term outcomes of various treatments, to improve management and psychological support and to learn from the past mistakes of secrecy and deception in communicating the diagnosis. We are learning that it is no longer acceptable to withhold the diagnosis from women with AIS. Although well intentioned, this deceit has led to a lack of genetic counselling, denial of access to the support groups and the considerable benefits they offer, and a life-time of doubt, uncertainty and fear for many patients.[35] A large body of medical opinion now exists that promotes truth disclosure as fundamental and essential clinical practice.

Partial androgen insensitivity syndrome (PAIS)

In PAIS, the basic problem is thought to lie again at the molecular level with the androgen receptor although, in contrast to CAIS, some function occurs. Depending on the amount of androgen receptor activity, the phenotype will vary in a spectrum from near complete AIS (severe androgen resistance) to near normal male (i.e. only very mild androgen resistance). Several classification systems have

Table 4 Sinnecker's classification of AIS[36]

AIS grade	Description of phenotype
Type 1	Normal male anatomy with impaired spermatogenesis (1a) and/or impaired virilisation at puberty (1b): also called minimal androgen resistance
Type 2	Male genitalia with hypospadius alone (2a) or combined with micropenis and a bifid scrotum (2b): also called Reifenstein syndrome
Type 3	Ambiguous genitalia
Type 4	Female genitalia with signs of virilisation, e.g. clitoromegaly or partial labial fusion
Type 5	Complete AIS, i.e. female genitalia with no signs of virilisation

been proposed to standardise description of the phenotypes (Table 4).[22,36] Due to the variation in genital appearance, the presentation of PAIS is extremely variable.[37] Some will present at birth with ambiguous genitalia, whereas others will present in puberty, either with lack of virilisation in a boy or signs of virilisation in a girl. PAIS grade types 1 and 2 (Table 4) may not present until adulthood, if at all.

Management is similar to CAIS in some aspects (see above); however, most clinicians will recommend prepubertal gonadectomy in those raised as girls, to avoid any virilisation at puberty. One of the most difficult decisions in the management of PAIS is often in assigning neonatal sex of rearing, especially in the middle grades (types 2b–4). As discussed earlier, there are many factors contributing to future gender identity, gender role and sexuality and for each PAIS baby currently, there is no accurate way to predict which gender assignment will be optimal.[38]. One approach is not to perform irreversible surgery in the neonatal and childhood periods, so that any gender is attainable in the long-term.[39,40] Others believe that gender should be assigned early on and reconstructive genital surgery (with gonadectomy for female assignment) should be performed before the age of 18 months.[41]

ENZYME ERRORS IN ANDROGEN PRODUCTION

The production of testosterone from the testes requires five enzymes encoded by four genes. As discussed above, testosterone acts on the internal genitalia (Woolfian structures) to lead development down the male pathway. Another enzyme, 5α-reductase, causes peripheral conversion of testosterone to DHT. It is this more potent androgen (DHT) that acts on the androgen receptors and causes virilisation of the external genitalia in utero. A loss of function abnormality in any of these six enzymes will cause autosomal recessive inheritance of male pseudohermaphroditism.

5α-Reductase deficiency

Mutations in the 5α-reductase type 2 isoenzyme gene on the short arm of chromosome 2 lead to this condition, which was previously called pseudovaginal perineoscrotal hypospadius (PPSH).[42] Testosterone and AMH production occur normally from the testes and cause development of the male internal ducts (i.e. seminal vesicles, vas deferens, epididymis and ejaculatory ducts) and regression of the Mullerian ducts. However, virilisation of the external genitalia does not take place as this testosterone cannot be converted into dihydrotestosterone (DHT).

This syndrome was first described in a large kindred in the Dominican Republic,[43] and later in populations in Papua New Guinea[44] and Turkey.[45] Affected individuals are born with predominantly female or ambiguous genitalia (often clitoro-phallus, bifid scrotum and vagina) and will usually be reared as female. Without any treatment, virilisation will occur at puberty, with growth of the phallus, and sometimes descent of inguinal testes into the scrotum. In the three large cohorts described in the literature,[43-45] affected individuals often change to a male gender role at puberty. Several patients have also successfully fathered children.[46,47] It is difficult to determine how far social and cultural pressures have affected these gender changes and to what degree prenatal, neonatal and pubertal hormone environments are important.[48,49] Standard UK treatment for babies diagnosed with 5α-reductase deficiency has been gonadectomy and feminising genital surgery. This management is now being reviewed, as potential fertility, sexuality and gender options are being removed from young infants who may want these options in their future.

Testosterone biosynthesis defects

Defects anywhere in the biosynthetic pathway from cholesterol to testosterone may lead to an XY female.[50] As other pathways producing aldosterone and/or cortisol may also be involved, some of these syndromes are types of congenital adrenal hyperplasia. Presentation is with variable degrees of genital ambiguity, usually in a severely ill neonate. Management is as for PAIS (see above).

The most common enzyme block in testosterone production affects the enzyme 17β-hydroxysteroid dehydrogenase (also called 17-ketosteroid reductase). Of the eight known isoenzymes, it is isoenzyme 3 that acts in the testes as the last step converting the inactive androgen androstenedione to testosterone. The biosynthetic pathways producing mineralocorticoids and glucocorticoids are unaffected, as this is exclusively a gonadal enzyme. The presentation at birth is similar to CAIS, with a predominantly female phenotype and absent uterus. Intriguingly, these women show signs of virilisation in puberty, and the mechanism causing this is unknown. It may be that peripheral conversion of androstenedione occurs at puberty due to the increased activity of other isoenzymes.[51] A proportion of affected individuals may opt to change from female to male gender at puberty.

STRUCTURAL ABNORMALITIES IN THE TESTES

Absent gonads

There are several reports in the literature of 46 XY individuals with completely absent gonads, some also associated with other abnormalities.[52-55] Either no development of the gonads (agenesis) has occurred or there has been loss of the gonads at some point in embryonic development.

In gonadal agenesis, the phenotype will be female with absent (not streak) gonads, and a uterus. This rare disorder may be caused by an abnormality in the earliest steps of gonadal development. Loss of the gonads in utero has been variously labelled familial anorchia, embryonic testicular regression syndrome and XY gonadal agenesis syndrome. The phenotype depends entirely on the timing of loss of the fetal or embryonic testicular tissue and can, therefore, range from completely female to an anorchic male. Theories of the aetiology range from sex limited autosomal recessive inheritance[55] (due to familial occurrence and consanguinity) to torsion of the testicular blood vessels in utero.[56]

Gonadal dysgenesis

Gonadal dysgenesis encompasses a range of conditions with abnormal or dysgenetic development of the fetal gonads. It can be subdivided into 45XO, 46XX or 46XY according to the sex chromosome complement and complete or partial according to the degree of dysgenesis.[57] Individuals with the complete form (whatever the sex chromosomes) have bilateral streak gonads with a female phenotype and Mullerian structures. The prefix 'pure' refers to the absence of any features associated with Turner's syndrome.

Partial 46XY gonadal dysgenesis, sometimes called mixed gonadal dysgenesis, in which there is incomplete testis determination, will often present with ambiguous genitalia and a mix of Woolfian and Mullerian structures. The gonads may have a mosaic 45X0/46XY karyotype, which might not be present in the karyotype from white blood cells. The gonads can sometimes be a streak on one side with a contralateral testis. True hermaphrodites, defined by the presence of both testicular and ovarian tissue with primordial follicles, may be related to the above disorders and share a common aetiology.[58]

The most common form of XY gonadal dysgenesis presenting to a gynaecologist is Swyer's syndrome or pure, complete 46XY gonadal dysgenesis. This condition was first described by Swyer, an endocrinologist in London, in 1955.[59] At that time, two types of 'male pseudohermaphrodites' were known and he described two cases that were clearly different from these and called them 'new type' male pseudohermaphrodites. They were new in that they had an XY karyotype along with a cervix, uterus and signs of poor oestrogenisation (such as poorly developed vaginal ruggae with hypo-oestrogenic vaginal smears and minimal breast development). In Swyer's syndrome, the gonads are small

---

Table 5 Features of Swyer's syndrome

Female external genitalia
46 XY karyotype
Bilateral streak gonads
Uterus and fallopian tubes that (with cyclical HRT with progesterone) will
    menstruate, and are able to conceive with IVF and donor oocytes
Absent Woolfian structures
Stature often taller than average
Poor breast development and lack of secondary sexual characteristics
    (without HRT)

Table 6 Chromosomal abnormalities known to cause isolated 46XY gonadal dysgenesis

Gene	Site	Abnormality
SRY	Yp11.3	Mutations or deletions
DAX1	Xp21.3	Duplication
Unknown (?DMT1)	9p21-24	Deletions
Unknown	10q	Deletions

dysgenetic streaks, and produced neither testosterone nor AMH in utero. It has been suggested that these gonads actually started fetal ovarian development and then underwent degeneration as occurs in Turner's syndrome.[60] Presentation will usually be with primary amenorrhoea and lack of secondary sexual characteristics (Table 5). Management is similar to CAIS. The main differences is that these women have a uterus and so require cyclical HRT with progesterone, will menstruate, and are able to conceive with IVF and donor oocytes. Also, the dysgenetic gonads are thought to have a higher risk of malignancy of around 30%.[24]

The aetiology of Swyer's syndrome is thought to be abnormalities in the genes controlling sexual differentiation. Investigation of cases of Swyer's syndrome have shown that mutations of the SRY gene account for approximately 15% of cases and a further 10–15% of cases are thought to be due to loss of the short arm of the Y chromosome that contains the SRY gene, occurring due to defective interchange between the X and Y in paternal meiosis.[61] The remaining 70% of individuals presumably have abnormalities in other elusive genes important in the pathway of gonadal determination (Table 6). Areas where these are suspected to lie are on chromosomes 9 and 10 as abnormalities in these areas also lead to Swyer's syndrome.[62,63] Other clues as to where the genes contributing to sexual differentiation may lie can be found in those syndromes which may include gonadal dysgenesis in their spectrum of abnormalities, e.g. campomelic dysplasia and Drash syndrome. Whatever the answers are, these cases of XY females present a unique opportunity to aid in unravelling the mysteries of human sexual determination.

LEYDIG CELL DYSFUNCTION

In Leydig cell hypoplasia, failure of virilisation occurs due to a defect in the Leydig cell receptor for luteinizing hormone (LH) and human chorionic gonadotrophin (hCG).[64] The gonads develop as testes but the inability of the Leydig cells to bind hCG causes a failure of testosterone secretion and hence a female phenotype. Later, during puberty, these receptors are again needed for male secondary sexual development this time under the stimulation of LH itself. Presentation is a spectrum, from female with primary amenorrhoea and poor secondary sexual characteristics to ambiguous genitalia. The diagnosis is suggested if gonadal histology shows an absence of Leydig cells[65] and confirmed with endocrine investigation prior to gonadectomy. Management is similar to CAIS (see earlier).

MISCELLANEOUS CONDITIONS

There are other conditions where male infants may have been re-assigned to a female sex of rearing and had feminising surgery along with a gonadectomy, hence producing an XY female. This diverse group contains; ambiguous genitalia of unknown aetiology, micropenis, traumatic loss of the penis in childhood and rare conditions with abnormal development of the urogenital sinus or cloaca (e.g. bladder extrophy). In the past, many of these infants were evaluated by the size of their phallus. If the genitalia were deemed inadequate for a male, the phallus and gonads were removed and a female sex of rearing assigned. The historical belief was that feminising surgery was more successful than masculinising surgery. With technical improvements in phalloplasty surgery and published poor long-term adult outcomes for both some of those who underwent female reassignment and for some vaginoplasty surgery, this approach is now under fierce debate. It has become clear that these infants are not psychosexually neutral at birth[13] and so irreversible surgery to remove precious gonadal and phallic tissue must be ethically re-examined.

KEY POINTS FOR CLINICAL PRACTICE

- There are a multitude of aetiologies that can lead to an XY female. These intersex conditions are complex with many management areas remaining highly controversial.

- Thorough review and investigation by experienced multidisciplinary teams is essential for optimal diagnosis and management.

- Objective long-term outcome studies of many areas including surgery, quality-of-life, gender identity, and gender role development and sexual function are urgently needed to help inform the current management debates.

- Clinicians involved in providing medical care for intersex patients need to remain open-minded to new management options and listen to the voices of those most closely involved, i.e. those who live with their intersex conditions.

References

1 Lascaratos J, Kostakopoulos A. Operations on hermaphrodites and castration in Byzantine times. Urol Int 1997; 58: 232–235
2 Bakan R. Queen Elizabeth I: a case of testicular feminisation? Med Hypotheses 1985; 17: 277–284
3 Berta P, Hawkins JR, Sinclair AH et al. Genetic evidence equating SRY and the testis determining factor. Nature 1990; 348: 448–450
4 Rey R, Picard J-Y. Embryology and endocrinology of genital development. Clin Endocrinol Metab 1998; 12: 17–33
5 Zhu Y-S, Katz MD, Imperato-McGinley J. Natural potent androgens: lessons from human genetic models. Clin Endocrinol Metab 1998; 12: 83–113
6 Capel B. Sex in the 90s: SRY and the switch to the male pathway. Annu Rev Physiol 1998; 60: 497–523

7 Voutilainen R. Differentiation of the fetal gonad. Horm Res 1992; 38 (Suppl. 2): 66–71

8 Parmley T. The embryology of the female genital tract. In: Verkauf BS. (ed) Congenital Malformations of the Female Reproductive Tract and Their Treatment. Norwalk, Connecticut: Appleton and Lange, 1993: 17–32

9 Jost A, Magre S. Control mechanisms of testicular differentiation. Philos Trans R Soc Lond B Biol Sci 1988; 322: 55–61

10 Wiener JS, Marcelli M, Lamb DJ. Molecular determinants of sexual differentiation. World J Urol 1996; 14: 278–294

11 Reiner W. To be male or female? – That is the question. Arch Pediatr Adolesc Med 1997; 151: 224–225

12 Hines M. Abnormal sexual development and psychosexual issues. Clin Endocrinol Metab 1998; 12: 173–189

13 Schober JM. Early feminising genitoplasty or watchful waiting. J Pediatr Adolesc Gynecol 1998; 11: 154–156

14 Newman K, Randolph J, Anderson K. The surgical management of infants and children with ambiguous genitalia. Lessons learned from 25 years. Ann Surg 1992: 215: 644–653

15 Woodhouse CR. The sexual and reproductive consequences of congenital genitourinary anomalies. J Urol 1994; 152: 645–651

16 Morris JM. The syndrome of testicular feminisation in male pseudohermaphrodites. Am J Obstet Gynecol 1953; 65: 1192–1211

17 Gottlieb B, Lehvaslaiho H, Beitel LK et al. The androgen receptor gene mutations database. Nucleic Acids Res 1998; 26: 234–238

18 O'Ahlquist JA. Gender identity in testicular feminisation. BMJ 1994; 308: 1041

19 Lubahn DB, Joseph DR, Sar M et al. The human androgen receptor: complementary deoxyribonucleic acid cloning, sequence analysis and gene expression in the prostate. Mol Endocrinol 1988; 2: 1265–1275

20 Brown CJ, Goss SJ, Lubahn DB et al. Androgen receptor locus on the human X chromosome: regional localisation to Xq11-12 and description of a DNA polymorphism. Am J Hum Genet 1989; 44: 264–269

21 Batch JA, Patterson MN, Hughes IA. Androgen insensitivity syndrome. Reprod Med Rev 1992; 1: 131–150

22 Quigley C, DeBellis A, Marschke KB et al. Androgen receptor defects: historical, clinical and molecular perspectives. Endocr Rev 1995; 16: 271–321

23 Rutgers JL, Scully RE. The androgen insensitivity syndrome (testicular feminisation): a clinicopathological study of 43 cases. Int J Gynecol Pathol 1991; 10: 126–144

24 Manuel M, Katayama PK, Jones Jr HW. The age of occurrence of gonadal tumours in intersex patients with a Y chromosome. Am J Obstet Gynecol 1976; 124: 293–300

25 Shah R, Wolley MM, Costin G. Testicular feminisation: the androgen insensitivity syndrome. J Pediatr Surg 1992; 27: 757–760

26 Jaffe RB. Disorders of sexual development. In: Yen SSC, Barbieri RL, Jaffe RB (eds) Reproductive Endocrinology: Physiology and Clinical Management. Philadelphia:Saunders, 1999: 363–387

27 VanGelderen H. Skeletal maturation in the XY female syndrome. Clin Genet 1986; 30: 199–201

28 Soule SG, Conway G, Prelevic GM et al. Osteopenia as a feature of the androgen insensitivity syndrome. Clin Endocrinol 1995; 43: 671–675

29 Goerzen JL, Gidwani GP, Bailez MM et al. Outcome of surgical reconstructive procedures for the treatment of vaginal anomalies. Adolesc Pediatr Gynecol 1994; 7: 76–80

30 Anon. Be open and honest with sufferers. BMJ 1994; 308: 1041–1042

31 Goodall J. Helping a child to understand her own testicular feminisation. Lancet 1991; 337: 33–35

32 Hall C. Girl born a boy wins new birth certificate. The Daily Telegraph 2nd December 1998; 3

33 BBC 1. QED Joella's Journey. 9th December 1998

34 Androgen Insensitivity Support Group (UK): PO Box 269, Banbury, Oxon OX15 6YT, UK (Tel: 01295 670140) Helpline – parent/patient support only <http://www.medhelp.org/www/ais>

35 Anon. Once a dark secret. BMJ 1994; 308: 542

36 Sinnecker GH, Hiort O, Nitsche EM, Holterhus PM, Kruse K. Functional assessment and clinical classification of androgen sensitivity in patients with mutations of the androgen receptor gene. Eur J Paediatr 1997; 156: 7–14

37 Batch JA, Evans BA, Hughes IA, Patterson MN. Mutations of the androgen receptor gene identified in perineal hypospadias. J Med Genet 1993; 30: 198–201

38 Slijper FM, Drop SL, Molenaar JC, de-Muinck-Keizer-Schrama SM. Long-term psychological evaluation of intersex children. Arch Sex Behav 1998; 27: 125–144

39 Diamond M, Sigmundson HK. Sex reassignment at birth: long-term review and clinical implications. Arch Pediatr Adolesc Med 1997; 15: 298–304

40 Schober JM. Feminising genitoplasty for intersex. In: Striger MD, Mouriquand PDE, Oldham KT, Howard ER (eds). Pediatric Surgery and Urology: Long-term Outcomes. Philadelphia:Saunders, 1998

41 Hughes IA, Malone P. Ambiguous genitalia and intersex. In: Atwell J. (ed) Paediatric Surgery. London:Arnold, 1998: 290–306

42 Cai LQ, Zhu YS, Katz MD et al. 5α-Reductase – 2 gene mutations in the Dominican Republic. J Clin Endocrinol Metab 1996; 81: 1730–1735

43 Imperato-McGinley J, Guerrero L, Gautier T, Petterson RE. Steroid 5-alpha-reductase deficiency in man. An inherited form of male pseudohermaphroditism. Science 1974; 186: 1213–1215

44 Herdt GH, Davidson J. The Sambia 'Turnim-Man': sociocultural and clinical aspects of gender formation in male pseudohermaphrodites with 5-alpha-reductase deficiency in Papua New Guinea. Arch Sex Behav 1988; 17: 33–56

45 Can S, Zhu YS, Cai LQ et al. The identification of 5α-reductase-2 and 17β-hydroxysteroid dehydrogenase-3 gene defects in male pseudohermaphrodites from a Turkish kindred. J Clin Endocrinol Metab 1998; 83: 560–569

46 Katz MD, Kligman I, Cai LQ et al. Paternity by intrauterine insemination with sperm from a man with 5α-reductase-2 deficiency. N Engl J Med 1997; 336: 994–997

47 Ivarsson SA. 5α-Reductase deficient men are fertile [Letter]. Eur J Paediatr 1996; 155: 425

48 al-Attia HM. Gender identity and role in Arabs with a pedigree of intersex due to 5α reductase-2 deficiency. Psychoneuroendocrinology 1996; 21: 651–657

49 Mendonca BB, Inacio M, Costa EM et al. Male pseudohermaphroditism due to steroid 5α-reductase-2 deficiency. Diagnosis, psychological evaluation and management. Medicine 1996; 75: 64–76

50 Miller WL. Early steps in androgen biosynthesis: from cholesterol to DHEA. Clin Endocrinol Metab 1998; 12: 67–81

51 Andersson S, Geissler WM, Wu L et al. Molecular genetics and pathophysiology of 17β-hydroxysteroid dehydrogenase deficiency. J Clin Endocrinol Metab 1996; 81: 130–136

52 Mendonca BB, Barbosa AS, Arnhold IJ et al. Gonadal agenesis in XX and XY sisters: evidence for the involvement of an autosomal gene. Am J Med Genet 1994; 52: 39–43

53 Sorgo W, Gortner L, Bartmann P et al. Gonadal agenesis in a 46XY female with multiple internal malformations and positive testing for the sex-determining region on the Y chromosome. Horm Res 1991; 35: 124–131

54 Josso N, Baird ML. Embryonic testicular regression syndrome: variable phenotypic expression in siblings. J Pediatr 1980; 97: 200–204

55 Rosenberg C, Mustacchi Z, Braz A et al. Testicular regression in a patient with virilised female phenotype. Am J Med Genet 1984; 19: 183–188

56 Abeyaratne MR, Aherne WA, Scott JE. The vanishing testis. Lancet 1969; 2: 822–824

57 Berkovitz GD, Fechner PY, Zacur HW et al. Clinical and pathological spectrum of 46 XY gonadal dysgenesis: its relevance to the understanding of sex differentiation. Medicine 1991; 70: 375–383

58 Berkovitz GD, Seeherunvong T. Abnormalities of gonadal differentiation. Clin Endocrinol Metab 1998; 12: 133–142

59 Swyer G. Male pseudohermaphroditism: a hitherto undescribed form. BMJ 1955: 1: 709–710

60 Brown S, Yu C, Lanzano P et al. A de novo mutation (Gln2stop) at the 5' end of the SRY gene leads to sex reversal with partial ovarian function. Am J Hum Genet 1998; 62: 189–192

61 Scherer G, Held M, Erdel M et al. Three novel SRY mutations in XY gonadal dysgenesis

and the enigma of XY gonadal dysgenesis cases without SRY mutations. Cytogenet Cell Genet 1998; 80: 188–192

62 Veitia RA, Nunes M, Murci-Quintana L et al. Swyer syndrome and 46XY partial gonadal dysgenesis associated with 9p deletions in the absence of monosomy 9p syndrome. Am J Hum Genet 1998; 63: 901–905

63 Wilkie AO, Campbell FM, Daubeney P et al. Complete and partial XY sex reversal associated with terminal deletion of 10q: report of 2 cases and literature review. Am J Med Genet 1993; 46: 597–600

64 Misrahi M, Beau I, Meduri G et al. Gonadotropin receptors and the control of gonadal steroidogenesis: physiology and pathology. Clin Endocrinol Metab 1998; 12: 35–66

65 Themmen AP, Brunner HG. Luteinizing hormone receptor mutations and sex differentiation. Eur J Endocrinol 1996; 134: 533–540

66 Imbeaud S, Carre-Eusebe D, Rey R et al. Molecular genetics of the persistent Mullerian duct syndrome: a study of 19 families. Hum Mol Genet 1994; 3: 125–131

Alexander Taylor

Current minimal access techniques for dysfunctional uterine bleeding

Dysfunctional uterine bleeding (DUB) affects 20–30% of women[1] and accounts for 12% of gynaecological referrals.[2] Within 5 years of referral, 60% of women will have undergone hysterectomy,[3] making it the commonest major gynaecological operation.[4] In a recent analysis of the Department of Health's *Hospital Episode Statistics* database, 22,543 hysterectomies were carried out for DUB in 1996.[5] However, hysterectomy has major socio-economic costs and is not without complications. The recent VALUE survey of over 35,000 hysterectomies reported the mortality rate was 0.38 per 1000 and the serious morbidity rate 3%.[6] Serious morbidity was defined as return to theatre to stop bleeding, visceral injury, or severe postoperative complications.

With the development of minimal access techniques, it has become possible to destroy the endometrium in situ, in a short, day-case operation. The first of these techniques, described in 1981, ablated the endometrium with a Nd:YAG laser.[7] Not long after, resection of the endometrium with the operative hysteroscope was described.[8] These techniques have since been extensively evaluated in randomised trials.[9–12] Based on these trials, endometrial ablative techniques have been given a grade A recommendation by The Royal College of Obstetricians and Gynaecologists for the treatment of heavy menstrual bleeding.[13] Even at 10 years, 75% of women who undergo transcervical resection of the endometrium (TCRE) will have avoided hysterectomy (Fig. 1; Magos, unpublished data). Unfortunately, these techniques require considerable surgical skill and a long learning curve. It has been suggested that a surgeon learning the technique of resection, should treat 200 cases before they are considered proficient.[14] In addition, though large audits of these techniques have shown them to be safe, they are still associated with a mortality of 2 per 10,000 and a serious complication rate of 2.1–6.4%.[15]

Mr Alexander Taylor MBBS MRCOG, Clinical Research Fellow, Minimally Invasive Therapy Unit and Endoscopy Training Centre, University Department of Obstetrics and Gynaecology, Royal Free Hospital, Rowland Hill Street, London NW3 2PF, UK

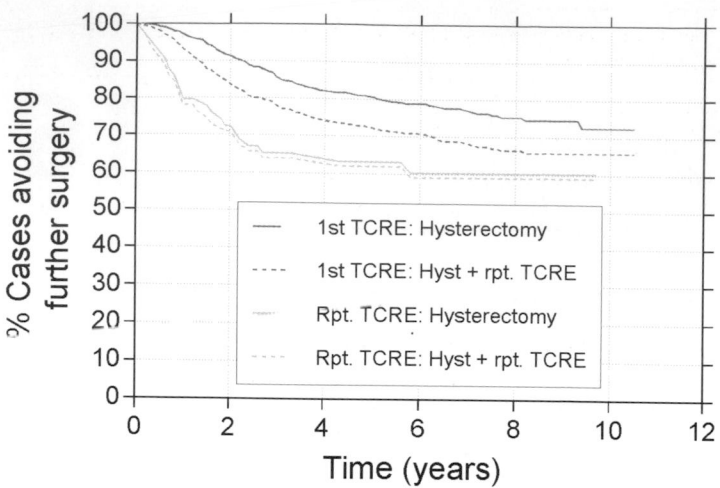

Fig. 1 Overall results of transcervical resection of the endometrium (TCRE) at 10 years.

Second generation ablative devices have, therefore, been developed with the aim of improving on these existing minimal access techniques. In the past 10 years, there has been an explosion of research in this field and it has yielded a plethora of devices all aimed at treating DUB, effectively, safely, quickly and easily and preferably in the out-patient setting. This article reviews the current available devices and techniques.

MICROWAVE ENDOMETRIAL ABLATION (MEA)

Microwaves lie in the radiowave part of the spectrum and have wavelengths that vary from 1 mm to 30 cm. Their properties have been utilised by the telecommunications industry and the domestic oven market. In the latter, by varying the frequency of the microwave and the power output of the micro-wave source, a heating effect can be created. It is this heating effect that destroys the endometrium raising the possibility of a role in the management of dysfunctional uterine bleeding.

The only current microwave device is produced by Microsulis PLC (Waterlooville, Hampshire, UK). It operates at a frequency of 9.2 GHz, chosen to generate a maximum depth of heating of 6 mm. At 30 W, energies of 1.5–9.3 kJ result. No earthing plate is required, unlike for radiofrequency electromagnetic waves or diathermy. The applicator is 8 mm in diameter and at the tip there is a thermocouple that records endometrial temperatures. The output from this is connected to a computer display to show the operator real-time endometrial temperatures throughout the procedure. The whole procedure takes about 3.5 min.

MEA has undergone in vitro and in vivo safety tests.[16] In vitro, four excised human uteri were used to determine the ideal parameters to achieve a 6 mm depth of thermal necrosis. No rise in serosal temperature was recorded and there was no leakage of microwaves. Similarly, in vivo no rise in serosal temperature was recorded in 16 women prior to hysterectomy and there was no leakage of microwaves. The Safety and Efficacy Registrar of New

Table 1 Safety and Efficacy Registrar of New Interventional Procedures (SERNIP): categories and definitions

Category	Definition
A	Safety and efficacy of the procedure established
B	Sufficiently close to an established procedure to give no reasonable grounds for questioning safety and efficacy; procedure may be used subject to continuing audit
C1	Safety or efficacy not yet established; procedure requires a fully controlled evaluation and may be used only as part of systematic research, consisting of an observational study in which all interventions and their outcomes are systematically recorded
C2	Safety and/or efficacy not yet established; procedure requires a fully controlled evaluation and may be used only as part of systematic research, consisting of a randomized controlled trial, and advising the UK Standing Group on Health Technology accordingly
D	Safety or efficacy shown to be unsatisfactory; procedure should not be used

Interventional Procedures (SERNIP)[17] has given MEA category B status which is defined as: 'sufficiently close to an established procedure to give no reasonable grounds for questioning safety and efficacy; procedure may be used subject to continuing audit'. SERNIP categories are depicted in Table 1.

MEA has been evaluated in a randomised trial comparing it with transcervical resection of the endometrium (TCRE).[18] The main outcome measures in this study were patients' satisfaction with the procedure and acceptability. The secondary outcome measures were effect on menstruation, quality-of-life and operative morbidity. To give an 80% power of detecting a 15% difference in the main outcome measure, 230 women were needed. Women were considered eligible for inclusion if the uterine size was ≤ 10 weeks' pregnancy and if they had no histological abnormality of the endometrium. Both groups underwent endometrial preparation with goserelin (3.6 mg). Those who underwent MEA had a gas hysteroscopy to confirm correct placement of the microwave device. A total of 129 women were randomised to MEA and 134 women were randomised to TCRE. There was no significant difference in satisfaction rates or acceptability between treatments. Both scored highly, MEA 77% and 94%, TCRE 75% and 90%, respectively. At 12 months' follow-up, both techniques had received significant reductions in menstruation ($P < 0.001$) but again there was no significant differences between the techniques. Both resulted in amenorrhoea rates of 40%. In this study, one blunt perforation occurred in each group resulting in hysterectomy. Four women in the MEA group underwent TCRE because the microwave equipment failed. Re-admission was required for four women in the MEA group and for six in the TCRE group. At 12 months, 10 (8%) women in the MEA group and 12 (9%) women in the TCRE group had undergone hysterectomy.

In the above trial, the MEA was conducted under general anaesthetic; more recently, the technique has been piloted under local anaesthesia where it was reported as feasible in 76% of unselected women.[19]

Though the initial description of insertion of the microwave probe was essentially blind in both the above studies to avoid inadvertent uterine perforation, hysteroscopy was performed prior to insertion.

THERMAL BALLOON ABLATION

Thermal balloon ablation of the endometrium involves inserting a balloon tipped catheter into the uterine cavity, inflating the balloon so it conforms to the shape of the cavity and then heating the fluid within it to 85°C. There are currently two available devices, the ThermaChoice system (Gynecare Ethicon, Menlo Park, CA, USA) and the Cavaterm system (Wallsten Medical, Morges, Switzerland).

The ThermaChoice system has been tested in human uteri in ex vivo and in vivo studies,[20,21] and has achieved a grade B classification from SERNIP. In the first of these studies,[20] two phases of experiments were described. In phase 1, the serosal, myometrial and endometrial temperatures were recorded on excised uteri during an 8 min treatment cycle and depth of necrosis examined. In phase 2, nine patients who were due to undergo hysterectomy agreed to undergo prior thermal balloon ablation. In these patients, the balloon was filled with 7–11 ml of 5% dextrose, to achieve a mean balloon start pressure of 166 mmHg. The mean uterine cavity depth was 8 ± 1 cm. Once again, thermocouples measured serosal temperatures and the depth of necrosis was assessed. The serosal temperatures in the phase 1 experiments remained below 45°C, except in a postmenopausal uterus and when one uterus was subjected to 24 min of heating. Here the serosal temperature reached 52°C. The mean myometrial depth of destruction was 3.4 ± 1.8 mm. In phase 2, the mean serosal temperatures were 33°C, lower than in phase 1 because of the heat sink effect of the uterus. The maximum depth of myometrial penetration was 3.4 mm. In the second study,[21] 8 women due to undergo hysterectomy had prior thermal ablation. Once again, a balloon pressure of 160 mmHg was used and the standard treatment time was 8 min. However, the investigators also undertook treatment times of 14, 15 and 16 min. The serosal temperature at 8 min was 36°C rising to 38°C at 16 min. The depth of coagulation in the body of the uterus varied from 0.1–7.9 mm. However, a coagulation depth of 11.5 mm was recorded at the fundus in one patient.

The ThermaChoice system has been evaluated clinically in a prospective comparative study with endometrial resection,[22] and also in a randomised multicentre trial with rollerball endometrial ablation.[23] In the randomised trial, 275 women with menorrhagia were recruited and randomised in a 1:1 allocation. Menstrual loss was assessed with diary-based pictorial charts.[24] No intra-operative complications were reported in the thermal balloon group, but 4 complications (3.2%) were reported in the rollerball group. These included two cases of fluid overload and one uterine perforation. The outcomes for operating times, menstrual diary scores, amenorrhoea, dysmenorrhoea and patient satisfaction at 1 year follow up are shown in Table 2. Of note in the comparative study with endometrial resection was the report of a 6.2-fold increase in failure after thermal balloon therapy in those women with a retroverted uterus.[22]

The Cavaterm thermal device, consists of a silastic balloon catheter, filled with 1.5% glycine compared to the 5% dextrose in the ThermaChoice system. The fluid is heated to 75°C and only a maximum of 30 ml of fluid can be used

Table 2 Outcomes at 1 year for ThermaChoice versus Rollerball

Measure	ThermaChoice (n = 125)	Rollerball (n = 114)	
Procedures completed in 30 min (%)	71	29	P < 0.05
Mean decrease in menstrual diary scores (%)	85.5	91.7	NS
Hypomenorrhoea, score ≤ 25 (%)	52.8	62.8	NS
Amenorrhoea (%)	27.2	15.2	P < 0.05
Decrease in dysmenorrhoea (%)	70.4	75.4	NS
Satisfaction (%)	96	99	NS

Significant differences between the groups are marked.

per case. Higher pressures (180–220 mmHg) are achieved with this device in an effort to tamponade the uterine vessels and reduce the heat-sink effect. In addition, the fluid is actively circulated in an effort to ensure a uniform temperature and, therefore, a uniform depth of endometrial ablation. The standard treatment time is 15 min, longer than the standard 8 min with the ThermaChoice system. The efficacy and safety of the Cavaterm device has been assessed in a study of 50 women with dysfunctional bleeding.[25] The authors did not carry out any ex vivo or in vivo experiments, but instead reported clinical outcomes. They did, however, refer to an early study[26] where experiments on pre-hysterectomy specimens resulted in a myometrial depth of destruction of 2–5 mm. Of the 50 women recruited, 36 had the procedure performed under general anaesthetic. No intra- or postoperative complications were reported. At 12 months' follow-up, subjective reported rates of amenorrhoea and hypomenorrhoea were 64% and 24%, respectively. However, only follow-up data on 25 women were available at this stage. At the time of writing, the Cavaterm system had only been awarded grade C status form SERNIP.

Clinical data on the Cavaterm system from randomised trials is not yet available, although there is a trial underway comparing it with Nd:YAG laser endometrial ablation.[25] A prospective study of 117 women treated for menorrhagia with the device has been published.[27] No immediate or peri-operative complications occurred. At the time of the final follow-up (mean 23 months, range 23–49 months), data were available on 51 women. Ten women had undergone hysterectomy, 12 reported amenorrhoea and 23 reported minimal menstrual loss.

ENDOMETRIAL LASER INTRA-UTERINE THERMOTHERAPY (ELITT)

The original work on endometrial ablation with lasers was done with a Nd:YAG laser.[28]. However, the Nd:YAG laser is cumbersome, expensive and requires fluid distension. The new ELITT, by contrast, uses a 830 nm diode laser powered by a 20 W source no bigger than a shoe-box and a disposable handset. The current machine on the market is called 'GyneLase' and it is manufactured by Sharplan ESC, Massachusetts, USA. Like the Nd:YAG it creates coagulation. The laser light is emitted from three integrated optical–light diffusers (6 mm in cross-section when folded) designed to conform to the shape of the cavity. This, it is alleged, allows a uniform distribution of laser light which is then absorbed by haemoglobin in the uterine wall, resulting in coagulation. The laser, therefore, does not need to be in contact with the endometrium, nor does the technique require fluid distension of the cavity. The cervix is dilated to 7 mm and the handset is inserted into the cavity in a blind manner. The laser is then activated for a 7-min preprogrammed cycle.

ELITT is reported as destroying the entire endometrium and 1–3.5 mm of the myometrium, leaving a 'safety buffer' of 67% of the myometrium. In vivo studies of temperature changes at the serosa have reported no significant variation.[29,30]

Currently, the clinical data on ELITT are sparse and it has not been evaluated in randomised trials. However, the US Food and Drug Administration has recently approved a study comparing it with Rollerball. The published data consist of series of patients studied prospectively.[31,32] In the first of these,[31] 100 premenopausal women with dysfunctional uterine bleeding were treated with ELITT; 38 of the women had the procedure carried out under local or regional anaesthesia. The main outcome measure was menstrual status which was based on the pictorial chart method.[24]. At 1-year follow-up, the reported rates of amenorrhoea and hypomenorrhoea were 71% and > 90%, respectively. No perforations were reported in this study and two patients underwent laparoscopic subtotal hysterectomy because of painful cornual hematometra. In the later prospective study,[32] 40 women with documented menorrhagia underwent ELITT. The same main outcome measure was used, but in addition the authors measured dysmenorrhoea scores and looked at satisfaction rates. At 1 year, the reported rates of amenorrhoea and hypomenorrhoea were 70% and 85%, respectively. The average dysmenorrhoea score decreased from 35 to 10, and 85% of the women were satisfied with their treatment. In this study, the investigators undertook hysteroscopic inspection of the cavity prior to insertion of the device. No perforations were reported. At 1 year, 5 women had undergone hysterectomy because of treatment failure.

INTRA-UTERINE SURGERY USING A COAXIAL BIPOLAR ELECTRODE

The first generation of resectoscopes were based on a monopolar circuit,[33] a design inherently more dangerous than a bipolar circuit for minimal access work.[34] Versapoint (manufactured by Gynaecare Inc, Johnson & Johnson) is a new coaxial bipolar system 1.6 mm in diameter that can be inserted into the operative channel of a 5 mm continuous-flow hysteroscope. There are currently three electrode tips configured as a spring, a 'twizzle', and a ball (Fig. 2).

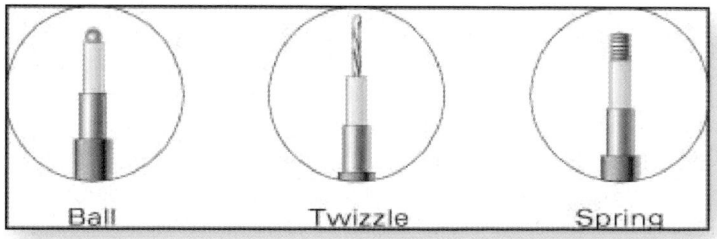

Fig. 2 Available electrode tips with Versapoint (from the J&J website at www.jnjgateway.com).

The electrosurgical generator is similar to other electrosurgical equipment. It provides power settings from 1–200 W, with a default setting of 50 W. The system requires uterine distension and this is achieved using normal saline rather than the non-physiological fluids that are used at traditional operative hysteroscopy. In use, the electrode does not extend more than 8 mm beyond the hysteroscope. When activated in the normal saline, a high resistance air pocket is created that effectively insulates the active electrode. It is only when contact is made with the tissue that the circuit is completed and cutting occurs.

Data on the system's safety and efficacy are scarce at the moment. Only two pilot studies and interim data from a randomised trial have been published to date.[35–37] Neither reported any in vitro or in vivo work verifying its safety or determining the depth of tissue destruction. In the first of these studies,[35] 15 women with menorrhagia were recruited and underwent hysteroscopic removal of submucous fibroids. Seven women in the study underwent concomitant endometrial ablation. Complete removal of the fibroids was achieved in all cases. No complications were reported. Two women became amenorrhoeic, and in the others menses returned to normal or less in the 2–16 month follow-up period. In the second study,[36] 8 women with intra-uterine lesions were recruited and one underwent endometrial ablation. No complications were reported, although the authors did highlight a death in 1997 in New York from fluid absorption during hysteroscopic myomectomy using the Versapoint system. The results of the interim data comparing the Versapoint system are shown in Table 3.

Table 3 Interim results of Versapoint versus Rollerball/resection

Measure	Vesta (n = 150)	Rollerball/resection (n = 126)
Mean decrease in menstrual score	94	91
Amenorrhoea (%)	31.8	39.6
Dysmenorrhoea (%)	Not reported	Not reported
Patient satisfaction (%)	Not reported	Not reported

HYDROTHERMAL ABLATION OF THE ENDOMETRIUM (HTA)

Hydrothermal ablation (HTA) involves instilling heated normal saline into the uterine cavity to achieve thermal coagulative necrosis of the endometrium. There are currently two devices on the market, the HTA (from BEI Medical Systems, Teterbro, NJ, USA) and the Enabl (from US Surgical Corp, Norwalk, CT, USA).

The HTA is a 7.8 mm continuous flow hysteroscope connected to a heater, a pump and a fluid chamber. Normal saline at a temperature of 90°C circulates continuously around the uterine cavity for 10 min at a pressure of 50 mmHg (less than the 70 mmHg opening pressure of the tubal ostia). Any leakage of fluid from the cervix is prevented with a tenaculum. If more than 10 ml of saline leaks from the system, the equipment automatically switches off to avoid inadvertent thermal injury.

Experiments in a pig's uterus demonstrated that, if a uterine cavity temperature of 85°C was maintained for 8 min, it resulted in a serosal temperature of 52°C and a depth of necrosis of 5 mm.[38] In humans, 14 patients with menorrhagia underwent the HTA procedure in a pilot study and were followed up for 9–18 months.[39] Eleven patients were amenorrhoeic at 9–18 months.

The Enabl device is a self-contained 5 mm thermal catheter that is inserted blindly into the uterine cavity. Normal saline is again heated to 90°C and circulated round the uterine cavity by a 'diffuser' device. It has been tested in vivo in sheep and ex vivo in human uteri.[40] In the ex vivo human uteri, temperatures of 80°C for 15–20 min resulted in serosal temperatures of 35–49°C and a 3 mm depth of myometrial destruction. The device has also been tested in 11 women prior to hysterectomy.[41] In this small study, the serosal temperatures were 35–37°C and the depth of necrosis into the myometrium was 1–2 mm.

At the time of writing, the hydrothermal devices had only achieved class C status from SERNIP.

CRYO-ABLATION OF THE ENDOMETRIUM

Destruction of the endometrium using freezing temperatures (cryo-ablation) was one of the first ablative techniques to be described.[42] However, its use was short-lived following reports of pelvic abscesses.[43] Recently, there has been renewed interest in the technology and data from in vitro and in vivo studies have been published.[44,45]

In the in vitro study,[44] the investigators experimented with different freezing parameters in ex vivo uteri, to determine the optimal settings for the Endocryo cryoprobe (Spembly Medical Ltd, Andover, UK). The cryoprobe was 9 mm in diameter and used carbon dioxide as the cryogen. It achieved temperatures of –55°C at the probe tip. A total of 84 experiments were carried out on fresh blocks of tissue. The minimum duration of freezing was 2 min and the maximum 10 min. Rates of freezing and thawing were examined, as was the use of distension media to improve tissue contact. The authors reported that freezing and thawing rates were of little importance, and that the most important feature was contact with the tissue – gaps of 1 mm or more rendered the device ineffective. A 2 min freeze–thaw cycle was reported as the safest, leading to a mean depth of cell death of 4.5 ± 0.6 mm.

In the in vivo study,[45] 10 women scheduled for hysterectomy agreed to undergo prior cryotherapy with the First Option device (Cryogen Inc., San Diego, CA, USA). The temperature at the tip of this probe was –90°C and the procedure was carried out under ultrasound control. Thermocouples were used to monitor the serosal temperature and no reduction in temperature was recorded. The depth of necrosis was 9–12 mm.

Cryotherapy of the endometrium may have been 're-discovered', but its use for the moment should be confined to a research setting.

PHOTODYNAMIC ENDOMETRIAL ABLATION

Photodynamic therapy (PDT) is based on the activation of a photosensitizer within tissues. This activation generates highly reactive oxygen molecules that are toxic to cell membranes. As a therapy, it has been used for a variety of benign and malignant conditions, most commonly in the field of dermatology.[46,47] A number of chemicals can have a photosensitizing effect and it is a recognised side-effect of a number of drug therapies.[48]

The effect of PDT on the endometrium has been studied in animal models,[49] including non-human primates.[50] Both studies investigated the effect of the photosensitizer 5-aminolevulinic acid (ALA). ALA is a precursor of haem and exogenous administration results in the preferential accumulation of proto-porphyrin IX in the endometrium rather than the myometrium.

In the non-human primate study, 18 rhesus monkeys were anaesthetised and the ALA instilled into the uterine cavity. After 4 h, light at a wavelength of 635 nm and an intensity of 300 mW was delivered for 60 min by a laser in either a continuous or fractionated manner. The experiments were performed in the early proliferative phase or, in 4 cases, in monkeys in whom a surgical menopause had been induced. The extent of the endometrial ablation was then assessed histologically following subtotal hysterectomy. The endometrial ablation was expressed as a percentage of endometrium and was most marked in the uteri of the menopausal monkeys, where the mean percentage ablation achieved was 72%. In contrast, only 29% was achieved in the uteri of monkeys in the proliferative phase at the time of exposure. Marked regional differences in ablation were noted in the uterine cavity with fundal rates of 41% compared to middle rates of 87%. The authors felt this was probably due to the perpendicular emission of light from the fibre axis. Continuous light was reported as being more effective than fractionated light. There was also a significant rise in the uterine endometrial temperature of up to 50°C. It is worth mentioning that the depth of penetration of visible light is 2–4 mm.[51]

Published work in human endometrium is scant. In a feasibility study,[52] three women underwent PDT with ALA. Two were suffering from menorrhagia and one from persisting postmenopausal bleeding. The procedure was carried out without general or local anaesthetic. At 6 months, the postmenopausal women had undergone hysterectomy, whilst the two premenopausal women reported a reduction in uterine bleeding.

Endometrial PDT at the time of writing has not been considered by SERNIP.

RADIOFREQUENCY-INDUCED THERMAL ENDOMETRIAL ABLATION

Radiofrequency ablation involves inserting a 10 mm diameter probe into the uterine cavity and generating electromagnetic radiation which causes irreversible tissue damage.[53] The probe is energised at 27 MHz with an incident power level of around 550 W, usually for 20 min. Reports of vesico-vaginal fistulae complicating the treatment[54] and of burns to bowel, fingers and thumbs (from radiofrequency energy at pulse-oximeters) has lead to the technique being discredited.[55]

THE LEVONORGESTREL INTRA-UTERINE SYSTEM

No review of the current management of dysfunctional uterine bleeding, would be complete, without mentioning the levonorgestrel intra-uterine system, more commonly known by its trade name, Mirena (Schering, Burgess Hill, UK). The Mirena intra-uterine system releases 20 μg of levonorgestrel daily into the uterine cavity, rendering the endometrium inactive. Not only is it one of the most effective forms of contraceptive,[56] it also reduces menstrual blood loss by 80%.[57] Compared to endometrial resection it is not as effective,[58] but its advantage over ablative techniques is that it is reversible. An important issue in cases where a woman wishes to preserve her fertility. Surprisingly, even at this low dose of levonorgestrel, a significant proportion of women suffer from progestogenic side-effects.[59] It has not been as rigorously evaluated as the surgical techniques and there is little long-term published data. One trial with a mean follow-up of 54 months reported that the Mirena failed in 50% of women.[60]

CONCLUSIONS

Dysfunctional uterine bleeding is a disabling condition for which many women seek medical help. Medical management often initiated in the community is only effective in around 50% of women.[61] The management options after failed medical therapy have tended to be surgical, although increasingly the levonorgestrel intra-uterine device is being tried before surgery is undertaken.

Hysterectomy is the definitive treatment and has high rates of patient satisfaction. However, it is a major operation with all the attendant morbidity and mortality.[6]

Less invasive minimal access techniques conserve the uterus, result in a shorter in-patient stay, and a quicker return to full activities. There is now overwhelming evidence that the first generation techniques of ablation and resection are a genuine alternative to hysterectomy.[9–12]

Unfortunately, the original techniques require considerable surgical skill and are still associated with a serious morbidity rate of 2.1–6.4%.[15] As a result, there has been a huge investment in the next generation of devices all aimed at improving on the old.

It is not yet clear which devices will prosper and which will fail and which will be approved by the National Institute of Clinical Excellence,[62] soon to take over from SERNIP. The picture will hopefully be clearer with the results of the randomised trials in progress. In the meantime, the existing evidence still favours the first generation techniques.

KEY POINTS FOR CLINICAL PRACTICE

- This review has identified seven different techniques and nine devices currently available to treat DUB. The evidence supporting the use of some of these is lacking at the moment.

- Of the current second generation devices, the Microsulis microwave device and the ThermaChoice balloon device are the most extensively researched and reported.

- Although safety is of paramount importance, the second generation devices are inserted 'blind' into the cavity, raising the possibility of incorrect placement. In addition, the devices have been designed to treat a normal size and shaped cavity, excluding a significant proportion of women.

- Most of the techniques use disposable probes; although the costs of these may be negated by treating in an out-patient setting, this has yet to be proved.

References

1   Cooper KG, Parkin DE, Garratt AM, Grant AM. A randomised comparison of medical and hysteroscopic management in women consulting a gynaecologist for treatment of heavy menstrual loss. Br J Obstet Gynaecol 1997; 104: 1360–1366

2   Cooke I, Lethaby A, Farquhar C. Anti-fibrinolytics for heavy menstrual bleeding (Cochrane Review). In: The Cochrane Library, Issue 3. Oxford: Update Software, 1999

3   Coulter A, Bradlow J, Agass M, Martin-Bates C, Tulloch A. Outcome of referrals to gynaecology outpatient clinics for menstrual problems: an audit of general practice records. Br J Obstet Gynaecol 1991; 98: 798–796

4   Vessey MP, Villard-Mackintosh L, McPherson K, Coulter A, Yeates D. The epidemiology of hysterectomy: findings in a large cohort study. Br J Obstet Gynaecol 1992; 99: 402–407

5   Bridgman S, Dunn K. Has endometrial ablation replaced hysterectomy for the treatment of dysfunctional uterine bleeding? National figures. Br J Obstet Gynaecol 2000; 107: 531–534

6   Maresh M, Metcalfe M, McPherson K et al. The VALUE national hysterectomy study: description of the patients and their surgery. Br J Obstet Gynaecol 2002; 109: 302–312

7   Goldrath MH, Fuller TA, Segal S. Laser photovaporisation of endometrium for the retreatment of menorrhagia. Am J Obstet Gynecol 1981; 140: 14–19

8   Magos AL, Baumann R, Turnbull AC. Transcervical resection of the endometrium in women with menorrhagia. BMJ 1989; 298: 1209–1212

9   Pinion SB, Parkin DE, Abramovich DR et al. Randomised trial of hysterectomy, endometrial laser ablation and transcervical resection of the endometrium for dysfunctional uterine bleeding. BMJ 1994; 309: 979–983

10 Aberdeen Endometrial Ablation Trials Group. A randomised trial of endometrial ablation versus hysterectomy for the treatment of dysfunctional uterine bleeding: outcome at four years. Br J Obstet Gynaecol 1999; 106: 360–366

11 Gannon MJ, Holt EM, Fairbank J et al. A randomised trial comparing endometrial resection and abdominal hysterectomy for the treatment of menorrhagia. BMJ 1991; 303: 1362–1364

12 Dwyer N, Hutton J, Stirrat GM. Randomised controlled trial comparing endometrial resection with abdominal hysterectomy for the surgical treatment of menorrhagia. Br J Obstet Gynaecol 1993; 100: 237–243

13 Royal College of Obstetricians and Gynaecologists. The Management of Menorrhagia in Secondary Care. Evidence-based Clinical Guidelines No.5. London: RCOG, 1995

14 Holt EM, Gilmer MD. Endometrial resection. Baillière's Clin Obstet Gynaecol 1995; 9: 279–297

15 Overton C, Hargreaves H, Maresh M. A national survey of the complications of endometrial destruction for menstrual disorders: the MISTLETOE study. Br J Obstet Gynaecol 1997; 104: 1351–1359

16 Hodgson D, Felberg I, Sharp N et al. Microwave endometrial ablation: development, clinical trials and outcomes at three years. Br J Obstet Gynaecol 1999; 106: 684–694

17. Anon. Safety and Efficacy Register of New Interventional Procedures. The Academy of Medical Royal Colleges, 1 Wimpole Street, London W1M 8AE (Tel: 0171 290 3917, Fax: 0171 495 2432)

18 Cooper K, Bain C, Parkin D. Comparison of microwave endometrial ablation and transcervical resection of the endometrium for treatment of heavy menstrual loss: a randomised trial. Lancet 1999; 354: 1859–1863

19 Bain C, Cooper K, Parkin D. A partially randomized patient preference trial of microwave endometrial ablation using local anaesthesia and intravenous sedation or general anaesthesia: a pilot study. Gynaecol Endosc 2001; 10: 223–228

20 Shah A, Stabinsk S, Klusak T et al. Measurement of serosal temperatures and depth of thermal injury generated by thermal balloon endometrial ablation in ex vivo and in vivo models. Fertil Steril 1998; 70: 692–697

21 Anderson L, Meinert L, Rygaard C et al. Thermal balloon endometrial ablation: safety aspects evaluated by serosal temperature, light microscopy and electron microscopy. Eur J Obstet Gynecol Reprod Biol 1998; 79: 63–68

22 Gervaise A, Fernandez H, Capella-Allouc S et al. Thermal balloon ablation versus endometrial resection for the treatment of abnormal uterine bleeding. Hum Reprod 1999; 14: 2743–2747

23 Meyer W, Walsh B, Grainger D et al. Thermal balloon and rollerball ablation to treat menorrhagia: a multicenter comparison. Obstet Gynecol 1998: 92: 98–103

24 Higham JM, O'Brien PMS, Shaw RW. Assessment of menstrual blood using a pictorial chart. Br J Obstet Gynaecol 1990; 97: 734–739

25 Hawe J, Phillips G, Chien P, Erian J, Garry R. Cavaterm thermal balloon ablation for the treatment of menorrhagia. Br J Obstet Gynaecol 1999; 106: 1143–1148

26 Friberg B, Persson BR, Willen R, Ahlgren M. Endometrial destruction by hyperthermia – a possible treatment of menorrhagia. An experimental study. Acta Obstet Gynecol Scand 1996; 75: 330–335

27 Friberg B, Ahlgren M. Thermal balloon endometrial destruction: the outcome of treatment of 117 women followed up for a maximum period of 4 years. Gynaecol Endosc 2000; 9: 389–395

28 Goldrath MH, Fuller TA, Segal S. Laser photovaporization of endometrium for the treatment of menorrhagia. Am J Obstet Gynecol 1981; 140: 14–19

29 Donnez J, Polet R, Mathieu PE et al. Nd-YAG laser ITT multifiber device (the Donnez device): endometrial ablation by interstitial hyperthermia. In: Donnez J, Nisolle M. (eds) Atlas of Laser Operative Laparoscopy and Hysteroscopy. Carnforth: Parthenon, 1994; 353–359

30 Donnez J, Polet R, Mathieu PE et al. Endometrial laser interstitial hyperthermy: a potential modality for endometrial ablation. Obstet Gynecol 1996; 87: 459–464

31 Donnez J, Polet R, Rabinovitz R et al. Endometrial laser intrauterine thermotherapy: the first series of 100 patients observed for 1 year. Fertil Steril 2000; 74: 791–796

32 Jones K, Abbott J, Hawe J et al. Endometrial laser intrauterine thermotherapy for the treatment of dysfunctional uterine bleeding: the first British experience. Br J Obstet Gynaecol 2001; 108: 749–753

33 Neuwirth RS, Amin HK. Excision of submucous fibroids with hysteroscopic control. Am J Obstet Gynecol 1976; 126: 95–99

34 Vilos GA, D'Souza I, Huband D. Genital tract burns during rollerball endometrial coagulation. J Am Assoc Gynecol Laparosc 1997; 4: 273–276

35 Vilos G. Intrauterine surgery using a new coaxial bipolar electrode in normal saline solution (Versapoint): a pilot study. Fertil Steril 1999; 72: 740–743

36 Loffer F. Preliminary experience with the VersaPoint bipolar resectoscope using a vaporizing electrode in a saline distending medium. J Am Assoc Gynecol Laparosc 2000; 7: 498–502

37 Corson SL, Brill AI, Brooks M et al. Interim results of the American Vesta Trial of Endometrial Ablation. J Am Assoc Gynecol Laparosc 1999; 6: 45–49

38 Goldrath M, Barrionuevo M, Husain M. Endometrial ablation by hysteroscopic instillation of hot saline solution. J Am Assoc Gynecol Laparosc 1997; 4: 235–240

39 Perlitz Y, Rahav D, Moshe B. Endometrial ablation using hysteroscopic instillation of hot saline solution into the uterus. Eur J Obstet Gynecol Reprod Biol 2001; 99: 90–92

40 Baggish M, Pariaso M, Breznock E, Griffey S. A computer-controlled, continuously circulating, hot irrigation system for endometrial ablation. Am J Obstet Gynecol 1995; 173: 1842–1848

41 Bustos-Lopez H, Baggish M, Valle R et al. Assessment of the safety of intrauterine instillation of heated saline for endometrial ablation. Fertil Steril 1998; 69: 155–160

42 Droegenmuller W, Makowski EL, Macsalka R. Destruction of the endometrium by cryosurgery. Am J Obstet Gynecol 1971; 110: 467–469

43 Burke L, Rubin HW, Kim I. Uterine abscess formation secondary to endometrial cryosurgery. Obstet Gynecol 1972; 41: 224–226

44 Kremer C, Duffy S. In vitro studies of cryoablation of the endometrium. Am J Obstet Gynecol 2000; 183: 22–27

45 Dobak JD, Willems J, Howard R, Shea C, Townsend D. Endometrial cryoablation with ultrasound visualisation in women undergoing hysterectomy. J Am Assoc Gynecol Laparosc 2000; 7: 89–93

46 Szeimes RM, Karrer S, Sauerwald A, Landthaler V. Photodynamic therapy with topical application of 5-aminolevulinic acid in the treatment of actinic keratoses: an initial clinical study. Dermatology 1996; 192: 246–251

47 Cairnduff F, Stringer MR, Hudson EJ, Ash DV, Brown SB. Superficial photodynamic

therapy with topical 5-aminolevulinic acid for superficial primary and secondary skin cancer. Br J Cancer 1994; 69: 605–608

48 Zehender M. Images in cardiovascular medicine. Amiodarone phototoxic reaction. Circulation 1995; 92: 1665

49 Wyass P, Tromberg J, Wyss M et al. Photodynamic destruction of endometrial tissue using topical 5-aminolevulinic acid in rats and rabbits. Am J Obstet Gynecol 1994; 171: 1176–1183

50 Van Vugt D, Krzemien A, Roy B et al. Photodynamic endometrial ablation in the non-human primate. J Soc Gynecol Invest 2000; 7: 125–130

51 Fehr MK, Madsen SJ, Svaasand LO et al. Intrauterine light delivery for photodynamic therapy of the human endometrium. Hum Reprod 1995; 10: 3067–3072

52 Wyss P, Fehr M, Van den Bergh, Haller U. Feasibility of photodynamic endometrial ablation without anesthesia. Int J Gynecol Obstet 1998; 60: 287–288

53 Phipps J, Lewis B, Roberts T et al. Treatment of functional menorrhagia by radiofrequency-induced thermal endometrial ablation. Lancet 1990; 335: 374–376

54 Phipps J, Lewis B, Prior M, Roberts T. Experimental and clinical studies with radiofrequency induced thermal endometrial ablation for functional menorrhagia. Obstet Gynecol 1990; 76: 876–881

55 Jones K, McGurgan P, Sutton C. Second generation endometrial ablation techniques. Curr Opin Obstet Gynecol 2000; 12: 273–276

56 Milson I, Anderson K, Andersch B, Rybo G. A comparison of flurbiprofen, tranexamic acid and levonorgestrel-releasing intrauterine contraceptive device in the treatment of idiopathic menorrhagia. Am J Obstet Gynecol 1991; 164: 879–883

57 Andersson JK, Rybo G. Levonorgestrel-releasing intrauterine device in the treatment of menorrhagia. Br J Obstet Gynaecol 1990; 97: 690–694

58 Istre O, Trolle B. Treatment of menorrhagia with the levonorgestrel intrauterine system versus endometrial resection. Fertil Steril 2001; 76: 304–309

59 Crosignani PG, Vercellini P, Mosconi P et al. Levonorgestrel-releasing intrauterine device versus hysteroscopic endometrial resection in the treatment of dysfunctional uterine bleeding. Obstet Gynecol 1997; 90: 257–263

60 Nagrani R, Bowen-Simpkins P, Barrington J. Can the levonorgestrel intrauterine system replace surgical treatment for the management of menorrhagia? Br J Obstet Gynaecol 2002; 109: 345–347

61 Serial and cross-over studies in the treatment of dysfunctional uterine bleeding with tranexamic acid, mefanamic acid and ethamsylate. In: Bonnar J, Smith SK. (eds) Dysfunctional Uterine Bleeding. London: Royal Society of Medicine Press, 1994; 102–103

62 National Institute of Clinical Excellence (NICE), 11 Strand, London WC2N 5HR, UK

Emeka Okaro George Condous Tom Bourne

The use of ultrasound in the management of gynaecological conditions

Out-patient assessment and investigation is changing the management of common gynaecological conditions. This has been driven by the demands of both patients and clinicians to provide a rapid, accurate diagnosis, with the minimum of investigations and invasive procedures. The need to avoid the unnecessary costs of multiple out-patient visits and in-patient admissions is also a major factor in this development.

Transvaginal ultrasonography (TVS) now has a pivotal role for the assessment of gynaecological patients in almost all areas of the specialty. Transvaginal probes provide high-resolution images of the pelvic organs, providing reliable and reproducible information. The use of a vaginal probe can be thought of as a natural extension of the conventional bimanual examination. The fact that a full bladder is not required improves patient acceptability.

Patients with early pregnancy problems and acute gynaecological conditions are ideally suited to assessment by ultrasonography at the time of presentation. A scan should be seen as a part of the overall clinical assessment of the patient and never looked at in isolation. Hence, we believe that a gynaecologist who can weigh up all the available information about the patient and place the scan findings in the correct context should carry out the scan. An accurate scan can enable the clinician to avoid surgery in some cases, and select the correct surgical approach in others. For women with menstrual disorders,

Mr Emeka Okaro MRCOG, Clinical Research Fellow, The Early Pregnancy, Gynaecological Ultrasound and Minimal Access Surgery Unit, St George's Hospital Medical School, London SW17 0QT, UK (for correspondence)

Mr George Condous MRCOG, Clinical Research Fellow, The Early Pregnancy, Gynaecological Ultrasound and Minimal Access Surgery Unit, St George's Hospital Medical School, London SW17 0QT, UK

Mr Tom Bourne PhD MRCOG, Consultant, The Early Pregnancy, Gynaecological Ultrasound and Minimal Access Surgery Unit, St George's Hospital Medical School, London SW17 0QT, UK

postmenopausal bleeding and chronic pelvic pain, TVS can be combined with out-patient endometrial sampling techniques as part of a 'one-stop' approach to diagnosis and management.[1,2]

This review aims to deal with the role of ultrasonography in the assessment of the patient presenting with acute or chronic symptoms, in which gynaecological pathology is suspected. Transvaginal ultrasonography is an extension of the clinical examination, it will not diagnose the cause of all presenting complaints; however, the failure to demonstrate pathology can be highly re-assuring and avoid the need for further investigation. The role of ultrasonography in the assessment of the infertile women is not included in this review.

HARDWARE AND PROCEDURES

The minimum requirements are a transvaginal probe (5–7.5 MHz), a 3.5 MHz transabdominal transducer and facilities for capturing images – either as a hard copy or digitally. The facility to perform Doppler studies or carry out three-dimensional ultrasonography is not required. Appropriate cleaning of the transducer using a germicidal (e.g. 70% alcohol) cloth or spray, after first wiping off the gel, is effective in preventing cross-infection. Hydrosonography (HS) is a simple technique involving the instillation of sterile saline into the uterine cavity as described by Parsons et al.[3] and Bourne et al.[4] Using a bi-valve speculum to view the cervix, a catheter is inserted into the uterine cavity. We use a 10 French paediatric nasogastric feeding tube. Alternatives to this include a modified Pipelle de Cornier (Prodimed, Neuilly-en-Thelle, France) and thin balloon catheters. The presence of a balloon helps to reduce back-flow of saline and maintain uterine distension. These devices tend to more expensive, are not readily available, and distension of the balloon at the internal cervical os can cause increased discomfort. Transvaginal ultrasonography is a well-tolerated procedure; even when HS is performed, the routine use of analgesia is not required in most cases.[5,6] HS should not be performed in the presence of overt pelvic infection. Although the risk of pelvic infection following HS is very small, we use prophylactic antibiotics in all potentially fertile women. One of the most important practical requirements is a database system for archiving ultrasound images and producing reports. This enables the operator to produce a report as soon as the scan has been completed and facilitates audit and clinical review.

EARLY PREGNANCY COMPLICATIONS

Early pregnancy units (EPUs) were introduced as a way of improving the efficiency of dealing with women with early pregnancy loss.[7] Admission can be avoided in about 40% of patients, with a further 20% of those admitted requiring a shorter stay. They provide an easily accessible, ultrasound-based assessment of pregnancy duration, viability and location. The EPU facilitates informed and individualised management, and appropriate counselling of the patient in a dedicated clinical area. Such clinics should run on a daily basis. Access to rapid serum β-human chorionic gonadotrophin (β-hCG) assays is essential. Scans should be performed transvaginally. In the UK, there is

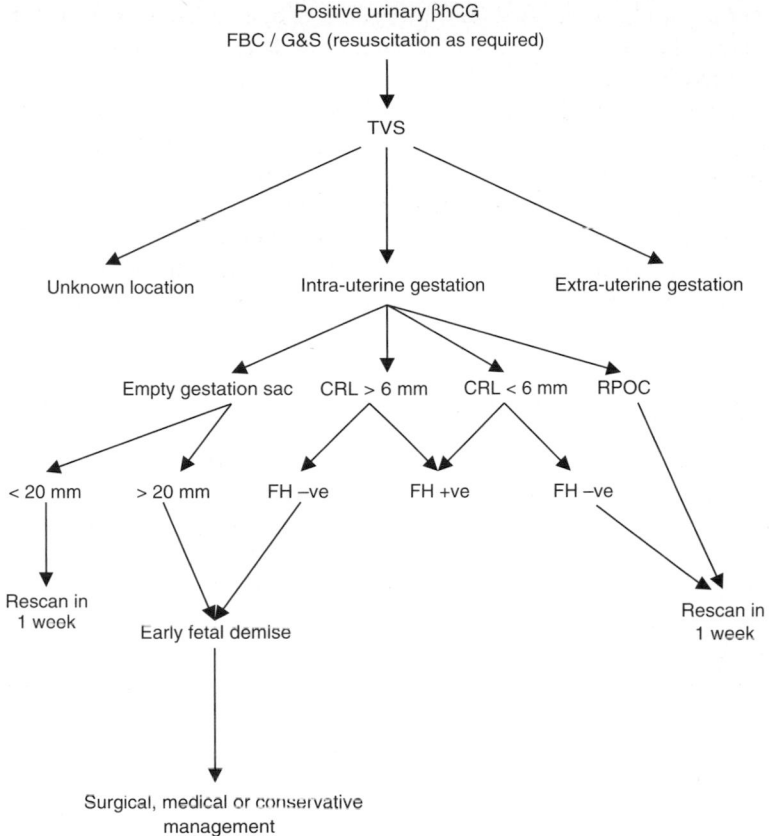

Fig. 1 TVS based assessment of early pregnancy. FBC, Full blood count, G&S, group and save serum; FH, fetal heart rate; CRL, crown rump length; RPOC, retained products of conception.

continuing debate about the preferred method of scanning in early pregnancy. Using transvaginal ultrasonography, a normal intra-uterine pregnancy can be identified at 4 weeks and 3 days' gestation in a woman with a regular 28-day cycle;[8] this is in comparison to 6 weeks' gestation by the transabdominal route.[9] It is important that all patients attending the unit receive a detailed information leaflet explaining the procedure. In our unit, we recently performed an audit to assess the acceptability of TVS. Of 180 consecutive patients, 99% underwent a TVS – 98% had no or mild discomfort during the scan and 96% said they found the procedure acceptable and would undergo another scan, if it were clinically indicated.

Normal intra-uterine pregnancy

An intra-uterine gestational sac can be seen from 4 weeks gestation on TVS. However, confirming pregnancy viability or failure is frequently dependent on changes over time or the presence or absence of fetal cardiac activity (Fig. 1). In early pregnancy, the gestational sac grows in diameter at approximately 1 mm/day.[10] The gestational sac usually has a thick echogenic ring surrounding

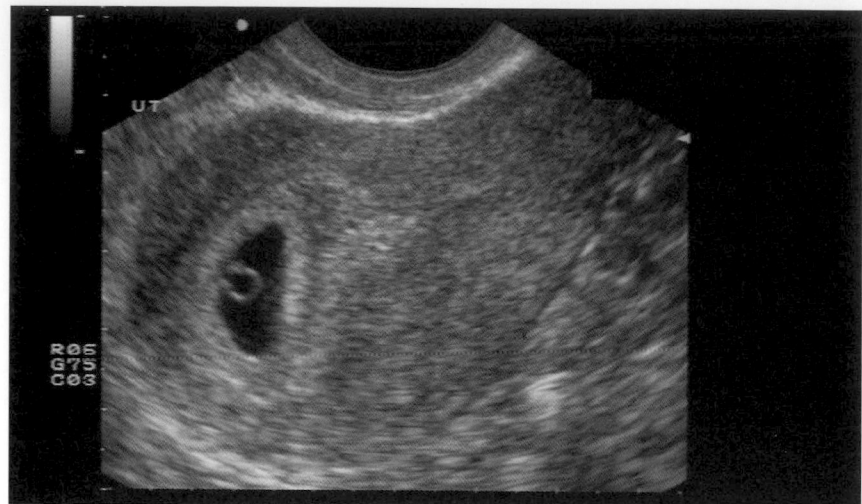

Fig. 2 TVS of an intra-uterine gestation sac and yolk sac; 5 weeks' gestation.

the echolucent central chorionic sac, and an eccentric location within the endometrial cavity. The concept of combining ultrasound with measurements of serum β-hCG levels is well described using a discriminatory zone.[11–13] When the serum β-hCG level is greater than 1000 IU, an intra-uterine gestation sac should be visible by transvaginal ultrasonography; however, visualisation is dependent upon a number of factors, including type of probe and ultrasound machine used, the presence of fibroids, operator experience and multiple gestations.[10,14] The yolk sac can be visualized from 5 weeks' gestation (Fig. 2), and the early embryonic pole from approximately 6 weeks. The embryonic pole is initially recognisable as a thickening along the yolk sac; it is linear to begin with, subsequently becoming curved. The embryonic growth rate is 1 mm/day and cardiac activity starts at approximately 5 weeks after the last menstrual period. Embryonic bradycardia can be associated with poor pregnancy outcome,[15] and a follow-up scan is warranted to confirm viability.

Miscarriage

Some 30% of women will complain of pain or bleeding during early pregnancy and approximately 15% of clinically recognisable pregnancies will result in miscarriage, the majority before the 13th week. The risk of miscarriage is reduced to 3% if a viable embryo is seen on ultrasound. Knowledge of the normal developmental parameters in early pregnancy is important. Of principal importance is not the earliest point at which a structure can be seen (threshold), but the point when a structure is always seen in a normally developing intra-uterine pregnancy (discriminatory level) and so its absence is diagnostic of pregnancy failure.

Early fetal demise

The diagnosis of early fetal demise by transvaginal ultrasound is based on a gestational sac with a mean sac diameter > 20 mm without a yolk sac or > 25 mm

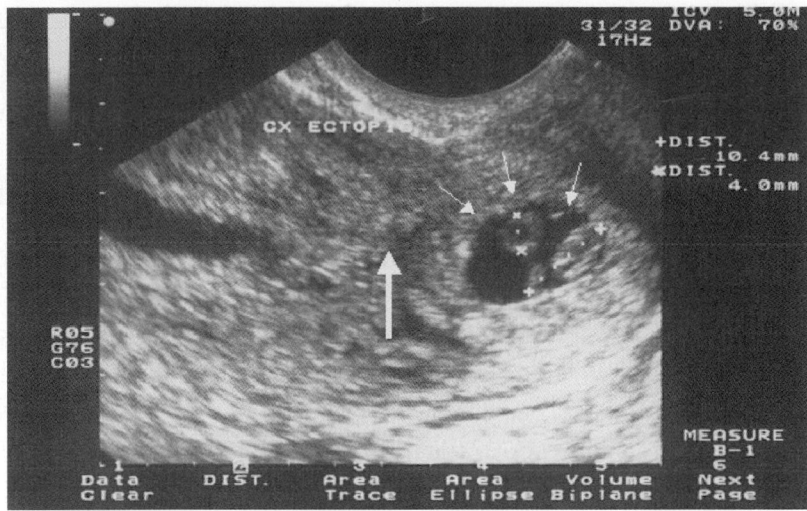

Fig. 3 TVS of an anteverted uterus, internal os (large arrow) with a viable cervical ectopic pregnancy (small arrows), the crown rump length is 10 mm with a 4 mm yolk sac.

without an embryo.[16,17] The diagnosis may only be made on the basis of an absent heart beat when the crown rump length is at least 6 mm, as about one-third of embryos with a crown rump length of less than 5 mm have no demonstrable cardiac activity.[18] Small or irregular gestational sacs, discrepancies between the crown rump length and gestational age, or an abnormal embryonic heart rate pattern are predictors of a poor pregnancy outcome.[15] When there is any uncertainty, a repeat scan with an interval of a week is necessary before a definite diagnosis can be made. Once a diagnosis of miscarriage has been made, the patient can be offered either surgical intervention or expectant management. The majority of women will choose expectant management.[19] Women with an incomplete miscarriage can be confidently offered expectant management in the expectation that over 80% will complete their miscarriage within 2 weeks; the likelihood of success does not necessarily relate to the ultrasound-based estimate of the amount of products left in the cavity.[20,21] For missed miscarriage and anembryonic pregnancy, miscarriage is often more painful and less likely to become complete in the same time span.[20]

Ectopic pregnancy

We were all taught that a patient presenting with abdominal pain and/or bleeding in early pregnancy has an ectopic pregnancy until proved otherwise. Nothing has changed. Whereas, previously, the role of ultrasound was to demonstrate an intra-uterine pregnancy, the use of TVS has substantially increased the possibility of demonstrating early ectopic pregnancies before major complications such as intraperitoneal bleeding occur. The number of laparoscopies carried out to exclude an ectopic pregnancy should be significantly reduced. A gestational sac of an ectopic pregnancy as small as 5 mm, and a complex adnexal mass as small as 10 mm in diameter can be seen with TVS (Fig. 3).[22,23] However, progress has been at a price, and an increasing number of women attend at very early stages of pregnancy when the pregnancy site cannot be demonstrated clearly. Various highly sensitive and specific diagnostic algorithms have been developed to clarify this situation based on TVS, β-hCG and/or serum progesterone.[24,25] In general, patients with symptoms and clinical findings suggestive of an ectopic gestation will fall into one of three categories:

1 An intra-uterine pregnancy will be diagnosed on scan: effectively this will exclude an extra-uterine location. The frequency of heterotopic pregnancy in spontaneous conceptions is estimated at between 1:10,000 and 1:50,000, but as high as 1:100 in assisted conceptions,[26] and should be suspected if there are persistent symptoms.

2 An extra-uterine gestation will be visualized by ultrasound; or features highly predictive of one (e.g. haemoperitoneum).

3 No evidence of an intra- or extra-uterine gestation will be found by ultrasonography: a pregnancy of unknown location (PUL).

Further management will be dependent upon the clinical status of the patient. In recent years, we have noted a significant reduction in those patients presenting with acute haemodynamic compromise due to a ruptured ectopic pregnancy. Ectopic pregnancies are detected earlier than before. This has meant that more conservative methods of treatment can be used, whether surgical (laparoscopic), medical (methotrexate), or expectant.

All non-surgical methods of treating ectopic gestations will need intensive follow-up with serial β-hCG values to ensure resolution. Patient compliance is essential for those being treated on an out-patient basis.

Pregnancy of unknown location

The earlier that patients present to the EPU the more women will have no sonographic features of either an extra or intra-uterine pregnancy. In this group, there will be patients who have a very early viable intra-uterine pregnancy, those with an ectopic gestation and those with a failing pregnancy – whether intra-uterine or extra-uterine. These women need to be managed on the basis of their serum β-hCG and progesterone values. In general, a rise in serum β-hCG of greater than 66% over 48 h is compatible with a viable intra-uterine pregnancy.[27] In ectopic pregnancy, the serum β-hCG tends to plateau or demonstrate an abnormal rise. High serum progesterone levels tend to be associated with a viable intra-uterine pregnancy.[28] However, there are exceptions, both 'sick' intra-uterine pregnancies and 'flourishing' ectopic pregnancies can give conflicting results.[29]

Co-existent pathology

Ovarian pathology is common in early pregnancy. One advantage of TVS is the ability to visualize the adnexa clearly in early pregnancy. The majority of adnexal pathology will be physiological in nature. Typically, these are luteal cysts, and will resolve spontaneously as the pregnancy advances. The need for surgical intervention is unusual. Some persistent symptomatic cysts will require either aspiration or surgical intervention,[30] although the management will depend on the ultrasound-based characterisation of the mass. Those patients with cysts managed expectantly should be re-scanned 6 weeks after delivery to check that the cyst has resolved or arrange surgical intervention if necessary.

THE ACUTE GYNAECOLOGY UNIT (AGU)

An ultrasound scan does not negate the need for a comprehensive history to be taken and physical examination carried out for the assessment of the acutely ill gynaecology patient. TVS can be seen as a natural extension of the clinical examination. In women with acute pelvic pain, TVS plays an important role in excluding and diagnosing pathology as well as mapping pelvic pain. A young woman with a negative pregnancy test, no pelvic tenderness on bimanual examination and with a normal pelvic scan is unlikely to have serious gynaecological pathology. Positive findings such as an ovarian cyst or tubal pathology can then be used as the basis for patient management (Fig. 4)

Adnexal masses

Even in postmenopausal women, the ovary can be seen in the majority of women. TVS has been shown to be accurate in the characterization of adnexal masses in different populations of women.[31,32] In premenopausal women, ovarian cysts are common (Fig. 5), and the majority of these are physiological and can be managed expectantly with a follow-up scan in 6 weeks. Knowledge of the last menstrual cycle will help indicate the most likely cause of the pain.

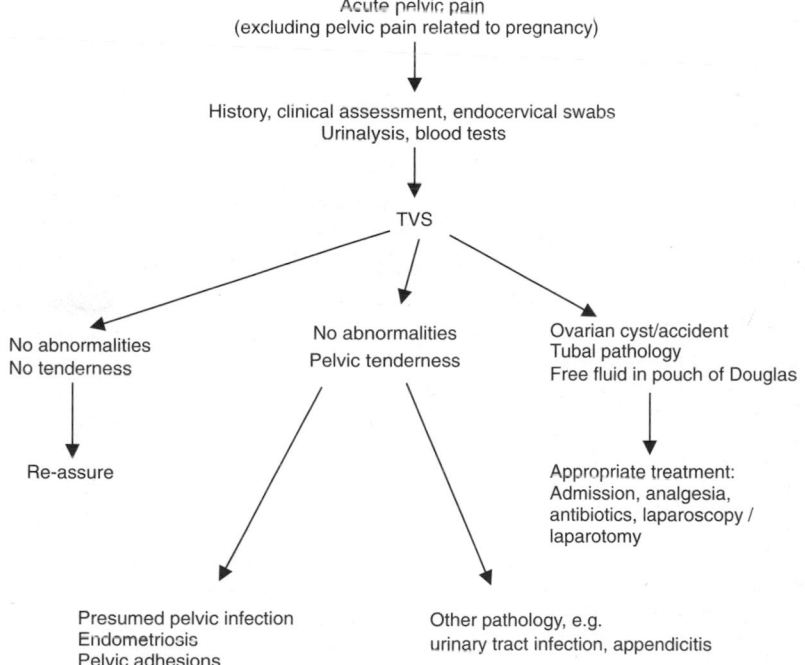

Fig. 4 The role of ultrasound in the triage of women with acute pelvic pain.

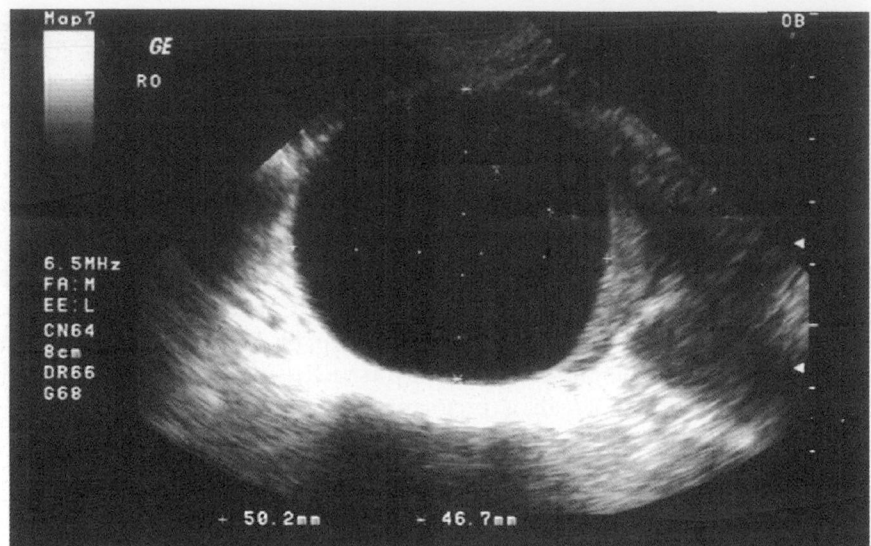

Fig. 5 TVS of a 50 x 46 mm unilocular ovarian cyst.

Mid-cycle pain 'Mittelschmerz' is caused by irritation of the peritoneum by fluid or blood at the time of ovulation, and on TVS there may be general pelvic tenderness and free fluid in the pelvis. Physiological (follicular or luteal) ovarian cysts are usually anechoic on TVS and vary in size. The majority will resolve spontaneously. Haemorrhage into a corpus luteum cyst has a characteristic 'web-like' appearance on ultrasound (Fig. 6), and is usually a self-limiting event that often responds to anti-inflammatory analgesia. Rupture of a physiological cyst may cause acute onset of lower abdominal pain

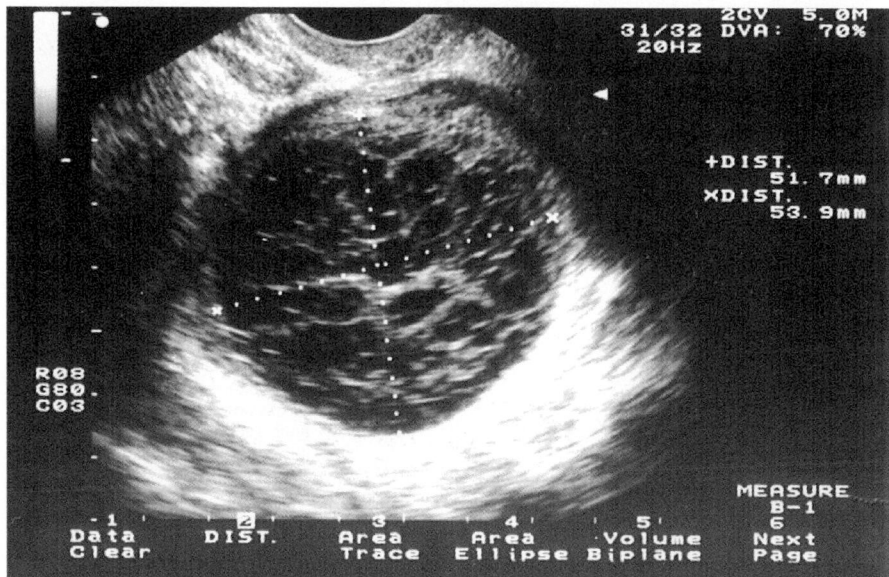

Fig. 6 TVS of a 50 x 50 mm haemorrhagic ovarian cyst, with a characteristic web-like appearance.

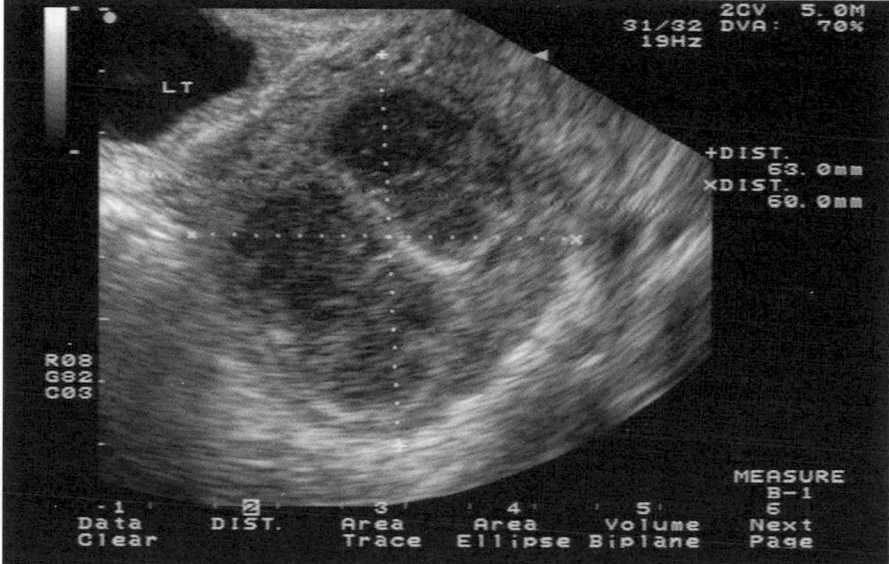

Fig. 7 TVS of a pyosalpinx: thick walled structure with loculated fluid.

and an ultrasound scan may demonstrate free fluid in the pouch of Douglas and a collapsed flaccid cyst with an irregular wall. In women with a history suggestive of endometriosis, a characteristic cyst (endometrioma) with low-level echoes may be seen. Although they are usually stuck in the pelvis and unlikely to undergo torsion, acute haemorrhage into the cyst can cause acute pelvic pain.

Adnexal masses < 5 cm in diameter are unlikely to undergo torsion. The diagnosis of torsion of an adnexal mass should be made on clinical grounds, as there are no typical ultrasound features. Colour Doppler has been used to investigate ovarian torsion; however, even in the presence of flow in the mass, ovarian blood flow may still be compromised.[33]

Tubal pathology

Sexually active young women between the ages of 16–25 years are particularly at risk of pelvic inflammatory disease (PID). The main cause is chlamydial salpingitis. PID can cause acute lower abdominal pain, vaginal discharge, a leukocytosis and systemic upset, but frequently presents as deep dyspareunia and non-specific abdominal pain. The Fallopian tubes are not routinely seen on grey-scale ultrasound; however, inflammation leads to fluid collecting in the tube as well as thickening of the walls (Fig. 7). The tube can then be seen as a cystic structure. Site-specific pelvic tenderness will also be apparent using the probe. The ultrasound appearance of an acutely infected tube can frequently be misdiagnosed as an endometrioma – both may have a thick wall and 'ground glass' contents. A chronic hydrosalpinx will be cystic with a thin wall (Fig. 8) and may be a coincidental finding.[34] Prompt diagnosis and treatment is important to reduce the incidence of tubal factor infertility and ectopic pregnancy, as these are proportional to the number of episodes of PID.

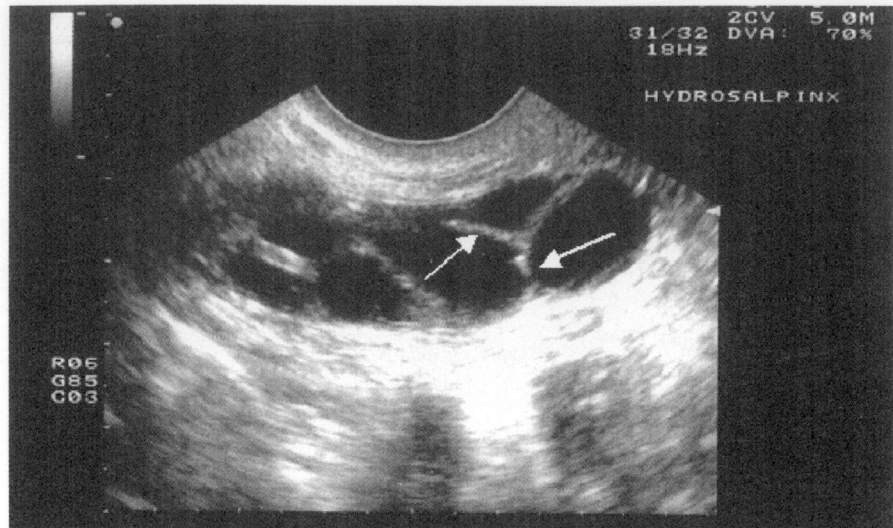

Fig. 8: TVS of a chronic hydrosalpinx. The thin-walled structure with incomplete septa (arrows) that are pathogenomonic of the dilated fluid filled tube.

ABNORMAL UTERINE BLEEDING – THE 'ONE-STOP' ULTRASOUND-BASED CLINIC

In-patient hysteroscopy under general anaesthesia is no longer considered acceptable practice as a first line strategy for the management of abnormal uterine bleeding. Currently, in the UK, patients with these problems often endure multiple hospital visits for assessment, investigations and treatment. Increasingly, out-patient-based management strategies are being established to avoid this situation.[35,36] These 'one-stop' clinics are generally based on flexible or rigid hysteroscopy, with directed or blind endometrial biopsies. We believe that the logical strategy is a 'one-stop' clinic based on TVS and HS as the primary diagnostic tools in combination with blind endometrial biopsy. Hysteroscopy is currently still the gold standard for uterine cavity evaluation;[37,38] however, TVS, with or without the addition of saline as a negative contrast agent, compares favourably.[5,6,39,40]

MENORRHAGIA

The role of a scan in this context is to exclude focal intracavity pathology in the form of fibroids or polyps. Furthermore, extra-uterine pathology such as endometriomas can be assessed. Data relating to endometrial thickness in pre-menopausal women are scanty, and no specific cut-off values exist to define normality. In general, however, the endometrium must be thought of as a dynamic structure that should change during the cycle. Persisting thick endometrium may be pathological.

Endometrial polyps

Polyps are echogenic structures with a fairly homogeneous texture without disruption of the myometrial–endometrial interface (Fig. 9). Recent evidence

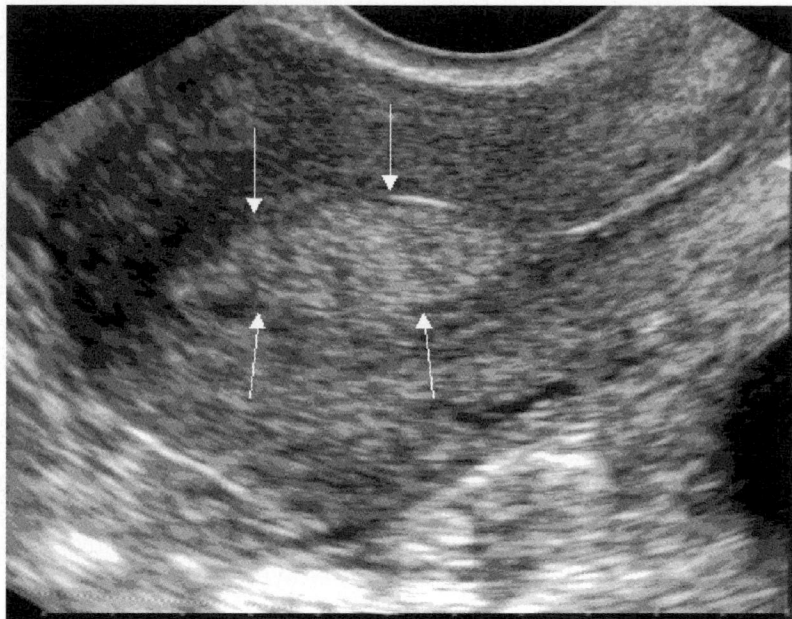

Fig. 9: TVS of an anteverted uterus, the hyperechoeic area (arrows) represents an endometrial polyp.

suggests that 10% of asymptomatic premenopausal women have ultrasound evidence of endometrial polyps.[41] In comparison to hysteroscopy, ultrasound with saline instillation is at least as good as hysteroscopy for detecting these lesions (Fig. 10).[5,6] Thus women with polyps can be selected for hysteroscopic resection. Problems may arise when distinguishing between larger polyps and submucous fibroids.[6]

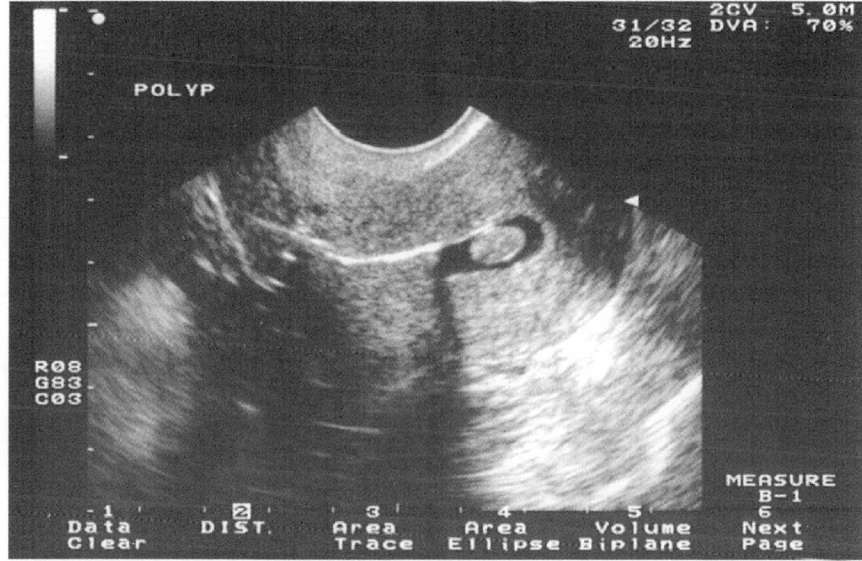

Fig. 10: TVS of a retroverted uterus with an endometrial polyp depicted by hydrosonography.

Uterine fibroids

The ultrasound appearances of fibroids are varied. Before the menopause, they tend to be a well-defined heterogeneous or hypoechoeic uterine mass in nature, and cystic areas may be visualized within the fibroid if it is degenerating. Areas of calcification tend to be seen more often in postmenopausal women. Submucosal fibroids distort the uterine cavity and have an inhomogeneous texture with possible continuity with the myometrium (Fig. 11). Their accurate classification with regard to size, number and location allows selection for transcervical resection in appropriate cases. They are classified according to the European Society of Gynaecologic Endoscopy Classification: type 0 (pedunculated submucous fibroid without intramural extension), type I (sessile and with an intramural part of less than 50%) and type II (with an intramural part of 50% or more). Fedele et al.[40] demonstrated the sensitivity and specificity of TVS for the diagnosis of submucosal fibroids to be 100% and 94%, respectively. Outpatient hysteroscopy performed on the same population had a sensitivity and specificity of 100% and 96%, respectively. The only criticism of TVS in this study was its apparent inability to differentiate between endometrial polyps and submucosal fibroids. The scans in this study were performed in the secretory phase of the cycle; endometrial polyps tend to be hyperechoeic structures, easily masked by a thick secretory endometrium. By performing the scans during the proliferative phase, the distinction between intracavity fibroids and polyps is easier to make.[5] Once again, the patients may be selected for hysteroscopic resection. Occasionally, a pedunculated fibroid may mimic a solid adnexal mass such as an ovarian fibroma; failure to visualise the ovary separate to the lesion may necessitate surgical intervention.

Adenomyosis

This is a common gynaecological disorder that affects women of reproductive age. Until recently, the diagnosis was rarely made prior to hysterectomy. TVS has

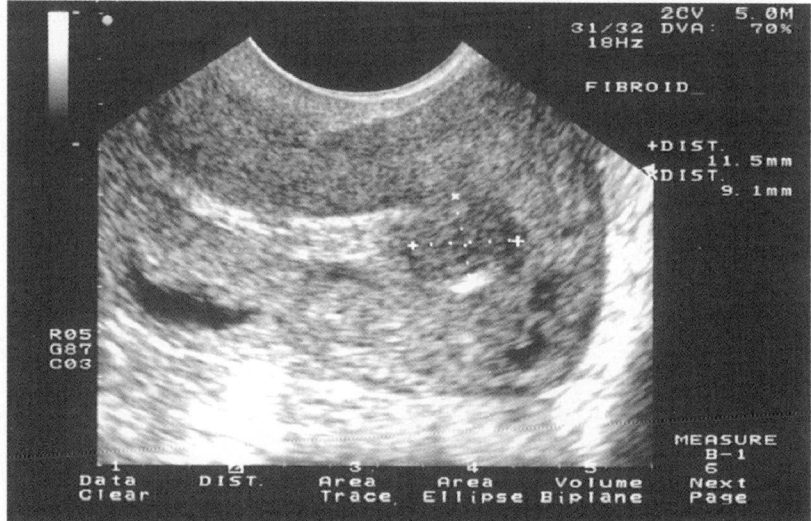

Fig. 11 TVS of a retroverted uterus, the endometrium is hyperechoeic, and there is an 11 x 9 mm submucous fibroid at the fundus. Note that the echo-texture of the fibroid and the myometrium are the same.

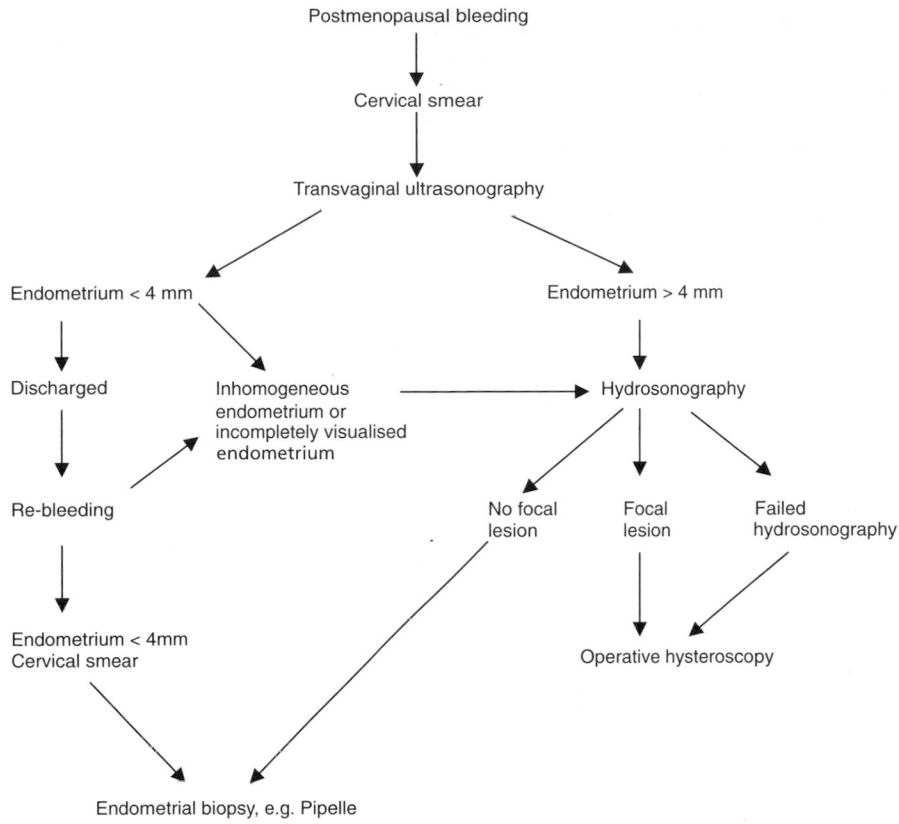

Fig. 12 TVS-based management of postmenopausal bleeding.

been shown to have a sensitivity and specificity of 86% and 86%, respectively, for the diagnosis of diffuse adenomyosis.[42] The most common appearance of the myometrium in diffuse adenomyosis is areas of hypo-echoic and heterogeneous texture; in 50% of cases, myometrial cysts may be visible.[42]

POSTMENOPAUSAL BLEEDING

There is almost universal agreement that, irrespective of hormone use, an endometrial thickness measurement of 4 mm or less is associated with endometrial atrophy.[43–47] Irrespective of HRT use, using a > 4 mm cut-off value to define an abnormal endometrium, 96% of women with endometrial cancer and 92% of women with endometrial disease (hyperplasia, polyps and fibroids) will have an abnormal result, with a false positive rate of 39% and 19%, respectively.[48]

The high sensitivity of TVS makes it an effective non-invasive test for selecting women with vaginal bleeding who do not require an endometrial biopsy (Fig. 12). Conversely, its relatively poor specificity means that an abnormal endometrial thickness measurement needs to be followed up by a second stage test in the form of an endometrial biopsy. Hydrosonography has a role in the assessment of PMB. When the endometrial echo obtained by ultrasonography is unclear, the instillation of sterile saline will outline the cavity and improve diagnostic performance. A normal scan in a woman with PMB is highly re-assuring. A negative TVS result can decrease pre-test odds of cancer by approximately 90% in women regardless of hormone use. A postmenopausal woman with vaginal bleeding has a pre-test probability of endometrial cancer of approximately 10%. Her probability of cancer is reduced to 1% following a normal transvaginal scan.[48] It is important to emphasize that endometrial sampling should be considered mandatory in women where the endometrium cannot be measured because endometrial pathology, and even endometrial cancer, is a common finding in these women. In women managed conservatively (i.e. endometrial thickness < 4 mm), re-bleeding occurs in 6–27% of cases, and endometrial pathology is rarely found in those with an endometrial thickness of < 5 mm on repeat TVS.[49,50] However, if the endometrium is > 5 mm on a repeat ultrasound scan, a biopsy is indicated to exclude endometrial pathology. Fluid in the endometrial cavity may be seen in postmenopausal women, but is not thought to be of significance.[51–53]

IRREGULAR BLEEDING ON HORMONE REPLACEMENT THERAPY

For a 4 mm endometrial thickness cut-off, the number of women with false positive results is higher among women using hormone replacement therapy (HRT; 23%) compared to non-users (8%).[48] The higher false positive results seen in HRT users are related to the day of the cycle when the scan is performed. For patients taking sequential HRT, the timing of an ultrasound scan suggested for optimal results is 5–10 days from the end of the progestogen phase.[51,54] In contrast, TVS can be performed at any time in women receiving continuous HRT. Omodei et al. have shown that the ET does not differ between women taking sequential compared to those on continuous combined HRT (3.6 mm versus 3.2 mm), if the measurement is taken on the days 5–10 day following the last progestogen tablet.[55] A woman with a 1% risk of cancer, which is the risk associated with vaginal bleeding in a postmenopausal woman using combined HRT, will have a 0.1% risk of cancer following a negative ultrasound examination result.

TAMOXIFEN AND THE ENDOMETRIUM

Tamoxifen is used as adjuvant therapy in women diagnosed with breast cancer and, more recently, its effectiveness as a chemoprevention agent has been established.[56] Tamoxifen use is associated with an increased risk of developing endometrial cancer (2/1000 tamoxifen treated women). The ultrasound appearances of the endometrium for women taking tamoxifen are often difficult to interpret. Many have an apparent thick cystic endometrium. Using HS, 50% of such cases have been shown to harbour large endometrial polyps.[57] The residues have subendometrial cystic changes with thin atrophic endometrium. For women who have abnormal bleeding on tamoxifen, the ultrasound data are unclear and it is advisable to seek histological confirmation that the cavity is normal.

TVS has also been proposed as a non-invasive means of screening for endometrial cancer in tamoxifen-treated women. Kedar et al. evaluated 111 asymptomatic, at-risk women randomly assigned to tamoxifen or placebo in a pilot chemoprevention study.[57] TVS was performed after a median time of 2 years and the mean endometrial thickness in the tamoxifen-treated group was nearly twice that of the placebo group. Although no cancers were detected in this study, 10 women had endometrial hyperplasia in the tamoxifen group. They concluded that an endometrial thickness > 8 mm had a 100% positive predictive value at detecting endometrial pathology. Other authors have published conflicting data questioning the efficacy of TVS as a surveillance method.[58-60] Timmerman et al. compared the ability of TVS with hydrosonography to office hysteroscopy, in detecting endometrial pathology in women on adjuvant tamoxifen therapy.[61] In this randomised cross-over study, there was no difference in the sensitivity and specificity of TVS/hydrosonography and hysteroscopy. However, two endometrial cancers were detected by ultrasound alone. TVS/hydrosonography was more acceptable to the patients.

Pretreatment screening has also been suggested. Berliere et al. screened 264 women with breast cancer and found that 17% (46/264) of asymptomatic postmenopausal had a thickened endometrial lining prior to tamoxifen therapy.[62] Hysteroscopy confirmed submucous myoma (7), benign polyps (34), simple hyperplasia (3), atypical hyperplasia (1), and endometrial cancer (1). Of the patients who subsequently developed premalignant or malignant conditions on tamoxifen therapy, 80% had had an endometrial lesion at pretreatment assessment. This would suggest that pretreatment assessment might identify women at risk of developing endometrial cancer. The small increase in risk of endometrial cancer is out-weighed by the benefits tamoxifen provides for women who have suffered from or who are at risk of breast cancer. Pretreatment assessment prior to tamoxifen therapy appears encouraging. However, its cost-effectiveness needs to be assessed prospectively as the majority of the premalignant and malignant endometrial lesions present with symptoms and the treatment of early stage endometrial cancer is quite successful. Only a large randomised trial with reduction in the mortality rate from endometrial cancer as the end point could prove that endometrial cancer monitoring in patients with breast cancer who are treated with tamoxifen is useful.

OVARIAN PATHOLOGY

Today, an ultrasound scan should not only demonstrate that ovarian pathology is present, but also give a reasonably accurate assessment of the likely pathology of the lesion. The likelihood of malignancy should be commented on and the probable histopathology. On the basis of subjective impression alone, this can be provided with a high degree of accuracy.[31] Ovarian pathology is common amongst young women, and the overwhelming majority of these lesions are physiological. In these cases, repeating the scan at an interval is important, as many ovarian masses are transient and will resolve without intervention. It is for persistent masses that characterisation has a role. The ability to differentiate between benign and malignant disease allows appropriate management to be selected, whether expectant, the use of minimal access surgical techniques, or open surgical procedures.

The majority of benign ovarian lesions are physiological in nature, and are frequently managed expectantly. In general, a benign cyst is simple and unilocular with no solid elements; for these lesions, a repeat scan at an interval will often demonstrate resolution. Persistent cysts of this type are most

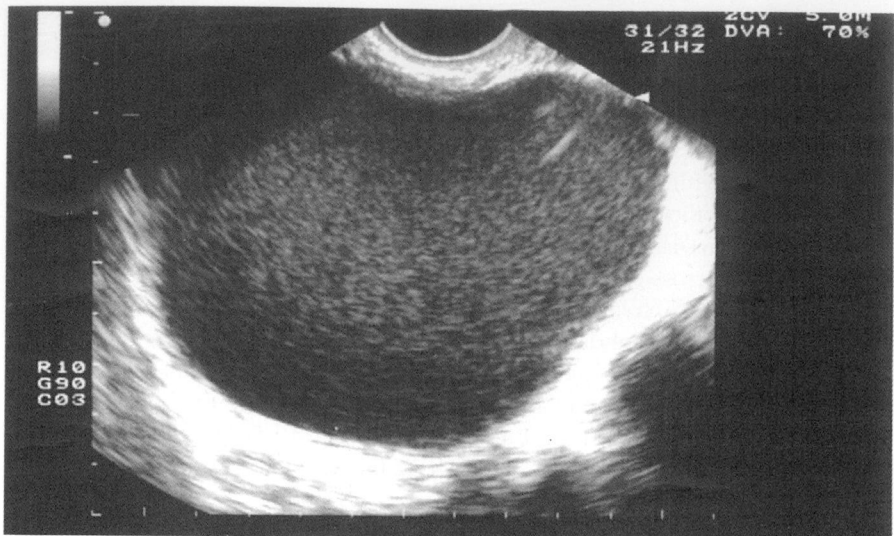

Fig. 13 TVS of a large endometrioma, with a characteristic 'ground glass' appearance.

frequently cystadenomas. Most pathology can be characterised on the basis of pattern recognition. Common examples are endometriomas (Fig. 13)[63,64] and dermoid cysts (Fig. 14).[32,65] These account for over two-thirds of persistent adnexal masses in premenopausal women.[66] These lesions can be particularly difficult to score using morphological scoring systems and, as angiogenesis is ubiquitous throughout the ovarian cycle, colour Doppler is of limited value.[67,68] Historically, dermoid cysts have created difficulties for morphological scoring systems designed to assign a risk of malignancy.[69] However, on the basis of subjective impression, Jermy et al. showed that the positive predictive value of

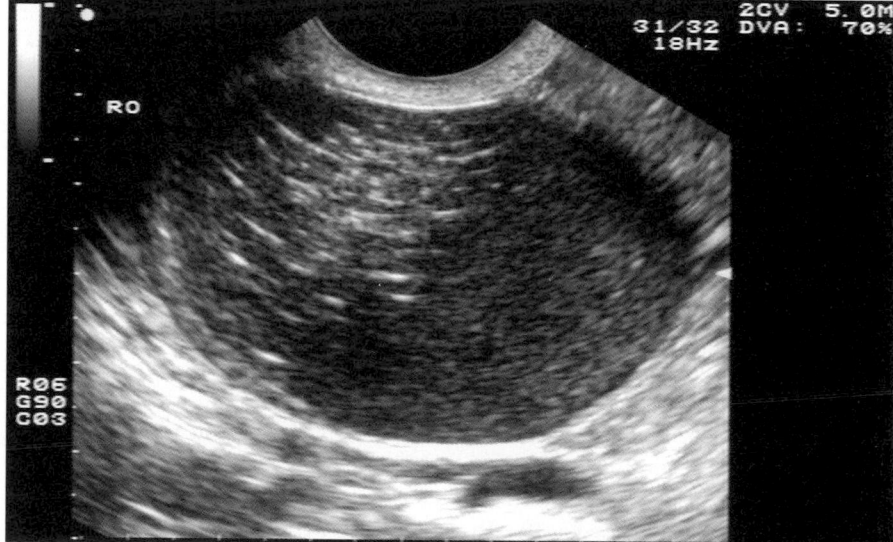

Fig. 14 TVS of a large dermoid cyst of the ovary. The echogenic strands represent hair and the speckled appearance is due to the sebaceous material within the cyst.

TVS for the diagnosis of endometriomas and dermoid cysts is 96.7% and 97.1%, respectively; the false positive rate was 3.8% and 3.0%, respectively.[32] This means that women can be confidently selected for appropriate surgery, as laparoscopic surgery has significant advantages compared with laparotomy for the treatment of benign adnexal masses.[70] More recently, sophisticated statistical algorithms have been employed to evaluate the nature of ovarian masses.[71,72] However, none of these models has been able to out-perform the opinion of an experienced operator. Timmerman et al. have shown that, based on subjective impression, the majority of adnexal masses are easy to characterise, with agreement between operators of varying experience in 65% of cases.[31] Approximately 10% of cases are difficult to classify and these are often tubo-ovarian masses and cyst-adenofibromas. It is on the classification of these difficult cases that mathematical models should concentrate; these models may then help to reduce the experience required to arrive at an accurate diagnosis.

A major problem that exists for the evaluation of ovarian masses is standardisation of terms. As a result, when applying any algorithm there may be a lack of reproducibility between different units.[71–74] This has led to the publication of agreed terms and definitions from the International Ovarian Tumour Analysis (IOTA) Group.[75] This may lead to a more useful application of future diagnostic models.

Clearly, for any patient presenting with an ovarian mass, the principal concern is the likelihood of malignancy. Several studies have now confirmed that the likelihood of malignancy in a simple unilocular cyst with no solid papillary projections is low (Table 1)

Any deviation from this is associated with an increasing risk of missing a malignancy. The main predictor for malignancy is the presence of solid papillary projections (Fig. 15). Based on the initial work of Granberg et al., risk of malignancy in a lesion containing a solid projection is as high as 50% (Table 2).[76]

The introduction of colour Doppler in addition to morphological assessment was initially felt to have significant promise.[77] However, as neovascularisation is present throughout the normal menstrual cycle, assessment of ovarian blood flow is not integral to the evaluation of an ovarian mass.[78]

Table 1 Positive predictive value of locularity in differentiating benign from malignant ovarian tumours

Reference	Population	n	Prevalence of malignancy (%)	Positive predictive value (%)		
				Uni-locular	Multi-locular	Solid
Granberg et al. 1989[76]	All ages	1017	22.4	1.0	40.3	39.2
Granberg et al. 1990[83]	All ages	180	21.7	1.8	37.4	12.5
Valentin et al. 1994[78]	All ages	149	18.8	5.8	17.9	57.9
Meire et al. 1978[84]	All ages	69	26.1	4.8	59.3	–
				Unilocular	Complex	
Deland et al. 1979[84]	All ages	60	28.3	2.6	72.7	
Luxman et al. 1991[85]	Postmeno-pausal	102	28.4	6.1	39.1	

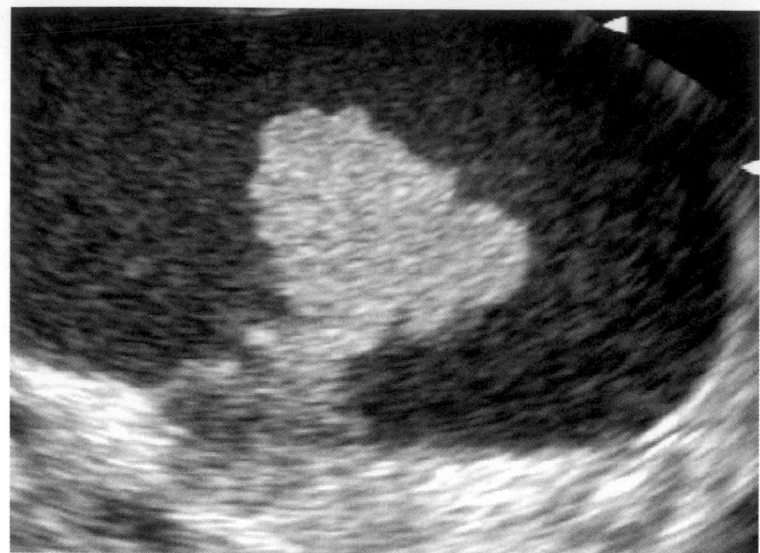

Fig. 15 Ovarian endometroid adenocarcinoma: stage 1A; note the large papillary projection from the cyst wall.

Table 2 Positive and negative predictive values of the presence of papillary projections in differentiating benign from malignant ovarian tumours

Reference	n	Number with papillary projections	PP	PPV	NPV
				Percentage of cystic tumours with	
Granberg et al. 1989[76]	1017	152	16.2	53.3	85.4
Granberg et al. 1990[83]	180	43	29.7	67.4	94.1
Meire et al. 1978[84]	69	18	26.1	83.3	94.1
Valentin et al. 1994[78]	149	42	32.3	40.5	89.7

Subsequently, Jacobs et al. introduced the concept of a 'risk of malignancy index'.[79] The risk of cancer for a given mass was assessed using a weighted score based on the presence of a mass, the patient's age, menopausal status and serum CA 125 level. This was the precursor to a number of studies that have tried to combine various ultrasound parameters, demographic data and serum CA 125 levels to assign a risk of cancer for any given lesion. Using a logistic regression model, Timmerman et al. have demonstrated that a mathematical approach can improve on the use of ultrasound parameters or CA 125 values alone.[71] More sophisticated modelling using neural networks may also enhance test performance.[80,81] However, none of these approaches can improve on the subjective impression of a mass by an experienced observer.[31,82] Using subjective impression, the majority of masses are relatively straightforward to characterise; however, certain lesions cause difficulties including cystadenofibromas, tubo-ovarian pathology and borderline tumours. Overall, the majority of ovarian pathology can be accurately characterised. In this way, appropriate patients can be referred to oncology units and the others selected for minimal access surgery or expectant management, as appropriate.

Transvaginal ultrasonography is now the ultrasound technique of choice for the investigation of many gynaecological disorders. The higher ultrasound frequencies used means that high-resolution images can be obtained, and this has led to an improvement in diagnostic accuracy for many conditions. The fact that a full bladder is not needed to carry out the procedure is a major practical advantage. Women with suspected gynaecological emergencies and early pregnancy complications can now be scanned at the point of admission, and immediate decisions made about management. This seems a more rational policy than having women waiting for departmental scans or experiencing delays because of a need to fill their bladders. Similar improvements in efficiency can be made when assessing women in the out-patients department, or in the context of cancer screening clinics. The desirability of gynaecologists performing their own scans in this context is clear from the point of view of patient management, the fact that the problems of training and quality control have yet to be grasped is another issue entirely. Notwithstanding such reservations, it seems certain that over the next few years the use of a small portable transvaginal ultrasound machine will become an intrinsic part of the gynaecological examination of most patients.

KEY POINTS FOR CLINICAL PRACTICE

Early pregnancy
- Early pregnancy complications should be seen in designated early pregnancy units. Transvaginal ultrasonography and 'same day' serum β-hCG levels should be available
- In case of doubt, a repeat scan should be performed at a 1-week interval
- The majority of women with an incomplete miscarriage will opt for expectant management and 80% will resolve the miscarriage within 2 weeks
- The diagnosis of ectopic pregnancy should be made with a degree of certainty in the majority of cases prior to operative procedures. In turn, a low false positive rate for the diagnosis of ectopic pregnancy will reflect the performance of an early pregnancy unit
- The management of pregnancies of unknown location (PULs) depends on monitoring the serum levels of hCG and progesterone

Acute gynaecology
- Transvaginal ultrasonography has a pivotal role in the assessment of women with acute lower abdominal pain
- An ultrasound scan is the natural extension of a comprehensive history and physical examination
- Ovarian cysts are common, frequently physiological and often transient
- Sexually active young (aged 16–25 years) women are particularly at risk of PID, which may have characteristic features on ultrasound; however, their absence does not exclude the diagnosis.

(Continued on next page)

KEY POINTS FOR CLINICAL PRACTICE• – Continued from previous page

- Adnexal torsion is a clinical diagnosis with no characteristic ultrasound features
- A young woman with a negative pregnancy test, normal physical examination and ultrasound scan is unlikely to have serious gynaecological pathology

The ovary

- A simple unilocular cystic lesion ≤ 5.0 cm is unlikely to be malignant, particularly in premenopausal women. In the absence of significant risk factors for cancer in the history, such cysts do not warrant surgical intervention
- It is very important that a repeat scan is performed on cysts to allow time for spontaneous resolution to take place. Assessments of morphology and blood flow should be seen as second stage tests to be carried out on persistent ovarian masses rather than as a primary investigation
- The application of more sophisticated second stage tests to evaluate a tumour will inevitably compromise the detection rate for early cancer. The more complex a tumour, the more likely it is to be malignant. The presence of papillary projections is a particularly ominous sign
- Some tumours such as benign teratomas (dermoids) and endometriomas have characteristic B-mode ultrasound appearances that may allow them to be characterised purely on the basis of pattern recognition.
- There is a prevalence effect that must be considered when evaluating masses in women at increased risk of ovarian cancer (e.g. strong family history). The odds of finding cancer at surgery in women with a persistent ovarian mass are high, irrespective of the morphology or Doppler findings
- Never just 'perform a scan'. An ultrasound scan should be a part of the evaluation of the whole clinical situation. Any scan can only be interpreted knowing the patient's menopausal status, day of cycle, and drug therapy, in order to know if the findings are appropriate

The endometrium

- It is important to be certain that the endometrium has been measured properly. An 'unmeasurable' endometrium should not be accepted as probably being normal. Hydrosonography should be performed to try to clarify the situation. If it is still unclear, in symptomatic patients this is an indication for an endometrial biopsy
- Overall, the data reviewed in this paper suggest that, in the assessment of symptomatic postmenopausal women, an endometrial thickness cut-off level of < 4 mm will have a high negative predictive value for the absence of cancer
- For women with PMB, if an endometrial thickness of > 4 mm returns a histological diagnosis of atrophy, the possibility of a sampling error should be considered

KEY POINTS FOR CLINICAL PRACTICE• – Continued from previous page

- There are no data to support the examination of asymptomatic postmenopausal women for the presence of pathology. For a disease of such low incidence such an approach is unlikely to be fruitful. However, in the 'real' world, given the data from the ROC curves we would perform an out-patient biopsy on an asymptomatic women not taking hormone therapy, whose endometrium measured more than 8.0 mm
- Women taking hormone replacement therapy have an increased endometrial thickness, and this will change according to the phase of cyclical therapy. In continuous combined regimens, the endometrium is likely to be relatively thin. It is probably best to evaluate such endometria just after the withdrawal bleed. Abnormal bleeding on HRT must still be investigated by biopsy, whilst thick endometrium on HRT is probably just a normal finding in the absence of symptoms
- B-Mode ultrasound imaging provides many answers to the evaluation of the pre- and postmenopausal uterus. For example, the endometrial thickness and echogenicity enable the presence or absence of significant pathology to be assessed in the majority of cases. The use of negative contrast agents introduced into the cavity may further enhance diagnostic confidence, and be of particular value in the recognition of polyps
- A thick endometrium in women taking tamoxifen is associated with the presence of pathology. For those with a cystic endometrium > 8.0 mm, 50% will have polyps that can be demonstrated with hydrosonography. Out-patient biopsy techniques will often miss focal pathology if present, and resection may be necessary.

References

1 Dueholm M, Laursen H, Knudsen UB. A simple one-stop menstrual problem clinic with use of hysterosonography for the diagnosis of abnormal uterine bleeding. Acta Obstet Gynecol Scand 1999; 78: 150–154

2 Jones K, Bourne T. The feasibility of a 'one stop' ultrasound-based clinic for the diagnosis and management of abnormal uterine bleeding. Ultrasound Obstet Gynecol 2001; 17: 517–521

3 Parsons AK, Lense JJ. Sonohysterography for endometrial abnormalities: preliminary results. J Clin Ultrasound 1993; 21: 87–95

4 Bourne T, Lawton F, Leather A, Granberg S, Campbell S, Collins W. Use of intracavity saline instillation and transvaginal ultrasonography to detect a tamoxifen associated endometrial polyp. Ultrasound Obstet Gynecol 1994; 2: 73–75

5 Schwarzler P, Concin H, Bosch H, Berlinger A, Wohlgenannt K, Collins WP, Bourne TH. An evaluation of sonohysterography and diagnostic hysteroscopy for the assessment of intrauterine pathology. Ultrasound Obstet Gynecol 1998; 11: 337–342

6 Widrich T, Bradley LD, Mitchinson AR, Collins RL. Comparison of saline infusion sonography with office hysteroscopy for the evaluation of the endometrium. Am J Obstet Gynecol 1996; 174: 1327–1334

7 Bigrigg MA, Read MD. Management of women referred to early pregnancy assessment unit: care and cost effectiveness. BMJ 1991; 302: 577–579

8 Fossum GT, Davajan V, Kletzky OA. Early detection of pregnancy with transvaginal ultrasound. Fertil Steril 1988; 49: 788–791

9 Nyberg DA, Laing FC, Filly RA. Threatened abortion: sonographic distinction of normal and abnormal gestation sacs. Radiology 1986; 158: 397–400

10 Nyberg DA, Filly RA, Mahony BS, Monroe S, Laing FC, Jeffrey Jr RB. Early gestation: correlation of HCG levels and sonographic identification. AJR Am J Roentgenol 1985; 144: 951–954

11 Barnhart KT, Simhan H, Kamelle SA. Diagnostic accuracy of ultrasound above and below the beta-hCG discriminatory zone. Obstet Gynecol 1999; 94: 583–587

12 Kadar N, DeVore G, Romero R. Discriminatory hCG zone: its use in the sonographic evaluation for ectopic pregnancy. Obstet Gynecol 1981; 58: 156–161

13 Peisner DB, Timor-Tritsch IE. The discriminatory zone of beta-hCG for vaginal probes. J Clin Ultrasound 1990; 18: 280–285

14 Bernaschek G, Rudelstorfer R, Csaicsich P. Vaginal sonography versus serum human chorionic gonadotropin in early detection of pregnancy. Am J Obstet Gynecol 1988; 158: 608–612

15 Martinez JM, Comas C, Ojuel J, Borrell A, Puerto B, Fortuny A. Fetal heart rate patterns in pregnancies with chromosomal disorders or subsequent fetal loss. Obstet Gynecol 1996; 87: 118–121

16 Goldstein SR. Early detection of pathologic pregnancy by transvaginal sonography. J Clin Ultrasound 1990; 18: 262–273

17 Cacciatore B, Tiitinen A, Stenman UH, Ylostalo P. Normal early pregnancy: serum hCG levels and vaginal ultrasonography findings. Br J Obstet Gynaecol 1990; 97: 899–903

18 Levi CS, Lyons EA, Zheng XH, Lindsay DJ, Holt SC. Endovaginal US: demonstration of cardiac activity in embryos of less than 5.0 mm in crown-rump length. Radiology 1990; 176: 71–74

19 Luise C, Jermy K, Collins WP, Bourne T. The outcome of expectant management of spontaneous first trimester miscarriage. An observational study. BMJ 2002; 324: 873–875

20 Luise C, Jermy K, Collins WP, Bourne T. Expectant management of incomplete, spontaneous first trimester miscarriage outcome according to initial ultrasound criteria and value of follow-up visits. Ultrasound Ostet Gynecol 2002; 19: 580–582

21 Schwarzler P, Holden D, Nielsen S, Hahlin M, Sladkevicius P, Bourne TH. The conservative management of first trimester miscarriages and the use of colour Doppler sonography for patient selection. Hum Reprod 1999; 14: 1341–1345

22 Cacciatore B, Stenman UH, Ylostalo P. Comparison of abdominal and vaginal sonography in suspected ectopic pregnancy. Obstet Gynecol 1989; 73: 770–774

23 Cacciatore B. Can the status of tubal pregnancy be predicted with transvaginal sonography? A prospective comparison of sonographic, surgical, and serum hCG findings. Radiology 1990; 177: 481–484

24 Stovall TG, Ling FW, Carson SA, Buster JE. Non surgical diagnosis and treatment of tubal pregnancy. Fertil Steril 1990; 54: 537–538

25 Ankum WM, Van der Veen F, Hamerlynck JV, Lammes FB. Laparoscopy: a dispensable tool in the diagnosis of ectopic pregnancy? Hum Reprod 1993; 8: 1301–1306

26 Ludwig M, Kaisi M, Bauer O, Diedrich K. Heterotopic pregnancy in a spontaneous cycle: do not forget about it! Eur J Obstet Gynecol Reprod Biol 1999; 87: 91–93

27 Lenton EA, Neal LM, Sulaiman R. Plasma concentrations of human chorionic gonadotropin from the time of implantation until the second week of pregnancy. Fertil Steril 1982; 37: 773–778

28 Radwanska E, Frankenberg J, Allen EI. Plasma progesterone levels in normal and abnormal early human pregnancy. Fertil Steril 1978; 30: 398–402

29 Banerjee S, Aslam N, Zosmer N, Woelfer B, Jurkovic D. The expectant management of women with early pregnancy of unknown location. Ultrasound Obstet Gynecol 1999; 14: 231–236

30 Lavery JP, Koontz WL, Layman L, Shaw L, Gumpel U. Sonographic evaluation of the adnexa during early pregnancy. Surg Gynecol Obstet 1986; 163: 319–323

31 Timmerman D, Schwarzler P, Collins WP, Claerhout F, Coenen M, Amant F et al. Subjective assessment of adnexal masses with the use of ultrasonography: an analysis of interobserver variability and experience. Ultrasound Obstet Gynecol 1999; 13: 11–16

32 Jermy K, Luise C, Bourne T. The characterization of common ovarian cysts in premenopausal women. Ultrasound Obstet Gynecol 2001; 17: 140–144

33 Rosado Jr WM, Trambert MA, Gosink BB, Pretorius DH. Adnexal torsion: diagnosis by using Doppler sonography. AJR Am J Roentgenol 1992; 159: 1251–1253

34 Timor-Tritsch IE, Lerner JP, Monteagudo A, Murphy KE, Heller DS. Transvaginal sonographic markers of tubal inflammatory disease. Ultrasound Obstet Gynecol 1998; 12: 56–66

35 Baskett TF, O'Connor H, Magos AL. A comprehensive one-stop menstrual problem clinic for the diagnosis and management of abnormal uterine bleeding. Br J Obstet Gynaecol 1996; 103: 76–77

36 Roman JD, Trivedi AN. Implementation of an outpatient hysteroscopy clinic at Waikato Women's Hospital report of the first 60 cases. N Z Med J 1999; 112: 253–255

37 Gimpelson RJ, Rappold HO. A comparative study between panoramic hysteroscopy with directed biopsies and dilatation and curettage. A review of 276 cases. Am J Obstet Gynecol 1988; 158: 489–492

38 Mencaglia L, Perino A, Hamou J. Hysteroscopy in perimenopausal and postmenopausal women with abnormal uterine bleeding. J Reprod Med 1987; 32: 577–582

39 Krampl E, Bourne T, Hurlen-Solbakken H, Istre O. Transvaginal ultrasonography sonohysterography and operative hysteroscopy for the evaluation of abnormal uterine bleeding. Acta Obstet Gynecol Scand 2001; 80: 616–622

40 Fedele L, Bianchi S, Dorta M, Brioschi D, Zanotti F, Vercellini P. Transvaginal ultrasonography versus hysteroscopy in the diagnosis of uterine submucous myomas. Obstet Gynecol 1991; 77: 745–748

41 Clevenger-Hoeft M, Syrop CH, Stovall DW, Van Voorhis BJ. Sonohysterography in premenopausal women with and without abnormal bleeding. Obstet Gynecol 1999; 94: 516–520

42 Reinhold C, Atri M, Mehio A, Zakarian R, Aldis AE, Bret PM. Diffuse uterine adenomyosis: morphologic criteria and diagnostic accuracy of endovaginal sonography. Radiology 1995; 197: 609–614

43 Goldstein SR, Nachtigall M, Snyder JR, Nachtigall L. Endometrial assessment by vaginal ultrasonography before endometrial sampling in patients with postmenopausal bleeding. Am J Obstet Gynecol 1990; 163: 119–123

44 Granberg S, Wikland M, Karlsson B, Norstrom A, Friberg LG. Endometrial thickness as measured by endovaginal ultrasonography for identifying endometrial abnormality. Am J Obstet Gynecol 1991; 164: 47–52

45 Varner RE, Sparks JM, Cameron CD, Roberts LL, Soong SJ. Transvaginal sonography of the endometrium in postmenopausal women. Obstet Gynecol 1991; 78: 195–199

46 Karlsson B, Granberg S, Wikland M, Ylostalo P, Torvid K, Marsal K, Valentin L. Transvaginal ultrasonography of the endometrium in women with postmenopausal bleeding – a Nordic multicenter study. Am J Obstet Gynecol 1995; 172: 1488–1494

47 Ferrazzi E, Torri V, Trio D, Zannoni E, Filiberto S, Dordoni D. Sonographic endometrial thickness: a useful test to predict atrophy in patients with postmenopausal bleeding. An Italian multicenter study. Ultrasound Obstet Gynecol 1996; 7: 315–321

48 Smith-Bindman R, Kerlikowske K, Feldstein VA, Subak L, Scheidler J et al. Endovaginal ultrasound to exclude endometrial cancer and other endometrial abnormalities. JAMA 1998; 280: 1510–1517

49 Epstein E, Valentin L. Rebleeding and endometrial growth in women with postmenopausal bleeding and endometrial thickness < 5 mm managed by dilatation and curettage or ultrasound follow-up: a randomised controlled study. Ultrasound Obstet Gynecol 2001; 18: 499–504

50 Gull B, Carlsson S, Karlsson B, Ylostalo P, Milsom I, Granberg S. Transvaginal ultrasonography of the endometrium in women with postmenopausal bleeding: is it always necessary to perform an endometrial biopsy? Am J Obstet Gynecol 2000; 182: 509–515

51 Levine D, Gosink BB, Johnson LA. Change in endometrial thickness in postmenopausal women undergoing hormone replacement therapy. Radiology 1995; 197: 603–608

52 Goldstein SR. Postmenopausal endometrial fluid collections revisited: look at the doughnut rather than the hole. Obstet Gynecol 1994; 83: 738–740

53 Gull B, Karlsson B, Wikland M, Milsom I, Granberg S. Factors influencing the presence of uterine cavity fluid in a random sample of asymptomatic postmenopausal women. Acta Obstet Gynecol Scand 1998; 77: 751–757

54 Doren M, Suselbeck B, Schneider HP, Holzgreve W. Uterine perfusion and endometrial thickness in postmenopausal women on long-term continuous combined estrogen and progestogen replacement. Ultrasound Obstet Gynecol 1997; 9: 113–119

55 Omodei U, Ferrazzia E, Ruggeri C, Patai N, Fallo L, Dordoni D et al. Endometrial thickness and histological abnormalities in women on hormonal replacement therapy: a transvaginal ultrasound/hysteroscopic study. Ultrasound Obstet Gynecol 2000; 15: 317–320

56 Fisher B, Costantino JP, Wickerham DL, Redmond CK, Kavanah M, Cronin WM et al. Tamoxifen for prevention of breast cancer: report of the National Surgical Adjuvant Breast and Bowel Project P-1 Study. J Natl Cancer Inst 1998; 90: 1371–1388

57 Kedar RP, Bourne TH, Powles TJ, Collins WP, Ashley SE, Cosgrove DO, Campbell S. Effects of tamoxifen on uterus and ovaries of postmenopausal women in a randomised breast cancer prevention trial. Lancet 1994; 343: 1318–1321

58 Bertelli G, Venturini M, Del Mastro L, Garrone O, Cosso M, Gustavino C et al. Tamoxifen and the endometrium: findings of pelvic ultrasound examination and endometrial biopsy in asymptomatic breast cancer patients. Breast Cancer Res Treat 1998; 47: 41–46

59 Cecchini S, Ciatto S, Bonardi R, Mazzotta A, Grazzini G, Pacini P, Muraca MG. Screening by ultrasonography for endometrial carcinoma in postmenopausal breast cancer patients under adjuvant tamoxifen. Gynecol Oncol 1996; 60: 409–411

60 Mourits MJ, Van der Zee AG, Willemse PH, Ten Hoor KA, Hollema H, De Vries EG. Discrepancy between ultrasonography and hysteroscopy and histology of endometrium in postmenopausal breast cancer patients using tamoxifen. Gynecol Oncol 1999; 73: 21–26

61 Timmerman D, Deprest J, Bourne T, Van den Berghe I, Collins WP, Vergote I. A randomized trial on the use of ultrasonography or office hysteroscopy for endometrial assessment in postmenopausal patients with breast cancer who were treated with tamoxifen. Am J Obstet Gynecol 1998; 179: 62–70

62 Berliere M, Galant C, Gillerot S, Charles A, Donnez J. [Endometrial evaluation prior to tamoxifen: preliminary results of a prospective study]. Bull Cancer 1998; 85: 721–724

63 Kupfer MC, Schwimer SR, Lebovic J. Transvaginal sonographic appearance of endometriomata: spectrum of findings. J Ultrasound Med 1992; 11: 129–133

64 Mais V, Guerriero S, Ajossa S, Angiolucci M, Paoletti AM, Melis GB. The efficiency of transvaginal ultrasonography in the diagnosis of endometrioma. Fertil Steril 1993; 60: 776–780

65 Mais V, Guerriero S, Ajossa S, Angiolucci M, Paoletti AM, Melis GB. Transvaginal ultrasonography in the diagnosis of cystic teratoma. Obstet Gynecol 1995; 85: 48–52

66 Koonings PP, Campbell K, Mishell Jr DR, Grimes DA. Relative frequency of primary ovarian neoplasms: a 10-year review. Obstet Gynecol 1989; 74: 921–926

67 Alcazar JL, Laparte C, Jurado M, Lopez-Garcia G. The role of transvaginal ultrasonography combined with color velocity imaging and pulsed Doppler in the diagnosis of endometrioma. Fertil Steril 1997; 67: 487–491

68 Bourne T. The use of transvaginal colour Doppler in gynaecology. Ultrasound Obstet Gynecol 1991; 5: 359–373

69 Sassone AM, Timor-Tritsch IE, Artner A, Westhoff C, Warren WB. Transvaginal sonographic characterization of ovarian disease: evaluation of a new scoring system to predict ovarian malignancy. Obstet Gynecol 1991; 78: 70–76

70 Yuen PM, Yu KM, Yip SK, Lau WC, Rogers MS, Chang A. A randomized prospective study of laparoscopy and laparotomy in the management of benign ovarian masses. Am J Obstet Gynecol 1997; 177: 109–114

71 Timmerman D, Bourne TH, Tailor A, Collins WP, Verrelst H, Vandenberghe K, Vergote I. A comparison of methods for pre-operative discrimination between malignant and benign adnexal masses: the development of a new logistic regression model. Am J Obstet Gynecol 1999; 181: 57–65

72 Alcazar JL, Jurado M. Using a logistic model to predict malignancy of adnexal masses based on menopausal status, ultrasound morphology, and color Doppler findings. Gynecol Oncol 1998; 69: 146–150

73 Aslam N, Banerjee S, Carr JV, Savvas M, Hooper R, Jurkovic D. Prospective evaluation of logistic regression models for the diagnosis of ovarian cancer. Obstet Gynecol 2000; 96: 75–80

74 Tailor A, Jurkovic D, Bourne TH, Collins WP, Campbell S. Sonographic prediction of malignancy in adnexal masses using multivariate logistic regression analysis. Ultrasound Obstet Gynecol 1997; 10: 41–47

75 Timmerman D, Valentin L, Bourne TH, Collins WP, Verrelst H, Vergote I. Terms, definitions and measurements to describe the sonographic features of adnexal tumors: a consensus opinion from the International Ovarian Tumor Analysis (IOTA) Group. Ultrasound Obstet Gynecol 2000; 16: 500–505

76 Granberg S, Wikland M, Jansson I. Macroscopic characterization of ovarian tumors and the relation to the histological diagnosis: criteria to be used for ultrasound evaluation. Gynecol Oncol 1989; 35: 139–144

77 Bourne T, Campbell S, Steer C, Whitehead MI, Collins WP. Transvaginal colour flow imaging: a possible new screening technique for ovarian cancer. BMJ 1989; 299: 1367–1370

78 Valentin L, Sladkevicius P, Marsal K. Limited contribution of Doppler velocimetry to the differential diagnosis of extrauterine pelvic tumors. Obstet Gynecol 1994; 83: 425–433

79 Jacobs I, Oram D, Fairbanks J, Turner J, Frost C, Grudzinskas JG. A risk of malignancy index incorporating CA 125, ultrasound and menopausal status for the accurate preoperative diagnosis of ovarian cancer. Br J Obstet Gynaecol 1990; 97: 922–929

80 Tailor A, Jurkovic D, Bourne TH, Collins WP, Campbell S. Sonographic prediction of malignancy in adnexal masses using an artificial neural network. Br J Obstet Gynaecol 1999; 106: 21–30

81 Timmerman D, Verrelst H, Bourne TH, De Moor B, Collins WP, Vergote I, Vandewalle J. Artificial neural network models for the preoperative discrimination between malignant and benign adnexal masses. Ultrasound Obstet Gynecol 1999; 13: 17–25

82 Valentin L, Hagen B, Tingulstad S, Eik-Nes S. Comparison of 'pattern recognition' and logistic regression models for discrimination between benign and malignant pelvic masses: a prospective cross validation. Ultrasound Obstet Gynecol 2001; 18: 357–365

83 Granberg S, Norstrom A, Wikland M. Tumors in the lower pelvis as imaged by vaginal sonography. Gynecol Oncol 1990; 37: 224–229

84 Meire HB, Farrant P, Guha T. Distinction of benign from malignant ovarian cysts by ultrasound. Br J Obstet Gynaecol 1978; 85: 893–899

85 Luxman D, Bergman A, Sagi J, David MP. The postmenopausal adnexal mass: correlation between ultrasonic and pathologic findings. Obstet Gynecol 1991; 77: 726–8

A.P. Hawkins C.L. Domoney J.W.W. Studd

Sexuality after hysterectomy

Hysterectomy is the commonest major gynaecological operation, being performed on 1 in 5 women in the UK at some stage in their lives. Research into the quality of women's sexual experience after hysterectomy is limited. The quality of research has been hampered by poor understanding of women's sexual response and the complicated interaction between the emotional, psychological and physiological factors involved. Our patients are now expecting more information on all aspects of any surgery they undergo, including what effects it may have on their sexual life. It is our duty to be able to provide them with as much evidence-based information as we can.

PSYCHOLOGICAL FACTORS

The psychological component of sexual response is a complex interplay of emotional responsiveness, sexual expectation and psychological history that have been poorly determined and evaluated and that are often individual and difficult to quantify.

Expectation and pre-operative sexuality

Postoperative sexual function is determined by pre-operative function, pre-operative expectations, particularly of sexuality,[1] and pre-operative symptomatology. Women

Ms A.P. Hawkins BSc MRCOG DFFP, Research Fellow, Academic Department of Obstetrics and Gynaecology, Chelsea and Westminster Hospital, 369 Fulham Road, London SW10 9NH, UK

Miss C.L. Domoney MA MRCOG, Research Fellow, Academic Department of Obstetrics and Gynaecology, Chelsea and Westminster Hospital, 369 Fulham Road, London SW10 9NH, UK

Prof. John W.W. Studd DSc MD FRCOG, Professor of Gynaecology and Consultant Gynaecologist, Academic Department of Obstetrics and Gynaecology, Chelsea and Westminster Hospital, 369 Fulham Road, London SW10 9NH, UK

who are continuing to enjoy sexual intercourse despite sometimes severe gynaeco-logical symptoms (e.g. menorrhagia, dyspareunia or premenstrual syndrome [PMS]) are more likely to have a fulfilling sexual life postoperatively.[2] The converse is also true, in that women with perceived limitations on sexuality pre-operatively are more likely to have problems postoperatively. There may be a psychological vulnerability in this group of women,[3] such that symptoms may lead to sexual problems or somatisation may be occurring even pre-operatively. A greater under-standing of this has led to improved counselling and selection of patients for surgery in recent years.[4]

Patients who have a better understanding of pelvic anatomy and who are better informed about the procedure and what to expect in the recovery phase post-hysterectomy are known to recover faster and have better postoperative sexual experience.[1]

Hysterectomy and depression

Depression is accompanied by low self-esteem and disinterest in life (anhedonia). Unsurprisingly, this is often associated with loss of libido, so it is important to address whether there is any association between hysterectomy and psychiatric disorders, particularly affective disorders such as depression.

Unfortunately the most common first-line treatment, selective serotonin re-uptake inhibitor antidepressants (SSRIs), often decrease sexual response, so while excellent at improving mood, may not be ideal in all women. Modell et al.[5] found 73% of patients to have negative side-effects on sexual function. Olah[6] found that 80% of his sample of 30 women showed some adverse sexual side-effects – 70% had decreased arousal, 53% had decreased orgasm intensity and 73% showed a delay in orgasm with 10% being anorgasmic altogether. In addition, 60% described decreased libido, which may or may not have been attributable to the drug. While it is of course important to treat clinical depression, this additional factor in the equation should not be overlooked.

Early studies seemed to show a strong link between hysterectomy and postoperative depression,[7] which was greater than that seen after other major surgical procedures. Richards' study from 1974[8] is often quoted, but is flawed in being retrospective. There was also no mention made of ovarian status or hormone replacement therapy (HRT) in use. He found 70% of women to suffer from depression in the 3 years after surgery, as opposed to 30% of the controls. In it he coins the phrase 'post-hysterectomy syndrome' to describe this post-operative depression. It appears that the significant symptoms his patients display (depression, tiredness, headaches and hot flushes) may be due to the hormone deficiency produced by surgical oophorectomy or premature ovarian failure when ovaries were conserved. This is often overlooked when this study is quoted.

Subsequent authors have performed prospective studies that have shown a surprising over-representation of depression amongst attenders of gynaecology clinics or patients with menorrhagia, pre-operatively and compared to the general population.[9,10] It has been considered[11,12] that this is psychological vulnerability combined with prolonged symptoms inducing severe emotional distress, which can lead to psychiatric illness, usually depression. A past history of psychiatric illness in general is the most important predictor for adverse

Table 1 Change in psychiatric morbidity in women undergoing hysterectomy in the same population over 15 years (after Gath et al.[18])

	Study 1[16]	Study 2[19]	Study 3[18]
Pre-operative psychiatric morbidity	58%	28%	9%
Postoperative psychiatric morbidity	26%	7%	4%

psychiatric outcome following gynaecological surgery.[13] In the gynaecological population this is largely affective disorders.

It must be remembered when assessing the studies looking at psychiatric morbidity pre- and postoperatively, not only may the gynaecological symptoms be so distressing that they are causing depression,[14] but the prospect of surgery itself may be frightening and lead to anxiety and depression.

Prospective studies have shown significant decrease in psychiatric illness after hysterectomy.[15] Gath et al. considered 59% of women with dysfunctional uterine bleeding fulfilled the criteria of a psychiatric 'case' pre-operatively and only 26% postoperatively.[16] Coppen et al.[17] showed women to have improved mood and vigour, with unaltered frequency of intercourse or orgasm 3 years post-hysterectomy. This was thought to be due to relief from gynaecological symptoms.

Comparison of three studies in a similar population in the Oxford area over 15 years showed the level of psychiatric morbidity in the gynaecology clinic to have fallen dramatically.[18] The studies were all in women having hysterectomy for benign reasons, and their psychiatric morbidity was measured pre-operatively and 6 months postoperatively. Psychiatric morbidity fell significantly across the three studies, both pre- and postoperatively. (Table 1) The authors postulate that clinicians are operating more appropriately and general practitioners may be better at identifying patients with emotional and psychological problems and treating them in primary care. It is certainly true that in recent years gynaecologists are frequently using more medical therapies, plus explanation and re-assurance before hysterectomy for benign conditions. This may enable the patient to understand her condition and be satisfied that surgery is necessary when that decision is made, leading her to be more comfortable with the outcome, and so encounter fewer psychological and sexual problems. However, it must be emphasised that removal of chronic disability and symptoms such as heavy painful periods, chronic anaemia, PMS, menstrual migraine, exhaustion, dyspareunia and pelvic pain will lead to a great improvement in depression, low-mood, well-being and libido, without any psychiatric component.

Hysterectomy and femininity

Human sexual behaviour is a complex mixture of emotional and physical factors and these are difficult to disentangle. It has been assumed that physical removal of the uterus should have no effect on desire or libido; however, hysterectomy may be associated with feelings of loss. This occurs when the womb is perceived as the centre of femininity leading to a reduced feeling of desirability in some women. It is important to be aware that the feelings surrounding hysterectomy vary widely from woman-to-woman and so exploring what loss of the uterus means to each woman is an important part of management and certainly pre-operative assessment. We would recommend that each woman's feelings on the subject are explored early in gynaecological assessment, in order to help in planning an individual management strategy.

Some women have reported feeling loss of youthfulness and attractiveness after hysterectomy; they have a change in self-image.[20] Some feel their partners are less attracted to them as non-fertile mates. Others have described feeling hollow or empty inside, and are certainly referring to feelings of loss. They may show frank grief and need to go through the stages of the bereavement reaction to resolve this. A few will have frank body fantasies, which can produce severe psychosexual difficulties if not discussed and resolved. The incidence of such psychosexual problems post-hysterectomy has not been quantified, and is difficult to assess with conventional medical models, but anecdotal reports are common. It is important for both gynaecologists and general practitioners to have an understanding of these possible psychological sequelae, so that they can be identified and addressed when they arise.[21]

Some authors describe the woman in her middle years as feeling a loss of role, as her children are leaving home and growing up, her years of mothering are complete. This is less pertinent in today's society where women have other roles outside the home, but there is no doubt that a sense of worthlessness, whatever its source, is a powerful dampener to libido. Many women, however, are relieved to be rid of the worry of contraception and the gynaecological symptoms such as heavy and irregular bleeding, plus premenstrual symptoms such as headaches and low mood. These women will feel a great benefit from surgery and, as long as they have appropriate hormone replacement therapy, are very likely to have an improved sexual life.

Post-hysterectomy sexuality

Indeed, Gath et al.[16] reported an increase in sexual activity and enjoyment 6 months after hysterectomy. At the 6-month follow-up visit, 56% of women reported an increase in sexual activity compared to pre-operatively, with 27% unchanged and 17% decreased. Reported enjoyment was improved in 39%, no different in 41% and decreased in 20%. This was statistically highly significant and remained constant at the 18-month follow-up assessment.

Dennerstein et al.[1] reported improved sexual outcome post-hysterectomy in their prospective study, with 56% women reporting improvement in their sexual lives, 30% saying there was no change and 14% a deterioration. Martin et al.[10] showed a non-significant improvement in sexual life, the only deterioration being seen in women with a previous psychiatric diagnosis. Helstrom et al.[22] prospectively studied sexuality after subtotal hysterectomy and found an improvement in sexual functioning in 50% of their patients, no change in 29% and a deterioration in 21%. Nathorst-Boos et al.[23] similarly found 39% of their sample experienced intercourse as improved or better, and 40% unchanged, 19% felt it was worse. They also asked about satisfaction with the surgery and found this to be very high at 84%. Interestingly, Alexander et al.[24] found no difference in sexual interest up to 1 year postoperatively in a group of women who were randomized to undergo either trans-cervical resection of the endometrium or hysterectomy

Table 2 Summary of psychological factors

Psychological factors	Identified factors to explore
Psycho-analytic theory on loss of uterus	Expectation
End of femininity, uterus defines female state	Assess pre-operative function
End of reproductive capacity, feeling worthless	Relationship
End of desirability, feels mutilated	Body image

for dysfunctional uterine bleeding. This finding was repeated by Crosignani et al.[25] with a longer 2-year follow-up.

In summary (Table 2), early research in this area was often flawed, for example by being retrospective or not considering hormonal factors and implied hysterectomy to be detrimental to women's mental health and sexuality. More recent research, which is more methodologically sound, has consistently shown an overall benefit to women's health and sexuality, where hysterectomy is appropriately performed for benign disease.[26]

SOCIAL FACTORS

Couple relationship

The relationship in which the woman is a partner is an important predictive factor in the quality of sexual life she can expect to enjoy postoperatively. Lalos et al.[27] found the couple relationship to be an important predictive factor for postoperative sexual function. They found that patients' partners, when interviewed, were anxious about the surgery. They were concerned about peri-operative complications and the possible diagnosis of malignancy. The main finding, however, was that post-hysterectomy there was a major beneficial effect on the couple's sexual life and overall quality of life.

Helstrom et al.[28] showed that women with either no relationship, or one which they were ambivalent about, were more at risk of deterioration of their sexuality after their hysterectomy than those in a pre-operative harmonious sexual relationship. Again, most of their sample showed an improvement or no change in their coital frequency and satisfaction.

Women are often married to men older than them, who may experience problems with arousal, erection or premature ejaculation. They may have medical conditions requiring treatment and many medications have adverse effects on sexual performance, for example β-blockers. They may have vascular disease, for example secondary to diabetes or smoking, that hinders erection. If there were problems before hysterectomy, then even though the woman's physical symptoms may be much improved postoperatively, her partner may have problems that prevent satisfactory intercourse.

As a relationship progresses there are many changes affecting both partners as individuals and as a couple. Familiarity and routine can reduce desire, resulting in a relationship of companionship only. Intercurrent illness, disability, immobility and difficulty with personal hygiene will all affect desire, and perceived desirability of both the affected person and their partner.

Table 3 Summary of social factors

Social factor	Suggested action
Partner anxiety	Include partner in pre-operative discussions and allow questions
Pre-existing sexual problem	Identify and clarify what operation can and cannot do
Relationship problem	Relationship counselling
Sexual problem in partner	Partner to seek change in medication or psychosexual counselling
Intercurrent illness or disability	Ensure optimally treated

There also may be relationship problems such that one or both partners do not want intercourse. By changing the woman's health status we may be changing a relationship that has developed to suit the problems of both partners. When enquiring about a woman's sexual life, it is necessary to remember both the partner and the relationship, either of which may be the source of difficulty, rather than the woman's libido or any physical or hormonal problem (Table 3).

PHYSICAL FACTORS

Anatomical

Pelvic surgery has the potential to disrupt both the anatomical relationships of the pelvic organs and their innervation. It is important for pelvic surgeons to try and understand not only the static anatomy of the pelvis, but the physiological, neurological and interactive nature of how these organs function in life, in order to preserve this function as far as possible.

Pelvic orgasm

The endopelvic fascia is a continuous sheet attaching the bladder, uterus and rectum to the pelvic side walls. It encompasses the cardinal and uterosacral ligaments, which anchor the cervix in place. The broad ligament drapes over the uterus and fallopian tubes, but provides no support, allowing movement of the uterus within the pelvis.

Masters and Johnson described how during intercourse the uterus moved upwards and the cervix 'dipped down' into the posterior fornix, which ballooned during arousal.[29] Some women described orgasm being invoked by stimulation of the cervix during penetration as different from clitoral orgasm.[30] Subtotal hysterectomy leaves the cervix and cervical supports intact and, in women who describe deep pelvic orgasm, has been thought to preserve it. Total hysterectomy, in contrast, was thought to remove the cervical component to pelvic orgasm. Research has both confirmed and denied these theories in turn.[31] It has also been mooted that removal of the cervix removes the cervical component of vaginal lubrication, although not all authors believe that this is significant. More modern authors no longer delineate between the clitoral and vaginal orgasm and deny any cervical contribution to it.

Remarkably, it its only in the last few years that there has been a greater understanding of the anatomy and neuro-anatomy of the female sexual response. Baskin et al.[32] describe the female anatomy as analogous to an unfolded penis, stretching back along the anterior vaginal wall. The small external structure we know as the clitoris is merely the outer part of a much larger interior structure. There are two cavernous bulbs, analogous to those in the penis, but separate and extending backwards. They fill with blood during arousal and cause the vagina and vulva to swell. O'Connell and colleagues[33,34] agree with this new version of female anatomy, after cadaveric dissection. Baskin et al.[32] have described the network of nerves supplying this area in the female embryo, with which the male is initially identical. It is postulated that the area anterior to the anterior vaginal wall which is rich in vasculature, erectile tissue and nerve supply is an area very sensitive to sexual stimulus and could be the source of internal orgasm and the perhaps mythical Graafenberg or 'G' spot. From this, it is clear that if internal and external clitoral structures are parts of a whole, the distinction between clitoral and vaginal orgasm is perhaps less important.

Studies of subtotal versus total hysterectomy can be used to assess the implications of surgery and aid our understanding of female sexuality. Kilkku et al.[35] questioned women who had undergone either total abdominal hysterectomy or subtotal hysterectomy and found no difference in libido between the groups pre- or post-surgery. They did find significantly decreased orgasm rates postoperatively in the group who had undergone total hysterectomy. This work led to a rise in the proportion of hysterectomies in which the cervix was left intact across Europe in the late 1980s, although the reasons for this decrease in orgasm frequency was not precisely defined. It could be removal of the cervix that was reducing the sexual response, some other neuronal damage or alternatively another non-anatomical cause.[36]

Pelvic nerves

Hysterectomy may potentially damage the pelvic autonomic plexus.[37] This plexus supplies the pelvic organs and controls the co-ordinated contractions of the smooth muscle of the bladder and bowel. It lies intimately related to the bladder, cervix and vagina and is at risk during four parts of the hysterectomy.

1 Nerves running beneath the uterine arteries are at risk during division of the cardinal ligaments.

2 The vesical innervation entering the bladder base to supply the detrusor muscle risks damage at the time of blunt dissection of the bladder from the anterior cervix and lower uterus.

This has been implicated in producing postoperative detrusor instability. Some studies have shown an increase in bladder symptoms postoperatively, but these are largely retrospective and so suffer from recall bias.[38] Another study has shown a significant decrease in stress incontinence frequency and nocturia post-surgery.[39] Evidence remains conflicting.

No difference has been proven between women who have undergone subtotal versus total hysterectomy in the incidence of bladder and bowel dysfunction postoperatively, despite the obvious lesser dissection necessary for the subtotal procedure. Kilkku reported improvement in his study of bladder function after subtotal or total hysterectomy.[38]

3 Paravaginal dissection may interrupt neurones passing out laterally.

4 Removing the cervix itself potentially removes a significant amount of the cervical plexus as they are so intimately related.

The autonomic nerve damage so produced has been implicated in denervation of the rectum and postoperative problems of constipation or irritable bowel syndrome, although some of the work is subjective and retrospective and there is work to dispute this. Quality studies attempting to assess the effect of hysterectomy on bladder and bowel function have shown no difference before and after hysterectomy.

Blood flow
Trauma to the vasculature of the ilio-hypogastric-pudendal arterial bed may result in diminished arterial blood flow to the vagina and clitoris following sexual stimulation.[40] Some women will prefer the option of subtotal hysterectomy if they are concerned about potential loss of deep pelvic orgasms or higher operative risk from the total hysterectomy. While there is logically increased risk of damage to the ureter, increased bleeding and a theoretical infection risk from opening the vagina at a total hysterectomy, there is no scientific evidence to support this.[41] Recent unpublished work from King's College Hospital, London (Thakkar R., personal communication) has shown no difference in complication rates between subtotal and total hysterectomy in the hands of experienced surgeons in uncomplicated cases. These factors should all be discussed pre-operatively with the patient and, if there are no other reasons why a particular form of hysterectomy should be chosen, she should be allowed to consider whether to keep her cervix.

Relief of symptoms
While all these are valid, if unproven, considerations, it must not be forgotten that the original indications for hysterectomy can be causing severe and disabling symptoms for the woman.[42] Removal of fibroids causing menorrhagia and pressure symptoms, endometriosis and endometriomas, adhesions and adenomyosis will all

Table 4 Improvement in dyspareunia after total and subtotal hysterectomy

	TAH ($n = 91$) within group (vertical)	Longitudinal comparison	STH ($n = 98$) within group (vertical) (horizontal)	Longitudinal comparison between groups	Statistical significance
Preoperatively	30.8%		28.6%		NS
6 months postoperatively	13.2%	$P = 0.01$	13.3%	$P = 0.01$	NS
12 months postoperatively	15.6%	$P = 0.05$	6.3%	$P = 0.001$	$P = 0.05$

Data from Kilkku.[43]

cause relief. Cyclical symptoms of premenstrual tension, cyclical migraine or cyclical depression will be relieved by bilateral oophorectomy at the time of hysterectomy. Relief of any or all of these is very likely to result in increased quality of life and so interest in and enjoyment of intimacy.

Deep dyspareunia is usually relieved by hysterectomy,[1] with little difference between subtotal hysterectomy (STH) and total hysterectomy (TAH). Kilkku[43] showed marked improvement in dyspareunia after both, but with significantly greater improvement in the subtotal group – although more of these women received postoperative hormone therapy (Table 4). In a follow-on study, Virtanen et al.[39] showed a significant decrease in dyspareunia 12 months after total abdominal hysterectomy (40% pre-operatively and 9% postoperatively) with no change in frequency of orgasm but a significant increase in libido.

New postoperative symptoms

Residual ovary syndrome

Ovarian conservation can lead to the 'residual ovary syndrome' of deep dyspareunia and chronic pelvic pain, due to the ovaries becoming adherent to the vaginal vault or pelvic side wall. This is more common if the ovarian pedicles are tied into the vaginal vault. This condition is under recognised and can lead to years of suffering, a difficult secondary bilateral oophorectomy procedure, or even psychological investigation. It is more common when the hysterectomy is performed for pelvic pain, endometriosis or pelvic inflammatory disease (PID).

Endometriosis

Ovarian conservation may also lead to recurrence of endometriosis and chronic pelvic pain, as endometriosis is dependent on ovarian function.[44] This occurs in up to 62% of women for whom endometriosis was the indication for hysterectomy,[45] with 25% requiring a second, often complicated, procedure.[46]

Ovarian cycle syndrome

Ovarian cycle syndrome can occur after ovarian conservation. Women who formerly had severe premenstrual syndrome, menstrual migraine or other cyclical symptoms will not be cured by hysterectomy alone as they are caused by cyclical fluctuations in ovarian hormones. It is imperative to consider carefully the indication before selecting the correct operation, and to counsel appropriately.

Prolapse post-hysterectomy

One group has shown an increase in colporrhaphy procedures after subtotal hysterectomy due to greater vault prolapse,[47] although not all authors agree with this increased prevalence.[48]

Ovarian cancer

Ovarian cancers are often diagnosed too late for cure, as they are asymptomatic until an advanced stage. In the UK, 4% of women will die of gynaecological cancer with half of these having ovarian cancer, so this cannot be overlooked in the decision making process.[49] However, there is also some evidence that the decrease in blood supply to conserved ovaries post-hysterectomy, not only causes their premature failure,[50] but may also decrease the ovarian cancer risk.[51]

Table 5 Summary of anatomical considerations

Anatomical considerations	Suggested action
TAH leading to loss of physiological cervical function, so reduced sexual response	Pre-operative discussion about orgasms
TAH leading to disruption of nervous pathways, so reduced sexual response	Pre-operative information and re-assurance
TAH leading to increased symptoms, e.g. urinary or bowel symptoms	Re-assurance Pre-operative urodynamics
Symptom relief	Appropriate choice of operation
Post-hysterectomy symptoms	Appropriate choice of operation
STH and risk of cervical carcinoma	Selection of patients Re-assure risk 0.3% only
Increased intra-operative complication rates in TAH versus STH	Appropriate case selection Current evidence

Cervical carcinoma

The justification for routine removal of the cervix has often been the future risk of cervical carcinoma. In women who have a history of normal smear test results, this is minimal (0.3%)[52] as the highest risk women are those who have never been screened. If women are prepared to continue screening, subtotal hysterectomy must remain an option. In the future, we may see a more accurate screening programme with the introduction of widespread screening for the human papilloma virus (HPV) which may decrease this risk even further.

Consideration of all these factors on a case-by-case basis along with a frank and open discussion about what we do and do not know about the female sexual response should occur pre-operatively in every case. This should ensure an individual and appropriate management plan is made to address that particular woman's gynaecological and emotional needs (Table 5).

HORMONAL FACTORS

Early studies showed decreased sexual function after hysterectomy, but did not differentiate between women who underwent oophorectomy or who had their ovaries conserved. Often there is no mention of, or fleeting regard to, whether hormone replacement was given postoperatively or what kind was used.[8] It is now recommended that women who have had a hysterectomy with ovarian conservation premenopausally, should have their FSH level estimated every year or so, especially if they become symptomatic of oestrogen deficiency, as it is understood that their ovaries are likely to fail earlier than normal.[53]

Oestrogen

We now recognise that adequate oestrogen replacement makes a huge difference to quality of life. Oestrogen has a secondary effect on libido, mediated

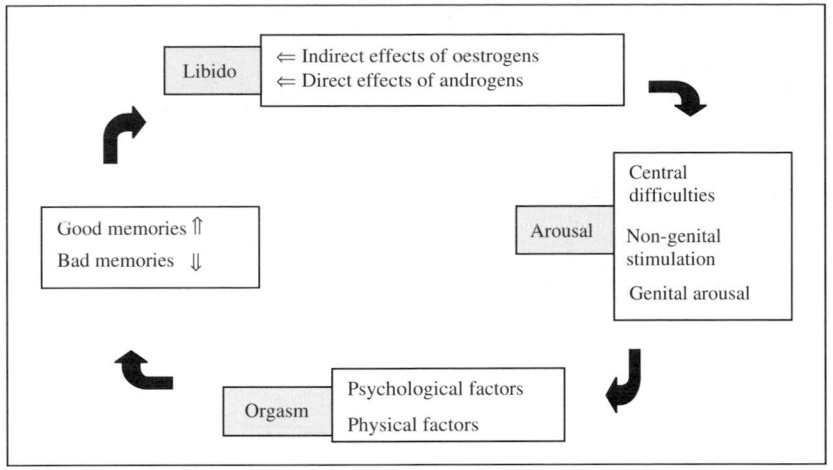

Fig. 1 Interplay of factors affecting sexuality. [Based on: Grazziottin A. Sexuality and the menopause. In: JWW Studd (ed). *The Management of the Menopause: Annual Review*. London:Parthenon, 1998: 49–58.]

through several different pathways. One of the most obvious effects is to reduce hot flushes, night sweats and insomnia, which will immediately improve quality of life, energy and libido. Oestrogen relieves tiredness and depression by acting as a mental tonic, again improving quality of life and so improving sexual desire. It will also significantly increase vaginal blood flow, thus decreasing vaginal dryness and so improve sexual responsiveness and enjoyment (Fig. 1).

Oestrogen deficiency leads to reduced blood flow to the sexual organs and, in turn, vaginal dryness and clitoral hyperaesthesia.[53] Intercourse may then become painful, leading to decreased enjoyment of (and so interest in) sex, producing a secondarily reduced libido. Similarly, there is increased mucosal dryness of other areas such as the eyes and mouth. Other effects of oestrogen on the body are equally important. Reduction in circulating oestrogens will lead to decreased peripheral vascular compliance and blood flow to the skin, producing hypo-elasticity. This will result in thinning and wrinkling of the skin and dryness of the skin, hair and nails.

Involution of the breast tissue occurs when there is a lack of oestrogen. Breasts are a highly visible secondary sexual characteristic, and their changes can be upsetting, as can the greying and thinning of pubic hair and atrophy of the external genitalia. The skin changes will produce altered sensation and decreased sensitivity, which can contribute to difficulty in arousal, with a negative feedback effect. There will also be altered olfactory function and pheromone secretion, which can both decrease attractiveness to and of a partner.

Finally, oestrogen is thought to have a role in the modulation of higher psychological function, which again can produce a secondary loss of desire.

These changes are perceived as ageing and so the patient's personal body image is diminished, which can make her feel less sexually attractive. This, in turn, contributes to her secondary loss of libido. Lack of enjoyment of her recent sexual experiences has a negative feedback effect in that it reduces the drive to have further sexual contact, so further reducing libido. It is essential

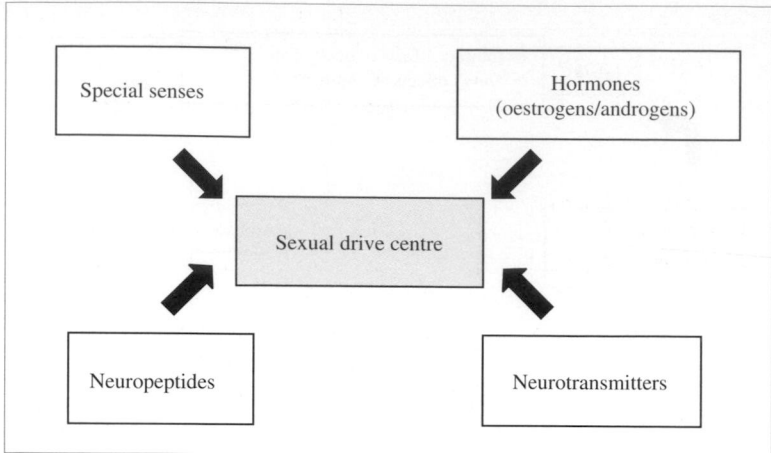

Fig. 2 Factors affecting the higher sexual drive centre.

for any person to perceive themselves as sexual and attractive sexually to enjoy sexual stimulation, with or without a partner.

Oestrogen replacement therapy can markedly reduce these signs and symptoms of oestrogen deficiency, which are perceived as ageing and so enhance the woman's body image, libido and hopefully her sexual life. Oestrogen therapy is most effective in arresting these changes, which it will markedly slow, although it cannot prevent them altogether. It can also partially reverse these changes when started after some years of oestrogen deficiency.[54] Factors affecting the higher sexual drive centre are summarised in Figure 2.

Testosterone

From the time of puberty, the thecal cells of the ovaries produce the hormones testosterone, dehydroepiandrosterone (DHEA) and androstenedione, which together comprise 50% of a woman's androgens. The other 50% of circulating testosterone is derived from peripheral conversion of adrenal androgens, primarily androstenedione.

In premenopausal women, testosterone levels peak mid-cycle. Most of the circulating testosterone is bound to sex hormone binding globulin (SHBG), which is a binding protein that is made in the liver and circulates in the plasma. Usually, only 1% of the total testosterone is free in the blood-stream and able to exert androgenic effects on the body. Anything that increases the level of SHBG in the blood will decrease free testosterone levels and directly affect libido and drive.

Thyroxine will increase SHBG, and it is commonly taken in middle life for the different hypothyroid states, or post-thyroidectomy or radio-active iodine treatment for hyperthyroidism. Once started, it is usually a life-long replacement therapy in itself and can, therefore, have a little-considered, indirect effect on libido. Oestrogen also increases SHBG and so can improve function while decreasing libido. Giving a woman oestrogen alone may have the effect of depleting her available testosterone still further.

Circulating androgens decline with age, and some women may be symptomatic for many years preceding the menopause, with tiredness, loss of drive, energy and libido. In most women, initially in the early post-menopause, the ovary ceases to produce oestrogens but continues to produce androgens, still producing up to 50% of circulating testosterone. In the later post-menopause, ovarian androgen production also declines.[55] At the time of bilateral oophorectomy, there is an immediate surgical menopause and loss of both the ovarian oestrogen and androgen production.

Nowadays, we are much better at replacing ovarian oestrogens, recognising their need, but too few women receive any testosterone replacement after bilateral oophorectomy. Removal of the ovaries can lead to the female androgen deficiency syndrome (FADS), characterised by lack of energy, headaches and depression, plus loss of sexual interest and libido.[56,57] All these have been shown to be significantly improved by adequate testosterone replacement.

It is difficult, but important to try and disentangle the effects of the different hormones on female sexuality. Oestrogen deficiency can lead to a marked and miserable secondary loss of libido for complex inter-related reasons as described above. In contrast, testosterone is thought to have a primary effect on libido and serum-free testosterone is correlated directly with sexual desire, in women as well as men.[58–60]

As far back as 1977, this distinction was clearly shown in two studies. The first[61] showed a high incidence of sexual dysfunction in the menopause clinic, with 136/300 (43.5%) women having at least one problem: 19 (6%) had dyspareunia, 59 (20%) had loss of libido and 58 (19%) had both. These women were given conjugated equine oestrogen (1.25 mg) and showed marked improvement in their dyspareunia, but no significant effect on libido. The same year, a study looking at the response to oestradiol and testosterone implants[67] showed that 80% of women had a marked improvement in libido and described their sexual response to be as good as before the menopause. Testosterone has been shown to improve not only sexual desire, but also arousal, frequency of sexual fantasies, pleasure, and satisfaction scores.[63]

Female sexuality is a difficult and complex area to research, but there have been repeated small studies that confirm and contribute to our understanding of the role of testosterone. Sands and Studd[56] showed, in an uncontrolled sample of 76 women with sexual problems, that an implant of 50 mg of oestradiol was effective at decreasing dyspareunia and increasing libido in 80% of patients. An additional implant of 100 mg testosterone significantly improved libido in 12/15 (80%) patients who had not responded to oestradiol alone.

Contra-indications to the use of low-dose testosterone therapy in women are few. These would include androgen insensitivity states, androgen secreting or dependent tumours or other proven states of excess, severe acne or hirsuitism, androgenic alopecia, pregnancy or lactation. In the UK, we are limited in our options for testosterone replacement in women.

In men androgens can be given as a tablet, a patch, a depot injection or an implant. Unfortunately, in women it is only licensed as an implant. The usual dose in women is 100 mg 6-monthly, although lower doses may be adequate. There have been studies looking at the use of transdermal patches of testosterone in women, but these are as yet unpublished. As with oestrogens, the non-oral routes are preferred to avoid first pass metabolism in the liver, so we may soon see the development of licensed androgen patches, transdermal gels and intra-vaginal rings.

Table 6 Summary of hormonal factors

Hormonal considerations	Suggested action
Ovarian conservation leading to premature ovarian failure and oestrogen deficiency symptoms	Yearly FSH levels
Oophorectomy and inadequate HRT l leading to oestrogen deficiency symptoms	Adjust ERT
Oophorectomy and inadequate HRT leading to female androgen deficiency syndrome	Ensure androgen replacement

The best oral option is the use of Tibolone, which is a unique compound combining oestrogenic, progestogenic and androgenic properties. Studies have shown it to improve significantly both mood and overall sexuality scores beyond that of comparable continuous combined HRT therapies.[64] It is the only oral HRT with a license for this use, and should be considered post-hysterectomy if the patient declines implant therapy.

The easiest way to achieve replacement of both hormones is with implants inserted at the time of bilateral salpingo-oophorectomy into the wound at closure. The usual dose is 50 mg oestradiol and 100 mg testosterone, although lower doses may be adequate. This is replaced in the out-patient clinic 6-monthly and monitored as necessary. The other great advantage of this route of administration is that this regimen shows excellent compliance rates, with 95% continuation rates at 5 years and 88% at 10 years in the studied population.[65] This also means that it is very effective at conferring the long-term benefits of protection against osteoporosis and cardiovascular disease, as the long-term compliance is so high (see Table 6).

KEY POINTS FOR CLINICAL PRACTICE (also see Tables in text)

- Women will not necessarily talk freely of the sexual problems they are experiencing unless they are asked. Once the subject is raised, they are often happy to discuss them and ask for help and advice.

- It is very easy to avoid offering women the opportunity to explain their problems, but only by listening and understanding can one understand more about female sexuality and what factors it may be important to consider when planning surgery.

- The primary aim is to improve quality of life, so it is imperative to consider the psychological, social, anatomical and hormonal implications of the planned surgery and ensure that the choices made are the best for the patient involved in each case.

- Patients must also be informed, as far as possible, about the implications of what is being proposed when surgery is suggested – both the beneficial and potentially harmful implications.

- It is essential that patients are not left in a hormone-deficient state after an iatrogenic menopause by providing adequate hormone replacement therapy, including testosterone as well as oestrogen.

1 Dennerstein L, Wood C, Burrows GD. Sexual response following hysterectomy and oophorectomy. Obstet Gynaecol 1997; 49: 92–96

2 Helstrom L, Weiner E, Sorbom D, Backstrom T. Predictive value of psychiatric history, genital pain and menstrual symptoms for sexuality after hysterectomy. Acta Obstet Gynecol Scand 1994; 73: 575–580

3 Ryan M, Dennerstein L. Psychosexual aspects of hysterectomy. In: Asch R, Studd JWW. (eds) Progress in Reproductive Medicine, vol. 2. London: Parthenon, 1995

4 Ryan MM. Hysterectomy: social and psychological aspects. Ballières Clin Obstet Gynaecol 1997; 11: 23–36

5 Modell JG, Katholi CR, Modell JD, DePalma RL. Comparative sexual side effects of bupropion, fluoxetine, paroxetine, and sertraline. Clin Pharmacol Ther 1997; 61: 476–487

6 Olah KS, The use of fluoxetine (prozac) in premenstrual syndrome: is the incidence of sexual dysfunction acceptable? J Obstet Gynaecol 2002; 22: 81–83

7 Zussman L, Zussman S, Sunley R, Bjornson E. Sexual response after hysterectomy – oophorectomy: recent studies and reconsideration of psychogenesis. Am J Obstet Gynecol 1981; 140: 725–729

8 Richards D. A post-hysterectomy syndrome. Lancet 1974: i: 983–985

9 Gath D, Osborn M, Bungay G et al. Psychiatric disorder and gynaecological symptoms in middle aged women: a community survey. BMJ 1987; 294: 213–218

10 Martin RL, Roberts WV, Clayton PJ. Psychiatric status after hysterectomy. A one year prospective follow-up. JAMA 1980; 244: 350–353

11 Gath D, Cooper P, Bond A, Edmonds G. Hysterectomy and psychiatric disorder: 2. Demographic psychiatric and physical factors in relation to psychiatric outcome. Br J Psychiatr 1982; 140: 342–350

12 Slade P, Anderton KJ. Gynaecological symptoms and psychological distress: a longitudinal study of their relationship. J Psychosom Obstet Gynecol 1992; 13: 51–63

13 Oates M, Gath D. Psychological aspects of gynaecological surgery. Ballières Clin Obstet Gynaecol 1989; 3: 734–749

14 Slade P, Anderton KJ. Gynaecological symptoms and psychological distress: a longitudinal study of their relationship. J Psychosom Obstet Gynaecol 1992; 13: 51–63

15 Ryan MM, Dennerstein L, Pepperell R. Psychological aspects of hysterectomy: a prospective study. Br J Psychiatr 1989; 154: 516–522

16 Gath D, Cooper P, Day A. Hysterectomy and psychiatric disorder. 1. Levels of psychiatric disorder before and after hysterectomy. Br J Psychiatry 1982; 140: 335–342

17 Coppen A, Bishop M, Beard RJ, Barnard GJR, Collins WP. Hysterectomy, hormones and behaviour, a prospective study. Lancet 1981; 1: 126–128

18 Gath D, Rose N, Bond A, Day A, Garrod A, Hodges S. Hysterectomy and psychiatric disorder: are the levels of psychiatric morbidity falling? Psychol Med 1995; 25: 277–283

19 Osborn M, Gath D. Psychological and physical determinants of premenstrual syndrome before and after hysterectomy. Psychol Medic 1990; 20: 565–572

20 Sloan D. The emotional and psychosexual aspects of hysterectomy. Am J Obstet Gynecol 1978; 131: 598–605

21 Field S. Psychosexual medicine in clinical practice: the gynaecology clinic. In: Skrine R, Montford H (eds). Psychosexual Medicine, An Introduction, 2nd edn. London: Arnold, 2001

22 Helstrom L, Lundberg PO, Sorbom D, Backstrom T. Sexuality after hysterectomy: a factor analysis of women's sexual lives before and after subtotal hysterectomy. Obstet Gynaecol 1993; 81: 357–362

23 Nathorst-Boos J, Fuchs T, Van Schoultz B. Consumer's attitude to hysterectomy. Acta Obstet Gynecol Scand 1992; 71: 230–234

24 Alexander DA, Atherton-Naji A, Pinion SB et al. Randomised trial comparing hysterectomy with endometrial ablation for dysfunctional uterine bleeding: psychiatric and psychosocial aspects. BMJ. 1996; 312: 280–284

25 Crosignani PG. Vercellini P. Apolone G. De Giorgi O. Cortesi I. Meschia M. Endometrial resection versus vaginal hysterectomy for menorrhagia: long-term clinical and quality-of-life outcomes. Am J Obstet Gynecol 1997; 177: 95–101

26 Helstrom L, Weiner E, Sorbom D, Backstrom T. Predictive value of psychiatric history,

genital pain and menstrual symptoms for sexuality after hysterectomy. Acta Obstet Gynecol Scand 1994; 73: 575–580

27 Lalos A, Lalos O. The partner's view about hysterectomy. J Psychosom Obstet Gynaecol 1996; 17: 119–124

28 Helstrom L, Sorbom D, Backstrom T. Influence of the partner relationship on sexuality after subtotal hysterectomy. Acta Obstet Gynecol Scand 1995; 74: 142–146

29 Masters W, Johnson V. Human Sexual Response. Boston, Mass, USA:Little Brown, 1966

30 Hite S. The New Hite Report: the revolutionary report on female sexuality updated. : London:Hamlyn, 2000

31 Domoney C, Studd JWW. Hysterectomy and sexuality. In: Sheth SS, Studd JWW. (eds) Vaginal Hysterectomy. London: Martin Dunitz, 2002

32 Baskin LS, Erol A, Li YW, Liu WH, Kurzrock E, Cunha GR. Anatomical studies of the human clitoris. J Urol 1999; 162: 1015–1020

33 O'Connell HE, Hutson JM, Anderson CR, Plenter RJ. Anatomical relationship between urethra and clitoris. J Urol 1998; 159: 1892–1897

34 Rees MA. O'Connell HE. Plenter RJ. Hutson JM. The suspensory ligament of the clitoris: connective tissue supports of the erectile tissues of the female urogenital region. Clin Anat 2000; 13: 397–403

35 Kilkku P, Gronroos M, Hirvonen T, Rauramo L. Supravaginal uterine amputation vs hysterectomy. Effects on libido and orgasm. Acta Obstet Gynecol Scand 1983; 62: 147–152

36 Thakar R, Manyonda I. Hysterectomy for benign disease – total versus subtotal. In: Studd JWW. (ed) Progress in Obstetrics and Gynaecology, vol 14. Edinburgh: Churchill Livingstone, 2000

37 Thakar R, Manyonda I, Stanton S, Clarkson P, Robinson G. Bladder, bowel and sexual function after hysterectomy for benign conditions. Br J Obstet Gynaecol 1997; 104: 983–987

38 Kilkku P. Supravaginal uterine amputation versus hysterectomy with reference to bladder symptoms and incontinence. Acta Obstet Gynecol Scand 1985; 64: 375–379

39 Virtanen H, Makinen J, Tenho P, Kiilholma P, Pitkanen Y, Hirvonen T. Effects of abdominal hysterectomy on urinary and sexual symptoms. Br J Urol 1993; 72: 868–872

40 Goldstein I, Berman JR. Vasculogenic female sexual dysfunction: vaginal engorgement and clitoral erectile insufficiency syndromes. Int J Impot Res 1998; Suppl 2: S84–S90, discussion S98–S101

41 Darnell-Jones DE, Shackelford P, Brame R. Supracervical hysterectomy: back to the future? Am J Obstet Gynecol 1999; 180: 513–515

42 Studd JWW, Shifting indications for hysterectomy. Lancet 1995; 345: 388

43 Kilkku P. Supravaginal uterine amputation vs. hysterectomy. Effects on coital frequency and dyspareunia. Acta Obstet Gynecol Scand 1983; 62: 141–145

44 Studd JWW. Prophylactic oopherectomy. Br J Obstet Gynaecol 1989; 96: 506–509

45 Namnoum AB, Hickman TN, Goodman SB, Gehlbach DL, Rock JA. Incidence of symptom recurrence after hysterectomy for endometriosis. Fertil Steril 1995; 65: 898–902

46 Zakaria FBP, Studd JWW. Hormone replacement therapy following hysterectomy for endometriosis. In: Mini symposium in endometriosis. Curr Obstet Gynaecol 1998; 8: 191–196. (Based on: Henderson AF, Studd JWW. The role of definitive surgery and hormone replacement therapy in the treatment of endometriosis: retrospective study of oestrogen replacement therapy following hysterectomy for endometriosis. In: Rock TE. (ed) Modern Approaches to Endometriosis. 1991, 275–290)

47 Bizette Y, Buzelin JM. Prolapse after a hysterectomy. A study of 70 cases. Rev Fr Gynecol Obstet 1984; 79: 687–692

48 Hasson HM. Cervical removal at hysterectomy for benign disease. Risks and benefits. J Reprod Med 1993; 38: 781–790

49 Office of National Statistics. Cancer Trends in England and Wales, 1950–1999. London: HMSO, 2000

50 Siddle N, Sarrell P, Whitehead MI. The effect of hysterectomy on age at ovarian failure. Identification of a subgroup of women with premature loss of ovarian function and literature review. Fertil Steril 1987; 47: 94–100

51 Parazzini F, Negri E, La Vecchia C, Luchini L, Mezzopane R. Hysterectomy, oophorectomy and subsequent ovarian cancer risk. Obstet Gynecol 1993; 81: 363–366

52 Storm HH. Clemmensen IH. Manders T. Brinton LA. Supravaginal uterine amputation in Denmark 1978–1988 and risk of cancer. Gynecol Oncol 1992; 45: 198–201
53 Riley AJ. Sexuality and the menopause. Sex Marit Ther 1991; 6: 135–146
54 Molander U, Milsom I, Ekelund P, Mellstrom D, Eriksson O. Effect of oral oestriol on vaginal flora and cytology and urogenital symptoms in the post-menopause. Maturitas 1990; 12: 113–120
55 Chakravarti S, Collins WP, Forecast JD, Newton JR, Oram DH, Studd JWW. Hormonal profiles after the menopause. BMJ 1976; 2: 784–787
56 Sands R, Studd J. Exogenous androgens in postmenopausal women. Am J Med 1995; 16: 98: 76S-79S
57 Bachmann G, Bancroft J, Braunstein G et al. Female androgen insufficiency: the Princeton consensus statement on definition, classification, and assessment. Fertil Steril 2002; 77: 660–665
58 Chakravarti S, Collins WP, Newton JR, Oram DH, Studd JW. Endocrine changes and symptomatology after oophorectomy in premenopausal women. Br J Obstet Gynaecol 1977; 84: 769–775
59 Bachmann GA, Leiblum SR. Sexuality in sexagenarian women. Maturitas 1991; 13: 43–50
60 Sherwin BB, Gelfand MM, Brender W. Androgen enhances sexual motivation in females: a prospective, crossover study of sex steroid administration in the surgical menopause. Psychosom Med 1985; 47: 339–351
61 Chakravarti S, Collins WP, Thom MH, Studd JWW. Relation between plasma hormone profiles, symptoms, and response to oestrogen treatment in women approaching the menopause. BMJ 1979; 1: 983–985
62 Studd JWW, Collins WP, Chakravarti S, Newton JR, Oram D, Parsons A. Oestradiol and testosterone implants in the treatment of psychosexual problems in the post-menopausal woman. Br J Obstet Gynaecol 1977; 84: 314–316
63 Khastgir G, Studd J. Patients' outlook, experience, and satisfaction with hysterectomy, bilateral oophorectomy, and subsequent continuation of hormone replacement therapy. Am J Obstet Gynecol 2000; 183: 1427–1433
64 Nathorst-Boos J, Hammar M. Effect on sexual life – a comparison between Tibolone and a continuous estradiol-norethisterone acetate regimen. Maturitas 1997; 26: 15–20
65 Domoney CL, Vashisht A, Kelma R, Studd JWW. HRT continuance 10 years after hysterectomy. Menopause 1999; 6: 338

David Nunns R.P. Symonds

Improving the prognosis in cervical cancer

Globally, cervical cancer remains an important cause of mortality among young women. Around 80% of women who present will have inoperable disease and around 300,000 will die from this disease each year. Non-industrialised countries account for the greatest number of cases. In India, cervical cancer is the commonest cause of death among women between the ages of 20 and 40 years.[1] Tragically, the inequities in healthcare and competition for scarce funds will mean that the incidence of this disease is unlikely to fall in incidence in the near future. There is currently an epidemic of human papilloma virus (HPV) infection and the prospect of a vaccine to this virus becoming available to non-industrialised countries in the next 10 years is small. In industrialised countries, however, the situation is very different with an overall decline in incidence and mortality from cervical cancer. In recent years, death rates were falling in the UK at a rate of 1.5%/year prior to the introduction of the 1988 NHS Cervical Screening Programme.[2] Since the introduction of population-based screening, death rates have fallen even further. Despite this good news, about 1000 women will still die from their disease each year and annually there are over 2500 new cases. How can we improve prognosis even further for these women? Clearly all aspects of the disease can be addressed from prevention with cervical screening, to improvements in imaging, surgery, chemo-irradiation and, most recently, the development of multidisciplinary teams.

CERVICAL SCREENING

The aim of screening is to prevent the development of cancer. There are three bases for any screening programme: (i) there is a long, latent interval in which

Mr David Nunns MD MRCOG, Consultant Gynaecological Oncologist, Nottingham City Hospital, Hucknall Road, Nottingham NG5 1PB, UK

Mr R.P. Symonds MD FRCP FRCR, Reader in Oncology, University of Leicester, Leicester Royal Infirmary, Leicester LE1 5WW, UK (for correspondence)

premalignant change or occult cancer can be detected; (ii) there is effective treatment for premalignant change and for cancer; and (iii) the screening programme is cost-effective.

Screening for cervical cancer certainly satisfies the first two criteria. There is usually a long, latent period in which cervical intra-epithelial neoplasia (CIN), can be detected. Treatment for CIN is effective, as is treatment for cervical cancer. The cost effectiveness of cervical cancer screening is debatable, but this is a political issue. By 1997, it was estimated that the UK screening programme was saving the lives of 800 women annually at a cost of £124 million per year.[2]

Effectiveness of cervical screening

Cervical screening was shown to be effective in several countries, although not by means of randomised controlled trials unlike with breast cancer where screening trials were carried out prior to its introduction. One of the earliest and arguably the most successful screening campaign originated in British Columbia in 1949.[3] Since 1970, the number of women screened at least has been maintained at about 85% of the population at risk. From 1975 to 1985, the incidence of invasive carcinoma of cervix has fallen by 78% and mortality by 72%. Another area of the world where mortality has fallen following an organised screening campaign is the Nordic countries. Mortality trends in Denmark, Finland, Iceland, Norway and Sweden are most instructive. These five countries have similar educational and socio-economic structures and share common factors in behaviour and life-style. The health care systems are also very similar, therefore comparison is valid. In Iceland, where the nation-wide programme had the greatest target range, the fall in mortality was greatest (50%). Nation-wide screening programmes also existed in Finland (50% reduction) and Sweden (34% reduction). The smaller reduction of mortality in Sweden in this time period was perhaps due to the narrow population age range screened compared to Finland. In Denmark, where only 40% of the population was covered by an organised screening campaign, overall mortality fell by 25% and in Norway, where only 5% were screened, there was the smallest reduction of cervical cancer deaths of only 10%.[4]

Screening for cervical cancer in the non-industrialised world

This disease is still the most important female cancer in South and South-East Asia, Latin America and sub Saharan Africa.[5] In these countries, there is neither the wealth nor the health resources to follow the Western model of taking smears 5-yearly or more often and intensive treatment for CIN. A large controlled trial from Zimbabwe containing almost 11,000 women points to an alternative strategy.[6] Cytology was compared to visual inspection of the cervix after acetic acid (VIA) was applied to demonstrate white areas containing potential premalignant areas. Women with abnormal smears by either test underwent colposcopy. The main findings were that VIA was abnormal in 20% of women and the sensitivity (76.7%) was greater than cytology (44.3%). The low sensitivity of cytology in this study may be due to the high incidence of sexually transmitted disease in the screened population. This may also explain the low specificity of VIA (64%) compared to cytology (90%). VIA in this study had a positive predictive value (PPV) of only 25.9%.

The second problem is how to treat CIN lesions on a large scale in non-industrialised areas. A review of randomised and non-randomised trials of treatment of CIN[7] concluded that recurrence and persistence rates following cryotherapy, laser and large loop excision were very similar. Cryotherapy, which requires only bottled gas to cool the cryoprobe, could be used to treat possible premalignant cervical abnormalities in non-industrialised areas. A test with the PPV of only 25.9% means that 3 out of 4 women were potentially over-treated. However, in view of the low morbidity associated with these treatments, in well-trained hands, the treatment of the cervix in all women with abnormal screening results could be judged to be ethical because of the huge reduction of risk of cervical cancer so achieved, especially without the complexity of colposcopy or other means of tissue diagnosis.

Screening for cervical cancer in the UK

If the target population is not adequately covered, screening may be less effective and this may be why screening in British Columbia prior to 1988 produced better results than in the rest of Canada.[8] The lessons learned from the British screening campaign are salutary. The British cervical screening programme started in 1964. With the exception of the highly successful screening programme in north-east Scotland,[9,10] overall the screening campaign was a failure. In a strongly worded editorial in *The Lancet*[11] entitled *Death by Incompetence* this failure was ascribed to inadequate use of resources. The British programme was extensively overhauled by the Department of Health and three major changes were instituted from 1988. The first was a computerised call and recall system to try to reach as many of the target population as possible. The laboratory service underwent a major quality assurance programme to ensure uniformity of reporting smears and screening targets were written into general practitioner's contracts. General practitioners are only paid for carrying out cervical smears when they have screened 50–80% of the target population within their practice over the preceding 5.5 years. During this period, the coverage of the target population in England increased from 41% to 83%.[12] This increased coverage of target population immediately translated into reduction of both incidence and mortality. By contrast, the incidence of carcinoma of cervix remained virtually constant between 1971 and 1988. The incidence of cervical cancer fell from 4467 new cases in 1985[12] to 2900 cases in 1995.[13] The age specific incidence fell by 35% from 16 per 100,000 in 1988 to 10 per 100,000 in 1995. Mortality has decreased even more than incidence. Owing perhaps to improvements in treatment and perhaps earlier diagnosis, mortality had been falling from 1950 to 1987 by about 1.5% per annum. Following the overhaul of the screening campaign in 1988, mortality had fallen to 3.7 per 100,000 (1150 deaths) by 1997.[13]

The real challenges for the cervical screening programme in the future are improving the predictive value of detecting CIN on a smear, reducing the false-negative rates and increasing the population uptake of the test. Progress is underway. There is currently a review of liquid based cytology within the National Health Service and HPV testing is in its early stages of development. Training of smear takers and cytoscreeners together with re-validation should help improve the accuracy of the cervical smear even further.

IMAGING

Recent improvements in cross-sectional imaging, in particular with magnetic resonance imaging (MRI), have led to improvements in pretreatment tumour assessment and assessing spread when surgery is being considered, either as a primary procedure or when a recurrence has occurred prior to pelvic exenteration. Better imaging has also resulted in optimal radiotherapy planning with more accurate assessments of the tumour target volumes used in planning.

Patients with cervical cancer are staged clinically according to FIGO. Accurate staging of cervical cancer is essential so that appropriate treatment can be planned. When patients are being considered for radical primary surgery, understaging the disease can lead to a need for postoperative adjuvant treatments. Ideally, multimodal treatment should be avoided to reduce morbidity. When a patient is felt to have early stage disease which may be potentially treated by radical surgery, then MRI has shown to be superior to clinical staging and computerised tomography (CT) in the identification of tumour extent, particularly with parametrial extension.[14] Hricak et al. examined the value of MRI detecting parametrial disease in 57 patients who had surgery and found a predictive value of 94% for determining the absence of disease.[15] MRI provides accurate staging information in 70–90% of cases when correlated to surgical findings compared to 60–70% with CT scanning. There are limitations of assessing lymph nodes with all cross-sectional imaging including MRI and CT and both techniques have an accuracy of 79–80% for detecting enlarged lymph nodes. MRI and CT can detect metastatic nodes on the basis of size, asymmetry and altered attenuation (e.g. cystic changes within the node), but overall sensitivity and specificity is reduced as it is difficult to distinguish between hyperplastic inflammatory nodes and small foci of disease within normal sized nodes.

The benefits of multiplanar imaging seen with MRI include better radiotherapy planning compared to clinical staging and CT in locally advanced disease. In a study by Russell et al., 25 patients undergoing primary radiotherapy for cervical cancer had treatment fields compared between MRI scanning with conventional bony landmarks and clinical examination.[16] In only 11 cases (44%) of patients clinically assessed would the treatment have adequately covered clinical tumour volume.

MANAGEMENT

Early disease

The term micro-invasive carcinoma was first defined in 1947 to include a group of patients who could perhaps be treated by less than radical means. Since 1961, the definition of micro-invasive disease underwent a number of changes. Currently, micro-invasive disease is sub-classified into two groups, stage 1a$_1$ and stage 1a$_2$. Micro-invasive disease by definition can only be diagnosed microscopically. All visible lesions, even if superficial, should be allocated to stage 1b. Cases of micro-invasive carcinoma should not extend more than 7 mm horizontally. In stage 1a$_1$, the depth of invasion is only 3 mm. In stage 1a$_2$, the depth of invasion is 3–5 mm.

Stage 1a₁

Prognosis is excellent for stage 1a₁ carcinoma of cervix and the problem is to avoid over-treatment. The incidence of nodal metastasis in this group is under 0.5%. A 100% 5-year survival was reported from patients treated in Dundee[17] and in the West of Scotland.[18] The very large American SEER study of 10% of all patients treated for gynaecological cancer in the US between 1973 and 1987 reported a 97% 5-year survival in this group.[19] The large series of 309 patients reported from Graz[20] suggested that a cone biopsy or simple hysterectomy is as effective as a radical vaginal abdominal hysterectomy if there is less than 3 mm stromal invasion. A radical hysterectomy in this group would be considered as overtreatment.

Stage 1a₂

When stromal invasion is 3–5 mm, the incidence of lymph node metastasis is 7% with an overall recurrence rate of 5%.[21] The optimal management of this group has not been defined. Clinical trials designed to address the optimal management in this group would need to recruit large numbers of patients, as recurrence and death rates in this group are low. Management options vary from cone biopsy, simple (extrafascial hysterectomy) and radical hysterectomy and pelvic lymph-adenectomy. In the past, the standard treatment has been a modified radical hysterectomy (Rutledge class 2) procedure, but there is little prospective evidence to support this and current opinion would class this procedure as overtreatment. Large retrospective series such as those of Burghardt et al.[20] certainly do suggest that more extensive treatment is more effective than simple hysterectomy or conisation, but even so the number of deaths associated with conservative treat-ment are small. Clearly a blanket approach to treatment should be discouraged and treatment should be individualised. An accurate histopathological assessment is crucial to help decide whether further treatment is necessary. The presence of tumour confluence, lymph-vascular space invasion and incomplete excision of CIN will help in decision making.

There is an increasing movement towards fertility conserving procedures using minimal access surgery in early stage disease. The primary tumour can be managed with loop biopsy or cone biopsy to remove the primary and any CIN. A repeat loop biopsy or cone biopsy can be performed if necessary for residual CIN. As an alternative, a simple hysterectomy can be suggested if there are con-current gynaecological problems. An assessment of the pelvic lymph nodes can be carried out using either the open retroperitoneal approach, or by performing a laparoscopic pelvic lymphadenectomy. This will identify those 7% of women in this group in whom adjuvant therapy is necessary. Vascular space involvement may be a useful predictor for possible nodal metastases and may distinguish which patients require more radical treatment. A retrospective series of 94 patients with stage 1a₂ disease found an incidence of lymph node metastases with or without lymph vascular space invasion of 16.1% and 3.2%, respectively.[21] Extension of CIN into the vaginal fornices should be identified prior to treatment and ideally excised at the time of surgery.

Stage 1B–2A

Population-based, retrospective studies show very similar results for radical surgery or radical radiotherapy in the treatment of potentially operable cervical cancer.[18] This may explain the lack of clinical trials over the years.

In 1975, Newton and colleagues[22] reported a study of 119 patients, randomised to receive either radical hysterectomy or radical surgery. The 10-year survival rates favoured surgery (75%) rather than radiotherapy (65%), but were not statistically different. It is noteworthy that 6 out of 12 patients who recurred after surgery were successfully cured by radiotherapy.

The definitive modern randomised study was carried out in North Italy.[23] A total of 343 patients with stage IB or IIA tumours fit for either modality were randomised to either radical surgery or radical radiotherapy. The 5-year overall and disease-free survival were identical for both surgical and radiotherapy groups (83% and 74%, respectively). A surprisingly large percentage of patients (64%) had postoperative radiotherapy following radical surgery for adverse pathological findings. This high frequency of postoperative radiotherapy does not explain the increased morbidity in patients treated by surgery. Of those treated by surgery alone, 31% had grade 2–3 morbidity. By comparison, only 12% of patients treated by radiation had grade 2–3 morbidity. The combination of both treatments increased morbidity; grade 2–3 morbidity was 29% for patients undergoing both surgery and radiotherapy. In this study, although the frequency of serious complications was greater in the surgical arm, these complications were easier to correct than those secondary to radiation. The conclusion of this study is that the optimum candidates for primary radical surgery were women with normal ovarian function and cervical diameters of 4 cm or smaller, whereas radiotherapy was preferable for post-menopausal women. It is noteworthy in this series that 88% of patients with tumours greater than 4 cm treated by primary surgery, required postoperative radiotherapy. Consideration should, therefore, be given to treating patient with stage 1B$_2$ tumours with primary chemoradiation because, following surgery for these tumours, there is a high chance of positive pelvic lymph nodes and incomplete/close margins when radiotherapy would be indicated.

If a surgical approach is to be considered, what is the procedure of choice? Piver et al.[24] reported on five classes of extended hysterectomy used in the treatment of cervical cancer (Table 1). The class III radical hysterectomy removes the central lesion with wide radical excision of the parametrial and

Table 1 Rutledge classification of extended hysterectomy for cervical cancer[24]

Class 1	Ensures removal of all cervical tissue: also called extrafascial hysterectomy
Class 2	Modified radical hysterectomy removing the medical half of the cardinal and uterosacral ligaments. The uterine vessels are divided medial to the ureter
Class 3	The classical Wertheim's radical hysterectomy with wide radical dissection of the parametrial and paravaginal tissue. The ureter is dissected down to the bladder. The uterosacral ligaments are divided at their origin and the cardinal ligaments are divided at the pelvic wall
Class 4	More radical than class 3. The ureter is completely dissected from the pubovesical ligament , the superior vesical artery is sacrificed and 75% of the vagina removed
Class 5	Removal of a central recurrence – likely to be an exenteration

paravaginal tissue. The uterine artery is ligated at its origin, the lateral and posterior parametria are resected to the pelvic side-walls and several centimetres of vagina are removed. It is considered the surgical standard for operable cervical cancers. The Rutledge classification, however, is useful as class III hysterectomy is likely to be overtreatment for some operable cervical cancers such as stage $1A_2$. In addition, morbidity in this group is high compared to class II. Evidence on the procedure of choice is scant. In a study by Landoni et al.,[25] 238 women with operable stage 1B/2A disease were randomised to class II or III radical hysterectomies. There were no differences between the overall survival, recurrence rates and disease-free survival between the two groups; however, morbidity was significantly higher among patients undergoing the class III procedure. This study did not show any survival benefit between the two classes of radical hysterectomies, but patients did not pre-operatively undergo any radiological imaging and there were a large number of patients with tumours greater than 4 cm in size. As a consequence, 54% of patients underwent adjuvant radiotherapy. Future trials could address the value of different classes of radical hysterectomy in appropriately staged $1B_1$ tumours where an MRI has been performed to detect parametrial involvement.

Since the development of laparoscopic assessment of pelvic lymph nodes, the vaginal radical hysterectomy, introduced by Schauta in 1901, has recently been revived as an alternative to the traditional abdominal procedure for operable cervical cancer. The procedure involved a radical excision of the cervix, parametria and proximal ligaments (Rutledge class 2) together with removal of the uterus. Its main benefits are its reduced morbidity over the abdominal procedure. Several studies have shown little difference in 5-year survival between the two procedures in early stage 1B disease.[26,27]

It is commonly said that radical surgery preserves sexual function compared to irradiation in the treatment of operable cervical cancer. There are no randomised trials to support this claim. A Swedish study comparing sexual function of women treated with early stage cervical cancer, compared to a control group randomly selected for age and region of residence, found that persistent vaginal changes compromised sexual activity and resulted in considerable distress.[28] The authors found treatment with surgery alone was associated with increased risks of insufficient vaginal lubrication, vaginal shortness and reduced vaginal elasticity. As compared with surgery alone, intracavity or external beam or both in addition or instead of surgery had a small effect if any on the risks of reduced vaginal lubrication, reduced genital swelling, vaginal shortness or vaginal inelasticity. The effect of treatment upon sexual function is a very poorly investigated topic and requires further study.

Fertility conserving surgery in early stage cervical cancer

Fertility conserving surgery can be considered in patients with small stage $1B_1$ cervical tumours using the radical vaginal trachelectomy procedure. Experience of this in the UK is limited and should still be considered as experimental with radical hysterectomy being the gold standard treatment. The procedure involves a radical (80%) excision of the cervix, upper vagina and proximal cardinal ligaments. A cervical suture is placed around the cervical isthmus.[29] This procedure is usually combined with a laparoscopic pelvic lymphadenectomy.

Suitable cases include small tumours less than 2 cm, either squamous or adenocarcinomas in well-informed, consented patients. Completion treatment may be necessary in 10% of patients because of either positive pelvic lymph nodes or close or incomplete excision margins. In Shepherd's series of 30 patients, there were no recurrences with a mean follow-up of 23 months.[29] Long-term follow-up is not known. Prior to trachelectomy, patients had undergone a loop biopsy to confirm the presence of invasive disease and had a pretreatment examination under anaesthetic and magnetic resonance imaging scan. The selection of patients appears appropriate, as 60% of cases had no residual tumour in the cervix. In the D'Argent's series, poor prognostic factors included tumours larger than 2 cm and the presence of lymphovascular space invasion where recurrences were reported.[30] In Shepherd's series, 9 live births were reported in 14 pregnancies and 7 of these were preterm with 4 of these being less than 30 weeks. Infertility occurred in 20% of patients.

Advanced disease

Radiotherapy is the treatment of choice for more advanced stage cancer (stages 2B–4). Treatment is usually a combination of external beam megavoltage radiotherapy to the pelvis plus a local boost to the pelvis using brachytherapy. There is no consensus on the best technique type of brachytherapy or even where and how to measure the radiation dose given to the tumour.[31] One reason may be that, in skilled hands, the 5-year survival at various stages are remarkably similar using conceptually different external beam schedules and types of brachytherapy. Typical results appear in Table 2. Recently, the fashion has been to treat fitter patients with chemotherapy along with radiotherapy.

Combined chemotherapy and radiation treatment

Both clinical studies and animal experiments have shown that radiation doses which will consistently eradicate small tumours will be only effective in a minority of large lesions. The maximum radiation dose that can be given to patients with carcinoma of cervix is limited by the tolerance of surrounding organs such as bladder or bowel. Even employing what are considered optimal

Table 2 Carcinoma of the cervix. Patients treated in 1990–1992. Survival by FIGO stage[39] ($n = 11,945$)

Stage	Patients (n)	Overall 5-year survival (%)
Ia$_1$	518	95.1
Ia$_2$	384	94.9
Ib	4657	80.1
IIa	813	66.3
IIb	2251	63.5
IIIa	180	33.3
IIIb	2350	38.7
IVa	294	17.1
IVb	198	9.4

external beam fractionation in combination with intracavity treatment, local control is seen in only approximately half of patients with stage III and stage IVa tumours. Theoretically, chemotherapy combined with radiotherapy may increase the therapeutic ratio by producing a greater tumour regression than either component alone without any increase in toxicity. Chemotherapy may act as a cytotoxic within its own right, killing cells within the irradiated pelvis, and by acting upon distant metastasis. Chemotherapy can also act as a radiation sensitiser leading to superadded cell kill.

Cisplatin is the most effective cytotoxic agent in the treatment of cervical cancer. Response rates of up to 72% have been seen in previously untreated patients when cisplatin-based chemotherapy has been given before radiotherapy,[32] but a meta-analysis of chemotherapy given before radiotherapy has not shown a consistent survival advantage.[33] However, chemotherapy given along with radiotherapy seems to be much more effective.

The magnitude of this effect led the National Cancer Institute of the US in February 1999 to propose that all patients with cervical cancer should be considered for concomitant chemotherapy and radiotherapy. This view was based on results of 5, of then unpublished, randomised clinical trials that showed a 30–50% reduction in the odds of death.

Five of the most influential studies are listed in Table 3. A meta-analysis has been carried out of 19 trials (17 published, 2 unpublished) performed between 1981 and 2000 using the Cochrane collaborative methodology.[34] These trials included 4580 randomised patients although due to patient exclusion and differential reporting, between 2865 and 3611 patients were available for different analyses. The trials differed in size, design, accrual period, and anticancer agent and schedule, Cisplatin being the most commonly employed agent. The review strongly suggests that chemo-radiation improves overall survival (HR = 0 71; $P >$ 0.00001) whether platinum was used (HR = 0.70; $P > 0.00001$) or not (HR = 0.81; $P = 0.20$). These effects were not modulated by the use of sequential chemo-therapy, use of hydroxyurea in the control arm or the timing of chemotherapy. There was some evidence that the beneficial effects were greater in trials including a higher proportion of stages 1 and 2 patients ($P = 0.009$). These relative effects translated into absolute survival benefit in progression free survival of 16% (95% CI 13–19%) and survival of 12% (95% CI 8–16%). There is evidence that chemotherapy reduced both local recurrence (OR = 0.61; $P \geq 0.0001$) and also distant metastasis. In addition to the expected improvement in local control, there was a highly significant reduction in the rate of distant metastasis (OR = 0.57; $P >$ 0.0001) in patients treated with platinum or non-platinum based chemotherapy, an effect that was not apparent in individual trials. This reduction was achieved with relatively short courses of chemotherapy combined with local treatment, yet currently there is no evidence that chemotherapy given before radiotherapy reduces the incidence of distant metastasis.

Combined chemo-radiotherapy seems to improve the therapeutic ratio. However, acute toxicity, particularly leukopenia and gastrointestinal, was increased in the combined arms of all trials. Acute side-effects are generally of short duration and resolve with medical management, whilst the late com-plications of radiotherapy lead to damage which can be difficult to reverse and may permanently impair quality-of-life. Unfortunately, late toxicity was recorded systematically in only three studies and the details of late morbidity reported

Table 3 Five of the most influential trials of radiotherapy and cisplatin-based chemotherapy

Trial	No. of patients	Stage	External beam R/T	LDR brachytherapy dose to point A	Chemotherapy	Survival	Reduction in risk of death	P
GOG 85[40]	368	IIB, III and IVa	As GOG 120	As GOG 120	Hydroxyurea or Hydroxyurea, cisplatin and 5-FU	43% / 55%	0.74	0.018
GOG 120[41]	575	IIb, III, IVa	40.8 Gy in 24 F (stage IIb); 51.0 Gy n 30 F (stage III, IVa)	40 Gy (stage IIb); 30 Gy (III or IVa) in 1 or 2 insertions	Hydroxyurea Hydroxyurea, cisplatin and 5-FU Weekly cisplatin	47% / 65% at 3 yr / 65%	0.58 / 0.61	0.004 / 0.002
RTOG 9001[42]	403	IIb III IVa or Ib/IIa > 5 cm or +ve pelvic nodes	Pelvic and para-aortic 45 Gy in 25 F; or Pelvic 45 Gy in 25 F	40 Gy (minimum total dose 85 Gy) in 1 or 2 insertions	None or Cisplatin and 5-FU	58% at 5 yr / 73%	0.52	0.004
GOG 123[43]	374	Bulky Ib (74 cm) (> 4 cm)	45 Gy in 25 F	30 Gy	None or Weekly cisplatin	74% at 3 yr / 83%	0.54	0.008
SWOG 8797[44]	243	Ia2, Ia2 Ib IIa, p.o. adverse path finding	49.3 Gy in 25 F	No brachytherapy	None or Cisplatin and 5-FU	71% at 4 yr / 81%	0.50	0.007

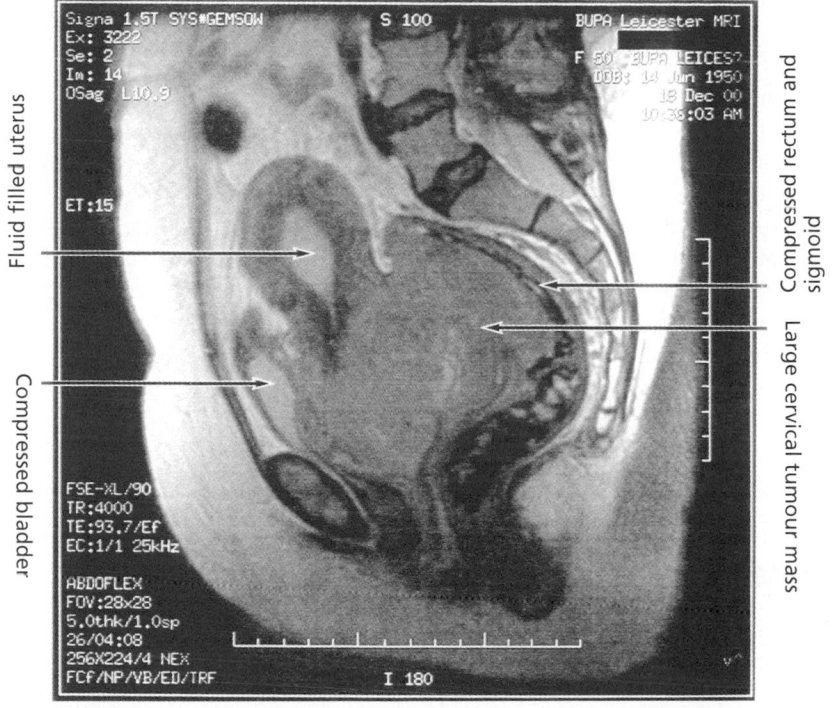

Fluid filled uterus

Compressed bladder

Compressed rectum and sigmoid

Large cervical tumour mass

Fig. 1 Before treatment. MRI scan of a patient with a stage III poorly differentiated carcinoma of cervix.

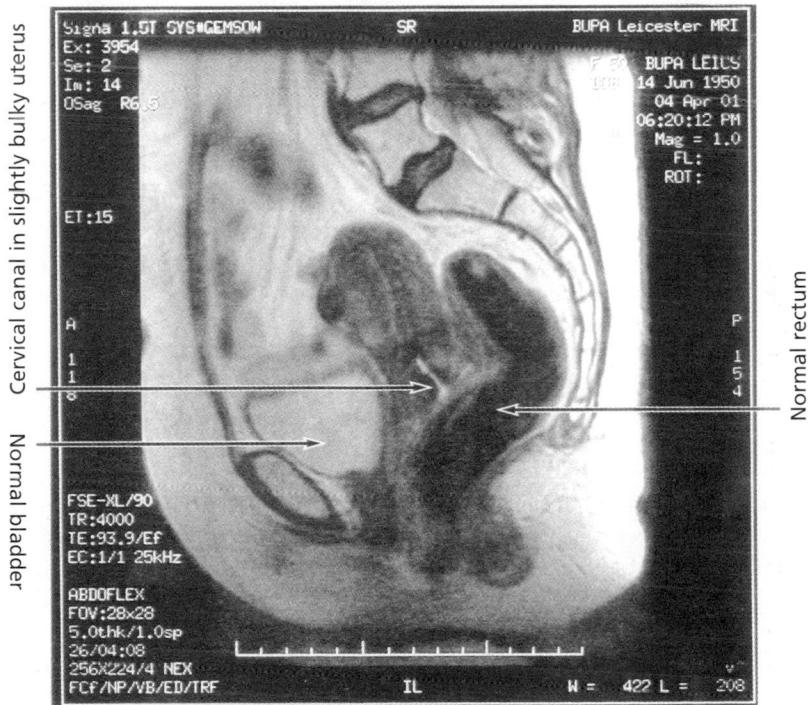

Cervical canal in slightly bulky uterus

Normal bladder

Normal rectum

Fig. 2 After treatment. MRI scan two months after treatment showed no evidence of tumour.

in other studies were sparse. Published information so far would indicate that there is no apparent increase in late complications but this question has not been fully answered.

Combined chemo-radiotherapy has become the current standard of care, but there still remains a number of outstanding issues, particularly the impact of radiation dose and the treatment duration plus the role of other cytotoxics in addition to cisplatin and drug scheduling.

Figure 1 is the MRI scan of a patient with a stage III poorly differentiated carcinoma of cervix filling the pelvis, compressing both the bladder and the rectosigmoid colon. She was treated with 6 pulses of cisplatin (40 mg/m^2) given weekly during pelvic radiotherapy. A dose of 45 Gy was given to the pelvic tumour using two 10 MV X-ray beams. This was followed by a single Selectron insertion of 26 Gy to point A at 1.46 Gy/h. An MRI scan two months after treatment (Fig. 2) showed no evidence of tumour. This was confirmed by an examination under anaesthetic, laparoscopy and biopsies of the cervix. She is disease-free 18 months after treatment.

MINIMAL ACCESS SURGERY

The current application of minimal access surgery (MIS) in gynaecological oncology relates to laparoscopic assessment of lymph nodes. In early disease, as mentioned previously, a laparoscopic pelvic lymphadenectomy can be carried out in patients with stage $1A_2/1B_1$ disease when either a cone biopsy or radical trachelectomy is being performed. This will help identify those patients where completion treatment is necessary and avoids the morbidity associated with the open extraperitoneal technique. The procedure is usually carried out as a day-case and the nodal counts between the two procedures are comparable.[35]

The technique of laparoscopic para-aortic lymphadenectomy is slowly evolving in the UK, but has its applications in the surgical staging of locally advanced cervical cancer.[36] The technique is performed as a day-case, usually extraperitoneally, and morbidity is minimal. Up to 30% of patients with stages 3–4 disease will have para-aortic nodal disease. There are benefits of knowing the para-aortic nodal status as it provides prognostic information, avoids unnecessary extended field irradiation, and avoids aborted exenterative surgery. In Querleu's series of 53 cases, there were two failures and the average node yield was 20.[37]

RECURRENCES

Pelvic exenteration is the preferred salvage treatment for patients with localised central recurrences following radiotherapy. With the improvements in radiotherapy techniques over recent years, the numbers of patients suitable for this procedure has fallen. In well-selected patients, exenteration can be curative with variable 5-year survival rates reported in the literature of up to 62%.[38] The procedure has mortality rate of 5% and postoperative morbidity is high including sepsis, small-bowel obstruction, and thrombosis. Prognosis in the group as a whole is likely to have improved over recent years with better patient selection, surgical techniques, and postoperative care.

KEY POINTS FOR CLINICAL PRACTICE

- Cervical cancer remains globally a major health problem. In non-industrialised countries, further research is necessary to confirm the value of visual inspection added to acetic acid (VIA) and to test other novel methods of screening. However, if the promise of VIA is realised, the incidence and mortality rate from this common disease may rapidly fall in the non-industrialised world.

- In the UK, the incidence of the disease is falling and patients are presenting at an earlier stage. Challenges for the future include tailoring the treatment according to the disease stage, avoiding overtreatment, and reducing treatment morbidity. Time has passed when a radical hysterectomy should be offered to all patients with operable disease.

- Fertility conservation remains an important issue in a disease which essentially affects young women.

- In advanced disease, the evidence for chemo-irradiation is convincing.

- Prognosis will clearly be a reflection of an accurate assessment of the tumour together with the most appropriate treatment.

- Integral to obtaining the best outcome is subspecialisation, the development of cancer centres and the input of the multidisciplinary team.

References

1 Pisani P, Parkin DM, Bray F, Ferlay J. Estimates of the world wide mortality from 25 cancers in 1990. Int J Cancer 1999; 83: 18–29
2 Shoell WMJ, Janicek MF, Mirhashemi R. Epidemiology and biology of cervical cancer. Semin Surg Oncol 1999; 16: 203–211
3 Anderson GH, Boyes DA, Benedet JL et al. Organisation and results of the cervical cytology screening programme in British Columbia, 1955–85. BMJ 1988; 196: 975–978
4 Laara E, Day NE, Hakama M. Trends in mortality from cervical cancer in Nordic countries. Association with organised screening programs. Lancet 1987; i: 1247–1249
5 Parkin DM, Pisani P, Ferlay J. Global cancer statistics. Cancer J Clin 1999; 49: 33–64
6 University of Zimbabwe/JHPIEGO Cervical Cancer Project. Visual inspection with acetic acid for cervical cancer screening: test qualities in a primary care setting. Lancet 1999; 353: 869–873
7 Cox JT. Management of cervical intra-epithelial neoplasia. Lancet 1999; 353: 857–859
8 Skrabanek P. Cervical cancer screening; the time for reappraisal. Can J Public Health 1988; 79: 86–89
9 MacGregor JE, Moss SM, Parkin MD et al. A case control study of cervical cancer screening in north east Scotland. BMJ 1985; 290: 1534–1536
10 Duguid HLD, Duncan ID, Currie J. Screening for cervical intra-epithelial neoplasia in Dundee and Angus 1962–81 and relation with invasive cervical cancer rates. Lancet 1985; ii: 1053–1056
11 Anon. Cancer of the cervix: death by incompetence [Editorial]. Lancet 1985; ii: 363–364
12 Austoker J. Screening for cervical cancer. BMJ 1994; 309: 241–248
13 Quinn M, Babb P, Jones J. Effect of screening on incidence and mortality from cancer of cervix in England: evaluation based on routinely collected statistics. BMJ 1999; 218; 904–908

14 Kim SH, Choi, Lee HP et al. Uterine cervical carcinoma: comparison of CT and MRI findings. Radiology 1990; 175: 45–51

15 Hricak H, Lacey CG, Sandles LG et al. Invasive cervical carcinoma: comparison of MR imaging and surgical findings Radiology 1998; 166: 623–631

16 Russell AH, Walter JP, Anderson MW, Zukowski CL. Sagittal magnetic Imaging in the design of lateral radiation treatment portals for patients with locally advanced squamous cells carcinomas from the human uterine cervix; the identification of prognostically different subgroups. Radiother Oncol 1991; 7: 249–258

17 Duncan ID, Walker J. Microinvasive squamous carcinoma of cervix in the Tayside region of Scotland. Br J Obstet Gynaecol 1977; 84: 67–70

18 Bisset D, Lamont DW, Nwabineli NJ, Brodie MM, Symonds RP. The treatment of stage I carcinoma of cervix in the west of Scotland 1980–1987. Br J Obstet Gynaecol 1994; 101: 615–620

19 Kosary CL. FIGO stage, histology, histologic grade, age and race prognostic factors in determining survival for cancers of the female gynecological system: an analysis of 1973–1987 SEER cases of cancers of the endometrium, cervix, ovary, vulva and vagina. Semin Surg Oncol 1994; 10: 31–46

20 Burghardt E, Giradi F, Lahousen M, Pickel H, Tamussino K. Microinvasive carcinoma of the uterine cervix (International Federation of Gynaecology and Obstetrics Stage IA). Cancer 1991; 67: 1037–1045

21 Buckley SL, Tritz DM, Van Le L et al. Lymph node metastases and prognosis in patients with stage Ia$_2$ cervical cancer. Gynecol Oncol 1996; 63: 4–9

22 Newton M. Radical hysterectomy or radiotherapy for stage I cervical cancer: a prospective comparison with 5 and 10 year follow up. Am J Obstet Gynecol 1975; 123: 535–542

23 Landoni F, Maneo A, Colombo A et al. Randomised study of radical surgery versus radiotherapy for stage Ib–IIa cervical cancer. Lancet 1997; 350: 28–33

24 Piver S, Rutledge F, Smith JP. Five classes of extended hysterectomy for women with cervical cancer. Obstet Gynecol 1974; 44: 264–272

25 Landoni F, Maneo A, Cormio G et al. Class II versus class III radical hysterectomy in stage 1B–IIA cervical cancer: a prospective randomised study. Gynecol Oncol 2001; 80: 3–12

26 Roy M, Plante M, Renaud MC, Tetu B. Vaginal radical hysterectomy versus abdominal radical hysterectomy in the treatment of early-stage cervical cancer. Gynecol Oncol 2001; 62: 336–339

27 Massi G, Savino L, Susini T. Schauta-Amreich vaginal hysterectomy and Wertheim-Meigs abdominal hysterectomy in the treatment of cervical cancer: a retrospective analysis. Am J Obstet Gynecol 1993; 168: 928–935

28 Bergmark K, Avall-Lundquist E, Dickman PW, Henningsohn L, Steineck G. Vaginal changes and sexuality in women with a history of cervical cancer. N Engl J Med 1999; 340: 1383–1389

29 Shepherd JH, Mould T, Oram D. Radical trachelectomy in early stage carcinoma of the cervix outcome as judged by recurrences and fertility rates. Br J Obstet Gynaecol 2001; 108: 882–885

30 D'Argent D, Martin X, Sacchetoni A, Mathevet P. Laparoscopic vaginal radical trachelectomy: a treatment to preserve the fertility of cervical carcinoma patients. Cancer 2000; 88: 1877–1882

31 Visscher AG, Symonds RP. Dose and volume specification for reporting gynaecological brachytherapy: time for a change. Radiother Oncol 2001; 58: 1–4

32 Sundfor K, Trope CG, Hogberg T et al. Radiotherapy for cervical carcinoma. Cancer 1996; 77: 2371–2378

33 Tierney JF, Stewart LA, Parmar MK. Can the published data tell us about the effectiveness of neoadjuvant chemotherapy for locally advanced cancer of the uterine cervix? Eur J Cancer 1999; 35: 406–409

34 Green JA, Kirwan JM, Tierney JF et al. Systematic review and meta-analysis of randomised trials of concomitant chemotherapy and radiotherapy for cancer of the uterine cervix: better survival and reduced distant recurrence rate. Lancet 2001; 358: 781–786

35 Childers JM, Hatch KD, Tran A, Surwill EA. Laparoscopic para-aortic lymphadenectomy in gynaecological malignancies. Obstet Gynecol 1993; 82: 741–747

36 D'Argent D, Ansquer Y, Mathevet P. Technical development and result of left extraperitoneal laparoscopic paraaortic lymphadenectomy for cervical cancer. Gynecol Oncol 2000; 77: 87–92

37 Querleu D, D'Argent D, Ansquer Y, Leblanc E, Narducci F. Extraperitoneal endosurgical aortic and common iliac dissection in the staging of bulky or advanced cervical carcinomas. Cancer 2000; 88: 1883–1891

38 Morley GW, Lindenauer SM. Pelvic exenterative therapy for gynecologic malignancy: an analysis of 70 cases. Cancer 1976; 38 (Suppl 1): 581–586

39 Benedet J, Odicino F, Maisonneuve P et al. FIGO 1990–92 annual report: results of treatment of carcinoma of the cervix uteri. J Epidemiol Biostat 1998; 3: 5–34

40 Whitney CW, Sause W, Bundy BN et al. Randomised comparison of fluorouracil plus cisplatin versus hydroxyurea as an adjunct to radiation therapy in Stage IIb–IVa carcinoma of cervix with negative para-aortic nodes; a Gynecologic Oncology Group and South West Oncology Group study. J Clin Oncol 1999; 17: 1339–1348

41 Rose PG, Bundy BN, Watkins EB et al. Concurrent cisplatin based radiotherapy and chemotherapy for locally advanced cervical cancer. N Engl J Med 1999; 340: 1144–1153

41 Morris M, Eiffel PJ, Lu JD et al. Pelvic radiation with concurrent chemotherapy compared with pelvic and para-aortic radiation for high risk cervical cancer. N Engl J Med 1999; 340: 1137–1143

42 Keys HM, Bundy BN, Stehman FB et al. Cisplatin, radiation and adjuvant hysterectomy compared with radiation and adjuvant hysterectomy for bulky stage Ib cervical carcinoma. N Engl J Med 1999; 340: 1154–1161

43 Peters WA, Liu PY, Barrett RJ et al. Concurrent chemotherapy and pelvic radiation therapy compared with pelvic radiation therapy alone as adjuvant therapy after radical surgery in high risk early stage cancer of the cervix. J Clin Oncol 2000; 18: 1606–1613

20

Raj Mathur Robert Fox

Bilateral oophorectomy and hormone replacement therapy for women with endometriosis

Endometriosis is the presence of tissue histologically similar to endometrium outwith the uterine cavity. It is a frequent finding even in asymptomatic women.[1] Endometriosis is generally thought of as being a common condition but its precise incidence as a cause of symptoms is not known, partly because different diagnostic criteria are used by different researchers, but also because the association between the finding of endometriotic tissue and a woman's symptoms is not necessarily causal. This latter point is of great importance for clinicians: there is a risk of advising radical surgery for so-called endometriosis when the symptoms might be due to another (occult) condition. Irritable bowel syndrome (IBS), the commonest cause of pelvic pain, is often overlooked.[2] In contrast, symptomatic endometriosis is comparatively rare and possibly overdiagnosed.[3]

The ectopic endometrial-like tissue is often responsive to endogenous oestrogen in ways similar to normally situated endometrium. Appreciation of this has allowed the development of endocrine therapies that suppress disease activity and alleviate symptoms. Pituitary suppression with GnRH analogues, which induces a reversible state of profound oestrogen deficiency, is associated with regression of lesions and improvement of symptoms. Treatment with hormones that have androgenic and/or progestagenic properties has similar effects.

Despite considerable advances in medical treatment of endometriosis in recent years, it is not possible to achieve a satisfactory degree of symptom control for all women with endometriosis with medical treatment alone. A proportion of women with endometriosis experience progression of their disease despite medical treatment.[4] Others, particularly those with endometriomas (Fig. 1) and extensive pelvic adhesions, present at a stage of endometriosis too far advanced to respond

Dr Raj Mathur MRCOG, Subspecialty Trainee (Reproductive Medicine), University Department of Obstetrics and Gynaecology, The Rosie Hospital, Cambridge CB2 2SW, UK (for correspondence)

Mr Robert Fox MD MRCOG, Consultant Gynaecologist, Maternity Unit, Directorate of Obstetrics, Gynaecology & Paediatrics, Taunton & Somerset Hospital, Musgrove Park, Taunton TA1 5DA, UK

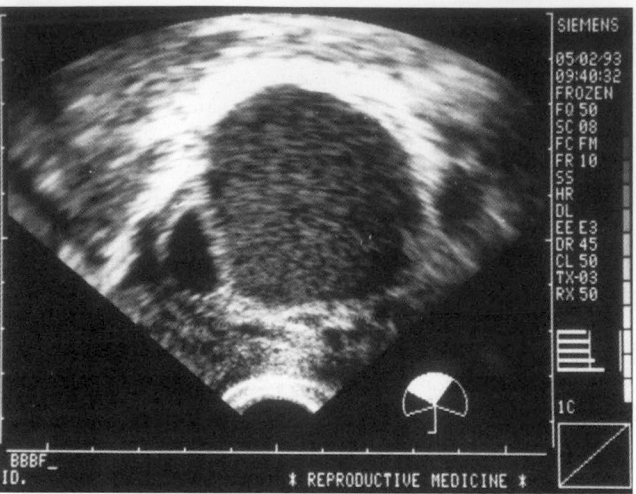

Fig. 1 A transvaginal ultrasound image of an ovary showing a circumscribed lesion with echogenic contents. At laparotomy, it was shown to be a small endometriotic (chocolate) cyst.

to medical treatment. Finally, some women are unable to tolerate the side-effects of any of the medical treatments available. Therefore, surgical treatment remains an important therapeutic option for the management of endometriosis. Conservative approaches are often employed, particularly for women who wish to retain their fertility, but for the small proportion of women with severe intractable symptoms, radical surgery with hysterectomy with ablation of all other pelvic disease is an important treatment option.

The role of bilateral oophorectomy in this situation remains unclear. Many clinicians have argued that optimum symptom control and prevention of recurrence requires the removal of both ovaries at the time of hysterectomy.[5] Set against this argument are the problems of hormone replacement therapy (HRT), particularly in younger women. Some women may find the thought of HRT from the age of 35 years a daunting prospect. Moreover, other women find that they cannot tolerate HRT and this may leave them to suffer severe menopausal-type symptoms (including loss of libido) after surgery and a significant chance of health problems in later life as a result of prolonged oestrogen deficiency. It is worth remembering that many women who choose surgery are exactly those who could not or would not tolerate the side-effects of hormonal treatments for their condition.

Clearly, the decision for or against bilateral oophorectomy is complex and each woman deserves a detailed and careful explanation. The purpose of this review, therefore, is to examine critically the available evidence for and against bilateral oophorectomy at the time of hysterectomy for women with endometriosis. In addition, we shall explore the value and safety of HRT in such cases.

EVIDENCE FOR AND AGAINST BILATERAL OOPHORECTOMY

The theoretical case for bilateral oophorectomy

The argument for bilateral oophorectomy as an adjunct to hysterectomy in women with endometriosis centres on the prevention of recurrent disease. It has long been recognised that women undergoing medical[4] or conservative surgical[6] treatments can experience a recurrence of their symptoms. This can be demoralising for the woman and frustrating for clinicians. Re-activation of endometriotic tissue after radical surgery is a doubly important issue because it may be precipitate a need for repeat surgery. One report revealed that repeat surgery after hysterectomy for endometriosis can be extremely difficult, with bowel involvement being common.[5] Complete removal of all ovarian tissue may prove difficult in these circumstances with the risk of further recurrence.

It is known that severe re-activation can occur regardless of whether the ovaries were removed or conserved at hysterectomy. Redwine[5] reported on symptomatic endometriosis requiring repeat surgery in 75 women who had had bilateral oophorectomy and in whom ovarian remnants were not detectable at the time of re-operation. The hypothesis that bilateral oophorectomy might provide improved symptom control probably arises from a number of separate observations: (i) the ovary is a common site of endometriosis; (ii) that intra-peritoneal oestrogen concentrations are very high in premenopausal women; and (iii) that endometriosis subsides after the menopause. However, it is important to examine critically whether, and to what extent, ovarian conservation increases the risks of recurrent symptoms and repeat surgery. The key questions in this regard are: (i) does bilateral oophorectomy reduce the recurrence of symptoms and the need for repeat surgery; and (ii) does the rate of problems justify it being undertaken routinely?

The nature of the published evidence

A literature search on the Medline database and a hand search of major fertility journals revealed no random-allocation trials comparing a policy of ovarian conservation with bilateral oophorectomy in women undergoing hysterectomy for endometriosis. Indeed, there are few studies on the subject at all and arguments for and against bilateral oophorectomy must of necessity be based on retrospective clinical data supplemented by our knowledge of the pathophysiology of endometriosis.

Critical review of individual articles

Cashman[7] followed up women treated surgically for endometriosis and found no significant differences in the incidence of recurrent/persistent symptoms between women undergoing bilateral oophorectomy and those who had some ovarian tissue conserved at hysterectomy. Importantly, they were able to contact only 155 of 271 women who had been treated during the 10-year study period. All patients in both groups reported some improvement in symptoms following surgery and none required repeat operation. Similarly, Sheets et al.[8] found recurrent endometriosis requiring treatment in only one woman out of 40 (2.5%) who had been treated with hysterectomy and ovarian conservation for significant symptoms thought to be related specifically to endometriosis. The average age of patients at hysterectomy was 36 years and the minimum duration of follow-up was 5 years. A significant limitation of this study was the lack of follow-up information on an additional 21 women, findings from whom may well have altered the results greatly as the numbers were small.

Moreover, in common with other early publications on this subject, a control group of patients who had undergone bilateral oophorectomy was not included in the analysis and the incidence of recurrent symptoms such as pain and dyspareunia, rather than simply re-operation, was not considered. In another early study,[9] a similarly low rate of recurrent problems was reported when ovarian tissue was conserved at hysterectomy for endometriosis. Of 86 women treated for endometriosis by hysterectomy with conservation of at least one ovary and a minimum duration of follow-up of 2 years, recurrent endometriosis needing re-operation was found in only 3 cases (4.1%). The length of follow-up in these studies was often quite short and so life-time risks cannot be calculated.

In 1994, Nezhat and colleagues reported a review of the case notes of 100 consecutive women presenting with chronic pelvic pain after total hysterectomy with or without bilateral oophorectomy. Laparoscopy performed between 8 months and 15 years after the hysterectomy showed the definite presence of endometriosis in 52% of cases and a possibility of endometriosis in a further 8%. Seven women with definite endometriosis on laparoscopy had no previous history of the disease, including presumably no disease at the time of hysterectomy. Women who had ovarian conservation were more likely to have endometriosis (30/36, 83%) than women in whom both ovaries had been removed (22/64, 34%). The overall incidence of endometriosis in patients in this study was quite high but there is no true denominator to calculate the incidence of recurrence.

A 'control' group of women in whom both ovaries were removed at the time of hysterectomy was included in the retrospective report by Hammond et al.[11] The average age at hysterectomy was 39 years. Forty-six·women underwent removal of the uterus, tubes and both ovaries and, in the majority, hormone replacement therapy was started prior to discharge after surgery. In 13 women, one or both ovaries were conserved. After a minimum duration of follow-up of only 1 year, as many as 11 of the 13 women (85%) who had ovarian conservation had undergone re-operation. It is not mentioned whether the extent of endometriosis was significantly different between the two groups of patients. It is possible that this may have been an important factor in the choice between ovarian conservation and bilateral oophorectomy and highlights the problems with using data from non-randomised patient populations in making a clinical judgement. Once again, follow-up was short in a significant proportion of patients.

A more recent study[12] followed up 138 women who had previously undergone hysterectomy for endometriosis at ≤45 years of age at Johns Hopkins Hospital over a 12-year time period, with the specific objective of determining the relative risks of symptom recurrence and/or re-operation following ovarian conservation. The analysis is potentially confounded by the 29 women who had any ovarian tissue conserved being significantly younger and having a significantly lower AFS endometriosis scores at the time of operation compared with than the 109 women who had bilateral salpingo-oophorectomy. The predominant indication for hysterectomy was pain. Hormone replacement therapy was used in 89% of women who had both ovaries removed. The mean length of follow-up was 58 months. Women who had any ovarian tissue conserved at hysterectomy had a relative risk of pain recurrence of 6.1 (95% confidence interval [CI] 2.5–14.6) compared to women who had bilateral salpingo-oophorectomy at the time of hysterectomy. The overall incidence of recurrent symptoms in this study was high (21%) and, even with bilateral salpingo-oophorectomy 10% of women developed recurrent pain, all of whom had received HRT. Nonetheless, it is significant that a much greater proportion of women with ovarian conservation had recurrent pain despite having had a lower stage of endometriosis at the time of hysterectomy. This increased risk of recurrent symptoms was matched by a greater risk of re-operation in the group with ovarian conservation (RR 8.1; 95% CI 2.1–31.3).

Interpretation of evidence

The details and findings of the five studies are summarised in Table 1. What seems clear is that there is very little substantive information on the rate of recurrence of symptoms. Moreover, the individual studies found very different rates of need for repeat operation. The reasons are not known for sure, but it should be noted that the older studies do not necessarily relate to current practice because of advances in the medical management of lesser forms of endometriosis. Equally, the reasons for these differences might relate to different referral practices (secondary versus tertiary centres) or the number of patients being lost to follow-up.

Table 1 Synopsis of studies reporting rates of recurrent symptoms and/or re-operation for endometriosis in women undergoing hysterectomy with or without conservation of at least one ovary

Author	Study design	Duration of follow-up	Method of follow-up	Recur/persist OC	BO	Re-op OC	BO
Cashman[7]	Retro-spective	Ovarian conservation group 3 yr; BSO group 52 months (average)	Patients contacted	42/85	14/33	0/85	0/33
Sheets et al.[8]	Retro-spective	Minimum 5 years	NS	NS	NA	1/40 (2.5%)	NA
Andrews & Larsen[9]	Retro-spective	Minimum 2 years	Review of case notes	NS	NA	3/86 (3.5%)	NA
Hammond et al.[11]	Retro-spective	Minimum 1 year	Review of case notes	NS	NS	11/13 (85%)	0/46
Namnoum et al.[13]	Historical pro-spective study	2–169 mth; average 57 mth	Review of case notes; question-naire if insufficient information	18/29 (62%)	11/109 (10%)	9/29 (31%)	4/109 (3.7%)

OC = Ovarian conservation
BO = Bilateral oophorectomy
Recur/persist = Recurrence/persistence of symptoms
Re-op = Re-operation
mth = months;　　　　　NA = Not applicable;　　　　NS = Not stated

The higher rate of recurrence of symptoms in the study by Namnoum and colleagues[11] appears to be easy to comprehend, but it should be interpreted with some caution and not necessarily extrapolated too readily from women with severe disease to those with more minor degrees of endometriosis. Furthermore, one should consider whether or not recurrence of symptoms following surgery always mean re-activation of endometriosis or is there another possible mechanism of effect in some cases? Given the difficulty in defining the cause of pelvic symptoms, it is possible that bilateral oophorectomy might be treating another condition such as IBS which, like endometriosis, varies with the menstrual cycle. It follows that an individual clinician could easily gain the impression from his/her own practice that bilateral oophorectomy is an effective treatment for minimal (co-incidental) endometriosis when it is IBS that is being ameliorated. There is a need for more specific data on the role of BSO with hysterectomy in women with minor degrees of endometriosis.

Regardless of the level of risk, what does seem clear is that ovarian conservation is probably associated with a higher chance of requiring further surgery. When considering the range of probability, it should not be forgotten that in two of the studies the chance of repeat surgery was less than 5%. If the chance were so low, would routine bilateral oophorectomy be justified particularly if the ovaries were not involved? Some women may think not.

HRT AFTER BILATERAL OOPHORECTOMY FOR ENDOMETRIOSIS

Rationale for use of HRT after hysterectomy for dysfunctional bleeding or fibroids

The practice of prescribing HRT for premenopausal women who have undergone prophylactic oophorectomy at the time of hysterectomy for dysfunctional uterine bleeding or fibroids is now widely accepted. In this circumstance, HRT alleviates the acute physical and psychological symptoms of a surgical menopause and it provides some protection against the long-term health problems of oestrogen deficiency. Oestrogen replacement has been shown to prevent loss of bone mineral mass and osteoporotic fractures and it may also prevent cardiovascular disease, colonic tumours and degenerative brain disease (Alzheimer's) though the available data on these potential effects are, as yet, less convincing.

Additional considerations of use in endometriosis

While these general considerations apply equally to women with endometriosis, there are additional specific concerns that must be taken into account. As indicated above, endometriotic tissue is usually hormone-sensitive and it follows that there is a theoretical possibility that HRT will stimulate any residual (microscopic) tissue which remains after radical surgery. It is important to consider the following questions, therefore:

1. Does HRT increase the risks of recurrent symptoms due to endometriosis?

2. What is the effect of HRT on malignant transformation of endometriotic tissue?

3. What is the best preparation to limit 1 and 2?

4. When should HRT be commenced after surgery?

Does HRT increase the risks of recurrent symptoms due to endometriosis?

It is clear that women with endometriosis who receive HRT after bilateral oophorectomy or a natural menopause may experience a recurrence of symptoms thought to be due to endometriosis. Severe symptoms attributed to endometriosis have also been described in oophorectomised women without detectable ovarian remnants and who had never received HRT.[5] A recent randomised trial[12] compared the recurrence rate of endometriosis in 115 women who received HRT following BSO with that in 57 women who did not receive HRT after BSO for endometriosis, with a mean follow-up time of 45 months. There were no recurrences in women who did not receive HRT, while 4 women (3.5%) in the group that received HRT developed recurrent endometriosis, of whom 2 required abdominal surgery. Peritoneal involvement > 3 cm and incomplete surgical clearance increased the risk of recurrent endometriosis. Further inferences may be drawn from reports of retrospective studies. Namnoum et al.[13] observed recurrent symptoms in 4 out of 97 (4.1%) women who received HRT after bilateral oophorectomy for endometriosis, compared with no recurrences in 12 oophorectomised women who did not receive HRT. Hickman et al.[14] reported recurrent symptoms in 11 out of 95 (11.6%) women receiving HRT after bilateral oophorectomy for endometriosis. Two of the 11 underwent repeat surgery. In contrast, an earlier report[11] found that none of 46 women developed recurrent symptoms during a 1-year follow-up despite 'prompt and adequate postoperative oestrogen replacement' following bilateral oophorectomy. At present, the extent of the risk of re-activation of endometriosis and the frequency with which any recurrence is severe enough to warrant re-operation or a discontinuation of HRT remain unknown. While the absolute risk of recurrence may be low, the consequences, in terms of difficult repeat surgery and severe symptoms, may be significant and patient counselling should include detail about this.

What is the effect of HRT on malignant transformation?

It has long been thought that oestrogen unopposed by progestagen will transform normal endometrium into hyperplastic tissue and ultimately into endometrial cancer. Given that the growth of endometriotic tissue is often oestrogen sensitive, it seems logical to suggest that hyperplasia and neoplasia are a possible consequence of oestrogen therapy if unopposed by progestagen. There are reports which describe the finding of endometriotic hyperplasia and endometrioid carcinoma[15,16] in women on oestrogen-only HRT suggesting that oestrogen may also promote tumour formation in ordinary endometriosis. Currently, there are insufficient data to indicate whether oestrogen-only HRT increases the propensity for malignant transformation of endometriosis or not. However, what does seem to be likely is that malignant transformation of endometriosis is a rare, though serious, event. Moreover, it is clear that to withhold HRT from young women who have undergone radical surgery for endometriosis is to inflict a life of severe menopausal symptoms and an increased chance of osteoporosis and possibly cardiovascular disease in years to come. Even a 0.5% increase in the chance of osteoporotic fractures or cardiovascular mortality because of oestrogen deficiency is likely to far outweigh any additional risk of endometrioid cancer from prescribing oestrogen-only HRT. Nevertheless, provided the woman can tolerate it, logic directs us to use a combined preparation rather than unopposed oestrogen (see below).

Which HRT preparation is most suitable for women with endometriosis?

In women without endometriosis who have had removal of both ovaries, oestrogen alone is sufficient to control hot flushes and protect bone density. The main rationale for the use of progestagen, namely the prevention of endometrial hyperplasia and malignant transformation, is not a concern in these women. In contrast, women who have bilateral oophorectomy for endometriosis, unopposed oestrogen may have significant effects on any residual disease, most notably re-activation but also the small risk of malignant transformation. Having stated that, it should be remembered that exogenous oestrogen therapy in HRT dosage will not produce the same intraperitoneal concentrations as the ovary and so oestrogen-only HRT may be no worse than combined preparations. Nevertheless, it remains an appealing notion that the addition of a progestagen would inhibit the re-activation of endometriotic tissue. It follows that women who have a pelvic clearance for endometriosis should be advised of the theoretical benefit of combined oestrogen/progestagen HRT rather than oestrogen alone.

If the clinician or patient chooses oestrogen-only HRT, careful thought should be given to the use of those preparations which give rise to supraphysiological levels of oestrogen – most notably oestrogen implants. On theoretical grounds alone, one might expect these to be more prone to activate endometriosis and they are more difficult to reverse in the event of re-activation. There is no evidence to show an increased risk, however. If an oestrogen-progestagen preparation is chosen, it would also seem to be logical to prescribe a continuous-combined formulation to avoid cyclical changes, but it must be emphasised that this is also based on our theoretical knowledge of endometriosis rather than clinical trials.

The use of combined oestrogen/progestagen HRT does have two theoretical disadvantages. First, there is a popular belief that the addition of progestogen to oestrogen HRT for women who have undergone hysterectomy is associated with reduced patient acceptability because of premenstrual-like side-effects and that this increases the discontinuation rate. A 2-year MRC study[17] has challenged this belief. The study looked at women who had undergone hysterectomy and compared a group given oestrogen alone with one given oestrogen and progestogen. Against expectation, the drug discontinuation rate was actually higher in the oestrogen-only group though the difference was not statistically significant. Second, it has been argued that the addition of progestogen to oestrogen-based HRT creates and adverse lipid profile. Siddle et al.[18] compared blood lipid profiles in women using oestrogen alone and oestrogen/progestogen in combination. This study used the more lipid-friendly progestogen dydrogesterone. There was little difference between the outcomes for both HRT formulations and it was concluded that non-androgenic progestogens cause little, if any, lipid or lipoprotein changes. It must be acknowledged that this study relied on surrogate markers rather than clinical end-points.

There is possibly a better alternative to combined oestrogen/progestogen formulations. Tibolone, a synthetic oestrogen, is converted to a progestagenic agent in endometrial tissue. It controls vasomotor symptoms and is licensed for

Table 2 Options for control of menopausal symptoms following hysterectomy and bilateral oophorectomy for endometriosis

Hormone-based therapy
Oestrogen-only (± testosterone implants)
Combined oestrogen and progestagen (± testosterone implants)
Cyclic
Continuous
Tibolone
Progestagen-only

Non-hormonal therapy for hot flushes
Clonidine
Venlafaxine

the prevention of osteoporosis. An additional feature of tibolone is that it enhances libido, an important effect in young women who have undergone bilateral oophorectomy, and it elevates mood. One small prospective, randomised study of women with **residual** endometriosis who had recently undergone oophorectomy compared symptoms according to type of HRT (transdermal oestradiol with oral medroxyprogesterone acetate versus tibolone).[19] Four of the 10 women receiving oestradiol and only 1 of the 11 women who received tibolone had moderately severe pelvic pain during the 12 months of follow-up. One patient in the oestradiol group suspended treatment due to severe dyspaerunia. The data are sparse, but fit with what is known of the use of tibolone for add-back therapy for women undergoing pituitary suppression with GnRH analogues for endometriosis. Clearly, tibolone has many features which makes it a potentially attractive option for women with endometriosis who undergo radical surgery but more information is needed (Table 2).

When should HRT be started following definitive surgery for endometriosis?

Hickman et al.[14] compared immediate with delayed introduction of HRT after bilateral oophorectomy for endometriosis in 95 women with pain as at least one of the indications for surgery. The average length of follow-up was 5 years. Information was obtained from a retrospective review of notes and follow-up questionnaires where needed. There was no significant difference between the two groups in the stage of endometriosis or the proportion of women in whom incomplete excision of endometriotic implants was documented. Women who started HRT within 6 weeks of surgery had a similar risk of recurrent pain (4/60, 7%) as women in whom the commencement of HRT was delayed till more than 6 weeks after surgery (7/35, 20%). Interestingly, the addition of medroxyprogesterone to oestrogen replacement made no difference to the risk of recurrent pain. Although this study was not randomised and did not have adequate power to answer effectively the question posed, the results suggest that there are insufficient grounds for delaying the start of HRT in women who undergo bilateral oophorectomy for endometriosis.

KEY POINTS FOR CLINICAL PRACTICE

- It seems likely that radical pelvic surgery will remain an important therapeutic option for women with symptomatic endometriosis for some years to come. It is clear that the issue of bilateral oophorectomy requires careful counselling with an in depth explanation of the advantages and disadvantages, especially so in the case of very young women with more minor disease. It is also important to counsel women about the need for, and potential problems with, HRT. Unfortunately, there are few good studies of the effects of radical surgery for endometriosis upon which to base this advice. Also, none of these studies have distinguished between severe and moderate disease.

- Current evidence tends to indicate that women with severe intractable symptoms should be advised to have their ovaries removed at the time of hysterectomy. This appears to lower the chance of symptom recurrence and also of repeat surgery. Ovarian conservation remains an option, nevertheless, perhaps especially so for women with mild/moderate disease whose main symptom is not pain and whose ovaries are not involved. Women who are considering ovarian conservation need to made aware of the possible need for repeat surgery and that this can be very difficult technically. If the ovaries are conserved, attempts should be made to lift them away from the vaginal vault and ureters so that any future surgery is easier. It is perhaps worth emphasising that the finding of minimal endometriosis at the time of hysterectomy for fibroids is not an indication to remove the ovaries if the woman had indicated that she preferred conservation.

- HRT after bilateral oophorectomy for endometriosis is an important consideration because menopausal symptoms are often more severe after a surgical menopause and there is the additional risk of long-term health problems. HRT appears to be associated with a low chance of re-activation of the disease, but the evidence base is poor. If re-activation does occur, it can have severe consequences, including ureteric obstruction and so women should be alerted to this possibility. There is a weak association between endometriosis and endometrioid cancer. It is not clear whether oestrogen-only HRT increases the risk of malignant transformation or not, but the absolute level of risk is low. Continuous combined oestrogen/progestagen formulations and tibolone offer the theoretical advantage over oestrogen-only HRT of being less likely to lead to re-activation or malignant transformation but more data are needed to confirm this view.

- Finally, when considering the therapeutic options in women with mild/moderate disease it is important to emphasise that there is a great onus on the clinician to be as certain as possible that endometriosis is the true cause of the woman's symptoms before undertaking the irreversible step of bilateral oophorectomy.

References

1 Farquhar C. Extracts from 'clinical evidence' endometriosis. BMJ 2000; 320: 1449–1451
2 Hogston P. Irritable bowel syndrome as a cause of chronic pain in women attending a gynaecology clinic. BMJ (Clin Res ed) 1987; 294: 934–935
3 Lim BH, Fisk NM, Templeton AA. Early endometriosis: does it cause symptoms? J Obstet Gynaecol 1989; 9: 332–333
4 Schmidt CL. Endometriosis: a reappraisal of pathogenesis and treatment. Fertil Steril 1985; 44: 157–173
5 Redwine DB. Endometriosis persisting after castration: clinical characteristics and results of surgical management. Obstet Gynecol 1994: 83: 405–413
6 Wheeler JM, Malinak LR. Recurrent endometriosis: incidence, management and prognosis. Am J Obstet Gynecol 1983; 146: 247–252
7 Cashman BZ. Hysterectomy with preservation of ovarian tissue in the treatment of endometriosis. Am J Obstet Gynecol 1945; 49: 484–493
8 Sheets JL, Symmonds RE, Banner EA. Conservative surgical management of endometriosis. Obstet Gynecol 1964; 23: 625–628
9 Andrews WC, Larsen D. Endometriosis: treatment with pseudopregnancy and/or operation. Am J Obstet Gynecol 1974; 118: 643–651
10 Nezhat D, Admon D, Seidman D, Nezhat CH, Nezhat C. The incidence of endometriosis in posthysterectomy women. J Am Assoc Gynecol Laparosc 1994; 4: S24–S25
11 Hammond CB, Rock JA, Parker RT. Conservative treatment of endometriosis: the effects of limited surgery and hormonal pseudopregnancy. Fertil Steril 1976; 27: 756–766
12 Matorras R, Elorriaga MA, Pijoan JI, Ramon O, Rodriguez-Escudero FJ. Recurrence of endometriosis in women with bilateral adnexectomy (with or without total hysterectomy) who received hormone replacement therapy. Fertil Steril 2002; 77: 303–308
13 Namnoum AB, Hickman TN, Goodman SB, Gehlbach DL, Rock JA. Incidence of symptom recurrence after hysterectomy for endometriosis. Fertil Steril 1995; 64: 898–902
14 Hickman TN, Namnoum AB, Hinton EL, Zacur HA, Rock JA. Timing of estrogen replacement therapy following hysterectomy with oophorectomy for endometriosis. Obstet Gynecol 1998; 91: 673–677
15 Heaps JM, Nieberg RK, Berrek JS. Malignant neoplasms arising in endometriosis. Obstet Gynecol 1990; 75: 1023–1028
16 Jimenez RE, Tiguert R, Hurley P et al. Unilateral hydronephrosis resulting from intraluminal obstruction of the ureter by adenosquamous endometrioid carcinoma arising from disseminated endometriosis. Urology 2000; 56: 331
17 MRC General Practice Framework Group. Randomised comparison of oestrogen versus oestrogen plus progestogen hormone replacement therapy in women with hysterectomy. BMJ 1996; 312: 473–478
18 Siddle N, Jesinger DK, Whitehead MI et al. Effect on plasma lipids and lipoproteins of postmenopausal oestrogen therapy with added dydrogesterone. Br J Obstet Gynaecol 1990; 97: 1093–1100
19 Fedele L, Bianchi S, Raffaelli R, Zanconato G. Comparison of transdermal estradiol and tibolone for the treatment of oophorectomized women with deep residual endometriosis. Maturitas 1999; 32: 189–193

Kevin Thomas Simon Wood D.I. Lewis Jones
C.R. Kingsland

Surgical options in the treatment of male infertility

The introduction of in vitro fertilisation in the late 1970s revolutionised the treatment of infertility and led to the development of an entire new field of assisted reproductive technology. Until the introduction of micromanipulative insemination techniques, the treatment of male infertility was limited and, in many cases, donor insemination (DI) was the only option available particularly in cases of azoospermia and severe oligozoospermia. However, micromanipulative techniques, of which intracytoplasmic sperm injection (ICSI) is the most widely practised, have changed this. ICSI has surpassed previous techniques, such as partial zonal dissection and sub-zonal insemination, because it overcomes both potential barriers to fertilisation – the zona pellucida and the oolemma. This technique has dramatically altered the options available in the treatment of the infertile male over the last decade,[1,2] and has been used world-wide to help couples with severe male factor infertility achieve conception and with their own gametes.[3] There are, however, some occasions when surgery may need to be performed either to obtain sperm, as in the case of germ cell failure or previous vasectomy, or in an attempt to improve sperm quality as in the case of varicoceles.

In this chapter, we shall review areas where surgery is indicated in the treatment of male infertility either to retrieve sperm for use in assisted reproduction or improve the sperm quality. Therefore, although surgical procedures

Dr Kevin Thomas MRCOG, Specialist Registrar, Liverpool Women's Hospital, Crown Street, Merseyside L8 7SS, UK

Dr Simon Wood MRCOG, Subspecialty Trainee in Reproductive Medicine, Liverpool Women's Hospital, Crown Street, Merseyside L8 7SS, UK

Dr D.I. Lewis Jones MD, Consultant Andrologist and Senior Lecturer, Department of Obstetrics and Gynaecology, Liverpool Women's Hospital, Crown Street, Merseyside L8 7SS, UK

Mr C.R. Kingsland MD FRCOG, Consultant Gynaecologist, Head of Reproductive Medicine Unit, Liverpool Women's Hospital, Crown Street, Merseyside, UK

can be performed for conditions such as impotence, this falls outside the scope of this chapter. There are four main procedures which can be used: (i) testicular/percutaneous epididymal sperm extraction (TESA/PESA) and testicular biopsy; (ii) reversal of vasectomy; (iii) varicocele ligation; and (iv) relief of epididymal obstruction.

SURGICAL SPERM RETRIEVAL

The first reported pregnancy achieved using aspirated epididymal sperm from azoospermic men in conventional IVF in 1985 predated ICSI by many years.[4] However, until the introduction of ICSI by Van Steirteghem in 1993,[2] fertilisation rates in IVF with epididymal sperm remained low and, although fertilisation had been reported in vitro, no pregnancies had been reported with testicular sperm.[5] The introduction of ICSI with the requirement of only one motile viable spermatozoon to achieve fertilisation led to the first pregnancy using testicular sperm in 1993.[6] It has now become a common treatment for azoospermic patients,[7-9] and has led to the rapid growth of many different techniques for extracting sperm, each accompanied by a new acronym. In essence, the techniques which are safe and well-tolerated[10] are essentially aspiration of sperm via a needle or extraction of tissue by an open biopsy technique.

It is important to differentiate between two distinct groups of azoospermic patients requiring surgical sperm retrieval. Obstructive azoospermia is by definition an absence of sperm in the ejaculate with normal spermatogenesis. The aetiology is varied, but is most commonly due to previous vasectomy either with or without failed reversal. Other significant causes include congenital bilateral absence of vas deferens (CBAVD) and a heterologous group of aetiologies due to unknown possibly developmental causes, post-infective, traumatic and surgical. In cases of obstructive azoospermia with normal spermatogenesis, sperm can be expected to be retrieved in 100% of cases,[12] and within our own unit all 73 patients undergoing retrieval for obstructive azoospermia achieved adequate sperm retrieval for treatment. Non-obstructive azoospermia is by definition an abnormality in spermatogenesis, often simply referred to as germ cell failure, but this is an over-simplification and includes patients with germ cell aplasia or Sertoli cell only syndrome to those with various stages of maturation arrest. Sperm retrieval rates are good for cases of non-obstructive azoospermia with recovery of sperm for treatment typically expected in over 50% of cases; within our own unit, retrieval rates are 65%. There is further evidence to suggest that the incidence of failed sperm retrieval can be reduced by a further 50% by careful fine mincing of tissue, prolonged examination of the sample (typically over 2 h) and finally by the digestion of testicular tissue with enzymes.[13] With incomplete maturation arrest, sperm is also expected to be recovered in 50% of cases of open biopsy.[10] Complete maturation arrest by definition indicates that surgery will be unsuccessful in achieving recovery of usable sperm. Yet, if the block of arrest occurs at meiosis, then spermatids both round and elongated can be recovered and injected to achieve pregnancy.[14,15] However, in the UK, the Human Fertilisation and Embryo Authority (HFEA) currently prohibits the use of spermatids in ICSI.

A true diagnosis of Sertoli cell only syndrome can only be made histologically, but even then diagnosis can be difficult as different histology can be found in different areas of the testes.[16] Biopsies from multiple sites will often lead to detection of sperm that a single biopsy may have missed.[17] True Sertoli cell only syndrome patients characteristically have high levels of follicle stimulating hormone (FSH) and small testes,[18] but most clinicians still find sperm in around 40–50% of patients with these clinical signs.[19]

A comparison of the results of ICSI treatment using sperm from either obstructive or non-obstructive azoospermia demonstrated significantly lower fertilisation rates (66% versus 45%) and implantation rates (12.1% versus 6.7%) in the non-obstructive cases.[20] Sperm has even been retrieved from patients with 47, XXY Klinefelter syndrome in 50% of cases,[21] and pregnancies have been achieved following ICSI with recovered sperm. The first babies were born in 1997 after utilising pre-implantation genetic diagnosis (PGD).[22,23]

Prior to embarking on surgical sperm retrieval, several important factors must be considered. If the diagnosis is one of CBAVD, then screening for cystic fibrosis in both partners is advised due to the high incidence of carriage for ΔF508 mutations in patients with CBAVD.[24] In non-obstructive azoospermia, the presence of abnormal karyotype should be screened for, as the incidence of karyotypic abnormalities are increased,[25,26] and Y chromosome deletions are more common.[27] In men with non-obstructive azoospermia, histology also reveals a high incidence of treatable testicular tumours (carcinoma *in situ*) from the recovered tissue with rates of carcinoma *in situ* reported at 0.7%.[28,29]

Surgical techniques for sperm retrieval

Although surgical sperm retrieval continues to develop as newer surgical and embryological techniques become available, most centres have simplified rather than expanded their treatment modalities and now the most widely used treatments are percutaneous epididymal sperm aspiration (PESA) and testicular sperm aspiration (TESA) or extraction (TESE). Microepididymal sperm aspiration (MESA) has become much less widely used as the alternatives provide simple and effective sperm retrieval.

Epididymal sperm retrieval

Although MESA predated ICSI and was the first successful form of surgical sperm retrieval,[4] its use has now declined dramatically with the introduction of the newer, less invasive techniques. MESA requires special microsurgical training and equipment that restricts its use to large, well-equipped centres with highly trained staff. MESA is usually performed under general anaesthesia or a cord block, using an operating microscope or binocular loupes and involves opening of the scrotum (scrototomy) and the delivery externally of the testes and epididymis which carries an increased risk of haematoma formation and fibrosis at the operating site with resulting reduction in chances of future sperm retrieval.[30] Proponents of MESA claim that it offers greater diagnostic accuracy with a full scrotal exploration and, if required, the performing of a vasoepididymostomy. Higher numbers of retrieved spermatozoa are usually reported.[31] Indeed, proponents of MESA claim that enough sperm can usually be recovered and stored for 20 future ICSI cycles,[32] although PESA proponents would claim that 20 cycles of ICSI should so very rarely be required by a patient that this is not a true benefit. In fact, MESA is not

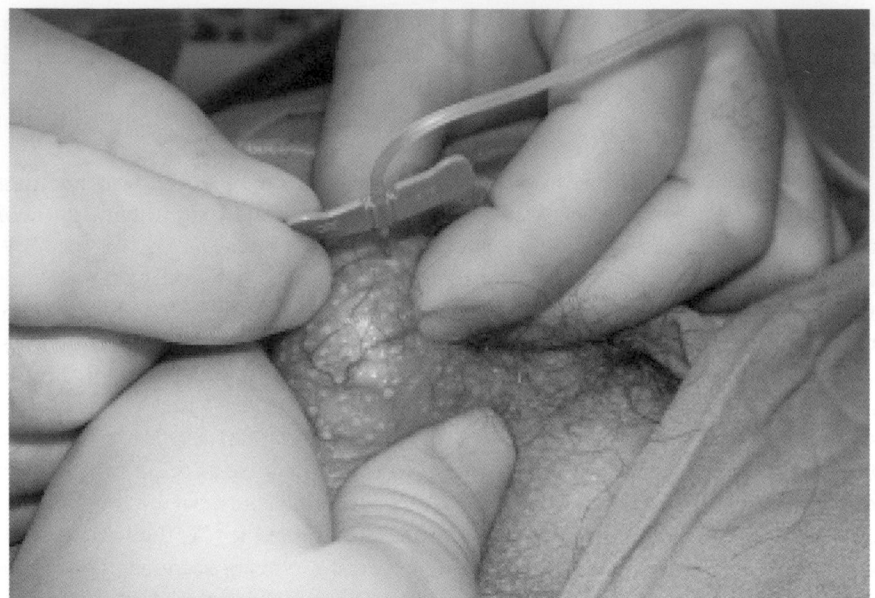

Fig. 1 Percutaneous epididymal sperm aspiration with 19G butterfly.

universally successful especially in cases of previous surgery, when success rates can fall to 77%.[30] This means that it remains as an alternative in some centres, especially in patients who have not had a full assessment by an andrologist or urologist.

The development of a less invasive method of sperm retrieval was first described by Craft in 1993.[33] Sperm was aspirated blindly from the epididymis via the percutaneous puncture of the epididymis with a 19-gauge needle with suction obtained using a 20 ml syringe under local or regional block. Since that first description, many different techniques have been tried successfully using needles or butterfly needles (venisystems) from 19 to 21 gauge either with aspiration via a syringe or using the instillation of saline with subsequent withdrawal with a 1 ml syringe. In all techniques, the epididymis is identified and secured between the thumb and index finger, whilst the remaining fingers and palm are use to cup and stabilise the testicle (Fig. 1). The major advantage of this technique is its non-invasive nature which means that it can be performed on an out-patient basis with general, regional, local and can even be used without any analgesia. It has fewer complications than MESA[34] and is well-tolerated by patients in terms of complications and satisfaction rates.[10] Fertilisation rates with PESA sperm are not different from MESA with most centres reporting fertilisation rates around 55%.[10,11,35] Although epididymal sperm freezes less well than testicular sperm, PESA will usually provide an adequate harvest of sperm to allow cryopreservation. Even if sperm is not able to be cryopreserved, repeated PESA procedures are usually successful. In some studies, up to 60% of patients[36] have repeat PESA and retain good sperm harvests[30] and patient satisfaction.

The major criticism of PESA is that it is a blind procedure and may cause inadvertent damage to the fine epididymal structures producing uncontrolled bleeding and resulting fibrosis.[37] However, many centres report better rates of repeat successful sperm recovery than with MESA including patients undergoing four successful procedures.[36]

Testicular sperm retrieval

Many techniques have been described for the percutaneous aspiration of sperm from the body of the testicle. If fine needle aspiration (FNA) is used using 21 gauge needles or smaller, then anaesthesia is not essential. If larger 19-gauge needles or biopsy guns[38] are used in testicular sperm retrieval, then general local or loco-regional anaesthesia is required.[39] While sperm recovery rates in patients with normal spermatogenesis using 21 gauge needles are quoted at 96%,[39] the sperm retrieved may not be suitable for treatment. Percutaneous biopsy with a 19-gauge needle will usually provide adequate spermatozoa for treatment, but does not give adequate tissue for histology.[40] However it should be noted that if sperm is obtained by TESA, fertilisation rates, cleavage rates and implantation rates do not differ between aspirated sperm (TESA) and sperm obtained from open extraction (TESE).[39] Of greater surprise considering that it is viewed as a much less traumatic method of sperm recovery, studies have shown greater stress rates and pain scores in patients undergoing aspiration (TESA) rather than extraction (TESE).[39]

TESE, as a method of sperm retrieval, is technically easier to perform than PESA and can be performed under general or local anaesthesia. Although trucut biopsy needles can be used, the most common method is by open excisional biopsy which is equivalent to a diagnostic testicular biopsy and this can be singular or multiple. While TESA may provide adequate sperm in most cases of obstructive azoospermia, with normal spermatogenesis TESE gives a

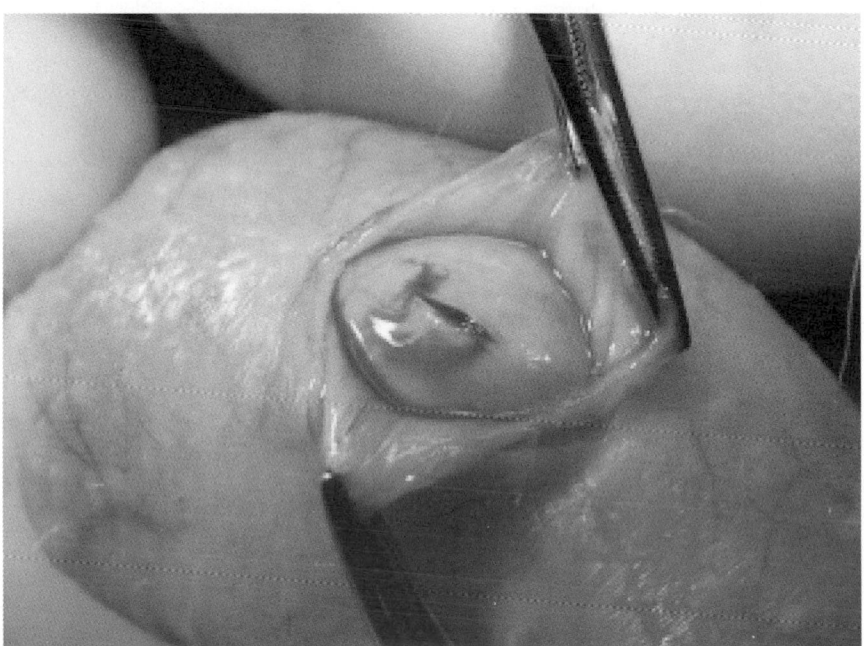

Fig. 2 Tunica albuginea displayed after reflexion of tunica vaginalis.

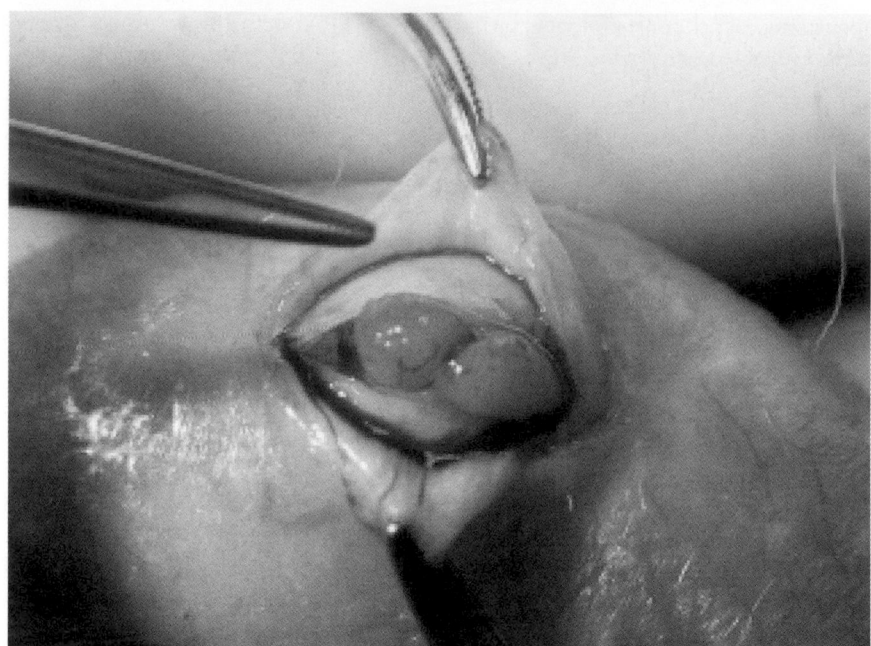

Fig. 3 Seminiferous tubules displayed after opening of tunica albuginea.

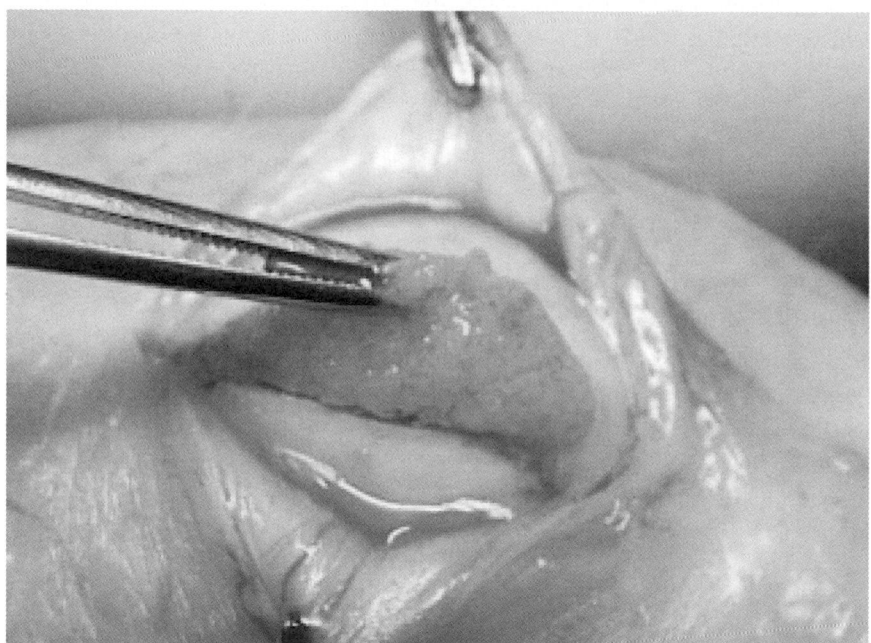

Fig. 4 Seminiferous tubules removed at open TESE.

100% recovery rate. Patients with testicular failure achieve much greater recovery rates with TESE and open biopsy can be expected to recover sperm in almost 50% of cases whilst TESA rates are 12.5%.[40] TESE also has the major advantage of providing tissue for freezing for future treatment. An open

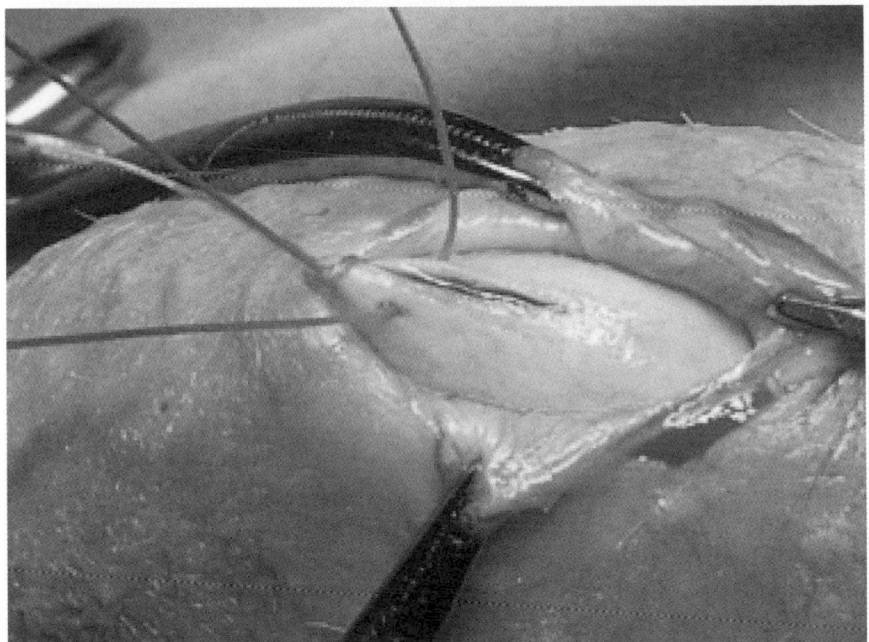

Fig. 5 Closure of tunica albuginea with Dexon.

biopsy either single or multiple is perhaps the method of choice, in which a small incision is made in the scrotal skin and the layers of tissue are opened through the spermatic fascia and the tunica vaginalis to the tunica albuginea (Fig. 2), after opening the tunica albuginea seminiferous tubules are removed (Figs 3 & 4). This procedure can be repeated with multiple incisions through the tunica albuginea or alternatively a single large incision can be made into the tunica albuginea and biopsies taken from various sites. In patients with incomplete Sertoli cell only syndrome, a refinement of this technique was proposed by Schlegel[41] whereby multiple small samples can be removed using x40–x80 magnification to select only the more distended tubules to improve sperm yield. In order to extract the usable spermatozoa from the tubules, the tissue can be minced and the tubes 'milked' with sterile needles[42] or digested by enzymes[13,43] to achieve the mechanical isolation of spermatozoa.

Immediate postoperative complications of TESE are both rare and usually minor. It is important that the layers of the scrotum are closed in layers to prevent postoperative haemorrhage (Fig. 5). Long-term follow-up of 64 patients having undergone TESE for non-obstructive azoospermia with physical examinations, serial ultrasonography, and repeat TESE has shown that 82% of patients had ultrasonographic abnormalities in the testes suggestive of resolving inflammation or haematoma.[44] At 6 months, these had resolved to a linear scar or calcification. The only report of any long-term abnormality showed a reported decrease in serum testosterone levels after TESE in azoospermic men.[45]

Isolated reports of sperm retrieved from various sites in the male genital tract have been described, including the vas deferens,[35,46] as an option if electro-ejaculation or vibrostimulation has failed in patients with anejaculation. PESA, TESA or TESE, however, have largely replaced these techniques.

Table 1 Sperm retrieval method and outcome

	PESA	TESE	Frozen sperm
Number of cycles	31	75	33
Fertilisation rate (%)	64.6	74.1	54.7
Embryo cleavage rate	95.8	87.4	94.1
No embryo transfers	28	62	26
Clinical pregnancies	6 (22%)	17 (28%)	6 (23%)

Table 2 Aetiology of azoospermia and its effects on surgical sperm retrieval

	Vasectomy	Congenital bilateral absence vas deferens CBAVD	Obstructive azoospermia	Germ cell failure
Patients (n)	74	17	39	32
Sperm retrieved	74 (100%)	17 (100%)	39 (100)	17 (53%)
Fertilisation rate (%)	65.9	60.4	67.8	55.2
Embryo cleavage rate (%)	93.6	92.7	91.4	98.4
Transfers (n)	62	13	24	12
Clinical pregnancies	13 (29%)	5 (38%)	7 (29%)	3 (25%)

The use of cryopreserved testicular or epididymal spermatozoa has increased dramatically over the last few years, initially as a by-product of successful sperm retrieval from previous cycles, but now increasingly as a first line treatment option. All the evidence confirms that there is no difference in terms of fertilisation rate, cleavage rate, implantation rate or pregnancy outcome using fresh or cryopreserved epididymal spermatozoa.[8,33,47] Indeed, there are even advocates for only using cryopreserved epididymal sperm.[48] The use of cryopreserved testicular sperm is more debatable in the fact that, although many studies have shown a small but significant reduction in fertilisation and implantation rates with a corresponding reduced live birth rate with ICSI using frozen thawed testicular sperm,[49] all these studies show high fertilising potential with testicular spermatozoa, many of around 70%. Our own success rates are shown in Tables 1 and 2.

VASECTOMY REVERSAL

Vasectomy is considered to be the most effective form of contraception[50] and it remains very popular, with some 100,000 men undergoing the operation each year in the UK.[51] More than 33 million couples now rely on vasectomy for contraception in the US, the UK, India and China, and it is the contraceptive method of choice in 4–15% of couples in Thailand, South Korea, Canada and New Zealand.[52] Vasectomy is a day-case procedure, usually carried out under local anaesthesia, and is considered a simple procedure. Conventionally, the operation involves a 1–2 cm incision on either side of the scrotal skin and division or excision of a segment of each vas is made. Excising a portion of the tube allows histological confirmation to be made, but makes reversal more difficult and probably does not increase the effectiveness of the operation. In China, the 'no-scalpel' technique (NSV) has been developed (already used in over 8 million cases) aimed at increasing the vasectomy uptake by reducing men's fear of incisions.[53] It makes use of specially designed instruments for isolating the vas through the scrotal skin and requires only a small puncture in the scrotal skin. The wound heals spontaneously without suturing, and the risks of haematoma and infection appear to be lower. However, this method is not widely used in the UK and the more conventional approach is usually performed.[54] Whichever method is used, the rate at which azoospermia is achieved depends on the frequency of ejaculation. When sperm are absent from two consecutive samples the vasectomy is considered complete. The failure rate for vasectomy, where azoospermia is not achieved, is around 3%.[55]

Complications of a vasectomy include wound infection, sperm granuloma, scrotal haematoma, the production of antisperm antibodies and late recanalisation. In a large series in Oxford,[56] 7.7% sought medical advise for local pain and 3.6% for bleeding. Scrotal haematoma developed in 0.9%. However, 80% returned to work in 3 days and 96% within 1 week. The NSV is quicker and is associated with a lower incidence of infection and haematoma.[53] Late recanalisation is very uncommon (less than 1 in 1000) but is well documented in the literature, first being reported 30 years ago.[57] There is also some concern about the long-term side-effects. Cale et al. showed a possible association with testicular cancer,[58] but a large cohort study of over 73,000 men in Denmark demonstrated no increased incidence following vasectomy.[59] There is also some evidence suggesting a link between prostatic cancer and vasectomy.[60]

Its increasing popularity as a method of birth control has, however, led inevitably to an increased demand for its reversal. Vasectomy reversal rates are about 8%.[61] This can be for a number of reasons including remarriage, death of children, a wish for further children within the same relationship or altered financial circumstances.[62] A survey in Australia showed that vasectomy-related infertility made up 9.3% of referrals to a general infertility clinic[63] of whom 91% had remarried and their new partners were on average 10 years younger. The median age of the men presenting at the clinic was 42 years, making it clear that male patients still wished to be parents at a relatively late age. Vasectomy reversal is possible because we know that sperm production remains well maintained after vasectomy and normal spermatogenesis has been observed in testicular biopsies taken from 1 month to 10 years following vasectomy.[64]

Techniques of reversal

Various techniques have been described in the literature although most debate revolves around whether macroscopic or microscopic methods should be used. The main objective of the operation is the establishment of a watertight anastamosis between the two divided ends of the vasa with no subsequent stricture formation. This is not easy to achieve, as the inner lumen of the thick walled vas deferens is less than 1 mm and the obstructed testicular portion is often dilated.[51] Initially, the operation was done with or without the aid of

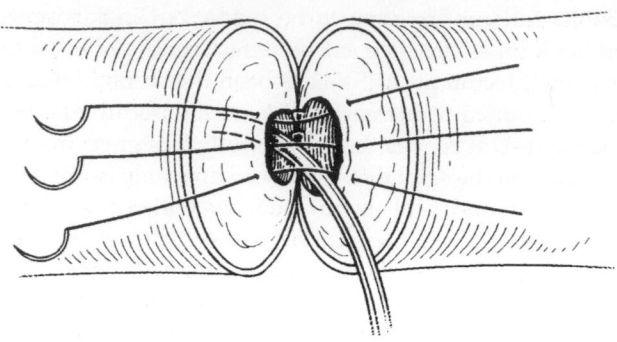

Fig. 6 First layer of sutures in two layered closure with nylon stent in place. Reproduced with kind permission of the *British Journal of Urology*.

magnifying spectacles (×2 or ×4) and 6.0 prolene. Results of vasovasostomy using this macroscopic technique have reported patency rates of 50% or higher with some quoting as high as 87%.[65,66] Other authors warn of a success rate as low as 20%,[67] and fertility rates of 5–25%.[68] There is a consensus that with microsurgery these results can be improved and this has been supported by results of several large series.[68–70] Sibler[72] pioneered a two-layer approach using a microscope, ultrafine suture material (9.0 nylon) and an exquisitely careful technique and reported a pregnancy rate of 71% in the first 42 patients followed for over 1 year. Most two-layered methods are a modification of this technique. Fox[51] showed patency rates of 83.5% and a 48% pregnancy rate using this method. These results are similar to those obtained in other series.[69–71] During the operation, very fine suture material (8/0 or 10/0) is used first approximating the mucosal edges with a small amount of muscle whilst the second comprises of muscle alone (Fig. 6). The operation is usually performed under general anaesthetic on a day-case basis. However, it is a lengthy operation with a bilateral vasovasostomy taking a minimum of 2 h to perform. Therefore, some surgeons prefer to use a modified single-layer anastamosis[73] as it reduces operating time and is quick, robust and reliable. Splints have been favoured by some surgeons but, with microsurgical techniques improving, comparative studies have shown an increased obstruction rate following the use of splints[74] with reduced pregnancy rates.[75]

Antisperm antibodies after reversal

Circulating antisperm antibodies (ASA) can be detected in the serum of 60–80% of men following vasectomy[76] and their presence may compromise fertility if reversal is attempted. There are several hypotheses for ASA formation in men. Theoretically, the blood–testis barrier may be breached by a variety of mechanisms resulting in exposure of immunogenic sperm antigens to the immune system. Extravasation of sperm is common in men after vasectomy.[77] Data suggest that IgM ASA develop within 2 weeks of a vasectomy.[78] IgM titres subsequently diminish over 4–8 weeks followed by increasing titres of ASA IgG between 8–12 weeks. There is, however, no evidence of increased incidence of other autoantibodies.[79]

Numerous methodologies are used to detect ASA. Each have their own advantages and disadvantages, the ideal assay being able to detect the presence of ASA, their location, and their isotype with high sensitivity and specificity. Most units would test using the immunobead assays (IBD) or mixed antiglobulin reaction (MAR) tests. An IBD assay is composed of polyacrylamide beads that are coated with specific anti-immunoglobulin. The coated beads are then mixed with fresh, viable, washed or unwashed sperm samples and ultimately bind to sperm-bound ASA. The test gives a semiqualitative score and is able to detect the isotype and physical location of the ASA with good sensitivity and specificity. It is, however, expensive and time-consuming and requires skilled staff. The MAR test uses group O Rh-positive erythrocytes coated with human IgG or IgA and subsequently mixed with washed or unwashed viable sperm. It is a quick test with good specificity, but is not able to give quantitative information about the ASA binding or location.

Patients with high levels of sperm antibody usually have severely suppressed fertility potential (< 0.5%/month pregnancy rate). The precise mechanism for ASA-mediated infertility is unclear. In either the male or female reproductive tract, ASA may have an adverse effect on sperm maturation and function or overall semen quality.[80] Antisperm antibodies may disrupt normal sperm function by damaging sperm motility or sperm concentration.[81] Following reversal of vasectomy, however, conceptions occur even when antisperm antibodies are present in the seminal plasma; this is most unusual in men with similar titres of such antibodies who are spontaneously infertile. This raises the question as to whether there is a difference between the ASA in the two groups. Parslow et al.[82] showed that the two groups had very similar amounts of IgG and IgM on the spermatozoa but infertile men had significantly more IgA and especially more secretory component than men who underwent vasectomy reversal. This was associated with significantly greater impairment of penetration of cervical mucus in the former group. One main question, therefore, is should reversal of vasectomy be performed if there are significant levels of ASA in the semen especially as studies have shown that there is a significant increase in ASA in patients who achieve patency following a reversal.[83] Carbone et al.[84] suggest that it is partial obstruction, not antisperm antibodies, that causes infertility after a vasovasostomy and that repeat reversal appears to be the most successful treatment option in these patients. They based this on the fact that men with a history of vasectomy and reversal had significantly lower sperm concentration, sperm motility and lower IgA binding than the control patients. If the sperm count is low, then IVF may be needed. ASA may reduce fertilisation rates in IVF cycles,[85] although other studies have shown no significant effect.[86] Intracytoplasmic sperm injection (ICSI) is used if the sperm quality is poor, but its use in all patients with ASA may help to avoid fertilisation failure.[87]

Pregnancy rates after reversal

Pregnancy rates after vasectomy reversal vary among different reporting surgeons. Sharlip[88] looked at patients who had a consistently normal postoperative semen analysis (sperm concentration > 20 × 10⁶/ml and sperm motility of > 50%). Of these patients, 61% achieved a pregnancy and the authors concluded that, allowing for some patients who would achieve a pregnancy after the study was complete, the maximum possible pregnancy rate would be 67%. It is known that the sperm count rises slowly after reversal reaching a plateau at 6 months, and there is also a direct relationship between time since vasectomy and success rates. Belker et al.[71] studied 1469 men and showed pregnancy rates of 76% after less than 3 years, 53% after 3–8 years, 44% after 9–14 years and 30% after more than 15 years. Success is also influenced by finding of sperms in the fluid from the testicular end of the vas which indicates a favourable prognosis as there can be no epidemiological blockage in such cases.[89]

The median length of time between vasectomy and reversal is about 10 years. It is not, therefore, possible to identify those patients who will undergo marital problems and ultimately end up regretting their decision to have a vasectomy. Regretted vasectomy is, therefore, a common cause of infertility and its treatment can be costly and unsuccessful. The debate about which treatment is best, reversal or ICSI with sperm aspiration, will continue but, in counselling patients prior to vasectomy, cryopreservation of spermatozoa should also be suggested.

VARICOCELE LIGATION

A varicocele is defined as a varicosity of the veins of the pampioform plexus. It may form a swelling that feels like a 'bag of worms', appearing bluish through the skin of the scrotum, but often can be small and only detected with the patient standing and performing a valsalva manoeuvre. It does not always cause symptoms and many are asymptomatic and constitute a chance finding in the investigation of the male partner of an infertile couple. There is a marked interobserver error in the assessment of a varicocele,[90] and further investigation by Doppler ultrasonography may be performed. However, no test will decide whether a varicocele is influencing fertility, as varicoceles are a common finding in all men. The World Health Organization (WHO) reported that, out of 3626 men with abnormal semen, 25.4% had a varicocele, whilst out of 3468 men with normal semen analysis, only 11.7% had a varicocele.[91] Kursh,[92] however, showed that using Doppler ultrasonography, 44% of men attending for a vasectomy had a varicocele. This has led to the diagnosis of subclinical varicoceles. There are a number of theories to explain the impairment of infertility in men with varicoceles including: (i) elevated testicular temperature; (ii) reflux of adrenal steroid catecholamines and renal metabolic waste products; (iii) venous stasis resulting in hypercapnia and acidosis; and (iv) changes in testicular perfusion and primary or secondary hypothalamo-pituitary-testicular hormonal abnormalities. There is, however, insufficient evidence for any of these theories.[93]

Methods of treatment

Operative
Various surgical approaches are used. The testicular vein may be tied above the internal inguinal ring (Palamo approach or high ligation), at the internal inguinal ring (inguinal ring) or at the scrotal neck. Increasingly, the operation is being performed laparoscopically with ligation of the internal spermatic veins.[94]

Non-operative

An alternative treatment is percutaneous varicocele embolisation which has the advantage that it can be performed on an out-patient basis and has the same outcome as surgical treatment.[95,96] Other non-operative ways have been tried, including the use of specially designed underwear which incorporates an irrigation system to keep the scrotum cool. However, people found these uncomfortable, especially in the cold weather!

Pros and cons of ligation

Ligation of varicoceles is, therefore, one of the most controversial areas in the management of male infertility because of the uncertainty in its value. The recommendation to treat varicocele by surgical ligation dates back to the early 1950s,[97] and there is a vast body of evidence in the literature suggesting a deleterious effect on fertility and recommending their ligation, either prophylactically or as a treatment of decreased fertility. There have been, however, very few randomised controlled trials done. Of these, Nieschlag et al.[98] randomised 125 patients to either spermatic vein ligation/occlusion or expectant management with counselling; 62 patients had either a surgical ligation or angiographic embolisation and 63 had no interventive treatment. Sperm concentration was significantly elevated in the intervention group after 9–12 months, whilst all other semen or hormonal parameters failed to show any significant difference. There was, however, no difference in the pregnancy rates between the two groups. Other studies have showed an improvement of semen quality after varicocele ligation,[99,100] but whilst Madger et al. showed a significant improvement in the pregnancy rate after ligation, most have showed no significant change.[98,100–102]

Varicocelectomy in adolescents

Varicoceles emerge at puberty and their management in this group is also controversial. Early treatment can lead to increased testicular volume and sperm density.[103] There is no consistent correlation between increase in testicular volume and improvement in sperm density. It remains unclear, therefore, whether preventative treatment of varicocele in young adolescents will have a positive effect on their future testicular function.

RELIEF OF EPIDIDYMAL OBSTRUCTION

Ejaculatory duct obstruction (EDO) is rare, but can be treated. The typical semen-related findings in patients with complete EDO include low ejaculate volume, no or low seminal fructose levels, and azoospermia. However, this typical clinical picture is complicated if the obstruction is partial; indeed, the clinical presentation of partial EDO is very variable.[104] The standard method of establishing the diagnosis is by vasography. With the advances in non-invasive diagnostic methods such as transrectal ultrasonography (TRUS),[105] the seminal apparatus can now be better identified making the diagnosis easier. The treatment of occlusive azoospermia is by microsurgical vasoepididymostomy, although results are poor because of difficulty in assessing the level of the obstruction intraoperatively and the quality of the sperm.[106] The standard procedure for partial EDO is transurethral resection (TUR) of the ejaculatory ducts, as originally described by Farley and Barnes.[107] Complications of this procedure, however, include rectal injury, external sphincter injury, bladder neck resection resulting in retrograde ejaculation, and urine reflux into the ejaculatory ducts.[104] Therefore, in this era of intracytoplasmic sperm injection, partial obstruction is probably best treated this way, although some urologists may argue against this. Also, with results being poor following surgery in the azoospermic group, surgical sperm retrieval may be the best treatment in these cases.

KEY POINTS FOR CLINICAL PRACTICE

- The treatment of male infertility has changed dramatically over the last decade and, whereas the outlook for many was very poor, this has totally changed.

- Even in cases of germ cell failure, pregnancies can now be achieved by surgical sperm retrieval.

- There will always be much debate between urologists and gynaecologists about the best form of treatment, especially in those patients who wish to have their vasectomy reversed.

- The main conclusion, however, is that there is a range of options which give real hope to all patients and that the patient should be made aware of these options.

References

1 Palmers G, Jons H. Derroey P, Van Steirteghem AC. Pregnancies after ICSI of a single sperm into an oocyte. Lancet 1992; 340; 17–18
2 Van Steirteghem AC, Nag Z, Jons H et al. High fertilisation and implantation rates after intracytoplasmic sperm injection. Hum Reprod 1993; 8: 1061–1066
3 Van Steirteghem AC, Nagy P, Jons H et al. The development of ICSI. Hum Reprod 1996: 11 (Suppl.); 59–72
4 Temple-Smith PD, Southwick GJ, Yates CA et al. Human pregnancy by in vitro fertilisation (IVF) using sperm aspirated from the epididymis. J In Vitro Fertil Embryo Transfer 1985; 2: 119–122
5 Hirsh A, Montgomery J, Mohan P et al. Fertilisation by testicular sperm with standard IVF techniques. Lancet 1993; 342: 1237–1238
6 Craft I, Benett V, Nicholson N. Fertilising ability of testicular spermatozoa [letter]. Lancet 1993; 342: 864
7 Devroey P, Liu J, Nagy Z et al. Pregnancies after testicular sperm extraction (TESE) and intracytoplasmic sperm injection (ICSI) in non-obstructive azoospermia. Hum Reprod 1995; 10: 1457–1460
8 Schoysman R, Vanderzwalmen P, Nijs M et al. Pregnancy after fertilisation with human testicular sperm. Lancet 1993; 342: 1237
9 Silber S, Van Steirteghem A, Liu J et al. High fertilisation and pregnancy rate after intracytoplasmic sperm injection with spermatozoa obtained from testicular biopsy. Hum Reprod 1995; 10: 148–152
10 Wood S, Thomas K, Sephton V et al. Patient satisfaction with surgical sperm retrieval. Hum Fertil 2000; 3: 146

11 Friedler S, Raziel A, Soffer Y et al. The outcome of intracytoplasmic injection of fresh and cryopreserved epididymal spermatozoa from patients with obstructive azoospermia-a comparative study. Hum Reprod 1998; 13: 1872–1877

12 Tournaye H, Verhayen G, Nagy P et al. Are there any predictive factors for successful testicular sperm recovery in azoospermic patients? Hum Reprod 1997; 12: 80–86

13 Crabbe E, Verhayen G, Silber S et al. Enzymatic digestion of testicular tissue may rescue the intracytoplasmic sperm injection cycle in some patients with non-obstructive azoospermia. Hum Reprod 1998; 13: 2791–2796

14 Fishel S, Green S, Bishop M et al. Pregnancy after intracytoplasmic injection of spermatid. Lancet 1995; 245: 1641–1642.

15 Tesarik J, Mendoza C, Testart Y. Viable embryos from injection of round spermatids into oocytes. N Engl J Med 1995; 333: 525

16 Sigg C, Hedinger C. Quantitative and ultrastructural study of germinal epithelium in testicular biopsies with mixed atrophy. Andrologia 1981; 13: 412–424

17 Tournaye H, Camus M, Goosens A et al. Recent concepts in the management of infertility because of non-obstructive azoospermia. Hum Reprod 1995; 10: 115–119

18 Del Castillo E, Trabucco A, De La Balze F. Syndrome produced by absence of the germinal epithelium without impairment of the Sertoli or Leydig cells. J Clin Endocrinol 1947; 7: 493–502

19 Tournaye H, Verhayen G, Nagy P et al. Are there any predictive factors for successful testicular sperm recovery in azoospermic patients? Hum Reprod 1997; 12: 80–86

20 Tournaye H, Liu J, Nagy Z et al. Correlation between testicular histology and outcome after intracytoplasmic sperm injection using testicular sperm. Hum Reprod 1996; 11: 127–132

21 Tournaye H, Staessen C, Liebars I et al. Testicular sperm recovery in 47, XXY Klinefelter patients. Hum Reprod 1996; 11: 1664–1649

22 Tournaye H, Camus M, Vandervorst M et al. Sperm retrieval for ICSI. Int J Androl 1997; 20 (Suppl. 3): 69–73

23 Reubinoff B, Abeliovich D, Werner M et al. A birth in non-mosaic Klinefelter's syndrome after testicular fine needle aspiration, intracytoplasmic sperm injection and pre-implantation genetic diagnosis. Hum Reprod 1998; 13: 1887–1892

24 Lissens W, Mercier B, Tournaye H et al. Cystic fibrosis and infertility caused by congenital bilateral absence of vas deferens and related clinical entities. Hum Reprod 1976; 11 (Suppl. 4): 55–80

25 Rivas F, Garcia-Esquival L, Diaz L et al. Cytogenic evaluation of 163 azoospermies. J Genet Hum 1987; 35: 291–295

26 Micic M, Micic S, Diklic V. Chromosomal constitution of infertile men. Clin Genet 1984; 25: 33–36

27 Reijo R, Lee T, Salo P et al. Diverse spermatogenic defects in humans caused by Y chromosome deletions encompassing a novel RNA-binding protein germ. Nat Genet 1995; 10: 383–393

28 Nieschlag E, Behre HM, Meschede D et al. Disorders at the testicular level. In: Nieschlag E, Behre HM. (eds) Andrology. Berlin: Springer, 1996; 131–159

29 Skakkebaek N. Carcinoma in situ of the testis; frequency and relationship to invasive germ cell tumours in infertile men. Histopathology 1978; 2: 157–170

30 Madgar I, Seidman S, Levran D et al. Micromanipulation improves in-vitro fertilisation results after epididymal and testicular sperm aspiration in patients with congenital absence of the vas deferens. Hum Reprod 1996; 10: 2956–2959

31 Devroey P, Liu J, Nagy Z et al. Ongoing pregnancies and birth after Intracytoplasmic sperm injection with frozen-thawed epididymal spermatozoa. Hum Reprod 1995; 10: 903–906

32 Silber S. Micoepididymal sperm aspiration or percutaneous epididymal sperm aspiration? The dilemma. Hum Reprod 1996; 11: 681

33 Craft I, Tsirigotis M, Benett V et al. Percutaneous epididymal sperm aspiration and intracytoplasmic sperm injection in the management of infertility due to obstructive azoospermia. Fertil Steril 1995; 63: 1038–1042

34 Tsirigotis M, Pelankos M, Yazdani N et al. Simplified sperm retrieval and intracytoplasmic sperm injection in patients with azoospermia. Br J Urol 1995; 76: 765–768

35 Tournaye H, Nagy Z, Devroey P et al. Microsurgical epididymal sperm aspiration and intracytoplasmic sperm injection; a new effective approach to infertility as a result of congenital bilateral absence of the vas deferens. Fertil Steril 1994; 61: 1045–1051

36 Godwin I, Meniru GI, Batha S et al. ICSI with epididymal sperm – percutaneous retrieval. In: Filicori M, Flamigni C (eds). Treatment of Infertility: The New Frontiers. New Jersey: Communications Media for Education, 1998; 363–372

37 Girardi S, Schlegel P. MESA; review of techniques, pre-operative considerations and results. J Androl 1996; 17: 5–9

38 Tournaye H, Clasen K, Aytoz A et al. Fine needle aspiration versus open biopsy for testicular sperm recovery: a controlled study in azoospermic patients with normal spermatogenesis. Hum Reprod 1998; 13: 901–904

39 Rosenlund B, Kvist U, Ploen L et al. A comparison between open and percutaneous needle biopsies in men with azoospermia. Hum Reprod 1998; 13: 1266–1271

40 Salzbrunn A, Benson D, Holstein A et al. A new concept for the extraction of testicular spermatozoa as a tool for assisted fertilisation (ICSI). Hum Reprod 1996; 11: 752–755

41 Schlegel P, Su L. Physiological consequences of testicular sperm extraction. Hum Reprod 1997; 12: 1688–1692

42 Tucker M, Morton P, Witt M et al. Intracytoplasmic sperm injection of testicular and epididymal spermatozoa for treatment of obstructive azoospermia. Hum Reprod 1995; 10: 486–489

43 Verhoyen G, De Croo, Tournaye H et al. Comparison of four mechanical methods to retrieve spermatozoa from testicular tissue. Hum Reprod 1995; 10: 2956–2959

44 Schlegel P, Palermo GD, Goldstein M et al. Testicular sperm extraction with intracytoplasmic sperm injection for non-obstructive azoospermia. Urology 1997; 49: 435–440

45 Manning M, Junemann K, Alken P. Decrease in testosterone blood concentrations after testicular sperm extraction for intracytoplasmic sperm injection in azoospermic men. Lancet 1998; 352: 37

46 Hirsh A, Mills C, Tan SL et al. Pregnancy using spermatozoa aspirated from the vas deferens in a patient with ejaculatory failure due to spinal injury. Hum Reprod 1993; 11: 89–90

47 Nagy Z, Liu J, Janssenswillen C et al. Using ejaculated, fresh and frozen-thawed epididymal and testicular spermatozoa gives rise to comparable results after intracytoplasmic sperm injection. Fertil Steril 1995; 63: 808–815

48 Oates R, Lobel S, Harris D et al. Efficacy of intracytoplasmic sperm injection using intentionally cryopreserved epididymal sperm. Hum Reprod 1996; 11: 133–138

49 De Croo I, Van der Elst J, Everaert K et al. Fertilization, pregnancy and embryo implantation rates after ICSI with fresh or frozen-thawed testicular spermatozoa. Hum Reprod 1998; 13: 1893–1897

50 Vessey M, Lawless M, Yeates D. Efficacy of different contraceptive methods. Lancet 1982; 1: 841–842

51 Fox M. Vasectomy reversal-microsurgery for the best results. Br J Urol 1994; 73: 449–453

52 Liskin L. Pile JM, Quillin WF. Vasectomy – safe and simple. Popul Rep 1983; 11: 61–99

53 Nirapathpongporn A, Huber DH, Kreeger JN. No scalpel vasectomy at the King's birthday vasectomy festival. Lancet 1990; 335: 894–895

54 Bottomley C, Wilkinson C. Male sterilisation: the procedure, complications and reversal. Trends Urol Gynaecol Sex Health 2000; 5: 22–27

55 Glasier A. Contraception, sterilisation and abortion. In: Shaw RW, Soutter WP, Stanton SL (eds). Gynaecology. Edinburgh: Churchill Livingstone, 1997; 403–404

56 Phillip T, Guillebaud J, Budd D. Complications of vasectomy: review of 16 000 patients. Br J Urol 1984; 56: 745–748

57 Pugh RCB, Hanley HG. Spontaneous recanalisation of the divided vas deferens. Br J Urol 1969; 41: 340–347

58 Cale AR, Farouk M, Prescott RJ, Wallace IW. Does vasectomy accelerate testicular tumour? The importance of testicular examination before and after vasectomy. BMJ 1990; 300: 370

59 Moller H, Knudsen LB, Lynge E. Risk of testicular cancer after vasectomy: cohort study of over 73 000 men. BMJ 1994; 309: 295–299

60   Rosenberg L, Palmer JR, Zauber AG, Warshauer ME, Stolley PD, Sharpio S. Vasectomy and the risk of prostate cancer. Am J Epidemiol 1990; 132: 1051–1055

61   Baker HWG. Failed vasectomy reversal: an epidemic of preventable infertility [Abstract No. 18]. In: Proceedings of the Annual Meeting of Fertility Society of Australia. Lorne, Victoria, Australia, 1990

62   Howard G. Who asks for vasectomy reversal and why? BMJ 1982; 285: 490–492

63   Jequier AM. Vasectomy related infertility: a major and costly medical problem. Hum Reprod 1998; 13: 1757–1759

64   Bagshaw HA, Mastres JRW, Pryor JP. Factors influencing the outcome of vasectomy reversal. Br J Urol 1980; 52: 57–60

65   Feber KM, Ruiz HE. Vasovasostomy: macroscopic approach and retrospective review. Tech Urol 1999; 5: 8–11

66   Mason RG, Connell PG, Bull JC. Reversal of vasectomy using a macroscopic technique: a retrospective study. Ann R Coll Surg Engl 1997; 79: 420–422

67   White AE, Sheridan WG, Crosby DL. Reversal of vasectomy and the general surgeon. Br J Clin Pract 1994; 48: 238–239

68   Derrick Jr FC, Yarbrough W, D'Agostino J. Vasovasostomy: results of questionnaire of members of the American Urological Association. J Urol 1973; 110: 556–557

69   Lee HY. Twenty years' experience with vasovasostomy. Br J Urol 1986; 136: 413–415

70   Sibler SJ. Microsurgery for vasectomy reversal and vasoepididymostomy. Urology 1984; 23: 505–523

71   Belker AM, Thomas Jr AJ, Fuchs EF, Konnak JW, Sharlip ID. Results of 1469 microsurgical vasectomy reversals by the vasovasostomy study group. J Urol 1991; 145: 505–511

72   Siber SJ. Microscopic vasectomy reversal. Fertil Steril 1997; 28: 1191–1202

73   Hendry WF. Vasectomy and vasectomy reversal. Br J Urol 1994; 73: 337–344

74   Thomas AJ, Pontes JE, Buddhdev H, Pierce JM. Vasovasostomy: evaluation of four surgical techniques. Fertil Steril 1979; 32: 342–348

75   Rothman I, Berger RE, Cummings P, Jessen J, Muller CH, Chapman W. Randomised clinical trial of an absorbable stent for vasectomy reversal. J Urol 1997; 157: 1697–1700

76   Hellema JWJ, Rumke P. Sperm autoantibodies as a consequence of vasectomy within 1 year post-operation. Clin Exp Immunol 1978; 31: 18–29

77   Wallach EE. Antisperm antibodies: aetiology, pathogenesis, diagnosis, and treatment. Fertil Steril 1998; 70: 799–810

78   Flickinger CJ, Howards SS, Bush LA, Baker LA, Herr JC. Temporal recognition of sperm autoantigens by IgM and IgG autoantibodies after vasectomy and vasovasostomy. J Reprod Immunol 1994; 27: 135–150

79   Rose NR, Lucas PL. Immunological consequences of vasectomy. II. Two year summary of prospective study. In: Leplow IH, Crozier B. (eds) Vasectomy: Immunologic and Pathophysiologic Effects in Animals and Man. New York: Academic Press, 1979; 533–560

80   Dimitrov DG, Urbanek V, Zverina J, Madar J, Nouza K, Kinsky R. Correlation of asthenozoospermia with increased antisperm cell-mediated immunity in men from infertile couples. J Reprod Immunol 1994; 27: 3–12

81   Dom J, Rudak E, Aitken RJ. Antisperm antibodies: their effect on the process of fertilisation studied in vivo. Fertil Steril 1981; 35: 535–541

82   Parslow JM, Poulton TA, Besser GM, Hendry WF. The clinical relevance of classes of immunoglobulins on spermatozoa from infertile and vasovasostimised men. Fertil Steril 1985; 43: 621–627

83   Matson PL, Junk SM, Masters JR, Pryor JP, Yovich JL. The incidence and influence upon fertility of antisperm antibodies in seminal fluid following vasectomy reversal. Int J Androl 1989; 12: 98–103

84   Carbone DJ, Shah A, Thomas AJ, Agarawal A. Partial obstruction, not antisperm antibodies, causing infertility after vasovasostomy. J Urol 1998; 159: 827–830

85   Yeh WR, Acosta A, Seltman HJ, Doncel G. Impact of immunoglobulin isotype and sperm surface location of antisperm antibodies on fertilisation in vitro in the human. Fertil Steril 1994; 62: 363–369

86   Pagidas K, Hemmings R, Falcone R, Miron P. The effect of antisperm antibodies in the male or female partners undergoing in vitro fertilisation-embryo transfer. Fertil Steril 1994; 62: 363–369

87   Lahteenmaki A, Reima I, Hovatta O. Treatment of severe male immunological infertility by intracytoplasmic sperm injection. Hum Reprod 1995; 10: 2824–2828

88   Sharlip ID. What is the best pregnancy rate that may be expected from vasectomy reversal? J Urol 1993; 149: 1469–1471

89   Sibler SJ. Epididymal extravasation following vasectomy as a cause for failure of vasectomy reversal. Fertil Steril 1979; 31: 309–311

90   Hargreave TB, Liakatas J. Physical examination for varicoceles. Br J Urol 1991; 62: 191–194

91   World Health Organization. The influence of varicocele on parameters of fertility in large groups of men presenting to infertility clinics. Fertil Steril 1992; 57: 1289–1293

92   Kursh ED. What is the incidence of varicocele in a fertile population? Fertil Steril 1987; 48: 510–511

93   Evers JLH. Varicocele. In: Templeton A, Cooke I, Shaugn O'Brien PM. (eds) Evidence Based Fertility Treatment. London: RCOG Press, 1998; 109–119

94   Ralph DJ, Timoney AG, Parker C, Pryor JP. Laparoscopic varicocele ligation. Br J Urol 1993; 72: 230–233

95   Nielsclag E, Behre HM, Schlinghider A, Nashan D, Pohl J, Fischedick AR. Surgical ligation vs angiographic embolization of the vena spermatica: a prospective randomised study for the treatment of varicocele related infertility. Andrologia 1993; 25: 233–237

96   Shlansky-Goldberg RD, VanArsdalen KN, Rutter CM et al. Percutaneous varicocele embolization versus surgical ligation for the treatment of infertility: changes in seminal parameters and pregnancy outcome. J Vasc Interv Radiol 1997; 8: 759–767

97   Tulloch WS. Consideration of sterility factors in the light of subsequent pregnancies: subfertility in the male. Edinb Med J 1952; 59: 29

98   Mordel N, Mor-Yosef S, Margolioth NM et al. Spermatic vein ligation as a treatment for male infertility. J Reprod Med 1990; 35: 123–127

99   Madgar I, Weissenberg R, Lunenfeld B, Karasik A, Goldwasser B. Controlled trial of high spermatic vein ligation for varicocele in infertile men. Fertil Steril 1995; 63: 120–124

100 Yamamoto M, Hibi H, Hirata Y, Miyake K, Ishigaki T. Effect of varicocelectomy on sperm parameters and pregnancy rate in patients with subclinical varicocele: randomised prospective controlled study. J Urol 1996; 155: 1636–1638

101 Nilsson S, Edvinsson A, Nilsson B. Improvement of semen and pregnancy rates after ligation and division of the internal spermatic vein: fact or fiction? Br J Urol 1979; 51: 591–596

102 Breznik R, Vlaisavjevic V, Borko E. Treatment of varicocele and male fertility. Arch Androl 1993; 30: 157–160

103 Laven JSE, Haans LCF, Mali WPTM et al. Effects of varicocele treatment in adolescents: a randomised study. Fertil Steril 1992; 58: 756–762

104 Paick JS, Kim SH, Kim SW. Ejaculatory duct obstruction in infertile men. Br J Urol Int 2000; 85: 720–724

105 Hellerstein DK, Meacham RB, Lipshultz LI. Transrectal ultrasonography and partial ejaculatory duct obstruction. J Urol 1992; 39: 449–452

106 Boeckx W, Van Helden S. Microsurgical vasoepididymostomy in the treatment of occlusive azoospermia. Br J Urol 1996; 77: 577–579

107 Farley S, Barnes R. Stenosis of ejaculatory ducts treated by endoscopic resection. J Urol 1973; 109: 664–666

Hassan N. Sallam

Embryo transfer –
the elusive step

Despite numerous developments in the field of assisted reproduction, the implantation rate of replaced embryos remains dismally low. It is estimated that 85% of the embryos replaced during in vitro fertilization (IVF) or intracytoplasmic sperm injection (ICSI) fail to implant.[1] The exact cause of this low implantation rate is unknown, but may reside in the technique of embryo transfer (ET), in the efficiency of endometrial receptivity, or in the ability of the embryo to invade the endometrium properly. This review will concentrate on the factors affecting the technique of ET in patients treated with IVF or ICSI and the alternative procedures available to deal with the difficult cases

THE TECHNIQUE OF EMBRYO TRANSFER

Embryo transfer (ET) is usually performed 48–96 h after oocyte retrieval. Although the knee chest position was originally recommended by some authors, most of the transfers are nowadays performed in the lithotomy position.[2,3] The procedure is performed under sterile conditions; the patient is draped, a speculum is inserted in the vagina and the cervix exposed. The cervical mucus is aspirated using a mucus aspirator and the cervix is then cleansed with a swab soaked with saline or culture medium.

Different types of plastic catheters are used for ET varying in length, diameter, stiffness and memory and are checked for embryo toxicity. Catheters are either pre-loaded or after-loaded depending on whether embryos are loaded directly into the catheter or whether the outer sheath is first placed in the uterine cavity using a guide wire or obturator.

At the time of transfer, the catheter is fitted with a 1 ml tuberculin-type syringe and flushed with culture medium. The embryos are then loaded in the distal end of the catheter in a volume of 15–25 µl of culture medium. If a pre-loading-type catheter is used, the catheter is passed through the cervix to approximately 1 cm

Prof. Hassan N. Sallam MD FRCOG PhD(Lond), Professor in Obstetrics and Gynaecology, The University of Alexandria in Egypt (For correspondence: 22 Victor Emanuel Square, Smouha, Alexandria, Egypt)

below the uterine fundus. This is determined by markings, 1 cm apart, on the catheter. The length of the uterine cavity should have been measured previously using a uterine sound or by ultrasonography. The embryos are then delivered into the uterine cavity by gently pressing the syringe plunger. The catheter is then left in situ for 10–60 s and then withdrawn gently. The catheter is finally checked under a dissecting microscope for retained embryos. If these are found, they are reloaded and transferred again.

If an after-loading catheter is used, the outer sheath is passed first through the cervix to approximately 1 cm above the internal cervical os. The inner catheter containing the embryos is then advanced inside the outer catheter to 1 cm below the uterine fundus. The embryos are then gently deposited into the uterine cavity.

Initially, the patients were asked to remain in bed for up to 12 h.[2,3] Nowadays, the patient usually rests for 30 min following the procedure, although recent studies have shown that this is not necessary.[4–6]

FACTORS AFFECTING EMBRYO TRANSFER

Despite its apparent simplicity, ET remains the most elusive and least understood step in assisted reproductive technology. Since the first description of the ET technique,[2,7] numerous refinements have been suggested and practised. These include:

Gentle and atraumatic technique

A gentle ET technique is thought to result in higher pregnancy and implantation rates. In particular, the presence of blood on the transfer catheter has been blamed as a cause for failure of implantation. In a retrospective study, Goudas et al.[8] studied the relationship between the presence of blood inside and outside the transfer catheter to pregnancy and implantation rates in 354 embryo transfers. They found that blood found outside, but not inside, the transfer catheter after ET was associated with decreased rates of embryo implantation and clinical pregnancy. Nabi et al.[9] studied 1204 ET procedures and found that embryos were significantly more likely to be retained when the ET catheter was contaminated with blood (3.3% versus 12%, $P = 0.00001$).

Performing the transfer on 2 consecutive steps if some or all of the embryos are retained in the transfer catheter has also been blamed for failure of implantation. However, Nabi et al.[9] found that there was no significant difference in the clinical pregnancy rate between those who had all their embryos transferred at the first attempt (24.7%) and those who required more than one attempt (23.2%).

Difficult transfers are also thought to compromise implantation. In the same study, Nabi et al.[9] found that embryos were significantly more likely to be retained when the transfer procedure was difficult compared with when it was easy (20.3% versus 0.8%, $P = 0.00001$). In a study by Abusheikha et al.,[10] cervical dilatation was performed in 57 women who failed to conceive after a previous attempt at IVF-ET. Of the 57 women, 18 (31.6%) achieved a clinical pregnancy after the cervical dilatation. In 40 patients (70.2%), the subsequent ET was classified as 'easy', whereas in the other 17 (29.8%) it remained difficult. The pregnancy rate was significantly higher when the ET was easy than when it was difficult (40% versus 11.8%, $P < 0.05$). Similarly, Mesrogli and Dieterle[11] measured the serum concentration of the early pregnancy factor (EPF) in 82 patients undergoing IVF treatment. The EPF is a marker of the development of the embryo before and during implantation. Clinical pregnancies occurred in 12 patients (15%) resulting in 9 deliveries. In patients with difficult ET, no EPF could be detected in the serum more frequently than in patients with easy transfers.

On the contrary, some studies have found no relationship between the difficulty of ET and implantation rates. Burke et al.[12] analyzed different variables present at the time of embryo transfer in 46 frozen and 159 fresh embryo transfers. They found that the two most important variables for predicting a clinical pregnancy were a first-time transfer and the number of high-grade embryos placed. In their small sample, the difficulty of the ET technique did not affect the pregnancy rate. Similarly, Tur-Kaspa et al.[13] studied a total of 854 consecutive ET procedures. Embryo transfer was easy in 734 cases (85.9%) and difficult in 72 (8.4%), cervical dilatation was required in 21 (2.5%), and one or two repeated attempts were needed in 27 cases (3.2%). There were no statistically significant differences in pregnancy rates between the easy and difficult transfers.

Difficult transfers are also thought to increase the incidence of extra-uterine pregnancies (EP). Lesny et al.[14] compared 18 patients with an EP after IVF to 314 patients with an intra-uterine pregnancy after transcervical ET performed during the same period. They found that a difficult ET significantly increases the risk of an EP. The risk was particularly high when the patient has a history of tubal damage or previous EP. Similarly, Khalifa et al.[15] reported a case of intramural pregnancy following a difficult embryo transfer in a 31-year-old woman. They suggested that the creation of a 'false passage' at a previous instrumentation of the cervix might be implicated in the ectopic placement of embryos. A similar case of intramural pregnancy was reported by Hamilton et al. following another difficult transfer.[16]

Performing a trial embryo transfer before the actual procedure

Performing a trial (mock or dummy) ET before the actual transfer has been shown to increases pregnancy and implantation rates. The trial transfer can be performed during the cycle preceding the treatment cycle, at the time of oocyte collection or immediately before the actual transfer. For example, Knutzen et al.[17] undertook a mock ET of 40 μl of radio-opaque dye during the cycle preceding the treatment cycle in 34 patients. They found that the dye remained primarily in the uterine cavity in 48–68% of cases. In these patients, the clinical pregnancy rate was 33%. They estimated that if the mock ET had been the actual ET, 32–52% of all patients would have lost their opportunity for pregnancy as a result of the ET procedure.

In another study, Sharif et al.[18] performed 113 ET procedures where a 'step-wise' mock ET protocol was performed with a full bladder immediately before the embryo transfer. They reported a pregnancy rate per ET of 45.1% and an intra-uterine implantation rate per embryo transferred of 20.6%.

In a larger study by Mansour et al.,[19] 335 patients undergoing ET were randomly divided into two groups. The first group (n = 167) was subjected to dummy ET before the start of IVF treatment to choose the most suitable catheter for each patient, while the second group B (n = 168) started their IVF treatment without dummy ET. The authors found that the ET technique was difficult in 50 cases (29.8%) in the no-dummy transfer group, whereas no

Table 1 Clinical pregnancy rates in selected studies using ultrasound-guided embryo transfer

Study	Type of trial	n	No U/S	U/S	P value
Prapas et al. 1995[22]	RCT	132	22.6%	31.6%	NS
Kan et al. 1999[23]	CCS	187	28.9%	37.8%	NS
Lindheim et al. 1999[21]	CCS	137	36.1%	63.1%	< 0.05
Wood et al. 2000[24]	CCS	518	25%	38%	< 0.002
Coroleu et al. 2000[25]	RCT	362	33.7%	50%	< 0.05
Sallam et al. 2002[26]	CCS	640	18.4%	26.3%	< 0.02

RCT, randomized controlled trial; CCS, case-control study; n, number of patients in the study; U/S, ultrasound-guided embryo transfer.

difficulty was met in the dummy transfer group. Pregnancy rate and implantation rate were significantly higher in the dummy transfer group (22.8% and 7.2%) compared to the no-dummy transfer group (13.1% and 4.3%).

Embryo transfer under ultrasound guidance

Performing ET under ultrasound guidance was found to improve pregnancy and implantation rates (Table 1). The technique was first suggested by Strickler et al.[20] who compared 16 abdominal ultrasound-guided transfers with 12 transfers guided by 'clinical feel' (Fig. 1). They found that ultrasound-guided

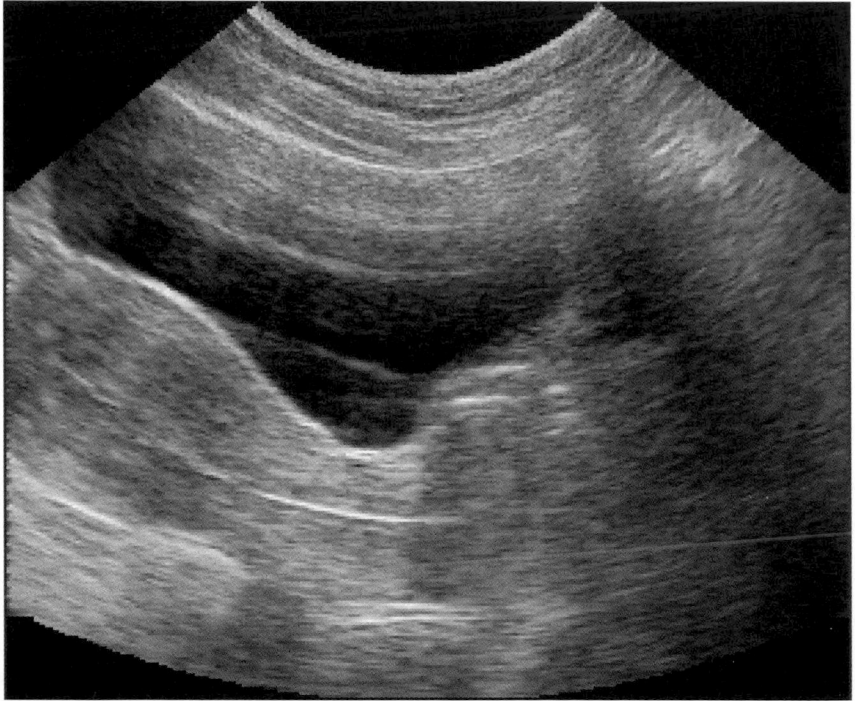

Fig. 1 Ultrasound-guided embryo transfer showing the catheter negotiating the cervical canal.

transfers were easier, and there was less catheter distortion. They concluded that with ultrasound guidance: (i) transfers can be done with the patient supine in the lithotomy position; (ii) the catheter tip can be accurately positioned in the fundus of the uterine cavity; (iii) the ejection of the transfer bubble into the uterus can be documented; and (iv) the observation of the bubble is comforting to the patient.

In a retrospective study, Lindheim et al.[21] studied 137 women undergoing ET of donated embryos. They found that abdominal ultrasound guidance significantly improved implantation and pregnancy rates in cycles with easy transfers (28.8% versus 18.4% and 63.1% versus 36.1%, respectively; $P < 0.05$).

In a randomized controlled trial, Prapas et al.[22] studied 132 consecutive ETs. The ET was performed under abdominal ultrasound control in 61 cases, whereas 71 cases were performed with the 'clinical feel' method. Ultrasound guidance yielded a significantly higher pregnancy rate than the blind method (36.1% versus 22.6%). In another prospective randomized controlled study, Kan et al.[23] compared the pregnancy and implantation rates between abdominal ultrasound-guided ($n = 93$) and clinical touch ($n = 94$) uterine ETs. Higher pregnancy and implantation rates of 37.8% and 20.4%, respectively, were achieved when ultrasound was used, compared to 28.9% and 16.2%, respectively, with clinical touch, although this difference was not statistically significant. In a larger study, Wood et al.[24] compared clinical pregnancy rates in 518 cycles in women undergoing ET. The clinical pregnancy rate in women having ET with abdominal ultrasound guidance was significantly higher than those without ultrasound guidance (38% versus 25%, respectively; $P < 0.002$). More recently, Coroleu et al.[25] studied 362 patients undergoing ET. The patients were prospectively randomized into two groups: 182 had abdominal ultrasound-guided ET, and 180 had clinical touch ET. The pregnancy rate was significantly higher among the ultrasound-guided ET group (50%) compared with the clinical touch group (33.7%; $P < 0.002$). There was also a significant increase in the implantation rate: 25.3% in the ultrasound group compared with 18.1% in the clinical touch group ($P < 0.05$).

The utero-cervical angle measured by ultrasound is also thought to affect the pregnancy and implantation rates (Fig. 2). We have recently conducted a prospective controlled study and found that acute utero-cervical angles ($> 60°$) are associated with lower pregnancy and implantation rates compared to mild angles ($< 30°$).[26]. Measuring the angle by ultrasound prior to ET and moulding the catheter accordingly resulted in a lower incidence of difficult transfers (8.4% versus 26.9%; $P < 0.0001$) as well as higher pregnancy (26.25% versus 18.43%; $P < 0.05$) and implantation rates (10.72% versus 7.55%; $P < 0.01$).

Transvaginal ultrasound-guided ET has also been described. In a controlled study, Hurley et al.[27] studied ET performed in 94 patients using transvaginal ultrasound guidance. They found that pregnancy rates were increased over a control group of 246 patients, although statistical significance was reached only in the subgroup of single ETs (i.e. the transfer of one embryo). In another study, Woolcott and Stanger[28] performed 121 consecutive transvaginal ultrasound-guided ET. They found that tactile assessment of ET catheter placement was unreliable: in 17.4% of transfers, the outer guiding catheter inadvertently abutted the fundal endometrium, the outer guiding cannula indented the endometrium in 24.8% and the transfer catheter embedded in the

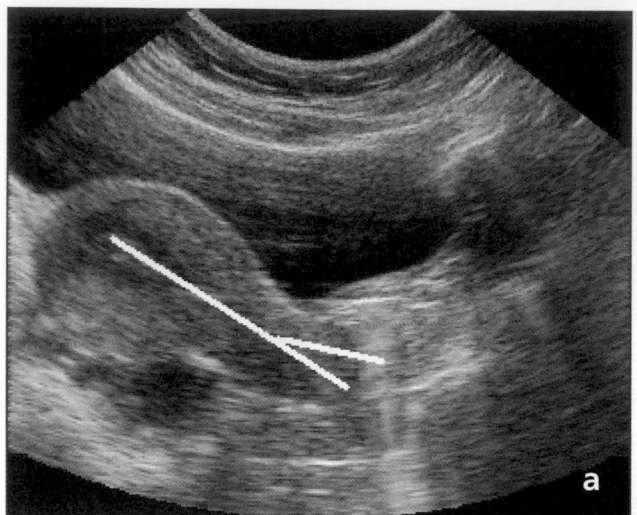

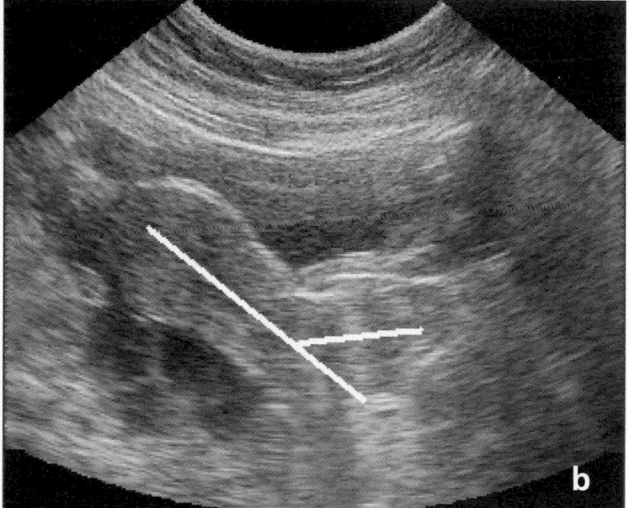

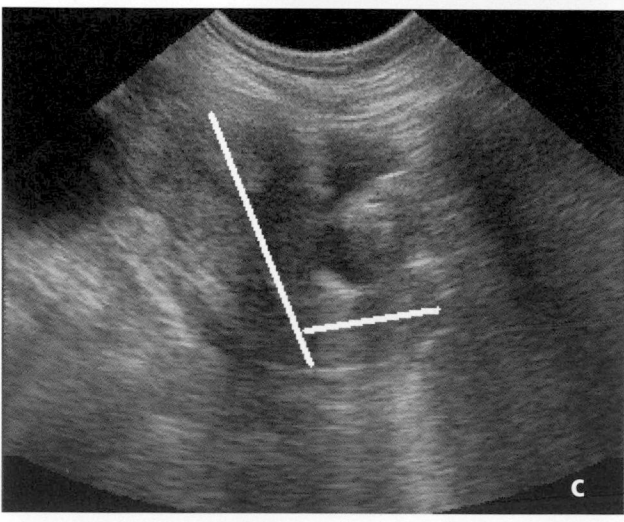

Fig. 2 Measuring the utero-cervical angle with abdominal ultrasound prior to embryo transfer. (a) mild angle (< 30°), (b) moderate angle (30–60°), (c) acute angle (> 60°). Reproduced with the kind permission of the Editor of *Human Reproduction*.

endometrium in 33.1%. Unavoidable sub-endometrial transfers occurred in 22.3% of transfers, but the technique had the advantage of avoiding accidental tubal transfer in 7.4% of instances.

Embryo transfer with a full bladder

Straightening the utero-cervical angle by performing ET with a full bladder improves pregnancy and implantation rates. In a study by Lewin et al.,[29] ET was performed in 796 patients. They were divided into 2 groups: 385 patients underwent ET with an empty bladder, and 411 patients underwent ET with a full bladder. In the empty bladder group, 64 pregnancies were achieved (16.6%) compared to 110 pregnancies in the full bladder group (26.8%, $P = 0.006$). The authors suggested that the higher pregnancy rate was probably attributable to the smooth and easy insertion of the ET catheter. Straightening the utero-cervical angle can also be effected by moderate traction with a tenaculum on the cervix. Johnson and Bronham,[30] using a radio-opaque guide wire, found that cervical traction in a caudal direction (force 2 N) reduced the median utero-cervical angle, from 75° to 10° ($P = 0.001$). However, other studies have shown that the use of a tenaculum leads to the initiation of uterine contractions and may diminish the pregnancy and implantation rates.[31,32] The method cannot, therefore, be advocated for use during ET.

Removing the cervical mucus prior to embryo transfer

The removal of the cervical mucus prior to ET is also thought to improve the pregnancy and implantation rates. In a study by Mansour et al.,[33] dummy ETs were performed in 35 patients. Each dummy transfer was performed twice in the same patient – before and after cervical mucus aspiration. The results showed that the dye was extruded at the external os in 57% of the cases when the cervical mucus was not aspirated compared to 23% when the mucus was aspirated ($P = 0.01$). In a study by Nabi et al.,[9] 1204 ET procedures were retrospectively analyzed. The authors found that embryos were significantly more likely to be retained when the ET catheter was contaminated with mucus (3.3% versus 17.8%, $P = 0.000001$). On the contrary, there was no significant difference in the clinical pregnancy rate between those who had all their embryos transferred at the first attempt (24.7%) and those who required more than one attempt (23.2%).

Flushing the cervical canal with culture medium prior to embryo transfer

Vigorous flushing of the cervical canal with culture medium prior to ET has been suggested as a method to improve implantation. In 1999, MacNamee[34] reported that vigorous flushing of the cervical canal and the use of a soft catheter improved the pregnancy (from 25.3% to 46.2%) and implantation rates (from 8.7% to 17.7%), respectively. However, these observation were based on a retrospective analysis and the authors did not study each factor separately (i.e. flushing the cervical canal or using a soft catheter). In a prospective randomized controlled study of 110 ETs, we have found no statistically significant difference with and without flushing in pregnancy rates (25.5% and 34.5 %, $P = 0.4053$) or implantation rates (15.4% and 17.5%, $P = 0.7687$).[35]

Avoiding the use of a tenaculum (volsellum)

The use of a tenaculum is thought to stimulate uterine junctional zone contractions affecting implantation of the transferred embryos. In a study by Lesny et al.,[31] the junctional zone contractility was assessed before and after ET in 20 patients at the time of mock ET during the mid-luteal phase (at commencement of down-regulation) using real-time transvaginal ultrasound and computer technology. When a tenaculum was applied, the total number of contractions, the number of cervico-fundal, random and opposing contractions all increased significantly ($P = 0.0003$, 0.005, 0.001 and 0.007, respectively). They concluded that the use of a tenaculum in the cervical area stimulates junctional zone contractions and is best avoided at the time of embryo transfer. In a comparable study, Dorn et al.[32] measured serum oxytocin concentration during ET in 10 women undergoing embryo transfer. They found an elevation in oxytocin level when the tenaculum was used (in 4 out of 5 patients) and remained elevated until of the end of ET procedure.

The type of catheter

The type of catheter used in ET was found to affect the pregnancy and implantation rates in many studies (Table 2). For example, Gonen et al.[36] compared the performance of two different transfer catheters in 193 consecutive ETs: the Frydman catheter and the Tomcat catheter. They found that the Tomcat catheter yielded a significantly higher pregnancy rate than the Frydman catheter (28% versus 16%; $P = 0.03$). In a prospective, randomized, clinical study, Meriano et al.[37] compared 32 patients who had embryo transfer using the Tomcat catheter to 34 patients using the TDT catheter. They found that the use of the Tomcat catheter resulted in significantly higher implantation (25.2% versus 8.4%) and clinical pregnancy rates (47% versus 14.7%) compared with the TDT catheter. Other studies reported less impressive results regarding the type of ET catheter used. For example, Burke et al.[12] analyzed different variables present at the time of ET to determine their effects on the clinical pregnancy rate in 46 frozen and 159 fresh embryo transfers. They found that

Table 2 Clinical pregnancy rates in selected studies comparing rigid to soft catheters used in embryo transfer

Study	Type of trial	n	Rigid catheter	Soft catheter	P value
Wisanto et al. 1989[38]	RCT	400	32.3%	19.2%	< 0.05
Al-Shawaf et al. 1993[41]	CCS	178	30.7%	30.3%	NS
Urman et al. 2000[40]	CCS	428	36.0%	41.6%	NS
Wood et al. 2000[24]	CCS	518	17%	36%	< 0.001
Ghazzawi et al. 2000[39]	RCT	320	30%	19%	NS

RCT, randomized controlled trial; CCS, case-control study; n, number of patients in the study.

the two most important variables for predicting a clinical pregnancy are a first-time transfer and the number of high-grade embryos placed, but the type of ET catheter used did not affect the pregnancy rate.

Some studies have shown that soft ET catheters are associated with higher pregnancy and implantation rates compared to rigid catheters. Mansour et al.[19] performed dummy embryo transfers in 40 patients using methylene blue dye. Each dummy transfer was performed twice in the same patient using two different catheters, the Wallace and the Craft catheters. The results showed that the dye was extruded at the external os in 25.5% of the patients when the soft Wallace catheter was used compared to 77.5% when the more rigid Craft catheter was used ($P > 0.05$). In another study, Wood et al.[24] compared clinical pregnancy rates in 518 cycles in women undergoing embryo transfer. The clinical pregnancy rate in women using soft catheters (Wallace and TDT) were significantly higher than in those using hard catheters (Tomcat or Tefcat) – 36% versus 17%, respectively.

On the contrary, Wisanto et al.[38] performed a prospective and randomized study on 400 consecutive ETs, and compared the performance of three different transfer catheters. They found that the (rigid) Frydman catheter yielded a pregnancy rate of 32.3% compared to 19.4% for the (rigid) TDT catheter, but the TDT catheter was better in cases of difficult transfer. The (soft) Wallace catheter showed similar performance, but the pregnancy rate was lower (19.2%) compared to the Frydman catheter. Similarly, Ghazzawi et al.[39] compared the (rigid) Erlangen catheter to the (soft) Wallace catheter in 320 patients in a randomized controlled trial. The pregnancy rate per ET was apparently higher in the Erlangen group than in the Wallace group, but this difference was not significant. In a similar study, Urman et al.[40] compared the (soft) Wallace catheter to the (rigid) TDT catheter in 428 patients undergoing ET. In this retrospective study, the authors found that both catheters performed similarly, although there was a slight, but non-significant, increase in clinical pregnancy and implantation rates with the Wallace catheter (41.6% versus 36.0% and 16% versus 14.4%, respectively). Similarly, Al-Shawaf et al.[41] found no significant difference in pregnancy rates when the (soft) Wallace catheter was used compared to the (rigid) Frydman catheter (30.3% versus 30.7%).

Special catheters have been devised and proposed by various groups for use in suspected or proven difficult transfers. For example, Yanushpolsky et al.[42] proposed the transcervical placement of a Malecot catheter after hysteroscopic evaluation in women with histories of difficult intra-uterine inseminations and/or ETs. They successfully used the method in 32 out of 36 patients with previously difficult transfers. Similarly, Zoll et al.[43] proposed the use of a new everting catheter and 'peel-back' technique and Patton et al.[44] devised a co-axial catheter system for use with difficult ETs. Finally, El Danasouri and Milki[45] proposed a new cervical introducer for ET with soft open-end catheters for use with the Tomcat catheter in difficult transfers.

Site of embryo deposition

The site of depositing the embryos during ET is thought to affect the pregnancy and implantation rates. The best site for depositing the embryos is thought to be 5–10 mm below the fundus. In a randomized prospective study,

Nazari et al.[46] compared the effects of a midfundal versus a deep fundal transfer technique on subsequent intra-uterine and ectopic pregnancies after IVF. The clinical pregnancy rate after the deep fundal transfer was 12.4% per cycle compared to 14.2% after midfundal transfers. The incidence of ectopic pregnancy was 1.5% after deep fundal transfers versus 0.4% after midfundal transfers. They concluded that the midfundal technique was superior to deep fundal procedures because of a lower percentage of EPs without any sacrifice of the intrauterine pregnancy rate.

The effect of the position and length of the uterine cavity on the success of ET has also been studied. In a prospective study of 807 consecutive women undergoing IVF or ICSI, Egbase et al.[47] measured the position and length of the uterine cavity in a pretreatment mock transfer procedure. They found no statistically significant differences in implantation and clinical pregnancy rates with respect to the length or position of the uterus. However, the incidence of ectopic pregnancy per reported clinical pregnancy was highest in women with small uteri (< 7 cm; 14.9%) compared to those with average uteri (7–9 cm; 1.8%) and those with large uteri (> 9 cm; 0%; $P < 0.0005$). This finding suggests that the size of the uterus is a critical factor in the aetiology of ectopic pregnancy in IVF/ICSI-embryo transfer.

Transcervical (fallopian) tubal ET was suggested by Yovich et al.[48] in 1990 as an alternative approach. This Australian group used ultrasound-guided transcervical tubal cannulation (TC-TEST) to replace embryos into the fallopian tubes in 17 women whose fallopian tubes were inaccessible by the abdominal route but where at least one tube was shown to be freely patent on hysterosalpingography. Three pregnancies resulted (17%): two went to term and the third resulted in an ectopic pregnancy. They concluded that the procedure has not shown a benefit over conventional IVF-ET. The same technique was used by Risquez et al.[49] in 28 patients treated with IVF. Five pregnancies occurred, a pregnancy rate of 9.8% per cycle. On the contrary, Van Voorhis et al.[50] compared pregnancy rates after fallopian tubal and uterine transfer of cryopreserved embryos in 40 patients in a prospective randomized trial. They found that tubal transfer of cryopreserved embryos resulted in statistically higher clinical (68% versus 24%) and on-going pregnancy rates (58% versus 19%) when compared with uterine transfer.

Subendometrial ET has also been reported. Asaad and Carver-Ward[51] performed transvaginal-transmyometrial-subendometrial ET in a patient with 7 previous failures in assisted conception cycles. The patient became pregnant and delivered healthy twin girls.

Slow withdrawal of the embryo transfer catheter

It has been suggested that gentle deposition of the embryos is necessary for implantation, and that the time during which the ET catheter remains in the cervical canal might lead to stimulation of uterine contractions. Martinez et al.[52] studied 100 women who were prospectively randomized into two groups: (i) slow withdrawal of the catheter immediately after embryo deposit ($n = 51$); and (ii) a 30 s delay before catheter withdrawal ($n = 49$). They found that the pregnancy rates for transfer in the two groups were 60.8% and 69.4%, respectively, with no significant differences. They concluded that either that the waiting interval was insufficient to detect differences, or that the retention time before withdrawing the catheter is not a factor that influences the pregnancy rate.

The use of a fibrin sealant

The addition of a fibrin sealant (glue) to the culture medium containing the embryos during ET was first suggested by Rodrigues et al.[53] who tested the system on mouse embryos. The method was subsequently used by Feichtinger et al.,[54] who used a two-component fibrin sealant to create a fibrin plug in the uterine cavity at the time of ET to decrease the possibility of embryo expulsion and ectopic pregnancy, and reported a 26% pregnancy rate. The same group subsequently conducted a prospective randomized study on 546 patients (270 with fibrin sealant and 276 conventional embryo transfers). The pregnancy rate was 18.9% in the fibrin sealant group compared to 17.0% in the control group. There were 6 ectopic pregnancies in the control group (2.2%) and no ectopic pregnancies in the fibrin sealant group and this difference was statistically significant ($P < 0.05$).[55]

A fibrin sealant was also used by Ben-Rafael et al.[56] in 211 patients undergoing IVF treatment in a randomized controlled trial. They found a significant increase in pregnancy ($P < 0.05$) and implantation ($P < 0.01$) rate in elderly patients (aged 39–42 years) using fibrin sealant for ET as compared with controls. These findings were recently confirmed by Bar-Hava et al.[57] who conducted a case-control study. A group of 265 women who underwent ET with fibrin sealant were matched for age and number of previous unsuccessful cycles to 1402 women who had ET without the fibrin sealant. The pregnancy rate was significantly higher in the fibrin sealant group (25.3% versus 14.9%). This also was true when the older women (> 35 years) and the women with ≥ 4 previous failed IVF attempts were analyzed separately (23.2% versus 9.8% and 26.1% versus 13.4%, respectively). They concluded that the use of fibrin sealant in ET appears to be beneficial in women of advanced reproductive age and in patients in whom IVF attempts repeatedly fail.

Bed rest after embryo transfer

Bed rest after ET has been found to have no effect on the pregnancy or implantation rates. In 1995, Sharif et al.[4,58] studied 103 women undergoing IVF treatment with no bed rest in hospital following ET and reported a clinical pregnancy rate of 40% per transfer. They subsequently compared 1019 IVF cycles performed in their unit with no bed rest following ET to 19,697 cycles reported in the UK national database that had bed rest following ET.[6] They found that the clinical PR per ET was significantly higher in their patients than in the national data (30% versus 22.9%), as was the pregnancy rate per cycle (23.5% versus 18.6%). Their implantation rate in their patients was 17.2%.

These findings were confirmed in a randomized controlled trial conducted by Botta and Grudzinskas[5] who studied 182 infertile patients undergoing IVF treatment. The patients were randomly assigned to two groups. The first group consisted of 87 patients who underwent 97 treatment cycles and had 87 ET procedures followed by a 24-h period of bed rest. The second group consisted of 95 patients who underwent 102 treatment cycles and had 93 ETs followed by a 20 min period of bed rest. There were no statistically significant differences between the groups regarding the pregnancy rates per ET (24.1% in the 24-h rest group, compared to 23.6% in the 20-min bed rest group).

In support to these studies, Woolcott and Stanger[59] investigated whether standing upright shortly after ET affects the position of embryos transferred to the uterine cavity during treatment with in vitro fertilization (IVF). In a prospective study of 93 patients undergoing 101 consecutive ETs, transvaginal ultrasound guided ET was performed with a second ultrasound in the standing position immediately after transfer, allowing the movement of embryo-associated air to be assessed. No movement occurred in 94.1% (95/101) of transfers, movement of < 1 cm in 4.0% (4/101) of transfers and movement of 1–5 cm in 2.0% (2/101) transfers. They concluded that standing shortly after ET does not play a significant role in the final position of the transferred embryos.

Routine administration of antibiotics following embryo transfer

Microbial infection was found to be a cause of diminished implantation after ET. Egbase et al.[60] studied 110 women at the time of transcervical ET following conventional IVF and ICSI procedures. Microbial cultures were performed on endocervical swabs and ET catheter tips. Positive microbial growths were observed from endocervical swabs in 78 (70.9%) women and from catheter tips in 54 (49.1%) women. The clinical pregnancy rates were 57.1% in the group of patients without growth and 29.6% in the group with positive microbial growth from catheter tips. Similarly, Fanchin et al.[61] performed microbial cultures from the catheter tips used in 279 ETs in women undergoing IVF treatment. In 143 (51%) women, cultures were positive. The clinical and on-going pregnancy rates as well as implantation rates were significantly lower in the positive culture group compared to the negative culture group (24% versus 37%, 17% versus 28%, and 9% versus 16%, respectively).

However, routine administration following ET is still a matter of debate. In a study by Moore et al.,[62] cultures were obtained from the vagina for aerobic and anaerobic bacteria at the time of both sonographic egg retrieval and ET and from the tip of the ET catheter from 91 women undergoing IVF. In all patients, doxycycline treatment was routinely started after egg retrieval. The authors found an increase in live-birth rate associated with the recovery of hydrogen peroxide-producing *Lactobacillus* from the vagina ($P = 0.01$) and from the ET catheter ($P = 0.01$). In contrast, they found a reduction in live-birth rate associated with recovery of *Streptococcus viridans* from the ET catheter tip ($P = 0.04$). Doxycycline had no substantial impact on the recovery of individual vaginal bacteria or on bacterial vaginosis. On the contrary, Egbase et al.[63] found that the routine administration of prophylactic antibiotics to women at the time of oocyte retrieval was associated with a reduction in positive microbiology cultures of embryo catheter tips 48 h later in 78.4% of patients. The implantation and clinical pregnancy rates were significantly lower (9.3% versus 21.6%, $P < 0.001$; 18.7% versus 41.3%, $P < 0.01$) in the women with positive microbial catheter-tip cultures.

Experience of the clinician

The experience of the clinician performing ET can also affect the pregnancy and implantation rates. For example, Hearns-Stokes et al.[64] evaluated the effect of individual providers on pregnancy outcome after ET in a retrospective data analysis of 670 patients undergoing IVF. They found that the clinical pregnancy rate varied significantly between clinicians performing the ET step (17.0% versus 54.3%, $P < 0.05$).

In addition, the incidence of ectopic pregnancy is related to the clinician performing ET. In a study by Yovich et al.,[65] the authors compared two techniques of ET. Four ectopic pregnancies occurred in a small group of 24 patients (16.7%) in whom the clinician attempted to deliver the embryos at the uterine fundus (mean distance of catheter insertion 62.9 ± 7.9 mm from the external cervical os), while only one ectopic pregnancy occurred in 56 patients (1.8%) whose embryos were transferred into the midcavity. They concluded that the ET catheter needs to be inserted only 55 mm as a routine and less in patients with a shortened cervix or a small uterus. They also suggested routine ultrasonic measurement of uterine length for this purpose.

In some units, ET is performed by trained nurses with a back up by clinicians. For example, Sinclair et al.[66] described their experience in Birmingham. After appropriate training, the nurses were allowed to perform the transfer. When they experienced difficulties during the mock transfer performed immediately before the real transfer, or if they were not available to do the procedure, a doctor performed it. Out of 522 embryo transfers, nurses performed 371 (71%) and doctors 151 (29%) of the procedures. The pregnancy rate per nurse transfer was 40.2% and per doctor transfer 41%. The corresponding implantation rates were 16.9% and 17%. None of these differences were statistically significant ($P > 0.05$). They concluded that, with appropriate training and medical backup, nurses can perform the majority of ETs with ease and outcome comparable to that of doctor ET.

DIFFICULT EMBRYO TRANSFERS

Despite all these precautions, in some patients ET cannot be accomplished due to the presence of a tight or closed cervix or due to anatomical distortion caused by fibromyomata or previous surgical interference. Different approaches have been described and practised in order to deposit the embryos inside the uterine cavity. These include:

Trans-abdominal trans-myometrial embryo transfer

Transabdominal ET has been tried by some clinicians with mixed results. For example, Lenz and colleagues[67] performed ultrasound-guided ET trans-abdominally in 10 patients. Although no complications or technical difficulties were experienced, none of the patients became pregnant. Similarly, Groutz et al.[68] compared ultrasound-guided transmyometrial and transcervical ET in 40 patients with cervical stenosis or in patients who failed to conceive after at least three previous IVF attempts in a prospective, randomized study. Transmyometrial ET was performed in 20 patients and resulted in one clinical pregnancy, while transcervical ET, performed in another 20 similar patients, resulted in three clinical pregnancies. They concluded that no benefit was derived by electing transmyometrial ET in preference to transcervical ET in patients who had failed to conceive in previous cycles.

Trans-vaginal trans-myometrial embryo transfer

In 1993, Kato et al.[69] performed ultrasound-guided transvaginal-transmyometrial ET in 104 patients and reported a clinical pregnancy rate of 36.5% per attempt. In 1996, Sharif et al.[58] performed the same procedure in 13 patients who had difficult or impossible mock transcervical ET immediately before the real transfer. Four patients became pregnant, including three with clinical pregnancies. More recently, Lai et al.[70] reported a successful pregnancy in a patient with congenital cervical atresia who had simultaneous transmyometrial and transtubal ET after IVF.

Cervical dilatation

Cervical dilatation has been performed in patients with cervical stenosis or with previously failed ETs. Abusheikha et al.[10] performed cervical dilatation at the initial visit in 57 patients with known cervical stenosis and who failed to conceive after a previous ET attempt and in whom the ET was classified as 'difficult'. Of the 57 women, 18 (31.6%) achieved pregnancy after cervical dilatation. In 40 patients (70.2%), the subsequent ET was classified as 'easy', whereas in the other 17 (29.8%) it remained difficult. The pregnancy rate was significantly higher when the ET was easy than when it was difficult (40% versus 11.8%, $P < 0.05$). Cervical dilatation can also be performed on the day of oocyte retrieval in patients with suspected cervical stenosis with unsatisfactory results. Groutz et al.[71] performed the procedure in 41 treatment cycles in 22 patients with a history of extremely difficult or impossible embryo transfer. Only one clinical and one extra-uterine pregnancy resulted. They concluded that cervical dilatation during the ovum pick-up session leads to easier ET in patients with cervical stenosis, but the pregnancy rate is low.

Hysteroscopic correction of cervical stenosis

Hysteroscopic cervical shaving to create a smooth passage for ET in patients with a history of difficult transfers has also been suggested. Noyes et al.[72] performed surgical correction of cervical stenosis in 8 patients with a history of extremely difficult ETs. Twelve postoperative IVF-ET in these women resulted in eight clinical pregnancies, six of which were multiple gestations. The embryo implantation rate of these cycles was 42.2%.

The use of laminaria tents

Slow dilatation of the cervical canal using laminaria tents has also been used in patients with a history of difficult transfers. Glatstein et al.[73] used the procedure in 2 patients with cervical stenosis and a history of multiple failed cycles of IVF. Both patients became pregnant. However, this work has not been repeated.

KEY POINTS FOR CLINICAL PRACTICE

- Embryo transfer remains an elusive step in assisted conception. Only two procedures have been shown by randomized controlled trials to

(Key points for clinical practice - continued)

improve implantation rates: performing a trial (dummy) ET before the actual ET and performing the ET under ultrasound guidance.

- Randomized controlled trials have also established that microbial infection diminishes implantation and that bed rest after ET is of no value.
- The value of routine administration of antibiotics after ET has not yet been established and no specific catheter has so far established its superiority over its competitors.
- More randomized controlled studies are needed to evaluate the numerous factors involved in this delicate and essential step of assisted reproduction.

References

1 Edwards RG. Clinical approaches to increasing uterine receptivity during human implantation. Hum Reprod 1995; 10 (Suppl 20): 60–66
2 Edwards RG, Steptoe PC, Purdy JM. Establishing full-term human pregnancies using cleaving embryos grown in vitro. Br J Obstet Gynaecol 1980; 87: 737–756
3 Jones Jr HW, Acosta AA, Garcia JE, Sandow BA, Veeck L. On the transfer of conceptuses from oocytes fertilized in vitro. Fertil Steril 1983; 39: 241–243
4 Sharif K, Afnan M, Lenton W et al. Do patients need to remain in bed following embryo transfer? The Birmingham experience of 103 in vitro fertilization cycles with no bed rest following embryo transfer. Hum Reprod 1995; 10: 1427–1429
5 Botta G, Grudzinskas G. Is a prolonged bed rest following embryo transfer useful? Hum Reprod 1997; 12: 2489–2492
6 Sharif K, Afnan M, Lashen H, Elgendy M, Morgan C, Sinclair L. Is bed rest following embryo transfer necessary? Fertil Steril 1998; 69: 478–481
7 Leeton J, Trounson A, Jessup D, Wood C. The technique for human embryo transfer. Fertil Steril 1982; 38: 156–161
8 Goudas VT, Hammitt DG, Damario MA, Session DR, Singh AP, Dumesic DA. Blood on the embryo transfer catheter is associated with decreased rates of embryo implantation and clinical pregnancy with the use of in vitro fertilization-embryo transfer. Fertil Steril 1998; 70: 878–882
9 Nabi A, Awonuga A, Birch H, Barlow S, Stewart B. Multiple attempts at embryo transfer: does this affect in vitro fertilization treatment outcome? Hum Reprod 1997; 12: 1188–1190
10 Abusheikha N, Lass A, Akagbosu F, Brinsden P. How useful is cervical dilatation in patients with cervical stenosis who are participating in an in vitro fertilization-embryo transfer program? The Bourn Hall experience. Fertil Steril 1999; 72: 610–612
11 Mesrogli M, Dieterle S. Embryonic losses after in vitro fertilization and embryo transfer. Acta Obstet Gynecol Scand 1993; 72: 36–38
12 Burke LM, Davenport AT, Russell GB, Deaton JL. Predictors of success after embryo transfer: experience from a single provider. Am J Obstet Gynecol 2000; 182: 1001–1004
13 Tur-Kaspa I, Yuval Y, Bider D, Levron J, Shulman A, Dor J. Difficult or repeated sequential embryo transfers do not adversely affect in vitro fertilization pregnancy rates or outcome. Hum Reprod 1998; 13: 2452–2455
14 Lesny P, Killick SR, Robinson J, Maguiness SD. Transcervical embryo transfer as a risk factor for ectopic pregnancy. Fertil Steril 1999; 72: 305–309
15 Khalifa Y, Redgment CJ, Yazdani N, Taranissi M, Craft IL. Intramural pregnancy following difficult embryo transfer. Hum Reprod 1994; 9: 2427–2428
16 Hamilton CJ, Legarth J, Jaroudi KA. Intramural pregnancy after in vitro fertilization and embryo transfer. Fertil Steril 1992; 57: 215–217

17 Knutzen V, Stratton CJ, Sher G, McNamee PI, Huang TT, Soto-Albors C. Mock embryo transfer in early luteal phase, the cycle before in vitro fertilization and embryo transfer: a descriptive study. Fertil Steril 1992; 57: 156–162

18 Sharif K, Afnan M, Lenton W. Mock embryo transfer with a full bladder immediately before the real transfer for in vitro fertilization treatment: the Birmingham experience of 113 cases. Hum Reprod 1995; 10: 1715–1718

19 Mansour R, Aboulghar M, Serour G. Dummy embryo transfer: a technique that minimizes the problems of embryo transfer and improves the pregnancy rate in human in vitro fertilization. Fertil Steril 1990; 54: 678–681

20 Strickler RC, Christianson C, Crane JP, Curato A, Knight AB, Yang V. Ultrasound guidance for human embryo transfer. Fertil Steril 1985; 43: 54–61

21 Lindheim SR, Cohen MA, Sauer MV. Ultrasound guided embryo transfer significantly improves pregnancy rates in women undergoing oocyte donation. Int J Gynecol Obstet 1999; 66: 281–284

22 Prapas Y, Prapas N, Hatziparasidou A et al. The echoguide embryo transfer maximizes the IVF results. Acta Eur Fertil 1995; 26: 113–115

23 Kan AK, Abdalla HI, Gafar AH et al. Embryo transfer: ultrasound-guided versus clinical touch. Hum Reprod 1999; 14: 1259–1261

24 Wood EG, Batzer FR, Go KJ, Gutmann JN, Corson SL. Ultrasound-guided soft catheter embryo transfers will improve pregnancy rates in in vitro fertilization. Hum Reprod 2000; 15: 107–112

25 Coroleu B, Carreras O, Veiga A et al. Embryo transfer under ultrasound guidance improves pregnancy rates after in vitro fertilization. Hum Reprod 2000; 15: 616–620

26 Sallam HN, Agameya AF, Rahman AF, Ezzeldin F, Sallam AN. Ultrasound measurement of the utero-cervical angle prior to embryo transfer – a prospective controlled study. Hum Reprod 2002; 17: 1767–1772

27 Hurley VA, Osborn JC, Leoni MA, Leeton J. Ultrasound-guided embryo transfer: a controlled trial. Fertil Steril 1991; 55: 559–562

28 Woolcott R, Stanger J. Potentially important variables identified by transvaginal ultrasound-guided embryo transfer. Hum Reprod 1997; 12: 963–966

29 Lewin A, Schenker JG, Avrech O, Shapira S, Safran A, Friedler S. The role of uterine straightening by passive bladder distension before embryo transfer in IVF cycles. J Assist Reprod Genet 1997; 14: 32–34

30 Johnson N, Bromham DR. Effect of cervical traction with a tenaculum on the uterocervical angle. Br J Obstet Gynaecol 1991; 98: 309–312

31 Lesny P, Killick SR, Robinson J, Raven G, Maguiness SD. Junctional zone contractions and embryo transfer: is it safe to use a tenaculum? Hum Reprod 1999; 14: 2367–2370

32 Dorn C, Reinsberg J, Schlebusch H, Prietl G, van der Ven H, Krebs D. Serum oxytocin concentration during embryo transfer procedure. Eur J Obstet Gynecol Reprod Biol 1999; 87: 77–80

33 Mansour RT, Aboulghar MA, Serour GI, Amin YM. Dummy embryo transfer using methylene blue dye. Hum Reprod 1994; 9: 1257–1259

34 MacNamee P. Vigorous flushing the cervical canal with culture medium prior to embryo transfer. Paper presented at the World Congress of IVF, Sydney 1999

35 Sallam HN, Farrag F, Ezzeldin A, Agameya A, Sallam AN. The importance of flushing the cervical canal with culture medium prior to embryo transfer. Fertil Steril 2000; 3 (Suppl 1): 64–65

36 Gonen Y, Dirnfeld M, Goldman S, Koifman M, Abramovici H. Does the choice of catheter for embryo transfer influence the success rate of in-vitro fertilization? Hum Reprod 1991; 6: 1092–1094

37 Meriano J, Weissman A, Greenblatt EM, Ward S, Casper RF. The choice of embryo transfer catheter affects embryo implantation after IVF. Fertil Steril 2000; 74: 678–682

38 Wisanto A, Janssens R, Deschacht J, Camus M, Devroey P, Van Steirteghem AC. Performance of different embryo transfer catheters in a human in vitro fertilization program. Fertil Steril 1989; 52: 79–84

39 Ghazzawi IM, Al-Hasani S, Karaki R, Souso S. Transfer technique and catheter choice influence the incidence of transcervical embryo expulsion and the outcome of IVF. Hum Reprod 1999; 14: 677–682

40 Urman B, Aksoy S, Alatas C et al. Comparing two embryo transfer catheters. Use of a trial transfer to determine the catheter applied. J Reprod Med 2000; 45: 135–138

41 Al-Shawaf T, Dave R, Harper J, Linehan D, Riley P, Craft I. Transfer of embryos into the uterus: how much do technical factors affect pregnancy rates? J Assist Reprod Genet 1993; 10: 31–36

42 Yanushpolsky EH, Ginsburg ES, Fox JH, Stewart EA. Transcervical placement of a Malecot catheter after hysteroscopic evaluation provides for easier entry into the endometrial cavity for women with histories of difficult intrauterine inseminations and/or embryo transfers: a prospective case series. Fertil Steril 2000; 73: 402–405

43 Zoll CC, Bauer O, al Hasani S, Kaisi M, Diedrich C, Diedrich K. Transcervical intrauterine embryo transfer (ET) with a new everting catheter and 'peel-back' technique. J Assist Reprod Genet 1996; 13: 452–455

44 Patton PE, Stoelk EM. Difficult embryo transfer managed with a coaxial catheter system. Fertil Steril 1993; 60: 182–183

45 El Danasouri I, Milki A. A new cervical introducer for embryo transfer with soft open-end catheters. Fertil Steril 1992; 57: 939–941

46 Nazari A, Askari HA, Check JH, O'Shaughnessy A. Embryo transfer technique as a cause of ectopic pregnancy in in vitro fertilization. Fertil Steril 1993; 60: 919–921

47 Egbase PE, Al-Sharhan M, Grudzinskas JG. Influence of position and length of uterus on implantation and clinical pregnancy rates in IVF and embryo transfer treatment cycles. Hum Reprod 2000; 15: 1943–1946

48 Yovich JL, Draper RR, Turner SR, Cummins JM. Transcervical tubal embryo-stage transfer (TC-TEST). J In Vitro Fertil Embryo Transf 1990; 7: 137–140

49 Risquez F, Boyer P, Rolet F et al. Retrograde tubal transfer of human embryos. Hum Reprod 1990; 5: 185–188

50 Van Voorhis BJ, Syrop CH, Vincent Jr RD, Chestnut DH, Sparks AE, Chapler FK. Tubal versus uterine transfer of cryopreserved embryos: a prospective randomized trial. Fertil Steril 1995; 63: 578–583

51 Asaad M, Carver-Ward JA. Twin pregnancy following transmyometrial-subendometrial embryo transfer for repeated implantation failure. Hum Reprod 1997; 12: 2824–2825

52 Martinez F, Coroleu B, Parriego M et al. Ultrasound-guided embryo transfer: immediate withdrawal of the catheter versus a 30 second wait. Hum Reprod 2001; 16: 871–874

53 Rodrigues FA, Van Rensburg JH, De Vries J, Sonnendecker EW. The effect of fibrin sealant on mouse embryos. J In Vitro Fertil Embryo Transf 1988; 5: 158–160

54 Feichtinger W, Barad D, Feinman M, Barg P. The use of two-component fibrin sealant for embryo transfer. Fertil Steril 1990; 54: 733–734

55 Feichtinger W, Strohmer H, Radner KM, Goldin M. The use of fibrin sealant for embryo transfer: development and clinical studies. Hum Reprod 1992; 7: 890–893

56 Ben-Rafael Z, Ashkenazi J, Shelef M et al. The use of fibrin sealant in in vitro fertilization and embryo transfer. Int J Fertil Menopausal Stud 1995; 40: 303–306

57 Bar-Hava I, Krissi H, Ashkenazi J, Orvieto R, Shelef M, Ben-Rafael Z. Fibrin glue improves pregnancy rates in women of advanced reproductive age and in patients in whom in vitro fertilization attempts repeatedly fail. Fertil Steril 1999; 71: 821–824

58 Sharif K, Afnan M, Lenton W, Bilalis D, Hunjan M, Khalaf Y. Transmyometrial embryo transfer after difficult immediate mock transcervical transfer. Fertil Steril 1996; 65: 1071–1074

59 Woolcott R, Stanger J. Ultrasound tracking of the movement of embryo-associated air bubbles on standing after transfer. Hum Reprod 1998; 13: 2107–2109

60 Egbase PE, al-Sharhan M, al-Othman S, al-Mutawa M, Udo EE, Grudzinskas JG. Incidence of microbial growth from the tip of the embryo transfer catheter after embryo transfer in relation to clinical pregnancy rate following in vitro fertilization and embryo transfer. Hum Reprod 1996; 11: 1687–1689

61 Fanchin R, Harmas A, Benaoudia F, Lundkvist U, Olivennes F, Frydman R. Microbial flora of the cervix assessed at the time of embryo transfer adversely affects in vitro fertilization outcome. Fertil Steril 1998; 70: 866–870

62 Moore DE, Soules MR, Klein NA, Fujimoto VY, Agnew KJ, Eschenbach DA. Bacteria in the transfer catheter tip influence the live-birth rate after in vitro fertilization. Fertil Steril 2000; 74: 1118–1124

63 Egbase PE, Udo EE, Al-Sharhan M, Grudzinskas JG. Prophylactic antibiotics and endocervical microbial inoculation of the endometrium at embryo transfer. Lancet 1999; 354: 651–652

64 Hearns-Stokes RM, Miller BT, Scott L, Creuss D, Chakraborty PK, Segars JH. Pregnancy rates after embryo transfer depend on the provider at embryo transfer. Fertil Steril 2000; 74: 80–86

65 Yovich JL, Turner SR, Murphy AJ. Embryo transfer technique as a cause of ectopic pregnancies in in vitro fertilization. Fertil Steril 1985; 44: 318–321

66 Sinclair L, Morgan C, Lashen H, Afnan M, Sharif K. Nurses performing embryo transfer: the development and results of the Birmingham experience. Hum Reprod 1998; 13: 699–702

67 Lenz S, Leeton J, Rogers P, Trounson A. Transfundal transfer of embryos using ultrasound. J In Vitro Fertil Embryo Transf 1987; 4: 13–17

68 Groutz A, Lessing JB, Wolf Y, Azem F, Yovel I, Amit A. Comparison of transmyometrial and transcervical embryo transfer in patients with previously failed in vitro fertilization-embryo transfer cycles and/or cervical stenosis. Fertil Steril 1997; 67: 1073–1076

69 Kato O, Takatsuka R, Asch RH. Transvaginal-transmyometrial embryo transfer: the Towako method; experiences of 104 cases. Fertil Steril 1993; 59: 51–53

70 Lai TH, Wu MH, Hung KH, Cheng YC, Chang FM. Successful pregnancy by transmyometrial and transtubal embryo transfer after IVF in a patient with congenital cervical atresia who underwent uterovaginal canalization during caesarean section: case report. Hum Reprod 2001; 16: 268–271

71 Groutz A, Lessing JB, Wolf Y, Yovel I, Azem F, Amit A. Cervical dilatation during ovum pick-up in patients with cervical stenosis: effect on pregnancy outcome in an in vitro fertilization-embryo transfer program. Fertil Steril 1997; 67: 909–911

72 Noyes N, Licciardi F, Grifo J, Krey L, Berkeley A. In vitro fertilization outcome relative to embryo transfer difficulty: a novel approach to the forbidding cervix. Fertil Steril 1999; 72: 261–265

73 Glatstein IZ, Pang SC, McShane PM. Successful pregnancies with the use of laminaria tents before embryo transfer for refractory cervical stenosis. Fertil Steril 1997; 67: 1172–1174

Adrian M. Lower

23

Laparoscopic myomectomy

Fibroids are benign tumours of the smooth muscle of the uterus. They are one of the most common tumours found in women during their reproductive years and are the single most common cause for hysterectomy prior to the menopause, being responsible for 20–77% of all hysterectomies performed. Fibroids can be found in up to half of all women undergoing a post mortem examination.[1] They are more common in nulliparous women, obese women and black women. Interestingly, fibroids seem to be less common in smokers. Only about a quarter of women with fibroids will experience any symptoms.[2]

Fibroids are oestrogen sensitive and tend to grow at a relatively slow rate although sometimes they can grow alarmingly quickly. The rate of growth seems to be semi-quantitatively linked to the number of oestrogen and progesterone receptors.[3] Rapid growth raises the possibility of malignant change within the fibroid although this is extremely rare. Leiomyosarcoma is the most common malignant tumour of the uterus. The diagnosis is usually made according to the number of mitotic figures seen per high power field at histological examination, as well as evidence of invasion or atypia. Such tumours displaying increased mitotic activity have been designated smooth muscle tumours of uncertain malignant potential (SMTUMP). However, recent evidence from Israel in which 20 women with mitotically-active tumours with 5–9 mitoses per 10 high power fields were followed for up to 11 years after surgical management with no sign of recurrence. Treatment was either by simple hysterectomy or by myomectomy depending on the woman's age and fertility status. These authors suggest the designation mitotically active leimyomas and stress that myomectomy is an appropriate treatment especially in young women wishing to retain their fertility.[4]

Fibroids are essentially avascular tumours and may undergo degeneration leading to cystic changes within the tumour. The most common type of

Mr Adrian M. Lower FRCOG, Consultant Gynaecologist, St Bartholomew's Hospital, London EC1A 2BE, UK

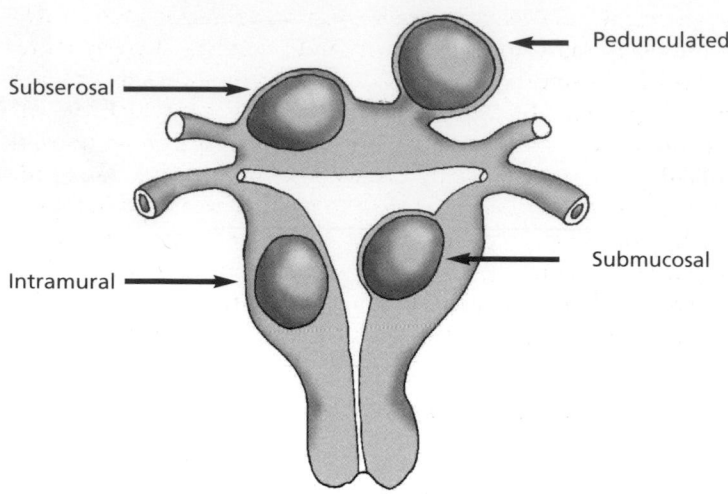

Fig. 1 Fibroids developing in the subserosal, pedunculated, submucosal and intramural positions

degeneration seen is hyaline degeneration, which is important in that it should not be mistaken for the coagulative tumour cell necrosis seen in leiomyosarcoma. Red degeneration (necrobiosis) is a form of degeneration that occurs characteristically, but not exclusively, in pregnancy, and the process is often the cause of pain and fever.[3]

Fibroids may be either submucosal, intramural, subserosal or pedunculated either protruding into the peritoneal cavity or developing in the broad ligament where they occasionally extend massively into the retroperitoneal space of the posterior abdominal wall. (Fig. 1) The symptoms they produce depend to some extent on the site and size of the fibroid. Submucosal fibroids tend to cause menstrual symptoms rather earlier including menorrhagia, intermenstrual bleeding and dysmenorrhoea. Submucosal fibroids are also more likely to cause early miscarriage and infertility. Intramural fibroids also cause dysmenorrhoea and fertility problems at relatively small size. Subserosal fibroids and pedunculated fibroids tend to be relatively asymptomatic, presenting rather later with symptoms due to their size and compression of the adjacent pelvic structures including the bladder and rectum. Often there are symptoms of frequency of micturition, tenesmus and dyspareunia. Larger fibroids also cause bloating and pelvic pain. In pregnancy, fibroids can present with acute abdominal pain and fever due red degeneration or torsion and infarction of pedunculated fibroids. Larger fibroids may also obstruct labour or cause post-partum haemorrhage.

DIAGNOSIS OF FIBROIDS

The diagnosis is usually made on the basis of a history of the symptoms described above or as an incidental finding at routine vaginal examination at the time of a cervical smear test. In women being investigated for infertility, fibroids are often found at a routine ultrasound scan. An ultrasound scan is an important investigation since it can also differentiate between an ovarian cyst or other pelvic tumour; however, there are limitations, particularly with larger fibroids where the size may limit adequate visualisation due to the limited penetration of ultrasound waves within the pelvis. Magnetic resonance imaging (MRI) is useful particularly for larger or multiple fibroids and to differentiate between fibroids and focal adenomyosis which may be much more difficult to treat, and can cause similar problems. Adenomyosis is much more difficult to remove since no clear plane of cleavage can be identified. Often, more damage is created by trying to remove areas of adenomyosis than by managing conservatively with gonadotrophin releasing hormone (GnRH) agonists. For this reason, it is the author's preference to manage adenomyosis conservatively wherever possible and promote early conception after treatment with GnRH agonists to shrink the lesions where appropriate.

MANAGEMENT OF FIBROIDS

Careful pre-operative assessment is especially important in women with fibroids, since in many cases the fibroids are asymptomatic and diagnosed as incidental findings at routine vaginal examination. Clearly, if the patient is symptomatic, the fibroids will need to be treated, but there is an argument for treating asymptomatic fibroids in younger women who may wish to have further children. Such fibroids may be relatively easily dealt with by minimal access techniques whilst they are still small and, therefore, there may be less risk of collateral damage or of hysterectomy.

For the woman with symptoms, there is a range of treatment available including medical management to control symptoms and reduce bleeding, in the hope that older women may reach a spontaneous menopause and the fibroids will then cease to be a significant problem. These include the use of tranexamic acid, mefenamic acid, progestagens and Mirena IUS or GnRH analogues. Surgical management offers longer term relief of symptoms and removal of fibroids prior to them causing more troublesome symptoms, particularly if growing rapidly. Most gynaecologists would recommend hysterectomy for women who have completed their families. There is no doubt that hysterectomy has a high rate of satisfaction and loss of all menstrual symptoms in most women;[5] however, there is an appreciable complication rate and currently has less popular appeal for many women who prefer to avoid what is considered by some to be mutilating and unnecessarily aggressive surgery.

Subtotal or supracervical hysterectomy may cause fewer intra-operative complications; however, the longer term complications following subtotal hysterectomy may negate this benefit.[6] It has also been suggested that subtotal hysterectomy may be associated with less impairment of the sexual response[7] because the cervix and its associated nerve supply are maintained. Open myomectomy has been the mainstay of management for women wishing to conserve the uterus for fertility. In larger and more complex cases, particularly where there are multiple fibroids associated with PID or previous surgery (often myomectomy), the procedure can be very demanding and there is a real risk of needing to perform a hysterectomy because of heavy bleeding or uncertain anatomy.

Uterine artery embolisation offers a non-surgical option although it is still subject to clinical evaluation and is not as efficacious as hysterectomy in terms of absence of menstrual symptoms. The advantages are that, for a number of women, open surgery and a prolonged convalescence are avoided and up to

90% experience relief from symptoms. Embolisation may be an appropriate treatment for larger fibroids or multiple fibroids where the risks from surgery are higher and there is a greater chance of hysterectomy being necessary at the time of attempted myomectomy.

Minimal access techniques are suitable for smaller fibroids. Submucosal fibroids are best dealt with by hysteroscopic resection or ablation using instruments such as Versapoint. In some cases, it may be necessary to perform a second-look procedure, particularly with larger type II fibroids in which the greater part of the diameter of the fibroid lies within the wall of the uterus. The long-term outcome for pregnancy and management of menorrhagia appears satisfactory and has been reviewed elsewhere.[8] Laparoscopic myomectomy is suitable for intramural or superficial subserosal fibroids of up to 10 cm in diameter. Larger pedunculated fibroids can be tackled depending on the site of the pedicle; the limitations here are access or difficulty in morcellation of larger fibroids. Laparoscopic procedures are best reserved for women with solitary fibroids of less than 10 cm in diameter or where three or less fibroids are present and the total combined diameter is less than 15 cm. Larger fibroids create difficulties with access and closure of the uterine defect.

PRE-OPERATIVE PREPARATION

There has been some debate regarding the value of pre-operative treatment with GnRH analogues. A *Cochrane Review* suggests that the use of GnRH analogues for 3–4 months prior to fibroid surgery reduces both uterine volume and fibroid size.[9] They are beneficial in the correction of pre-operative iron deficiency anaemia, if present, and reduce intra-operative blood loss. The reduction in fibroid size may be important to allow the procedure to be completed laparoscopically. The disadvantage is that a dense fibrosis occasionally develops around the fibroid following GnRH therapy. For this reason, the author tends not to use GnRH agonists routinely and reserves their use for larger fibroids, which might other wise be too large to deal with laparoscopically.

It is important to take a clear and informed consent. The patient should be made aware of the alternative treatments available for the condition and the reasons for recommending a laparoscopic approach. She must be warned of the risk of damage to the bowel, bladder and blood vessels at laparoscopy and the risk of proceeding to laparotomy should excessive bleeding or other technical difficulty be encountered. The risk of hysterectomy is extremely small, but should be mentioned. Some authorities put the risk as high as 1 in 100 for myomectomy in general. The risk should be much lower than this for laparoscopic myomectomy since multiple fibroids and the massively enlarged uterus are excluded.

OPERATIVE TECHNIQUE

The patient is placed in the lithotomy position and the bladder catheterised. In the early stages of the learning curve, where the duration of surgery exceeds 2 h, it is helpful to leave the bladder on free drainage using a Foley catheter. A four portal technique is used. The primary 10 mm trochar is introduced through the umbilicus using a standard blind technique after establishment of a 15 mmHg CO_2 pneumoperitoneum using a Veress needle with saline test. Two 5 mm secondary trochars are usually inserted under direct vision, one to each iliac fossa lateral to the inferior epigastric arteries. A further 10–12 mm trochar is placed suprapubically in the midline at a level just above the fundus of the uterus.

Intra-operative haemorrhage is decreased by the use of a solution of pitressin (20 units in 20 ml saline). This is injected around the insertion of each round ligament, 10 ml to each side, and leads to a rapid blanching of the uterus caused by spasm of the uterine vasculature. Pitressin can induce a profound systemic hypertension and deaths have occurred following local administration. For this reason, pitressin is banned in France and some other countries. Care should, therefore, be exercised to avoid intravenous administration and the anaesthetist must be aware of its use.

The most important part of the procedure is planning the incision in the uterus; this must be done to facilitate suturing with the dominant hand once the fibroid has been removed. For a right-handed surgeon, posterior wall fibroids are most easily removed through longitudinal midline incisions so that the needle holder can be introduced through the midline trochar. Anterior wall fibroids are more easily removed through an oblique incision made from top right to bottom left of the uterus so that the needle holder can be introduced through the trochar in the right iliac fossa and lie parallel to the incision. Some authorities prefer to use two 5 mm trochars introduced in the left side so that suturing can be done in a more relaxed fashion without the need to stretch the right hand across the patient. In these circumstances, a transverse incision is better.

The incision is made using diathermy armed scissors or needle electrode or harmonic scalpel. The serosa and myometrium is incised until the pseudo capsule is identified and then extended as far as is necessary to allow the fibroid to be stripped away from the myometrium. The fibroid is manipulated using a 10 mm claw grasping forceps or a myoma screw and carefully stripped away from the myometrium. This process is usually surprisingly bloodless, even without pitressin, provided the correct plane is chosen.

The defect is then repaired in two layers using interrupted 2/0 vicryl to the myometrium to obliterate the dead space and 3/0 monocryl to the serosa. The sutures can be tied using intracorporeal instrument ties or extracorporeally tied knots advanced with a knot pusher. With practice, the former technique is simpler, quicker, and gives better tissue approximation. If the endometrial cavity is inadvertently entered, it can be repaired by a further layer of 3/0 vicryl before the myometrial repair.

Myomectomy has a reputation for being a very adhesiogenic procedure. Reports of laparoscopic myomectomy suggest that adhesions also represent a significant problem.[10] Careful surgical technique goes some way to reducing adhesion formation. It is important to keep the operative field irrigated and some surgeons advocate the use of humidifiers and warmers for CO_2 insufflators to further reduce the drying effect the gas has on the peritoneal surface. Two commercially available barriers have been shown to be effective in reducing postoperative adhesion formation following myomectomy. Interceed is an absorbable mesh of oxidised regenerated cellulose and polytetrafluoroethylene (PTFE, GoreTex) is a non-absorbable membrane which is sutured in place to mask

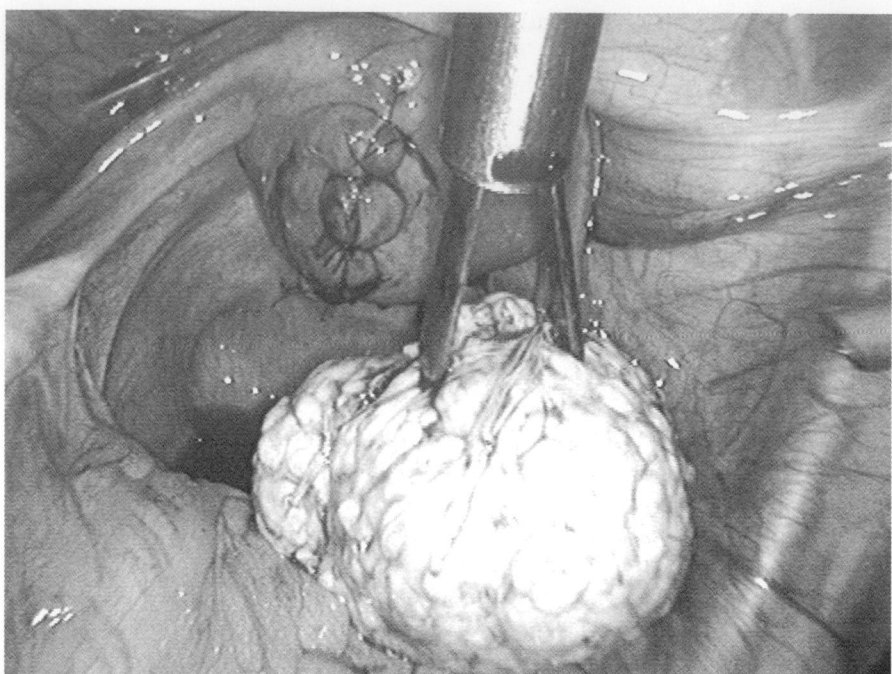

Fig. 2 Fibroid being removed using a 10 mm morcellator and grasping forceps.

the myomectomy incision site on the uterus. GoreTex may be superior to Interceed in preventing adhesion formation but its usefulness is limited by the need for suturing and later removal.[11]

REMOVAL OF THE FIBROID FROM THE PERITONEAL CAVITY

There are two possibilities for removal of the fibroid. The most elegant involves the use of a tissue morcellator (Fig. 2). This consists of two concentric cylinders with a motor drive causing the inner cylinder to rotate relative to the outer. The inner cylinder has a sharpened blade at its end and this cuts into the specimen coring it out or cutting peripheral strips similar to peeling an apple. The original design by Steiner is marketed by Storz and has an outer diameter of 10 mm. More recently, a single-use morcellator has been developed by Gynaecare. This has a similar principle of operation but an outer diameter of 15 mm. The single-use instrument has a definite advantage in that it is always sharp and the extra 5 mm means that tissue is removed more quickly; however, there are cost implications. The morcellator is introduced with relative ease through the 10–12 mm suprapubic incision after suturing the uterus. This port site must of course be closed in two layers using an instrument such as the Phipps J-shaped needle to ensure separate closure of the rectus sheath to prevent later hernia formation.

The alternative to the morcellator is to use the CCL pelvic extraction kit also marketed by Storz. This consists of a sphere of around 3 cm in diameter mounted on a 10 mm laparoscopic trochar with gas valve. The sphere is introduced into the vagina and pushed up into the posterior fornix between the uterosacral ligaments. Diathermy armed scissors are then used to perform a posterior colpotomy through which quite large fibroids can be removed due to the elasticity of the posterior fornix compared with the rectus sheath. The gas valve on the trochar attached to the sphere prevents loss of pneumoperitoneum and allows a 10 mm claw grasping forceps to be introduced to the peritoneal cavity from below to remove the specimen without the need for morcellation. The colpotomy is easily closed using vicyl sutured either from above or below. This technique is only dangerous if the pouch of Douglas is obliterated, as in the case of severe adhesions or endometriosis.

ANTIBIOTIC AND THROMBOPROPHYLAXIS

All laparoscopic procedures performed by the author are covered by a single dose of intravenous antibiotics. Generally cefuroxime (750 mg) and metronidazole (500 mg) are given at the commencement of surgery. If the procedure is long or complicated or the endometrial cavity is inadvertently opened, two further doses are given postoperatively. TED stockings are routinely used and patients receive clexane (20 mg) daily by subcutaneous injection whilst in hospital.

COMPLICATIONS

Concern has been expressed that there may be a higher complication rate following laparoscopic myomectomy than with open surgery. The available data do not support this. Seracchioli and colleagues published the results of a 5-year study in which 131 women with significant fibroids of at least 5 cm in diameter underwent myomectomy either by laparotomy or laparoscopy.[12] They found that women undergoing laparoscopic myomectomy had a lower incidence of febrile morbidity of > 38 C (12.1% versus 26.2%; $P < 0.05$), a less pronounced drop in haemoglobin (1.33 ± 1.23 versus 2.17 ± 1.57; $P < 0.001$). Three patients received a blood transfusion after laparotomy and none after laparoscopy. The postoperative hospital stay was shorter in the laparoscopic group (142.80 ± 34.60 h versus 75.61 ± 37.09 h; $P < 0.001$).

Further speculation has suggested that the tissue apposition following laparoscopic myomectomy is less accurate than at open myomectomy. Dubuisson and colleagues reported a relatively high rate of spontaneous uterine rupture following laparoscopic myomectomy of 3 cases in 100 deliveries although only one of these was in the line of the myomectomy repair and none occurred during formal trials of labour.[13] Provided the myometrial defect is closed with the same degree of care as it would be at open myomectomy, there appears to be no clear reason why the rate of uterine rupture should be higher after laparoscopic myomectomy than at open surgery. Some surgeons use a single layer closure of the defect. It is interesting to note that in reported series the rate of uterine rupture after caesarean section (0.1%) is much higher than the rate of rupture after myomectomy (0.002%).[5] It may be that the risk of rupture is related to the size of the myometrial defect. Larger fibroids would, therefore, be expected to result in rupture more frequently, making the risk of rupture less likely after laparoscopic treatment, which is restricted to smaller diameter fibroids.

KEY POINTS FOR CLINICAL PRACTICE

- Fibroids are a common condition and may cause symptoms of menorrhagia, dysmenorrhoea, infertility and pelvic compression although the majority are asymptomatic.

- Laparoscopic management is suitable for subserosal and intramural fibroids of up to 10 cm in diameter.

- The procedure is quite demanding, but can be mastered by most surgeons with adequate training in laparoscopic procedures.

- Further prospective trials are required to determine whether myomectomy will have a substantial effect on improving pregnancy rates in women with fibroids.

References

1 Hillard PA. Benign diseases of the female reproductive tract: symptoms and signs. In: Berek JS, Adashi EY, Hillard PA. (eds) Novak's Gynecology, 12th edn. Baltimore: Williams & Wilkins, 1996; 331–397

2 Buttram VC, Reiter RC. Uterine leiomyomata: etiology, symptomatology and management. Fertil Steril 1981; XX: 433–445

3 Robboy SJ, Bentley RC, Butnor K, Anderson MC. Pathology and pathophysiology of uterine smooth-muscle tumors. Environ Health Perspect 2000; 108 (Suppl 5): 779–784

4 Dgani R, Piura B, Ben-Baruch G et al. Clinical pathological study of uterine leiomyomas with high mitotic activity. Acta Obstet Gynecol Scand 1998; 77: 74–77

5 Lumsden MA. Embolization versus myomectomy versus hysterectomy: which is best, when? Hum Reprod 2002; 17: 253–259

6 Ewies AA, Olah KS. Subtotal abdominal hysterectomy: a surgical advance or a backward step? Br J Obstet Gynaecol 2000; 107: 1376–1379

7 Ewen SP, Sutton CJ. Advantages of laparoscopic supra-cervical hysterectomy. Baillière's Clin Obstet Gynaecol 1995; 9: 707–715

8 Ubaldi F, Tournaye H, Camus M, Van der Pas H, Gepts E, Devroey P. Fertility after hysteroscopic myomectomy. Hum Reprod Update 1995; 1: 81–90

9 Lethaby A, Vollenhoven B, Sowter M. Pre-operative GnRH analogue therapy before hysterectomy or myomectomy for uterine fibroids. Cochrane Database Syst Rev 2002; (1)

10 Dubuisson J-B, Fauconnier A, Chapron C et al. Second look after laparoscopic myomectomy. Hum Reprod 1998; 13: 2102–2106

11 Farquhar C, Vandekerckhove P, Watson A, Vail A, Wiseman D. Barrier agents for preventing adhesions after surgery for subfertility. Cochrane Database Syst Rev 2000; (2)

12 Seracchioli R, Rossi S, Govoni F et al. Fertility and obstetric outcome after laparoscopic myomectomy of large myomata: a randomized comparison with abdominal myomectomy. Hum Reprod 2000; 15: 2663–2668

13 Dubuisson JB, Fauconnier A, Deffarges JV, Norgaard C, Kreiker G, Chapron C. Pregnancy outcome and deliveries following laparoscopic myomectomy. J Reprod Med 2000; 45: 23–30

Index